The Nurse's Role in Promoting Optimal Health of Older Adults:

Thriving in the Wisdom Years

The Nurse's Role in Promoting Optimal Health of Older Adults:

Thriving in the Wisdom Years

Jean W. Lange, PhD, RN, FAAN
Founding Dean and Professor
Quinnipiac University School of Nursing
Hamden, Connecticut

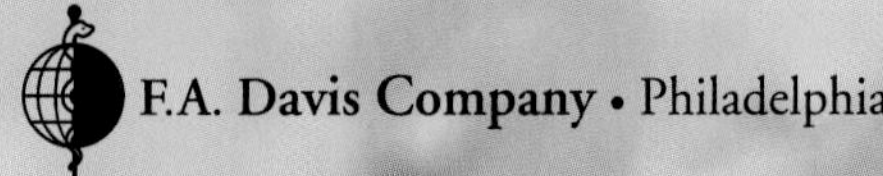
F.A. Davis Company • Philadelphia

F. A. Davis Company
1915 Arch Street
Philadelphia, PA 19103
www.fadavis.com

Printed in the United States of America

Last digit indicates print number: 10 9 8 7 6 5 4 3 2 1

Publisher, Nursing: Joanne Patzek DaCunha, RN, MSN
Director of Content Development: Darlene Pedersen
Project Editor: Elizabeth Hart
Illustration and Design Manager: Carolyn O'Brien

ISBN: 978-0-8036-2245-6

I dedicate this book to the many mentors I have had across my career. These individuals are too numerous to name, but they have been instrumental to my professional growth and achievements. I am forever grateful for their encouragement, wise counsel, and readiness to open new doors to opportunity.

No accomplishment is achieved without the support of family, and so I also dedicate this book to them: To my parents, Sandra and W. Beverly White who taught me to be the best I can be; to my husband, Bill, who keeps me grounded and is always by my side; to my two sons, Jeffrey and Eric, who have taught me much about what is important in life; and to my sister, Cheryl Lotz, who supports me as only a sister can.

Finally, I dedicate this book to the many wise elders from whom I have learned, and to the nurses who, every day, advocate for older adults.

About the Author

Dr. Jean W. Lange has made seminal contributions as one of the few nursing faculty nationally to bridge the science of geriatrics and palliative care nursing. As principal investigator for a 3-year grant from the John A. Hartford Foundation, Dr. Lange led curricular reform to enhance gerontology in the undergraduate nursing program at Fairfield University and develop expertise among its nursing faculty. Student attitudes and superior knowledge about the care of older adults on a nationally benchmarked exam prompted the American Association of Colleges of Nursing to highlight Dr. Lange's leadership in its publication, *Caring for an Aging America: A Guide for Nursing Faculty*, and for recognizing Fairfield University with its "Model of Gerontology Curricular Excellence" award in 2005.

As a certified trainer in end-of-life care, Dr. Lange and colleagues created one of the first programs in the country to integrate the End-of-Life Nursing Education Consortium (ELNEC) curriculum at graduate and undergraduate levels. Her leadership in refining the ELNEC-Knowledge Assessment Tool (ELNEC-KAT) has been adopted for use by educators across care settings nationwide.

Dr. Lange has a long history of funding to support her work. She was a 2002 Hartford Scholar, received a 2003 National Institute of Aging training grant, and has secured more than $1 million from federal, state, and foundation sources. Her passion to improve care for older adults has touched providers across the continuum of care. A program with area hospitals to educate nursing staff about geriatric best practices led to reduced fall rates and national certification in gerontology by the majority of participants. As principal investigator on a 6-year, federally funded ELDER Project (Expanded Learning Dedicated to Elders in the Region), Dr. Lange currently partners with home health and long-term care agencies to enhance provider knowledge about geriatric best practices and palliative care and to promote team-building and cultural sensitivity across disciplines.

Dr. Lange's work is well known through numerous publications and presentations regionally, nationally, and internationally. Her reputation in leading curriculum reform led to an invitation by the AACN to serve on the National Task Force that revised the standards for baccalaureate nursing education. In 2010, she was honored with a national award for outstanding contributions to palliative care and inducted into the American Academy of Nursing in recognition of her contributions to improving the care of older adults.

Foreword

With Baby Boomers passing age 65 and seeking ways to stay active and healthy in their old age, publication of *The Nurse's Role in Promoting the Health of Older Adults: Thriving in the Wisdom Years* is extremely timely. The book's focus on the nurse's role in promoting healthy aging, what it means to age successfully, and how to optimize patients' well-being during the later years of life is well aligned with the goals and aspirations of today's older adults.

In addition, this book reflects a "coming of age" for geriatric nursing. The past 30 years have been spent ensuring that nurses graduate with basic competencies in the care of older adults. We are now ready to impart to nurses a broader set of values related to their role in helping older adults live vibrant, rich, and eclectic lives. This book is an important resource in helping faculty, students, and practicing nurses accomplish this goal.

The intent of this book and its contents and language reflect a newly vital understanding of the importance of thriving in old age. As our population ages and life expectancy lengthens, this focus becomes increasingly timely and important. Also important is the book's adherence to evidence-based, critical thinking standards based on such authorities as the 2010 American Association of Colleges of Nursing *Recommended Baccalaureate Competencies and Curricular Guidelines for the Nursing Care of Older Adults,* the Hartford Institute for Geriatric Nursing Education Consortium program, the Quality and Safety Education for Nurses competencies, the Geriatric and End-of-Life Nursing Education Consortia, and recent recommendations of the Institute of Medicine in both geriatrics and nursing.

The combination of sensitive and timely instruction in helping older adults age well with the most up-to-date theoretical and clinical expertise make this book a valuable resource for nursing students, faculty, and their clinical partners. I recommend it heartily.

Mathy Mezey, EdD, RN FAAN
Professor Emerita, Senior Research Scientist
Associate Director, the Hartford Institute for Geriatric Nursing
New York University College of Nursing

Preface

It's an exciting time to be aging. Many older adults are living longer and staying healthier than ever. In fact, most of the patients you care for throughout your nursing career will likely be over age 65—a proportion that will continue to increase and age as the worldwide population of older adults expands.

Nurses have a central role as educators, advocates, and caregivers for older adults. This role, when fully filled, extends well beyond the single goal of caring for older adults during illness. Instead, it asks nurses to help patients move through their older years with vigor and satisfaction, knitting all the parts of life into a whole that promotes wellness at every age and level of ability and disability.

Holistic Focus

Many resources are available to help nurses provide excellent physical care to elders in need. But rarely do these resources cover all aspects of the older patient's life and health. This new text fills that gap. Based on a bedrock theory of successful aging, the book takes a holistic approach that addresses physical, psychosocial, and spiritual aspects of the older adult's life, focusing on the nurse's role in promoting healthy aging, what it means to age successfully, and what tools, skills, resources, and knowledge can be used to optimize well-being during the later years of life.

Helping older adults age well is a complex, multifaceted task that requires wide-ranging, evidence-based knowledge on the part of health care professionals. That's why this book is built on key recommendations and best practices from such authoritative sources as the Hartford Institute of Geriatric Nursing, the American Association of Colleges of Nursing's *Recommended Baccalaureate Competencies and Curricular Guidelines for the Nursing Care of Older Adults,* the Geriatric and End-of-Life Nursing Education Consortia, and recommendations from the Institute of Medicine as embedded in the six Quality and Safety Education for Nursing (QSEN) competencies. These six seminal competencies include patient-centered care, teamwork and collaboration, evidence-based practice, quality improvement, safety, and informatics.

Special Features

The book's 25 chapters have been written by an interdisciplinary team of health care professionals with expertise in such areas as exercise physiology, nutrition, pharmacy, elder law, social work, mental health, occupational therapy, finance, and home care in addition to nursing. Throughout, the book emphasizes quality of care, patient safety, patient-centered care, and collaborative practice—all in an accessible, easy-to-read style.

Case studies and patient vignettes appear throughout the book to add personal experience to the clinical content, bringing to life the successes and challenges of aging. The book also highlights key studies, explaining each study's implications for successful nursing practice. Breakout quotes highlight important concepts in each chapter, along with learning objectives at the start of the chapter and key points at the end.

Wide-Ranging Coverage

The book is arranged in four units meant to cover all the major components of holistic care. Unit I lays a foundation for understanding the demographic and personal aspects of growing older. It contains chapters on successful aging, characteristics of older adults, the importance of collaborative geriatric care, and the need to engage and empower older adults in their own well-being. Providing comprehensive interdisciplinary care means being able to coordinate personalized and evidence-based services with others on the health care team.

Unit II helps readers understand normal aging, the importance of staying physically fit, and the common physical changes and challenges of aging, including such key quality-of-life issues as sleep, intimacy, nutrition, assistive devices, and the safe use of medications. As more people choose to "age in place" at home, nurses need to know how to optimize the older adult's independence and access to needed resources.

Unit III turns to the economic, legal, and social aspects of life so often neglected in the care of older adults. Chapters in this section review important legal and economic considerations and ways to promote safely in the older adult's environment. The section also discusses older adults as both givers and receivers of care and the unique needs of an increasingly diverse older population that includes more visible cohorts of veterans and of lesbian, gay, bisexual, and transgender patients.

Unit IV addresses the crucial topics of mental wellness, spirituality, and the end of life. Health care providers with sensitivity, knowledge, and skills can do much to improve these qualitative aspects of life, not just for patients but also their loved ones. Experts acknowledge a worldwide need for improvement in these areas of care, and particularly in end-of-life care. Indeed, the book closes with a chapter written by nursing experts from developed and developing countries around the world. As they describe so clearly, optimization of health among older citizens is a global challenge.

Sensitive and Timely

It has been said that all nurses are gerontology nurses because of the great number of older adults who need nursing care now and who will need it in the future. Unlike other books that focus heavily on disease and disability, this book shows nurses how to help older adults maintain health and vigor in all areas of their lives, not just physical but also emotional, social, and economic. Further, this book helps readers appreciate the rich life experiences of older adults and, with sensitive and timely advice, shows readers how to help patients live out their older years with meaning, purpose, spiritual connectedness, and self-acceptance.

Acknowledgments

I wish to acknowledge the editorial staff at F.A. Davis Company without whom this book would not have been written: To Joanne DaCunha, for her belief in my ability to write the book, her willingness to plant its seeds several times over a 2-year period, her suggestions for the book's contents, her continued advocacy on my behalf, and her encouragement and support, especially during the critical early stages; to Elizabeth Hart, who kept this project on task; and to Catherine Harold, whose editorial assistance, advice, and support throughout the process were invaluable. I thank you all for this opportunity.

Contributors

Kathryn A. Blair, PhD, FNP-BC, FAANP
Professor
Beth El College of Nursing and Health Sciences
University of Colorado
Colorado Springs, Colorado

Pamela Pitman Brown, MA
Doctoral Candidate
Miami University
Oxford, Ohio

Patricia Burbank, DNSc, RN
Professor
College of Nursing
University of Rhode Island
Kingston, Rhode Island

Dympna Casey, PhD, RGN
Senior Lecturer
PhD Programme Director
School of Nursing and Midwifery
National University of Ireland
Áras Moyola, Galway, Ireland

Ronni Chernoff, PhD, RD
Associate Director, GRECC for Education/Evaluation
Geriatric Research Education and Clinical Center
Central Arkansas Veterans Healthcare System;
Director, Arkansas Geriatric Education Center
Reynolds Institute on Aging
University of Arkansas for Medical Sciences
Little Rock, Arkansas

Leanne Clark-Shirley, MGS
Doctoral Candidate
UMB/UMBC Program in Gerontology
University of Maryland, Baltimore County
Baltimore, Maryland

Heather L. Connors, PhD
Instructor, Management in Aging Services
Masters in Gerontology Program
University of Massachusetts
Boston, Massachusetts

Adeline Cooney, PhD, RGN, RNT
Deputy Head, Master of Health Sciences (Nursing/Midwifery Education)
Programme Director, School of Nursing and Midwifery
National University of Ireland
Áras Moyola, Galway, Ireland

Lorri B. Danzig, MS
Certified Sage-ing® Leader
Woodbridge, Connecticut

Susan Fisher, EdD, APRN, BC, AOCN, ACHPN
Clinical Nurse Specialist, Oncology Services
Hospital of St. Raphael
New Haven, Connecticut

Carol D. Gaskamp, PhD, RN
Assistant Professor of Clinical Nursing
Division Chair
Family, Public Health Nursing, & Nursing Administration Division
University of Texas School of Nursing
Austin, Texas

Sally Gerard, DNP, RN, CDE
Assistant Professor
Fairfield University School of Nursing
Fairfield, Connecticut

Kerstin Gerst, PhD
Institute of Gerontology
Assistant Professor, Department of Health Policy & Management
College of Public Health
University of Georgia
Athens, Georgia

Philip Greiner, DNSc, RN
Associate Dean for Faculty Development in Scholarship & Teaching
Lienhard School of Nursing
Pace University
Pleasantville, New York

Ruth E. Johnston, MS, RD, LD
GRECC Education Specialist
Geriatric Research Education and Clinical Center
Central Arkansas Veterans Healthcare System
Little Rock, Arkansas

Mary Keys, PhD
Lecturer, School of Law
National University of Ireland
Galway, Ireland

Priscilla M. Koop, PhD, RN
Associate Professor
University of Alberta
Edmonton, Alberta, Canada

Alison Kris, PhD, RN
Assistant Professor
Fairfield University School of Nursing
Fairfield, Connecticut

Roni Lang, LCSW
Clinical Social Worker, Center for Healthy Aging
Greenwich Hospital
Adjunct Faculty, University of Connecticut
Stamford, Connecticut

Jean W. Lange, PhD, RN, FAAN
Professor
Program Director, Doctor of Nursing Practice
Fairfield University School of Nursing
Fairfield, Connecticut

Philip Larkin, PhD
Joint Chair, Associate Professor and Director of Clinical Academic Liaison
School of Nursing Midwifery and Health Systems and Our Lady's Hospice and Care Services
College of Life Sciences
University College Dublin
Dublin, Ireland

Joan Lindsay, PhD
Adjunct Professor
Department of Epidemiology and Community Medicine
University of Ottawa
Ontario, Canada

Doris Troth Lippman, APRN, EdD, FAAN
Professor
VA Nursing Academy Project Director
Fairfield University School of Nursing
Fairfield, Connecticut

Diana DeBartolomeo Mager, DNP, RNc
Assistant Professor and Director
Robin Kanarek Learning Resource Center
Fairfield University School of Nursing
Fairfield, Connecticut

Kinsuk Maitra PhD, OTR/L
Associate Professor and Associate Chairperson
Department of Occupational Therapy
Rush University Medical Center
Chicago, Illinois

Martha Meraviglia, PhD, RN, ACNS-BC
Associate Professor of Clinical Nursing
School of Nursing
University of Texas
Austin, Texas

Denise Miner-Williams, PhD, RN, CHPN
Geriatrics Research Fellow, Geriatric Research Education and Clinical Center
Audie L. Murphy Veterans Hospital
Assistant Research Professor
School of Nursing
University of Texas Health Science Center
San Antonio, Texas

Christina E. Miyawaki, MA, MSW
Doctoral Student
School of Social Work
University of Washington
Seattle, Washington

Kathy Murphy, PhD, RGN
Professor
Head of School of Nursing and Midwifery
National University of Ireland
Áras Moyola, Galway, Ireland

Dagfinn Nåden, RN, HVD (Doctor in Health Care)
Professor of Nursing
Oslo University College
Oslo, Norway

Ellen Z. Navarro, MA
Consultant
Honduran Alzheimer's Association
Tegucigalpa, Honduras

Timothy C. Okeke, PhD, PLCSW
Assistant Professor
Director of the Social Work Program
Department of Education/Psychology/Social Work
Livingstone College
Salisbury, North Carolina

Eamon O'Shea, PhD
Professor
Head of the Economics Department
The Irish Centre for Social Gerontology
National University of Ireland
Áras Moyola, Galway, Ireland

Paula E Papanek, PhD, MPT, LAT, FACSM
Associate Professor of Physical Therapy
Program Director, Exercise Science
Marquette University
Milwaukee, Wisconsin

Margaret A. Perkinson, PhD
Associate Professor
Department of Occupational Science & Occupational Therapy
Doisy College of Health Sciences
St. Louis University
St. Louis, Missouri
and
Director of Gerontology
NAPA-OT Field School
Antigua, Guatemala

Terry Tavella Quell, PhD, RN
President, Connecticut Nurses Association
Assistant Dean for Undergraduate and Graduate Program Management
Fairfield University School of Nursing
Fairfield, Connecticut

Chris Shea, PharmD, CGP
President, IntegriCare Clinical Associates
Reno, Nevada

Åshild Slettebø, PhD, RN
Professor in Health Science
Department of Health and Sport Sciences
University of Agder, Grimstad, Norway
Oslo University College, Norway

Rebecca Sutter, RN, CNS
Instructor of Clinical Nursing, Retired
School of Nursing
University of Texas
Austin, Texas

Gloria Messick Svare, PhD, LCSW
Associate Professor and MSW Coordinator
School of Social Work
Division of Health Sciences
University of Nevada
Reno, Nevada

Debbie Tolson, RGN, PhD, BSc, MSc
Professor
Director, Centre for Evidence-Based Care of Older People
Glasgow Caledonian University
Scotland, United Kingdom

Mary C. Toole, JD
Attorney at Law—Elder Law
Toole & Saxby, P.A.
Portland, Maine

Heather Townsend, PharmD, CGP, BCPS
Clinical Pharmacist
Renown Regional Medical Center
Reno, Nevada

Meredith Troutman, PhD, PMHCNS-BC
Assistant Professor
Gerontology Program Affiliate
School of Nursing
University of North Carolina
Charlotte, North Carolina

Leana R Uys, D Soc Sc, ASSAf
Professor of Nursing
University of KwaZulu-Natal
Durban, South Africa

Dr. Jeanne Wendel
Professor
Department of Economics
College of Business
University of Nevada
Reno, Nevada

Erin Wert, BSN, RN
Vanderbilt University Medical Center
Staff Nurse
Neurology/Neurosurgery ICU
Nashville, Tennessee

Reviewers

Carl Christensen, RN, PhD
Northwest University
Kirkland, Washington

Gretchen R. Cornell, PhD, RN, CNE
Utah Valley University
Orem, Utah

Theresa Marie Delahoyde, EdD, RN
BryanLGH College of Health Sciences
Lincoln, Nebraska

Carmela Theresa De Leon, RN,BSN, MAN, PhD (c)
PIMA Medical Institute
Mesa, Arizona

Mary E. Donahue, MS, RN, CNE
Finger Lakes Health
Geneva, New York

Tanya Drake, RN, MSN
Rockland Community College
Suffern, New York

Rowena W. Elliott, PhD, RN, CNN, BC, CNE
University of Southern Mississippi
Hattiesburg, Mississippi

Mary Fabick, MSN, Med, RN-BC, CEN
Milligan College
Milligan College, Tennessee

Yvonne J. Fast, MSN, ARNP
Wichita State University School of Nursing
Wichita, Kansas

Gail Freeman-Campbell, LPN
Assiniboine Community College
Brandon, Manitoba

Linda H Garrett, PhD., FNP-BC
East Tennessee State University
Johnson City, Tennessee

Sheryl R. Gombert, BSN, MSN, CNM
Eastern Idaho Technical College
Idaho Falls, Idaho

Phyllis Graves, BSN
Waynesville School of Practical Nursing
Waynesville, Missouri

Kris Hale, RN, MSN
San Diego City College
San Diego, California

Melissa A. Hanson, MSN, RN
Medcenter One College of Nursing
Bismarck, North Dakota

Corlis Hayden, RN, MSN
Nebraska Methodist College
Omaha, Nebraska

Kimberly D. Helms, RN, MSN
Jacksonville State University
Jacksonville, Alabama

Peggy Hernandez, MSN, RN, CNE
Aurora University
Aurora, Illinois

Ardyce F. Hill, MSN, RN
Western Wyoming Community College
Evanston, Wyoming

Cathy Horinouchi, MS, RN
Loma Linda University School of Nursing
Loma Linda, California

Marlene Huff, MSN, PhD, RN
The University of Akron College of Nursing
Akron, Ohio

Carolyn Hulsen, RN, MSN
Black Hawk College
Moline, Illinois

Tatiana Isaeff, EdD, MSN, RN
College of San Mateo
San Mateo, California

Georgina Julious, MSN
Florence Darlington Technical College
Florence, South Carolina

Helen H. W. Lach, PhD, RN, GCNS, BC
Saint Louis University
St. Louis, Missouri

Susan J. Lamanna, RN, MA, MS, ANP, CNE
Onondaga Community College
Syracuse, New York

Kristen L. Mauk, PhD, DNP, RN, CRRN, GCNS-BC, GNP-BC, FAAN
Valparaiso University
Valparaiso, Indiana

Lori Schindel Martin, RN, PhD
Ryerson University
Toronto, Ontario

Ellen F. McCarty, PhD RN PMHCNS- BC
Salve Regina University
Newport, Rhode Island

Linda Miles, RN, MSN
BryanLGH College of Health Sciences
Lincoln, Nebraska

Diane Monsivais, PhD, CRRN
University of Texas at El Paso
El Paso, Texas

Cecilia Mukai, PHD, APRN, FNP-BC
University of Hawaii at Hilo
Hilo, Hawaii

Robbie L. Murphy, RN, BSN
San Jacinto College North Campus
Houston, Texas

Theresa Petersen, RN, MSN
Montana State University-Northern
Havre, Montana

Christine Pilon-Kacir, PhD, RN
Winona State University
Winona, Minnesota

Cynthia Ploutz, RN, MS, FNP
Hartwick College, Department of Nursing
Oneonta, New York

Gina Qualls, RN, MSN
Baptist Health Schools Little Rock
Little Rock, Arkansas

Eleanor Joyce Roland, MSN, CNE, PhD
North Carolina Central University
Durham, North Carolina

Donna F. Richards, RN, PhD
University of Utah
Salt Lake City, Utah

Jean Rubino, EdD, RN, PMHCNS-BC
Seton Hall University
South Orange, New Jersey

Deborah S. Rushing, DNP, RN
Troy University School of Nursing
Troy, Alabama

Debra L. Sanders, PhD, RN, GCNS-BC
Bloomsburg University
Bloomsburg, Pennsylvania

Elaine Schow, RN, BScN, MN
Mount Royal College
Calgary, Alberta

Tenna Roxanne Schumacher, RN, MSN
NMSU School of Nursing
Las Cruces, New Mexico

Mary Anne P. Shannon, PhD, RN, GCNS-BC
Lake Superior State University
Sault Ste. Marie, Michigan

Christie Shelton, RN, PhD
Jacksonville State University
Jacksonville, Alabama

Ingrid Sheets, EdD, MS, RN-BC, CNS
Dominican University of California
San Rafael, California

Lara Jean Sheppa, RN, MSN
Wake Tech Community College
Raleigh, North Carolina

Sally D. Schmidt, MSN, RN
Fort Hays State University
Hays, Kansas

Cheryl D. Slack, RN, MS
Valparaiso University
Valparaiso, Indiana

Kathy A. Stolfer, EdD, RN, C
Waynesburg University
Waynesburg, Pennsylvania

Jeanine Tweedie, MSN, RN, CNE
Hawaii Pacific University
Kaneohe, Hawaii

Constance Twyman, RN, MSN, CNE
Alvernia University
Reading, Pennsylvania

Jeanette Vincent, RN, MSN
Central Community College
Grand Island, Nebraska

Margie Washnok, APRN, MS, DNP
Presentation College
Aberdeen, South Dakota

Molly Westland, BScN MN RN
Trent Fleming School of Nursing
Peterborough, Ontario

Jacqueline Willetts, RN, MSN, GNP
California State University, East Bay
Newark, California

Judith A. Williams, ABD, RNC
Northampton Community College, Monroe Campus
Tannersville, Pennsylvania

Mamie Williams, MPH, MSN, RN
Tennessee State University
Nashville, Tennessee

Table of Contents

Unit I

Thriving in Old Age

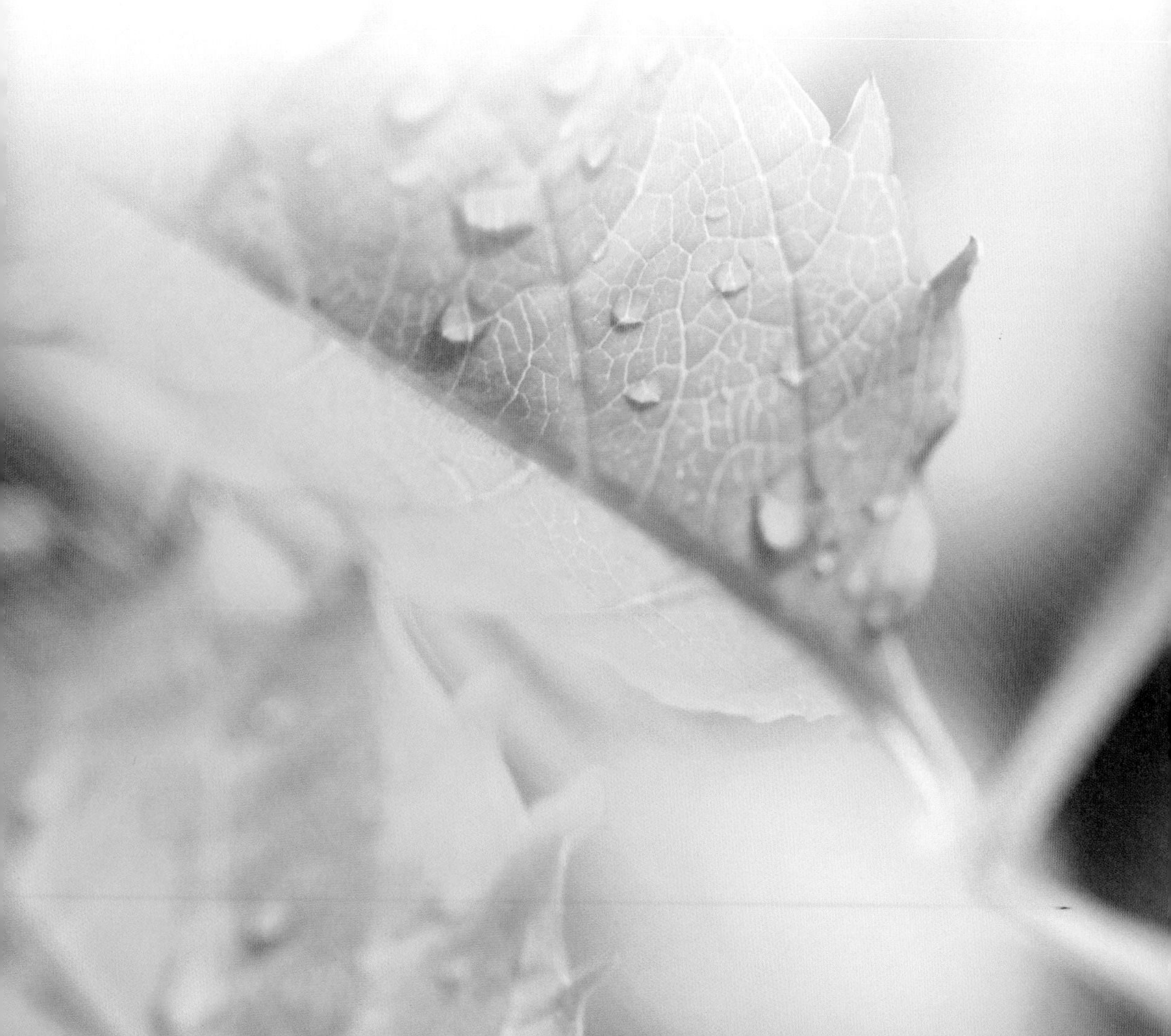

Chapter 1

What Does It Mean to Age Successfully?

Jean W. Lange, RN, PhD, FAAN

LEARNING OBJECTIVES

- Explore personal experiences and attitudes about aging.
- Discuss the ethical implications of ageism.
- Compare theories of aging from the perspective of psychosocial, biological, and nursing disciplines.
- Describe evidence-based qualities that contribute to successful aging.

What does it mean to age successfully? Is it to live to our 100th birthday? To have enough time and money to do most of the things we dream about throughout our lives? To share the wisdom gained through life's experiences? To lead a life that others will remember after we are gone? To be active and productive until the end of our days? To be healthy enough to take care of ourselves? Or is successful aging something so personal that each of us must define its meaning for ourselves?

Aging is a process that involves physical, psychological, and social changes. We can easily identify some of the outward physical signs of aging as hair lightens, weight begins to redistribute, and skin begins to wrinkle. Physiological changes that occur internally will affect the way the body continues to function and are mediated by the life habits we choose. Psychological changes happen over time as we form new relationships, seek out new opportunities and experiences, and learn new ways of coping with everyday stresses. Societal roles, such as worker, parent, partner, volunteer, retiree, or grandparent, also shift as we move through life, but not necessarily in a linear order. Many retired individuals today pursue life-long passions that were put on hold in earlier years. Older adults also may resume a parenting role as they take on the care of grandchildren in support of working parents. The physical, psychological, and social changes experienced throughout life present new growth opportunities as well as challenges. We will discuss some of these changes, opportunities, and challenges in detail in the following chapters in this book.

Defining Aging

How we define or think about aging can lead to very different assumptions about older adults. Age can be thought of chronologically (time since birth), biologically (the physical functioning of our bodies), or psychologically (how old we feel) (Stuart-Hamilton, 2006). Consider an 80-year-old gentleman who decides to audit a health promotion class. If we think of anyone over the chronological age of 60 as old, we might imagine that an 80-year-old would not have the cognitive capacity to remember what was said in class. We might wonder whether this person could benefit from new information about exercise, for example, to design his own walking program. Yet from a psychological point of view, this person clearly believes that he is capable of learning new things and perhaps has something to offer the other students in this class as well. Biologically, we would be making an inaccurate assumption that cognitive decline is a natural part of aging.

How we define or think about aging can lead to very different assumptions about older adults.

Let's consider another example of a 90-year-old woman who teaches low-impact aerobics at her local senior center. From a biological viewpoint, we might think that this is an unsafe activity that puts someone of her chronological age at risk for injury. Embedded in our concern is the assumption that all older adults become frail with age. Is this necessarily true, or is it a commonly held misconception? A purely chronological definition of age does not tell the whole story.

Although the physical and intellectual pursuits of these individuals perhaps defy what we expect of someone in their 80s or 90s, clearly there is a psychological attitude present in both scenarios that shows their desire to stay mentally and physically engaged with others. The phrase "you're as young as you feel" gets at the heart of the idea that attitude has much to do with our overall feeling of well-being, or satisfaction with living. This attitude may have as much to do with how we age as the actual time we have lived, or the physical capabilities of our bodies.

Often, we are unaware of our attitudes or expectations until we are faced with someone else's views that conflict with our own. If you are interested in discovering your personal beliefs about older adults, several self assessment tools are available to provide some insight (Table 1-1). Our expectations can be deceiving. Most of us as young, college-aged adults have had at least a limited exposure to what aging is like through our experiences with relatives. Perhaps you had a favorite great aunt who always seemed to notice you during big holiday gatherings, or a grandfather who lived with gusto and died suddenly of a myocardial infarction (MI) or stroke at 88.

Or perhaps your experiences with aging were very different. You watched the sadness of your parent as she or he made faithful visits but went unremembered by your grandmother in the dementia unit of a nursing home, or you witnessed your grandfather become increasingly dependent and depressed as he succumbed to the debilitating and progressive effects of emphysema. Our experiences shape our views and expectations about what it means to age. Based on those experiences, we may think old age is something to look forward to, as a time when we have fewer demands and more

TABLE 1-1 Tools That Measure Beliefs and Attitudes About Older Adults

TOOL	AUTHOR	DESCRIPTION
Attitudes Toward Old People Scale	Kogan	34 paired questions measure attitudes about older adults.
Reactions to Ageing Questionnaire (RAQ)	Gething et al.	23 questions measure attitudes toward personal aging.
Refined Aging Semantic Differential (ASD) Attitude Scale	Polizzi	24 paired adjectives measure attitudes about older adults.
Aged Inventory	Knox, Gekoski, & Kelly	14 questions measure age-related stereotypes and attitudes.
Fraboni Scale of Ageism	Fraboni, Saltstone, & Hughes	29 questions measure age-related stereotypes and attitudes.
Ageism Survey	Palmore	20 questions measure older adults' experience of ageism.
Perspectives Toward Caring for Older Patients Questionnaire	Burbank, McCool, & Burkholder	20 questions provide insight into nurse caring attitudes, with a focus on health-promoting behaviors.
Anxiety about Aging Scale	Lasher & Faulkender	17 questions measure fears about aging.

choices. On the contrary, we may view old age as a time to be feared, characterized by illness and decline and is full of unknowns. Because we cannot really know what it means to become old until we reach that point in our lives, most of us form expectations based on our rather narrow experiences. We develop beliefs and suppositions about the elderly and apply these assumptions broadly to others we don't know.

What Is Ageism?

Generalizing one's beliefs to an entire population can lead to societal biases or myths about aging. Such negative views are known as *ageism.* Salzman (2006) defines ageism as "a term that describes the negative stereotyping of older adults and discrimination because of older age" (p. 141). The health care literature has abundant citations on this topic and reveals that ageism is most prevalent in western nations of the world. In these societies, researchers report that older adults are less valued and often seen as a burden to society (Bowling, 2007). Widely held myths reportedly include believing that senility, loneliness, poor heath, and lack of interest in sexual activity are to be expected, along with ending up in a nursing home, being poor, and becoming more religious (Wilken, 2002). Another commonly held belief is that genetics is the most important determinant of sustained health. However, research shows that choices about exercise, diet, and active engagement produce health benefits regardless of how late in life we make them (Rowe & Kahn, 1997). Thus, genetics alone does not tell the whole story about how we age.

Negative views about aging can be found not only among the general population, but also among health care professionals. Surveys of physicians and nurses reveal that they also tend to have negative attitudes about caring for older adults. Ageism was particularly evident with respect to people over age 85 or those living in nursing homes (Gunderson, Tomkowiak, Menachemi, & Brooks, 2005). Salzman (2006) cautions that attitudes of ageism among health care providers can have serious consequences, such as discounting complaints about health as merely due to the aging process. This dismissive tendency has been blamed for the failed recognition of significant but treatable illnesses such as depression, cognitive impairment, and substance abuse (Salzman, 2006).

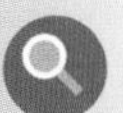

EVIDENCE FOR PRACTICE
Attitudes about Aging

Purpose: This study compared attitudes about older adults among young people from Germany and the United States. Fears about changes in appearance, functional losses, and loss of significant others were explored, as well as how each group defined the term *old.*

Sample: Participants included 254 undergraduate, Caucasian students from middle-income families (157 German and 97 U.S.). German students were somewhat older on average than American students (25 vs. 22 years old). The proportion of male and female participants was nearly equal in the two groups.

Methods: Participants completed the Anxiety about Aging Scale (Lasher & Faulkender, 1993), and indicated the age at which participants would define themselves as being old.

Results: Significant differences between U.S. and German participants were found. German students tended to be more fearful about being around older adults and to believe they would be more unhappy in their old age than American students did. Both groups worried about changes in their physical appearance. This was especially true for women. However, Americans considered themselves to be old on average by age 53 for males and 48 for females. German students tended to report higher ages (age 64 for males, 60 for females).

Implications: This study suggests that aging is viewed negatively by younger adults in Germany and the United States. Such negative views may impact the extent to which young adults seek employment that places them in contact with older adults. Studies are needed to explore the role of culture in how aging is viewed, and whether negative views impact work choices. Additional research is needed to determine whether these findings are similar in other ethnic, age, or socioeconomic groups.

Reference: McConatha, J. T., Schnell, F., Volkwein, K., Riley, L., & Leach, E. (2003). Attitudes toward aging: A comparative analysis of young adults from the United States and Germany. *Int J Aging Hum Dev, 57*(3), 203–215.

Does ageism really affect how older adults are treated and cared for? Evidence suggests that attitudes do indeed influence policy formation, insurance reimbursement, and treatment regimens. Policies that support rationing of health care services to elderly people suppose that older adults are likely to die sooner and thus benefit less from expensive diagnostic tests and treatment modalities (Bowling, 2007). Examples of this practice include withholding screening and diagnostic tests for cardiac, gastrointestinal, and respiratory diseases (Bond et al., 2003; Peake, Thompson, Lowe, & Pearson, 2003; Yoong & Heymann, 2005). An example of treatment rationing is evident in policies that prioritize candidates needing an organ replacement. Organ recipient guidelines typically include an age qualifier, so older citizens are less likely to receive, for example, a kidney transplant than younger adults (Curtis, 2006). Adults over age 65 are also excluded from most new drug trials. Reasons cited include the possibility of cognitive decline that impedes the ability to give informed consent, an increased likelihood of dying before the study concludes, and an increased risk of drug-related adverse effects from multiple health problems. But studies that exclude older adults offer no information about how effective or safe a new drug will be for that age group. The unfortunate consequence is that these medications may be prescribed based on insufficient evidence of safety or efficacy, or they may be withheld to the patient's detriment (Godlovitch, 2003). Although older adults do typically receive treatment for most medical conditions, cost versus benefit plays a role in allocating resources to older adults.

Another issue affecting equitable care to older adults is the lack of education about gerontology (the study of older adults) in the educational programs of most health care professions. Adults over age 60 are the fastest growing population in most countries throughout the world (World Health Organization [WHO], 2007). It stands to reason, therefore, that most health professionals will be working with older adults at some point in their practice. Effective health care by knowledgeable professionals is fundamental to promoting health, preventing disease, and managing chronic illness. Therefore, many organizations and foundations have provided leadership and funding to rectify this gap (e.g., WHO, John A. Hartford Foundation, Institute of Medicine, National Institute on Aging, American Association of Colleges of Nursing). We will discuss the role of some of these organizations in Chapter 5.

Thriving in the Wisdom Years

What does "thriving in the wisdom years" mean? Haight, Barba, Tesh, and Courts (2002) state that thriving consists of a balance among three important elements: the person, his or her interpersonal relationships, and the physical environment. If you looked up the word *thrive* in the dictionary, you would see adjectives such as *prosper, flourish, grow,* and *success* used in its definition. When we think about what qualities we would like to experience in later life, all of these adjectives may sound desirable. This gets at the heart of what is a central premise of this book: Aging is an unfolding process that can be enriching, satisfying, and fulfilling.

Wisdom

What about this notion of *wisdom years?* Is wisdom something we can look forward to when we are older? Does everyone who is old become wise? Suppose you suspect that a faculty member is grading you unfairly because an older sibling did poorly in that same course. How would you decide from whom to seek advice? Would your choice be your best friend? Another student in your class? A parent? Your academic advisor? Another faculty member? Would you consider the person's experience with academia, your trust that they will keep your communication in confidence, how realistic you believe their advice is likely to be, or your sense that the person can objectively listen to your point of view? Most of us would consider all of these qualities in making our decision.

Some might characterize a person who has the right balance of experience, reflection, practicality, interpersonal skills, and judgment to creatively solve problems as a wise person. A popular author on wisdom defines it as being able to use intelligence and experience to inform well-considered actions that promote the common good (Sternberg, 2004). Sternberg writes that *common good* should reflect generally held values such as human dignity, justice, and equality. Sternberg also says that wisdom involves knowing how to keep a balance among ourselves, others, and our environment. Other authors agree that wisdom involves translating experience into just actions, but also suggest that a wise person exhibits understanding of or empathy toward others (Peterson & Seligman, 2004).

Age certainly exposes us to an accumulation of experiences, but this is only one ingredient of wisdom. We all know people who seem not to learn from their experiences, have poor interpersonal skills, cannot maintain a confidence, or seem "book smart" but not "street smart." How do we know wisdom when we see it? According to Peterson and Seligman (2004), five qualities associated with wisdom include the ability to get to the heart of an issue, sincerity, forthrightness, knowing when to seek counsel, and acting in a way that is consistent with one's own values. Although we have opportunities to master each of these ingredients as we age, and wisdom is acquired over time, we would probably agree that not all older adults are wise. Research suggests that there is also a connection between wisdom and life satisfaction. Ardelt (1997, p.15), investigator for the Berkeley Guidance Study, surveyed 120 older men and women and concluded that wisdom has a profoundly positive influence on life satisfaction.

How do we acquire wisdom? Although there is much disagreement about the relationship between wisdom and age in the literature, most scholars agree that openness to reflective learning from our experiences is essential to its development (Sternberg, 2005). This book takes the position that the potential for wisdom grows as we age, and that thriving is related to living and aging successfully.

Ingredients of Successful Aging

According to Hansen-Kyle (2005), successful aging is a consequence of healthy aging. Successful aging also is sometimes referred to as *active aging*, implying that people are involved in making choices that can affect how they age. According to the World Health Organization (WHO, 2009, p. 1), active aging is "the process of optimizing opportunities for health, participation, and security to enhance quality of life as people age." Active aging implies that people participate in achieving the best possible health outcomes for themselves. According to WHO, staying engaged physically, mentally, and socially is a critical part of optimizing health as we age.

Do we have any say in how we age? Or will we wind up in the same place no matter how we live our lives? Is genetics the primary driver of our health, or do we have some degree of control through our lifestyle choices? Scientists have made clear connections between the development and progression of disease and lifestyle habits such as physical activity, diet, and the use of substances such as illegal drugs, alcohol, or tobacco (Gaziano, Galea, & Reddy, 2007; Jetha et al., 2008; Kruk, 2007; Rowe & Kahn, 1997; Tapsell & Probst, 2008). We discuss healthy lifestyles that reduce the likelihood of developing chronic diseases in later chapters of this book. But physical health is only part of the story.

The MacArthur Foundation Study of Successful Aging was conducted from 1988 to 1996, with nearly 1,200 highly functioning adults (Berkman et al., 1993). The researchers concluded that adults who were functioning at higher levels not only had fewer risk factors for chronic illnesses such as diabetes or heart disease, but study participants also tended to be more social and likely to engage in mentally stimulating activities. In another study of patients recovering from MIs, Seeman (1996) reported that those who were more socially connected had a better recovery. Likewise, Gruenewald, Karlamangla, Greendale, Singer, and Seeman (2007) reported that older adults who felt useful had lower mortality and morbidity rates than those who rarely felt useful. It seems that psychosocial conditions as well as physical health are closely linked to aging well.

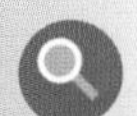

EVIDENCE FOR PRACTICE
Effects of Functional Level

Purpose: To explore factors that influence and distinguish physical and cognitive capabilities among low- to high-functioning older adults.

Sample: Participants included 1,354 volunteers ages 70 to 79 living in three communities in the northeastern and southeastern United States. Most (1,192) of the volunteers were classified as highly functional. Of the remaining participants, 162 were classified as low- ($n = 80$) or medium-functioning ($n = 82$) based on their degree of impaired cognition or inability to perform basic self-care activities (e.g., bathing, dressing, or feeding oneself).

Methods: Data were collected over a 7-year period by interviewing participants about their lifestyle patterns and by conducting physical and mental status examinations. Examination of physical functioning included balance, gait, and upper body strength. Cognitive tests measured memory recall, language (ability to name objects from pictures), abstraction (comparing similar but distinct objects), and praxis (copying geometric designs).

Results: Lower-functioning participants were poorer, less educated, and more likely to be sedentary and smoke cigarettes than higher-functioning participants. High-functioning participants were more likely to perceive themselves to be healthy and satisfied with life, participate in volunteer activities, and report fewer psychiatric symptoms than lower-functioning participants. Exercise, work or volunteer activities, or regular socialization with friends were associated with improved physical functioning, even among participants who had chronic diseases. Physical activity and socialization were also related to better cognitive functioning.

Implications: Lifestyle behaviors can play a role in the quality of life experienced with aging. Active engagement and moderate levels of exercise, such as walking, contribute to successful aging by stimulating mental functioning and reducing disability.

Reference: Berkman, L.F., Seeman, T.E., Albert, M., et al. (1993). High, usual and impaired functioning in community-dwelling older men and women: Findings from the MacArthur foundation research network on successful aging. *J Clin Epidemiol, 46*(10), 1129–1140.

How to age successfully is a popular topic today in both the media and professional literature, in part because the percentage of adults over age 65 is growing rapidly. Gilmer and Aldwin (2003) define successful aging as the absence of physical or mental disability, having a strong social network, and making favorable ratings about eight aspects of one's own health (marriage, work, children, friendship and social contacts, hobbies, community service activities, religion, and recreational activities). Clearly, aging is not simply physical changes; it also has complex psychological, social, and biological dimensions. Numerous theories have been written in an attempt to more fully explain these dimensions.

Aging is not simply physical changes. It also has complex psychological, social, and biological dimensions.

Theories about Aging

Humankind has been fascinated with the aging process for centuries. Mystical notions about how to forestall the aging process, find the fountain of youth, or live forever have appeared in writings across the ages. The first ideas or theories to explain *how* we age were credited in the late 1800s to Weismann (1889), who proposed that the more we use our bodies, the more they wear out and eventually die. It wasn't until the 1950s that sociologists, biologists, and psychologists attempted to explain aging more fully (Table 1-2). Biologists proposed that chemical processes, life stressors, and genetically programmed events cause cellular damage, which leads to a gradual deterioration of body systems. Sociologists proposed that changing roles, relationships, social status, and key events of a generation or cohort (e.g., wars, natural disasters, terrorist events, or social movements) impact how older adults adapt to growing old (Fig. 1-1). Psychologists believed that aging is about need fulfillment and navigating predictable stages of personality development across the lifespan, such as adolescence, parenting, and productivity in mid-life (Lange & Grossman, 2006).

Erikson's (1963) theory is one example of a psychological theory commonly used by nursing to explain the varied stages of personality development throughout our lives. Erikson proposed that life is an unfolding set of challenges to be mastered. In the final challenge, ego integrity versus despair, older adults judge their life accomplishments to have been either meaningful and worthwhile (integrity), or to have somehow fallen short of the mark (despair). Other theorists in the 1960s agreed that reflecting about life and death within the context of one's experience is an important part of the aging journey (Cumming & Henry, 1961; Jung, 1960).

More recently, theorists have expanded on the idea that the search for meaning involves just our personal experiences in the natural world. They suggest that understanding how we fit within the larger universe is also an important challenge in later life. For example, Tornstam (1994), one of the first nurses to propose a theory about aging, suggests that feeling connected to something greater than ourselves (spirituality) helps us come to terms with our eventual death. She believes that striving for unity with a larger universe instead of focusing on the materialistic aspects of life can transform one's fears about dying. This transformation replaces fears about death with feelings of connectedness to a larger universe, and to past and future generations. Tornstam's theory suggests that spirituality is, therefore, a critical aspect of the aging process.

TABLE 1-2 Theories of Aging

YEAR	AUTHOR	THEORY	SUMMARY
Psychosocial theories of aging			
1953	Havighurst & Albrecht	Activity	Satisfaction in old age is related to being engaged and involved.
1954	Maslow	Human Needs	Behavior is motivated by five basic needs (physiologic, safety and security, love and belonging, self-esteem, and self-actualization). Need fulfillment is a lifelong process.
1960	Jung	Individualism	Older adults search for the meaning of life from an internal or external perspective and learn to adjust to both functional and social loss.
1961	Cumming & Henry	Disengagement	As we age, it is normal to slowly withdraw from relationships and social involvement to make time for self-reflection.
1963	Erikson	Stages of Personality Development	Life is a series of challenges to be mastered. "Ego integrity versus despair" is the last challenge, where individuals judge whether their lives were meaningful or not. Learning to let go, accept help as function declines, and detach from relationships are central tasks of aging adults.
1965	Rose	Subculture	Older adults form a societal subculture in response to negative attitudes held by society in general about the elderly. Social status is affected by health and functional ability.
1968	Havighurst et al.	Continuity	Personality tends to be stable throughout life. Consistent coping patterns are used to adapt to the physical, financial, and social challenges of aging. Personality affects roles in later life as well as satisfaction. Key challenges include connecting with others, coping with limitations, assuming new roles, and contemplating death.
1972	Riley et al.	Age Stratification	We acquire resources, roles, status, and deference from others based upon our age group. Age cohorts share similar experiences and beliefs that shape their attitudes and expectations about living.
1980	Back	Life Course/ Lifespan Development	Older adults must adjust to altered roles and relationships as they move through life's stages. Expectations about older adults affect one's life course or development.
1982	Lawton	Person-Environment Fit	Our self-concept, physical health, mental and sensory status, and environment affect our ability to function and adapt to environmental demands.

Continued

TABLE 1-2 Theories of Aging—cont'd

YEAR	AUTHOR	THEORY	SUMMARY
Psychosocial theories of aging			
1987	Baltes	Selective Optimization with Compensation	Older adults deal with loss by choosing activities and roles with optimal benefits. Dealing with disability, impending death, and satisfaction in living are challenges to be mastered. Learning to compromise facilitates life satisfaction.
1994	Tornstam	Gero-transcendence	Older adults transition from a materialistic/rational perspective toward unity with the universe. An external focus, coming to terms with death, and strong relationships facilitate successful transformation.
Biological theories of aging			
1889	Weismann	Wear & Tear Theory	Internal and external stressors cause a decline in cellular function over time.
1956	Harman	Free Radical Theory	Free radicals produced by cellular oxidation accumulate over time and disrupt normal cell function.
1956	Verzar	Cross-Link Theory	Abnormal bonding of glucose and proteins causes breakdown of collagen, which leads to physical alterations and developing disabilities.
1963	Orgel	Protein Error Theory	Protein synthesis becomes increasingly flawed with age, leading to cellular compromise and death.
1979	Kay	Immunological Theory	Atrophy of the thymus gland with age impedes immune functioning and increases vulnerability to disease.
1981	Hayflick & Moorehead	Programmed Theory	Cells have a genetically determined, preprogrammed code that determines aging.
1986	Walford	Metabolic Theory	Caloric restriction and enriched nutrient foods hasten DNA repair and reduce production of biochemicals associated with disease development.
1996	Hayflick	Neuroendocrine/Pacemaker Theory	Aging is due to changes in endocrine production and functioning, which impair the body's ability to adapt to internal and external stressors.
1998	Keys & Marble	Genetic Telomere Theory	Chromosomal telomeres shorten with each replication. Disappearance of telomeres results in cellular death and contributes to aging.

TABLE 1-2 Theories of Aging—cont'd

YEAR	AUTHOR	THEORY	SUMMARY
Nursing theories of aging			
1990	Miller	Functional Consequences Theory	Ability to function is influenced by environmental and bio-psycho-social consequences. Nurses minimize these consequences to reduce disability and enhance safety and quality of life.
2002	Haight et al.	Theory of Thriving	Disharmony between individual and environment or relationships leads to a failure to thrive. Nurses help to identify and remove sources of disharmony.
2005	Flood	Theory of Successful Aging	Successful aging is the positive adaptation to physical and functional changes as we grow older, while maintaining spiritual connectedness and a sense of meaning and purpose in our lives. Nurses support patients' adaptation to change and search for meaning.

Flood (2005) wrote a nursing theory about successful aging in which spirituality is also a central concept. The author proposes that to age successfully, we must adapt to the physical and functional changes that occur as we grow older and believe that our lives have meaning and purpose. The sections of this book, Thriving in Old Age, Optimizing Physical Health and Functioning, Optimizing Economic and Social Well-Being, and Optimizing Mental Well-Being and Spiritual Fulfillment, are based on Flood's theory of successful aging. No single theory of how we age is accepted by everyone as the one correct theory. However, each perspective provides insight into the complex dimensions of aging. These insights can inform nursing practice by guiding our assessment, planning, and interventions in the care of older adults.

KEY POINTS

- Aging is a process that involves physical, psychological, and social life changes.
- Physiological changes affect the way the body continues to function and are mediated by life habits.
- Psychological changes include forming new relationships, seeking out new opportunities and experiences, and learning new ways of coping with everyday stresses.
- Societal roles held in earlier life may recur. Age can be thought of chronologically, biologically, or psychologically.
- Attitude has much to do with feelings of well-being and life satisfaction.
- Experiences shape our beliefs and assumptions about older adults.
- Ageism, or generalizing one's beliefs to an entire population, can lead to unwarranted discrimination.
- Studies show that ageism occurs among health professionals, as well as among society in general.
- Ageism can influence policy formation, insurance reimbursement, and treatment regimens.
- Lack of education about gerontology contributes to ageism.
- Aging is an unfolding process that can be enriching, satisfying, and fulfilling.
- Wisdom is acquired by reflecting on life's experiences. The opportunity to acquire wisdom grows as we age.
- Thriving is related to living and aging successfully.
- Active aging is "the process of optimizing opportunities for health, participation and security in order to enhance quality of life as people age" (WHO, 2009, p. 1).

The Historical Experience of Three Cohorts of Older Americans: A Timeline of Selected Events 1923–2008

1943 Cohort	1933 Cohort	1923 Cohort	Year	Historical Events	Legislative Events
		Born	1923		
		5 years old	1928	**1929**—Stock market crashes	
	Born		1933		**1934**—Federal Housing Administration created by Congress **1935**—Social Security Act passed **1937**—U.S. Housing Act passed, establishing Public Housing
	5 years old	15 years old	1938	**1941**—Pearl Harbor; U.S. enters WWII	
Born			1943	**1945**—Yalta Conference; Cold War begins **1946**—Baby Boom begins	
5 years old	15 years old	25 years old	1948	**1950**—U.S. enters Korean War	
			1953	**1955**—Nationwide polio vaccination program begins	**1956**—Women age 62–64 eligible for reduced Social Security benefits **1957**—Social Security Disability Insurance implemented
15 years old	25 years old	35 years old	1958		**1959**—Section 202 of the Housing Act established, providing assistance to older adults with low income **1961**—Men age 62–64 eligible for reduced Social Security benefits **1962**—Self-Employed individual Retirement Act (Keogh Act) passed
			1963	**1964**—U.S. enters Vietnam War; Baby Boom ends	**1964**—Civil Rights Act passed **1965**—Medicare and Medicaid established; Older Americans Act passed **1967**—Age Discrimination in Employment Act passed
25 years old	35 years old	45 years old	1968	**1969**—First man on the moon	**1972**—Formula for Social Security cost-of-living adjustment established; Social Security Supplemental Security Income legislation passed
			1973		**1974**—Employee Retirement Income Security Act (ERISA) passed; IRAs established **1975**—Age discrimination Act passed
35 years old	45 years old	55 years old	1978	**1980**—First AIDS case is reported to the Centers for Disease Control and Prevention	**1978**—401(k)s established
			1983		**1983**—Social Security eligibility age increased for full benefits **1984**—Widows entitled to pension benefits if spouse was vested **1986**—Mandatory retirement eliminated for most workers **1987**—Reverse mortgage market created by HUD Home Equity Conversion Program
45 years old	55 years old	65 years old	1988	**1989**—Berlin Wall falls **1990**—U.S. enters Persian Gulf War	**1990**—Americans with Disabilities Act passed
			1993		**1996**—Veterans' Health Care Eligibility Reform Act passed, creating access to community-based long-term care for all enrollees
55 years old	65 years old	75 years old	1998	**2001**—September 11—Terrorists attack U.S.	**1997**—Balanced Budget Act passed, changing Medicare payment policies **2000**—Social Security earnings test eliminated for full retirement age
			2003	**2003**—U.S. enters Iraq War	**2003**—Medicare Modernization Act passed **2005**—Deficit Reduction Act passed, realigning Medicaid incentives to provide noninstitutionalized long-term care **2006**—Medicare prescription drug benefit implemented; Pension Protection Act passed
65 years old	75 years old	85 years old	2008	**2008**—First Baby Boomers begin to turn 62 years old and become eligible for Social Security retired worker benefits	

Figure 1-1 *(From Federal Interagency Forum on Aging-Related Statistics. (2008). Older Americans 2008: Key indicators of well-being (p. 161). Federal Interagency Forum on Aging-Related Statistics, Washington, DC: U.S. Government Printing Office. March 2008. Retrieved October 22, 2010, from http://www.aoa.gov/agingstatsdotnet/Main_Site/Data/2008_Documents/OA_2008.pdf)*

- The MacArthur Foundation Study of Successful Aging concluded that highly functioning older adults had fewer risk factors for chronic illnesses and tended to be more socially and mentally active (Berkman et al., 1993).
- Psychosocial conditions as well as physical health are closely linked to aging well.
- Theories about aging have been written from biological, sociological, and psychological perspectives.
- Recent theories expand on the idea of a search for meaning based on experiences in the natural world to include a person's fit within the larger universe.
- Spirituality, transformation, and transcendence are central concepts in nursing theories about aging.
- Flood's theory of successful aging, the framework for this book, includes three central themes: thriving in old age, optimizing economic and social well-being, and optimizing mental well-being and spiritual fulfillment.
- Theories provide insight into the complex dimensions of aging and inform nursing assessment, planning, and interventions in the care of older adults.

CRITICAL THINKING ACTIVITIES

1. Draw a picture of yourself when you are old. What is your age? Where will you be? Are others with you? What, if any, health problems do you have?
2. Discover your own thoughts about aging by answering the questions on one of the tools in Table 1-1. Share the reasons for your answers with a partner. Can you discover any assumptions you have about older adults?
3. Consider an older adult that you know personally, or perhaps a famous person that exhibits how you would like to be when you are old. What qualities do you desire? Are these qualities consistent with what the research says about how to age successfully? Would you need to make any lifestyle changes to achieve these qualities in later life?
4. Go to the drugstore and find a product that makes anti-aging claims. Determine the active ingredient(s), and research what evidence exists to support the anti-aging claims.
5. Discuss how aging is portrayed in the television sitcom, "The Simpsons." Then consider the perspectives suggested in this article: Blakeborough, D. (2008). "Old people are useless": Representations of aging on The Simpsons. *Canadian Journal on Aging/La Revue Canadienne du Vieillissement, 27*(1), 57–67.

REFERENCES

Ardelt, M. (1997). Wisdom and life satisfaction in old age. *The Journals of Gerontology: Series A Biological Sciences and Medical Sciences, 52A*(1), 15–27.

Back, K. (1980). *Life course: Integrated theories and exemplary populations.* Boulder, CO: Westview Press.

CASE STUDY | *MARIA ESPOSITO*

The eldest of five children, Maria Esposito is 28 years old, single, and working full-time as a dental hygienist. She is concerned about her mother's future because her father passed away last month. Maria's mother, Mrs. Esposito, is 68 years old and lives alone in a suburban neighborhood where she has many friends. She is active in a nearby Catholic church and walks the few blocks to Mass and choir practice three times each week.

Mrs. Esposito has high blood pressure and diabetes that are well controlled with medication. Maria worries that her mother will be unable to manage living alone and wonders whether she should move in with her mother. In sharing her concern with a coworker, the coworker responds, "Most older adults live alone anyway. I'm sure your mother will be able to take care of herself. The only problem is that she is still driving a car. At her age and with her diabetes, she might start getting forgetful and having problems with her eyesight. If I were you, I'd talk to her doctor about whether she ought to stop driving."

1. What behaviors does Mrs. Esposito exhibit that contribute to successful aging?
2. Are Maria's concerns justified? Which theories of aging support your views?
3. What myths about older adults does the coworker exhibit?

Baltes, P. B. (1987). Theoretical propositions of life-span developmental psychology: On the dynamics between growth and decline. *Developmental Psychology, 23,* 611–626.

Berkman, L. F., Seeman, T. E., Albert, M., Blazer, D., Kahn, R. L., Mohs, R. . . . McClearn, G. (1993). High, usual and impaired functioning in community-dwelling older men and women: Findings from the MacArthur foundation research network on successful aging. *Journal of Clinical Epidemiology, 46*(10), 1129–1140.

Bond, M., Bowling, A., McKee, D., Kennelly, M., Banning, A. P., Dudley, N. . . . (2003). Does ageism affect the management of ischaemic heart disease? *Journal of Health Services Research & Policy, 8*(1), 40–47.

Bowling, A. (2007). Honour your father and mother: Ageism in medicine. *The British Journal of General Practice, 57*(538), 347–348.

Burbank, P., McCool, J., & Burkholder, G. (2005). *Perspectives Toward Caring for Older Patients Questionnaire.* Retrieved November 8, 2010, from http://www.aacn.nche.edu/Education/Hartford/ShowcasingInnovations/UofRIShowcase.htm

Cumming, E., & Henry, W. (1961). *Growing old.* New York, NY: Basic Books.

Curtis, J. (2006). Ageism and kidney transplantation. *American Journal of Transplantation, 6*(6), 1264–1266.

Erikson, E. (1963). *Childhood and society.* New York, NY: Norton.

Flood, M. (2005). A mid-range nursing theory of successful aging. *Journal of Theory Construction and Testing, 9*(2), 35–39.

Fraboni, M., Saltstone, R., & Hughes, S. (1990). The Fraboni scale of ageism (FSA): An attempt at a more precise measure of ageism. *Canadian Journal on Aging, 9*(1), 56–66.

Gaziano, T. A., Galea, G., & Reddy, K. S. (2007). Scaling up interventions for chronic disease prevention: The evidence. *Lancet, 8,* 1939–1946.

Gething, L., Fethney, J., McKee, K., Persson, L., et al. (2004). Validation of the reactions to ageing questionnaire: Assessing similarities across several countries. *Journal of Gerontological Nursing, 30*(9), 47–54.

Gilmer, D. F., & Aldwin, C. M. (2003). *Health, illness, and optimal aging: Biological and psychosocial perspectives.* Thousand Oaks, CA: Sage.

Godlovitch, G. (2003). Age discrimination in trials and treatment: Old dogs and new tricks. *Monash Bioethics Review, 22*(3), 66–77.

Gruenewald, T. L., Karlamangla, A. S., Greendale, G. A., Singer, B. H., & Seeman, T. E. (2007). Feelings of usefulness to others, disability, and mortality in older adults: The MacArthur study of successful aging. *Journals of Gerontology Series B: Psychological Sciences and Social Sciences, 62*(1), 28–37.

Gunderson, A., Tomkowiak, J., Menachemi, N., & Brooks, R. (2005). Rural physicians' attitudes toward the elderly: Evidence of ageism? *Quality Management in Health Care, 14*(3), 167–176.

Haight, B. K., Barba, B. E., Tesh, A. S., & Courts, N. F. (2002). Thriving: A life span theory. *Journal of Gerontological Nursing, 28*(3), 14–22.

Hansen-Kyle, L. (2005). A concept analysis of healthy aging. *Nursing Forum, 40*(2), 45–57.

Harman, D. (1956). Aging: A theory based on the free radical and radiation chemistry. *Journal of Gerontology, 11,* 298–300.

Havighurst, R. J., & Albrecht, R. (1953). *Older people.* New York, NY: Longmans-Green.

Havighurst, R. J., Neugarten, B. L., & Tobin, S. S. (1968). Disengagement and patterns of aging. In B. L. Neugarten (Ed.), *Middle age and aging: A reader in social psychology* (pp. 67–71). Chicago, IL: University Press.

Hayflick, L. (1996). *How and why we age.* New York, NY: Ballantine Books.

Hayflick, L., & Moorehead, P. S. (1981). The serial cultivation of human diploid cell strains. *Experimental Cell Research, 25,* 585–621.

Jetha, N., Robinson, K., Wilkerson, T., Dubois, N., Turgeon, V., & DesMeules, M. (2008). Supporting knowledge into action: The Canadian Best Practices Initiative for Health Promotion and Chronic Disease Prevention. *Canadian Journal of Public Health, 99*(5), I1–18.

Jung, C. G. (1960). *The structure and dynamics of the psyche. Collected works* (Vol. VIII). Oxford, England: Pantheon.

Kay, M. B. (1979). The thymus: Clock for immunological aging? *Journal of Investigative Dermatology, 73*(1), 29––38.

Keys, S.W., & Marble, M. (1998, May). In vivo data demonstrate critical role for telomeres. *Transplant Weekly,* 11.

Knox, V. J., Gekoski, W. L., & Kelly, L. E. (1995). The age group evaluation and description (aged) inventory: A new instrument for assessing stereotypes of and attitudes toward age groups. *International Journal of Aging and Human Development, 40*(1), 31–55.

Kogan, N. (1961). Attitudes toward older people: The development of a scale and examination of correlates. *Journal of Abnormal and Social Psychology, 62,* 44–54.

Kruk, J. (2007). Physical activity in the prevention of the most frequent chronic diseases: An analysis of the recent evidence. *Asian Pacific Journal of Cancer Prevention, 8,* 325–338.

Lange, J. W., & Grossman, S. C. (2006). Aging theories. In K. L. Mauk (Ed.), *Gerontological nursing: Competencies for care* (pp. 57–84). Sudbury, MA: Jones & Bartlett.

Lasher, K. P., & Faulkender, P. J. (1993). Measurement of aging anxiety: Development of the anxiety about aging scale. *International Journal of Aging and Human Development, 37*(4), 247–259.

Lawton, M. P. (1982). Competence, environmental press, and the adaptation of older people. In M. P. Lawton, P. G. Windley, & T. O. Byerts (Eds.), *Aging and the environment: Theoretical approaches* (pp. 33–59). New York, NY: Springer.

Maslow, A. H. (1954). *Motivation and personality.* New York, NY: Harper & Row.

McConatha, J. T., Schnell, F., Volkwein, K., Riley, L., & Leach, E. (2003). Attitudes toward aging: A comparative analysis of young adults from the United States and Germany. *International Journal of Aging and Human Development, 57*(3), 203–215.

Miller, C. A. (1990). *Nursing care of older adults: Theory and practice.* Glenview, IL: Scott, Foresman/Little, Brown Higher Education.

Orgel, L. E. (1963). The maintenance of the accuracy of protein synthesis and its relevance to ageing. *Proceedings of the*

National Academy of Sciences of the United States of America (0027-8424), 49, 517–521.

Palmore, E. (2001). The ageism survey: First findings/ Response. *Gerontologist, 41*(5), 572–575.

Peake, M. D., Thompson, S., Lowe, D., & Pearson, M. G. (2003). Ageism in the management of lung cancer. *Age and Ageing, 32*(2), 71–77.

Peterson, C., & Seligman, M. (2004). *Character strengths and virtues: A handbook and classification.* Cary, NC: Oxford University Press.

Polizzi, K. G. (2003). Assessing attitudes toward the elderly: Polizzi's refined version of the aging semantic differential. *Educational Gerontology, 29*(3), 197–216.

Riley, M. W., Johnson, M., & Foner, A. (1972). *Aging and society: A sociology of age stratification* (Vol. 3). New York, NY: Russell Sage Foundation.

Rose, A. M. (1965). The subculture of the aging: A framework for research in social gerontology. In A. M. Rose & W. A. Peterson (Eds.), *Older people and their social worlds* (pp. 3–16). Philadelphia, PA: Davis.

Rowe, J. W., & Kahn, R. L. (1997). Successful aging. *Gerontologist, 37*(4), 433–440.

Salzman, B. (2006). Myths and realities of aging. *Care Management Journals, 7*(3), 141–150.

Seeman, T. E. (1996). Social ties and health: The benefits of social integration. *Annals of Epidemiology, 6*(5), 442–451.

Sternberg, R. J. (2004). What is wisdom and how can we develop it? *Annals of the American Academy of Political and Social Science, 591*(1), 164–174.

Sternberg, R. J. (2005). Older but not wiser? The relationship between age and wisdom. *Ageing International, 30*(1), 5–26.

Stuart-Hamilton, I. (2006) *The psychology of ageing: An introduction* (4th ed.). London, England: Kingsley.

Tapsell, L. C., & Probst, Y. C. (2008). Nutrition in the prevention of chronic diseases. *World Review of Nutrition and Dietetics, 98,* 94–105.

Tornstam, L. (1994). Gerotranscendence: A theoretical and empirical exploration. In L. E. Thomas & S. A. Eisenhandler (Eds.), *Aging and the religious dimension* (pp. 203–226). Westport, CT: Greenwood.

Verzar, F. (1956). Aging of collagen fibres. In *Experimental research on aging. Experientia, Supplement 4:35,* 35-41. Basel: Birkauser Verlag.

Walford, R. L. (1986). *The 120-year diet: How to double your vital years.* New York, NY: Pocket Books.

Weismann, A. (1889). On heredity. In A. Weismann, *Essays upon heredity and kindred biological problems* (Vol. 1, pp. 67–105). Oxford, U.K.: Clarendon Press.

Wilken, C. S. (2002). *Myths and realities of aging.* (University of Florida IFAS Extension. FCS2193). Department of Family, Youth and Community Sciences, Florida Cooperative Extension Service, Institute of Food and Agricultural Sciences, University of Florida, Gainesville.

World Health Organization. (2007). *10 facts on ageing and the life course.* Retrieved October 22, 2010, from http://www.who.int/features/factfiles/ageing/en/index.html

World Health Organization. (2009). *What is "active ageing"?* Retrieved October 22, 2010, from http://www.who.int/ageing/active_ageing/en/print.html

Yoong, K., & Heymann, T. (2005). Colonoscopy in the very old: Why bother? *Postgraduate Medical Journal, 81*(953), 196–197.

Chapter 2

Mid-Range Theory of Successful Aging

Meredith Troutman, PhD, PMHCNS-BC

LEARNING OBJECTIVES

- Define successful aging.
- Describe the importance of a multidimensional conceptualization of successful aging.
- Identify major concepts of the mid-range theory of successful aging.
- Identify clinical implications related to promotion of successful aging in older adults.

Significance of Successful Aging

The subject of aging is an increasingly important topic in research, theory development and refinement, policy development, and clinical practice. Professionals and lay people alike are concerned with aging successfully. There are many reasons for this interest, including growing life expectancies, increasing diversity of our elderly population, rising health care costs, the nursing shortage, the smaller number of nurses interested in gerontological nursing as compared with other specialties, and health care consumer needs.

Life expectancy has risen dramatically since 1900. On average, White men have experienced an increase of 29 years; Black men, 37 years, White women, 32 years; and Black women, 43 years in life expectancy during this time (Arias, 2007). As of 2006, life expectancy was 77.7 years (Heron et al., 2009). People age 65 or older numbered 35 million in 2000 and made up 12.4% of the U.S. population, about 1 in every 8 Americans (Administration on Aging, 2001). As of 2008, 12.8% of the population was 65 or older (U.S. Census Bureau, 2009). By the year 2040, the United States will have more people over age 65 than under 20 (U.S. Census Bureau, 2000). Older adults from all racial/ethnic groups will experience more rapid population growth than Whites, with non-White elders increasing from 16% to 26% of the total aged population by 2030 (US Bureau of the Census & National Institute on Aging, 1993). (See Chapter 3 for more on the demographics of older adults.)

By 2018, national health care expenditures are expected to reach $4.4 trillion, more than double the spending of 2007 (Siska et al., 2009). The cost of caring for aging U.S. residents by 2030 will add 25% to the nation's overall health care costs (Centers for Disease Control and Prevention, 2007). Of concern is who will provide nursing care for tomorrow's older adults. Nationally, the shortage of registered nurses is expected to reach 29% by 2020, and of the 2.56 million registered nurses in the United States, fewer than 15,000 (0.005%) are certified gerontological nurses (Carter, 2009). Older adults are acutely aware of issues such as these that affect or may impact their lives; vast numbers have identified aging with dignity and purpose as being vital to them, and they support advocacy for health and financial security, livable communities, community services efforts, and ongoing research on aging through their membership in AARP, formerly the American Association for Retired Persons (AARP, 2009).

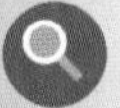

EVIDENCE FOR PRACTICE
Defining Successful Aging

Purpose: To understand how older adults define successful aging and to examine relationships among physical health, functional ability, well-being, and subjective assessment of successful aging.

Sample: 53 community-dwelling adults age 60 and older.

Methods: Surveys were administered at local senior centers. They included a checklist of illnesses, measurement of activities of daily living and instrumental activities of daily living, assessment of depressive symptoms, measurement of life satisfaction, measurement of social support, an open-ended question that asked their definition of successful aging, and a Likert format self-assessment of one's success at aging.

Results: Participants defined successful aging as including activity/exercise, physical health, social relationships, and psychological/cognitive health. Successful aging, as assessed by the open-ended question, was positively related to social support, life satisfaction, and subjective health.

Implications: Researchers can begin to develop interventions for successful aging if they understand older adults' perceptions of the phenomenon. Clinicians can facilitate goal setting with older adults, based on the older adult's description and perception of what successful aging is.

Reference: Ferri, C., James, I., & Pruchno, R. (2009). Successful aging: Definitions and subjective assessment according to older adults. *Clin Gerontol, 32,* 379–388.

It is thus clear that there are a number of stakeholders when it comes to the health and well-being, and the potential for successful aging of our older adult population. The two overarching goals of *Healthy People 2010,* which lays out national health objectives, are increasing quality and years of healthy life and eliminating health disparities (U.S. Department of Health and Human Services, 2008). Accordingly, the body of research on successful aging has grown over the past 20 years, and it continues to expand. Research has shown that health is predictive of successful aging (Duay & Bryan, 2006; Ford et al., 2000; Vaillant & Mukamal, 2001). However, disparities between older adult ethnic and racial groups are increasing (Agency for Healthcare Research and Quality and the Centers for Disease Control and Prevention, 2002; Wilmoth & Longino, 2006). People with lower incomes often experience worse health, have reduced access to high-quality health care (Agency for Healthcare Research and Quality and the Centers for Disease Control and Prevention, 2002), and are more likely to die prematurely (Adler & Newman, 2002). Inadequately managed chronic disease also presents challenges to aging successfully, in terms of quality of life, individual finances, and longevity. More than 80% of people over age 65 have at least one chronic health condition, and the average 75 year old has at least three (Mezey & Gray-Miceli, 2007). Further, growing life expectancies mean that more older adults are living with multiple chronic illnesses. Thus, chronic disease presents a major hurdle that must be overcome to age successfully. It is unrealistic to consider only those with good physical health as successful agers because clearly many older adults do not fit the traditional descriptions of successful aging.

Therefore, a useful theory must have an inclusive approach to successful aging. Such theory will be more applicable to the real-life older adults and will provide a more relevant context for research involving increasingly diverse older adults of multiple age strata (the old, the old old, and the oldest old).

Background of Successful Aging

Though there has been some research and theory development involving older adults of countries other than the United States (e.g., Baltes & Baltes, 1999; Litwin, 2005; Roos & Havens, 1991; Tornstam, 1996,1997; von Faber et al., 2001), much of the research on successful aging has been conducted with White, educated, middle- or upper-class, relatively healthy American-born participants (e.g., Bryant, Corbett, & Kutner, 2001; Crowther et al., 2002; Lamond et al., 2008; Rowe & Khan, 1998; Tate, Leedine, & Cuddy, 2003; Wong, 2000). Thus, theory development has been informed by research with older adults from select ethnic, regional, racial, and demographic backgrounds.

Depp and Jeste's (2006) review of the literature on successful aging identified 28 studies with 29 different definitions of successful aging. Based on existing research and theoretical literature on successful aging, several themes can be identified.

- Having some degree of physical health and mobility is included repeatedly (Chodzko-Zajko, Schwingel, & Park, 2009).
- Better self-reported health status is linked with higher successful aging scores (Young et al., 2009).

- Sustained personal autonomy has been suggested as indicating successful aging (Ford et al., 2000).
- Cognitive and emotional health have also been described as essential features of successful aging (Depp, Vahia, & Jeste, 2007).
- Social engagement and/or leisure activity are also often described as vital for successful aging (Brown, McGuire, & Voelkel, 2008; Bryant, Korbet, & Kutner, 2001; Nimrod & Kleiber, 2007).

While there are important health- and action-oriented features, previous work also points to the subjective components of successful aging, those elements that are related to the older adult's perceptions. Equal to or perhaps more important than the objective elements is one's attitude, outlook on life, and personality traits (Bryant, Corbett, & Kutner, 2001; Fisher & Specht, 1999). Some authors have identified various combinations of these features as key ingredients of successful aging, suggesting that the phenomenon is multidimensional (Duay & Bryan, 2006; Inui, 2003; Knight & Ricardelli, 2003; Ko et al., 2007; Li et al., 2005; Litwin, 2005; Marquez, Bustamante, Blissmer, & Prohaska, 2009; Phelan, Anderson, LaCroix, & Larson, 2004; Reichstadt et al., 2007; Rowe & Khan, 1987, 1998; Vaillant & Mukamal, 2001).

Bowling and Dieppe (2006) concluded from a systematic literature review that the main constituents of successful aging include several important areas for the nurse to assess (Box 2-1). Thus, successful aging involves many facets of health and lifestyle, including those that are objective (externally and impartially measurable) as well as subjective (reliant upon the person's perception of something). Therefore, a comprehensive assessment of multiple health domains is essential.

Some authors have worked to capture both the subjective and objective perspectives of successful aging to compare and contrast these. Strawbridge, Wallhagen, and Cohen (2002) investigated a sample of 867 older adults and compared self-assessed successful aging with Rowe and Khan's (1998) objective (neutral or unbiased) criteria of absence of disease, disability, and risk factors; maintaining physical and mental functioning; and active engagement with life. Participants were asked to respond to a single item that asked how strongly they agreed or disagreed with the statement "I am aging successfully (or aging well)." Consequently, the percentage of participant self-reports of aging successfully was 50.3% compared with 18.8% classified according to Rowe and Kahn's criteria. Thus, the literature suggests that successful aging is a complex and multidimensional phenomenon, with important subjective (things that older adults report feeling or thinking) and objective (measurable by another person, such as blood pressure) features. There appear to be some universal as well as culture-specific aspects as well (Litwin, 2005).

BOX 2-1 Constituents of Successful Aging

- Life expectancy
- Life satisfaction
- Mental and psychological health
- Cognitive function
- Personal growth and learning new things
- Physical health and functioning, and independent functioning
- Psychological characteristics and resources, including perceived autonomy, control, independence, adaptability, coping, self-esteem, positive outlook, goals, sense of self
- Social, community, and leisure activities, integration, and participation
- Social networks, support, participation, and activity
- Accomplishments
- Enjoyment of diet
- Financial security
- Neighborhood
- Physical appearance
- Productivity and contribution to life
- Sense of humor
- Sense of purpose
- Spirituality

From Bowling, A., & Dieppe, P. (2006). What is successful ageing and who should define it? BMJ, 331, 1548–1551.

> *Successful aging is a complex and multidimensional phenomenon with important subjective and objective features.*

Earlier theories

Earlier theories of successful aging, such as those of Rowe and Khan (1998), have been important contributions to the body of knowledge about successful aging, though there seems to be some fragmentation and lack of accounting for the aging person's perceptions (of their aging). Some well-known theories and models include those of

Baltes and Baltes (1999); Bryant, Corbett, and Kutner (2001); Crowther et al. (2001); and Rowe and Khan (1998).

Baltes and Baltes

Baltes and Baltes' (1999) theory is based on the premise that individual aging is a process involving selection, optimization, and compensation. This theory originated from the work of Roman philosopher and statesman, Cicero, who believed old age was not a phase of decline and loss. Rather, Cicero argued that if approached properly, old age afforded many opportunities for positive change and productive functioning. Rooted in psychology, Baltes and Baltes' framework deals with cognitive adaptation, rather than actual biological change, Their work is based on the three processes of selection, optimization, and compensation.

Selection (of various alternative domains of functioning) indicates an increasing restriction of one's life world to fewer domains of functioning because of an age-related loss in the range of adaptive potential. Optimization suggests that people engage in behaviors to enrich and enhance their general reserves and to maximize their chosen behaviors with regard to quality and quantity. Compensation results from restriction in the range of adaptive potential, becoming operative when specific behavioral capacities are lost or reduced below a standard needed for adequate functioning (Baltes & Baltes, 1999). While this theory offers an explanation about the roles of cognition and adaptation in successful aging, Bryant and colleagues' (2001) theory describes how adaptation combined with social components contribute to successful aging.

Bryant, Corbett, and Kutner

Bryant, Corbett, and Kutner (2001) suggest a psychosocial model of "healthy or successful aging" (p. 928), in which health means going places and doing something meaningful. Their model was developed from semistructured interviews with older adults and a regression model from older adults' responses to an insurance company's health status questionnaire. These authors define healthy aging as having a level of health and adaptation to the aging process that is acceptable to the individual.

Well-being encompasses physical condition, financial and mental security, the ability to do things and be with people, and personal internal characteristics such as positive attitude. Healthy agers have something worthwhile and desirable to do, possess the required abilities to meet perceived challenges, have the necessary resources, and the will to go places and do things. These components each play a role in health or successful aging, interact to supplement each other, and contribute to adaptation to change (Bryant, Corbett, & Kutner, 2001).

Rowe and Kahn

Perhaps the most widely recognized theory of successful aging is that of Rowe and Khan (1998), based on the MacArthur Aging Studies. Rowe and Khan define successful aging as the ability to maintain a low risk of disease-related disability, high mental and physical function, and active engagement with life. Rowe and Khan's theory is entrenched in a conceptualization of successful aging in which both physical and mental factors enable individuals to continue to function effectively into old age.

The ordering of these components is hierarchical, with an absence of disease and disability facilitating maintenance of physical and mental function. Maintaining physical and mental function enables active engagement with life. The combination of these three components represents the concept of aging most fully. Maintaining a high level of overall functioning requires both physical and mental abilities, which are significantly independent of each other. The significance of a "just keep on going" attitude (Rowe & Khan, p. 40) explains the independence of physical and mental abilities necessary for high-level overall functioning.

Crowther and Colleagues

After the development of Rowe and Khan's theory, Crowther and colleagues (2002) suggested adding positive spirituality as a fourth factor to enhance the theory. Spirituality is a personal quest for understanding answers to ultimate questions about life, its meaning, and a relationship to the sacred, which may or may not lead to or arise from the development of religious rituals and the formation of community (Crowther et al., 2002). "Positive spirituality involves a developing and internalized personal relation with the sacred or transcendence that is not bound by race, ethnicity, economics, or class, and promotes the wellness and welfare of self and others" (Crowther et al., 2002, p. 614). Positive spirituality may decrease the sense of loss of control that accompanies an illness and provide a cognitive framework that reduces stress and increases purpose and meaning in the face of illness, they note.

Crowther and colleagues (2002) contend that their addition of positive spirituality to Rowe and Khan's theory provides many opportunities for community-based health promotion interventions. Crowther and colleagues' theory suggests that spirituality is vital to successful aging. Similarly, the search to find meaning through relating to a sacred power is also reflected in Wong's (2000) theory.

Wong

Wong believes personal meaning is the hidden dimension of successful aging. Originating from existential philosophy, Wong's theory asserts that when many sources of meaning, such as social status and work, are threatened, one's life satisfaction depends on whether the existential need (for personal meaning) is met. The challenge of successful aging is thus to discover a positive meaning of life and death even when one's physical health is failing. Zest for life, positive attitude, and a clear sense of meaning and purpose are criteria for successful aging. The successfully aging person experiences a spiritual and existential quest, and personal growth in wisdom and spirituality (Wong, 2000).

From this perspective, successful aging is attainable for anyone with positive meaning, regardless of his or her physical condition. Positive meanings of life and death provide the necessary motivation for pursuing healthy lifestyles and worthy life goals. Individuals who age successfully exhibit neutral acceptance of death, realizing their personal mortality and making the most of life, or they demonstrate acceptance, looking forward to a rewarding afterlife after completing their mission in life (Wong, 2000).

Limitations and Needs

While each of these theories or models has been a significant and meaningful contribution to the body of knowledge, they tend to focus on or emphasize one or two aspects of successful aging (Table 2-1). Although some allude to the relevance of the older adult's perception of aging, none defines successful aging from this frame of reference. Further, none fully integrates the physical, mental, spiritual, and existential health or well-being of older adults or attempts to describe the interrelationships among these four dimensions of successful aging. It is not only one's physical body and abilities that change over time, but the mind and spirit are subject to change as well. Young,

TABLE 2-1 Theories of Successful Aging

TYPE OF THEORY	AUTHORS	SUMMARY AND CONCEPTUAL UNDERPINNINGS
Cognitive/psychological	Baltes & Baltes (1999)	Emphasis is on cognitive adaptation. Individual aging is a process involving selection, optimization, and compensation. Successful aging encompasses *selection* of functional domains on which to focus one's resources, *optimizing* developmental potential, and *compensating* for losses, thus ensuring the maintenance of functioning and a minimization of losses (Freund, 2008). The model is a metamodel that attempts to represent scientific knowledge about the nature of development and aging, with the focus on successful adaptation (Baltes & Carstensen, 1996).
Existential philosophical	Wong (2000)	Personal meaning is the hidden dimension of successful aging. When many sources of meaning, such as social status and work, are threatened, one's life satisfaction depends on whether the existential need for personal meaning is met. The challenge of successful aging is to discover a positive meaning of life and death even when one's physical health is failing.

TABLE 2-1 Theories of Successful Aging—cont'd

TYPE OF THEORY	AUTHORS	SUMMARY AND CONCEPTUAL UNDERPINNINGS
Psychosocial	Bryant et al. (2001)	Emphasis is on reducing the risk of negative events, but includes the concept of bolstering the positive aspects of aging as well. Older adults may have one or more chronic illnesses but still consider themselves healthy. Health means going and doing something meaningful, which requires four components: something worthwhile to do, balance between abilities and challenges, appropriate external resources, and personal attitudinal characteristics (Bryant et al., 2001). This model encourages interdisciplinary support of desired goals and outcomes rather than only medical approaches to deficits and challenges (Bryant et al., 2001).
Biopsychosocial and spiritual	Crowther et al. (2001)	In addition to the concepts of Rowe and Khan's theory, positive spirituality may enhance one's ability to adapt, by decreasing the sense of loss of control that accompanies an illness and providing a cognitive framework that reduces stress and increases purpose and meaning in the face of illness. Spirituality is a vital foundation for successful aging.
Biopsychosocial	Rowe & Kahn (1998)	Successful aging is lower risk of disease/disability, greater mental and physical function, and active engagement with life. The theory is based on the assumption that both physical and mental factors enable individuals to continue to function effectively into old age.

Frick, and Phelan (2009) note that most constructs of successful aging have been unidimensional, though a few have been multidimensional. They further observe that no definition has incorporated all the dimensions (physical, functional, social, and psychological) endorsed by older adults as important to successful aging.

As people live longer, and the older adult population becomes more culturally and ethnically diverse, it is increasingly important that we consider successful aging from the perspective of the aging person. Those perspectives are likely to vary, influenced in part by culture, race, and ethnicity. Indeed, there are divergences in successful aging, based on gender, for example (Hsu, 2005). Rossen, Knafl, and Flood's (2008) female sample described comportment, presentation of self to the outside world in a way that conveys regard for self and interest in others, as a key attribute of successful aging. Litwin (2005) identified variation according to whether participants were Jewish Israelis, Arab Israelis, or new immigrants. Thus, it is important to be aware of the variations in successful aging that are influenced by variables such as gender, race, and culture.

Perhaps of utmost importance is the need for a theory from which interventions can be derived to promote successful aging. If successful aging is influenced by gender, race, culture, and thus, the older adult's perception of his or her aging, then interventions aimed at enhancing successful aging must take into consideration what the older adult considers more important (physical, mental, spiritual, existential well-being, etc.), and target these. Interventions are more likely to be accepted if one believes they will be beneficial and finds them reasonable and realistic to adopt.

Nursing is widely recognized as a discipline concerned with patient advocacy, emphasis on patient education, communication skills, and health promotion. Because of nursing's concern with holistic care of the person, successful aging is quite relevant to nursing theory and research. Therefore, nursing is in an ideal role to encourage successful aging.

Nursing and Successful Aging

Despite the appropriateness of nursing's involvement in successful aging, there has been limited theoretical work (or research) from the discipline. A review of the nursing literature in HealthSource, CINAHL, and PsycInfo on the topic of successful aging yielded 22 papers and 1 book, dating back as far as 1973. In contrast, there were 1,416 nonnursing sources. In other words, nursing research on successful aging is minimal.

Imperio (2006) conducted a grounded theory study of older women's strategies to age successfully and identified three paths of transcendence in successful aging. These were sedulous transcendence, spiritual transcendence, and sanguine transcendence. The general strategies used by these women to manage age- and health-related change and age successfully included

- Accepting by being positive
- Surveying the options and following the path
- Adjusting by charting the options
- Acting by preserving interest and continuing involvement (Imperio, 2006)

The participants described successful aging strategies specific to each type of transcendence. The outcome of transcendence in successful aging was identified as personal satisfaction with life course (Imperio, 2006). These participants described adaptive coping mechanisms to age successfully, rather than things such as good nutrition or physical health. Imperio's work highlights the need to consider older adults' perceptions and variables that influence these, such as gender.

Rossen, Knafl, and Flood (2008) examined older women's perceptions of successful aging. This qualitative study used naturalistic inquiry to examine older women's perceptions of the characteristics and components of successful aging. Three themes were identified: acceptance (of physical, environmental, personal change), engagement (in social and self-care activities), and comportment (positive attributes toward life and demeanor toward others).

Jenerette and Lauderdale (2008) conducted a qualitative pilot study using life review with six women with sickle cell disease. Their analysis resulted in identification of three themes: vulnerability factors (number of pain crises, overprotection, limitations), self-care management resources (religion/spirituality coping behaviors, social support, assertiveness, self-care activities), and health outcomes (living beyond expectations, enjoying life, doing well in spite of sickle cell disease). These findings point toward a more action-oriented set of strategies for successful aging, in contrast to Imperio's findings. However, an orientation toward coping mechanisms seems apparent in the nursing research and theory development on successful aging.

The nursing research and theoretical literature on successful aging remains rather limited as of present. In light of U.S. population trends, the narrow range of nursing research and theoretical work on this topic signals a need for further research inquiry and theoretical development, if nurses are to adequately understand and foster successful aging in older adults.

A Concept Analysis of Successful Aging

Direct clinical care of older adults experiencing various mental and physical illnesses spurred this author's inquiry into successful aging. Two people of the same age, gender, and similar demographic and socioeconomic backgrounds might share the same chronic health conditions. One might manage to maintain a hopeful attitude and positive outlook, striving to maintain his independence and "keep on going," while the other might experience hopelessness and despair. Why could some older adults overcome acute (psychiatric and physical) illnesses, adequately manage their chronic health conditions, and thrive, while others remained mired in hopelessness, focusing on their limitations, narrowing their social interactions and physical activity, and experiencing despair? Perhaps readers have encountered patients such as these. What accounts for the differences? What is it that makes the former individual keep on going while the latter struggles through older adulthood?

These questions proved to be monumental. This author's quest to answer and explain them has unfolded a decade-long path of inquiry and discovery. Careful observation of older adults over the course of their nursing care stimulated the author's initial theoretical work, a concept analysis. How would one describe what made such older adults disparate? Specifically, what features were present in the older adults who seemed to be doing better, and what term(s) best described these people?

It was important to develop a starting point from which to understand these differences in older adults and aging. Finding a name for the phenomena of interest was therefore a fundamental step. With the help of a small group of colleagues, the author engaged in a brainstorming session in which all terms and ideas associated with the older adults who seemed to be "doing well" were listed. This group of nurse colleagues (who were doctoral classmates and a professor) critically discussed each of the terms or phrases identified. After a careful evaluative process, the descriptors were narrowed down to a single term, which captured the traits this author repeatedly saw in those older adults who seemed to fare better: *successful aging.*

Concept analysis helps define the attributes of a concept, in this case successful aging, and is a useful tool to understand successful aging from a multidimensional perspective consistent with the author's clinical observations (Box 2-2). Thus, the initial concept analysis was done to establish a more holistic understanding of successful aging from a nursing perspective (Flood, 2002).

Uses of the Concept

To age means to grow aged or become old (Webster Dictionary, 2009) and refers to one of the periods or stages of human life; or means to mature (Dictionary.com, 2009). A more biological definition of aging is the cumulative changes in an organism leading to a decrease in functional capacity (Columbia Encyclopedia, 2004). Another meaning is to acquire a desirable quality (as mellowness or ripeness) by standing undisturbed for some time, as in cheese or wine, or to bring to a state fit for use or to maturity (Webster Dictionary, 2009). These definitions suggest that the process of aging could be viewed as something desirable or as a series of damaging events that ultimately impair an organism.

To be successful means to to have a degree or measure of succeeding, a favorable or desired outcome, the attainment of wealth, favor, or eminence (Merriam-Webster, 2009). Thus, successfulness is associated with achievement of a preferred or favorable outcome, goal, or consequence. Using a generic definition based on popular dictionary references, successful aging can be defined as *a favorable outcome as perceived by the individual, and his ability to adapt to the cumulative changes associated with the passage of time, while experiencing meaning or purpose in life* (Flood, 2002, p. 105). This explanation is appropriate for the concept of successful aging because it allows for consideration of multiple dimensions of the aging person. This definition was later refined to *an individual's perception of a favorable outcome in adapting to the cumulative physiologic and functional alterations associated with the passage of time, while experiencing spiritual connectedness, a sense of meaning and purpose in life* (Flood, 2006a, p. 36). This conceptual definition more clearly reflects the multidimensionality of successful aging, with the specific inclusion of spirituality.

To establish a thorough and clear conceptual description of successful aging, it was then necessary to identify defining attributes of successful aging. Recurrent themes from the literature that were noteworthy and applicable included

- Desired or favorable outcomes
- Cumulative changes associated with physical deterioration
- Purpose and meaning in life (Flood, 2002)

The literature on aging is consistent with the conceptual definition. Multiple chronic health conditions associated with aging can impact the older adult's ability to function independently. Functional status characterizes a person's ability to provide for the necessities of life, that is, the activities that people do in the normal course of their lives to meet basic needs, fulfill usual roles, and maintain their health and well-being, making functional status an important variable related to successful aging. Multiple authors have found functional status to play a critical role in the lives of older adults (Kivett, Stevenson, & Zwane, 2000; Poon, Gueldner, &

BOX 2-2 Steps in a Concept Analysis

Walker and Avant (1995) suggest eight steps for a concept analysis:

- Selection of a concept
- Determination of the aims or purpose of the analysis
- Identification of all uses of the concept
- Determination of the defining attributes
- Construction of a model case
- Construction of borderline, related, contrary, invented, and illegitimate cases
- Identification of antecedents and consequences
- Definition of empirical referents

Adapted from Walker, L., & Avant, K. (1995). Strategies for theory construction in nursing (3rd ed.). Norwalk, CT: Appleton & Lange.

Sprouse, 2003; Rowe & Khan, 1998). Life satisfaction and meaning in life also have been associated with successful aging (Bearon, 1996; Bowling & Dieppe, 2006; Bryant, Korbett, & Kutner, 2001; Depp & Jeste, 2006; Fisher, 1995; Palmore, 1995; Roos & Havens, 1991; Tornstam, 1997).

Model Cases

Based on these three defining attributes, model cases of successful aging can be illustrated. Examples of the defining attributes in a clinical scenario can help you assess your own understanding of successful aging.

Mr. P. is 73 years old. He attends a remembrance ceremony that his children host in honor of his wife, whom he lost 1 year ago. He expresses his thanks for their support and that of his congregation, stating that although his wife is gone he feels her presence and knows he must take care of his own health now. His goal was to remain independent in the home after his wife died. So far, he has done this with the help of his five children, despite daily arthritic pain and macular degeneration. Mr. P. surrounds himself with neighbors and family and stays as involved as he can in his church, where he used to be the pastor. "My purpose in life is doing for others, reaching out as best I can," he states.

Mrs. B. leads the local senior lunch group at her church in weekly exercise and devotionals. She describes this circle of friends as "the reason I get up and go every day." She stays active delivering meals to other adults in the neighborhood. She is pleased that, at age 80, she takes only two cardiac medicines. She is followed by a local cardiologist, who performed her heart valve surgery last year. Mrs. B. recovered quickly from the surgery and states, "Yes, I don't like to exercise particularly. But I have to keep going and to eat right for my heart." She is asymptomatic now and with a blood pressure in the normal range.

Additional Cases

Developing some additional cases helps elucidate the defining characteristics that have the best fit for the concept (Walker & Avant, 1995). Two of these cases could apply when considering successful aging. A borderline case is an instance that contains some, but not all, of the critical attributes of a concept. Consider the following case.

Mrs. G. is a 96-year-old resident of Pine Haven rest home, where she has lived for 10 years since her son abandoned her there. The staff has a difficult time keeping her at Pine Haven because she often wanders. She has fallen several times, sustaining a hip fracture on one of these occasions. She is not on any medications and surprisingly has no chronic physical health problems. When asked about her health, she says, "I'm great! I just celebrated my 36th birthday. Someone must keep the troops entertained!" Three years into Alzheimer's disease, Mrs. G. believes she is still a United Services Organization volunteer. Her cognitive impairments prevent her from being completely oriented or involved in activities involving much cognitive skill.

In this instance, the older adult feels she has achieved a favorable outcome and has experienced cumulative changes that have resulted in physical deterioration. She also reports a sense of purpose, believing she keeps others entertained. These factors are consistent with the criteria established for successful aging; however, Mrs. G. has cognitive impairment to the degree that she does not know her age, the time, or situation. Although she reports a sense of purpose, her mental status is such that she is not capable of experiencing a more existential transcendent dimension than "keeping the troops entertained."

A contrary case is a clear example of what is not the concept (Walker & Avant, 1995).

Mr. E. is 47, widowed, and a bilateral amputee. He has three children who refuse to be involved in his care. He is very angry, unpleasant, and usually irritable. Even his paid sitter argues with him. He regularly employs passive-aggressive tactics to manipulate the sitter and often refuses to perform self-care. He sometimes deliberately urinates on furniture to anger the sitter. He cries daily and expresses hopelessness and anger at his family, who will not spend time with him because of a lifetime of abuse from him. Mr. E has poorly controlled diabetes and eats sweets to get his family's attention by creating diabetic emergencies that require hospitalizations.

This is an obvious case of unsuccessful aging; Mr. E has not yet even reached old age, is dissatisfied with the outcome of his life thus far, and can find no purpose or meaning in his existence.

Antecedents and Consequences

Antecedents are the events that must occur before successful aging. To age successfully, one must have the opportunity to age, which is to live long enough to experience the elder years. Without living into old age, a person can neither experience the cumulative changes of aging nor have the possibility of achieving a favorable outcome (Flood, 2006a). One must also have the cognitive ability to evaluate life and determine whether aging has been successful.

The consequences of successful aging are acceptance of one's life; the ability to remain actively engaged physically, psychologically, and socially to the extent desired by the person; and the ability to comfortably anticipate what lies beyond (Flood, 2006a). Aging successfully allows one to confront the prospect of death without fear; thus, a spiritual dimension is elemental.

Consequences of successful aging are acceptance of one's life; the ability to remain actively engaged physically, psychologically, and socially to the extent desired by the person; and the ability to comfortably anticipate what lies beyond.

Empirical Referents

Empirical referents permit one to determine the presence of successful aging in the real world. Successful aging can be operationalized by measuring one's achievement of a desirable outcome, ability to cope with cumulative changes that have resulted in physical and functional decline, spiritual connectedness, and sense of meaning and purpose in life. Such a measure should capture the aging person's perception because the existence of what is desirable to the person is subjective, as is meaning and purpose in life.

Measures of successful aging include the Life Satisfaction Index for the Third Age (LITSA) (Barrett & Murk, 2006), Successful Aging Inventory (SAI) (Flood, 2008); Successful Aging Scale (SAS) (Reker, personal communication, December 1, 2008); and the Successful Aging Questionnaire (Tate, Leedine, & Cuddy, 2003). Each of these instruments captures various aspects of successful aging.

- A 35-item, 6 response forced choice Likert format scale, the LITSA is based on the theoretical framework that Neugarten, Havighurst, and Tobin (1961) used to design the Life Satisfaction Index-Form A (LSI-A).
- The SAI is a 20-item Likert format instrument derived from the theory of successful aging (Flood, 2006a).
- The SAS is a 14-item Likert format instrument that is based on four well-known models of aging (Reker, personal communication, December 1, 2008).
- The Successful Aging Questionnaire (Tate, Leedine, & Cuddy, 2003) is composed of questions adapted from the Canadian National Population Health Survey (Statistics Canada, 1994); Short Form—36 items describing physical, mental, and social functioning (Ware & Sherbourne, 1992); self-rated health compared with others of the same age and current satisfaction with life rated on an ordinal 5-point Likert scale; questions regarding living arrangements, marital status, type of housing; ability to perform nine basic activities of daily living such going up and down stairs, bathing, dressing, grooming, and eating; and questions concerning the ability to perform 16 instrumental activities of daily living such as ability to do housework, meal preparation, and laundry. Two key open-ended questions were asked: "What is your definition of successful aging?" and "Would you say you have 'aged successfully"?" (Tate, Leedine, & Cuddy, 2003).

Thus, successful aging is empirically accessible via several methods. Although several well-known theories were used as the basis for the SAS (Reker, personal communication, December 1, 2008), the SAI is the only other measure with a specifically identified theoretical basis. The SAI was derived from Troutman's (formerly Flood's) theory of successful aging, which was developed subsequent to the (Flood, 2002) concept analysis.

Theory Development

A logical step following the concept analysis is theory development, with the ultimate goal of identifying intervention strategies to promote successful aging. Perhaps readers have cared for patients like Mrs. G or Mr. E. These are key illustrations of people who could benefit from interventions to facilitate successful aging to enhance the quality of their lives. A nursing theory of successful aging could provide a useful framework for identifying interventions. There are a number of nonnursing theories of successful aging, but these do not provide clear indications for nursing intervention. Well-known nursing theories are somewhat restricted in their attention to aging.

Nursing Theories

Wadensten and Carlsson (2007) reviewed 17 well-known nursing theories and found that none had a description of human aging. They noted that only five theories (Benner & Wrubel, 1989; King, 1981; Roy, 1997; Travelbee, 1971; Watson, 1997) deal with some aspects of human development toward old age and indirectly affect attitudes toward care of older adults. None of these theories provides practical nursing guidelines on care of older adults.

Therefore, building upon the concept analysis and guided by the literature on successful aging, this author developed a mid-range nursing theory of successful aging using a variation of deductive reformulation, a process involving the derivation of existing knowledge from a nonnursing theory, and reformulation, using knowledge obtained deductively from a nursing conceptual model (Reed, 1991).

A mid-range theory is one with more limited scope and less abstraction that addresses specific phenomena or concepts and reflects practice (Meleis, 1997). Mid-range theories are more focused than grand theories. They have fewer concepts and variables in their structure, are presented in a more testable form, have a more limited scope, and have a stronger relationship with research and practice (McKenna, 1997). Merton (1968) maintained that mid-range theories were particularly important for practice disciplines. He stated that mid-range theories identify a few key variables, present clear propositions, have limited scope, and can easily lead to the derivation of testable hypotheses. Therefore, the phenomenon of successful aging is fitting for the focus of a mid-range theory.

Roy Adaptation Model

Existing knowledge obtained deductively from the Roy Adaptation Model (Roy & Andrews, 1999) was integrated with ideas from Tornstam's (1996) sociological theory of gerotranscendence and the literature on the concepts found in the definition for successful aging. The following assumptions were proposed

- Aging is a progressive process of simple to increasingly complex adaptation.
- Aging may be successful or unsuccessful, depending upon where a person is along the continuum of progression from simple to more complex and extensive use of coping processes.
- Successful aging is influenced by the aging person's choices.
- The self is not ageless (Tornstam, 1996); aging people experience changes, which uniquely characterize their beliefs and perspectives as different from those younger adults (Flood, 2006a).

The Roy Adaptation Model was used in the development of the theory of successful aging because of the theoretical fit of the successful aging assumptions in the Roy model. The Roy Adaptation Model is based on Helson's (1964) adaptation theory and von Bertalanffy's (1968) general systems theory. Roy (1997) referenced Erikson's developmental theory and stated that specific medical problems may arise with age and consideration should be given to the age of the patient. Scientific and philosophical assumptions underlie the Roy Adaptation Model (Box 2-3).

BOX 2-3 Assumptions in the Roy Adaptation Model

The Roy Adaptation Model includes a number of scientific and philosophical assumptions.

Scientific Assumptions

- Systems of matter and energy progress to higher levels of complex self-organization.
- Consciousness and meaning are constitutive of person and environment integration.
- Awareness of self and environment is rooted in thinking and feeling.
- Humans by their decisions are accountable for the integration of creative processes.
- Thinking and feeling mediate human action.
- System relationships include acceptance, protection, and fostering of interdependence.
- Persons and the earth have common patterns and integral relationships.
- Persons and environment transformations are created in human consciousness.
- Integration of human and environment meanings results in adaptation.

Philosophical Assumptions

- Persons have mutual relationships with the world and God.
- Human meaning is rooted in omega point convergence of the universe.
- Persons use human creative abilities of awareness, enlightenment, and faith.
- Persons are accountable for the processes of deriving, sustaining, and transforming the universe (Roy, 2010).

Source: Roy, C. (2010). The Roy Adaptation Model: Assumptions. Retrieved October 27, 2010 from http://www.bc.edu/schools/son/faculty/featured/theorist/Roy_Adaptation_Model.html

The Nursing Metaparadigm

Troutman's assumptions about successful aging are congruent with Roy's conceptualizations of nursing's metaparadigm and reflect the concepts of the nursing metaparadigm as well. Each of these is discussed next.

Person and Adaptation

The person is a holistic adaptive system with coping processes and is a whole composed of parts (Roy, 1997). Roy conceptualizes the person from a holistic perspective: Individual aspects of parts act together to form a unified being (Roy & Andrews, 1999). As living systems, people are in constant interaction with their environments. Between the living system and the environment, an exchange of information, matter, and feedback occurs.

As adaptive systems, people have inputs of stimuli and adaptation level, outputs as behavioral responses that serve as feedback, and control processes known as coping mechanisms (Roy & Andrews, 1999). The adaptation level of the person, in addition to stimuli, acts as input to that person as an adaptive system (Roy & Andrews, 1999). Focal, contextual, and residual stimuli combine and interface to set the adaptation level of the person at a particular point in time. Significant stimuli that comprise the focal, contextual, and residual stimuli include attributes such as past experiences, knowledge level, and strengths and limitations (Galbreath, 1995). The range of response is unique to the individual, and each person's adaptation level is constantly changing. Outputs of the person as a system are that individual's internal and external responses (Roy & Andrews, 1999). Thus, output responses are the person's behaviors; these responses become feedback to the person and to the environment. Roy classified outputs of the person (system) as either adaptive responses or ineffective responses. Adaptive responses are those that promote the integrity of the person (Roy & Andrews, 1999).

Roy (1997) describes the control processes of the person (as an adaptive system) as coping processes. Some coping processes are inherited or genetic; for example, immune system integrity. Other mechanisms are learned, for example, engaging in physical exercise as a health promotion activity. "The adaptation level of the person as an adaptive system is influenced by the individual's development and use of these coping mechanisms. Maximal use of coping mechanisms broadens the adaptation level of the person and increases the range of stimuli to which the person can positively respond" (Roy & Andrews, 1999, p. 258). Roy defines adaptation as the process and outcome through which thinking and feeling people, as individuals, use conscious awareness and choice to create human and environmental integration (Roy & Andrews, 1999). Aging may be successful or unsuccessful, depending upon where the person is along the continuum from simple to more complex and extensive use of coping processes. Someone with more highly developed and frequently used coping mechanisms would be closer to the successful end of the aging continuum. This person would have reached a more complex adaptation level than someone with poorly developed or infrequently used coping mechanisms, who is more likely to be an unsuccessful ager.

Environment

Environment includes "all conditions, circumstance, and influences that surround and affect the development and behavior of persons and groups" (Roy & Andrews, 1999, p. 18). Stimuli from within and around the person are environment. Altering environmental stimuli that contribute to situations of health and illness can facilitate a person's adaptation.

Health

Health is both a state and process of being and becoming integrated and whole that reflects person and environmental mutuality (Roy, 1997). An individual's integrity is expressed as the ability to meet the goals of growth, survival, reproduction, and mastery (Roy & Andrews, 1999). Health can be promoted by promoting adaptive responses.

Nursing

Nursing is the science and practice that expands adaptive abilities and enhances person and environmental transformation (Roy, 1997). Adaptive responses positively affect health; the goal is promotion of adaptive responses in the four adaptive modes, as "the person's adaptation level determines whether a positive response to internal or external stimuli will be elicited" (Galbreath, 1995, p. 261).

Adaptation levels represent the condition of the life processes described on three different levels: integrated, compensatory, and compromised (Roy, 1997). The term *integrated* describes the structures and functions of the life process working as a whole to meet human needs (Roy & Andrews, 1999).

Someone who is aging successfully has integrated adaptation levels. He or she has effectively functioning coping mechanisms and experiences a state of physical, mental, and spiritual well-being. *Compensatory* adaptation levels occur when the subsystems of the person have been activated by a challenge to the integrated processes (Roy & Andrews, 1999). A compensatory adaptation level (in someone who is aging successfully) might be seeking social support from friends and family after experiencing a mild stroke. *Compromised* adaptation levels occur when both integrated and compensatory processes are inadequate (Roy & Andrews, 1999). For example, an older adult who sustains a hip fracture might refuse physical therapy or social support from family and become hopeless and depressed.

Roy's conceptualizations of environment, health, and nursing provide a logical context within which this author's assumptions about successful aging are relevant. Environmental exchanges occur through the interrelationships among theory concepts, some of which involve interactions with other people and environmental resources. The integration and wholeness present with health are reflected in a successfully aging person. Moreover, nursing by Roy and Andrews' (1999) definition, promotes successful aging.

The Theory of Successful Aging

Troutman's theory is composed of three "levels" of *coping processes,* the complex dynamics within the person according to Roy and Andrews (1999), seen in Figure 2-1. Three coping processes make up the foundation of the theory

- (Adaptation of) functional performance mechanisms
- Intrapsychic factors
- Spirituality

These coping processes describe the ways that the person responds to the changing environment (Flood, 2006a). Constructs within each of these coping processes are empirically accessible output responses. These responses provide feedback to the person (and to the environment) and are thus interconnected by arrows. Solid arrows denote those exchanges that occur initially and broken arrows indicate exchanges that occur subsequently (Flood, 2006a).

The dimensions of successful aging (physical, mental, spiritual, and existential) were derived from

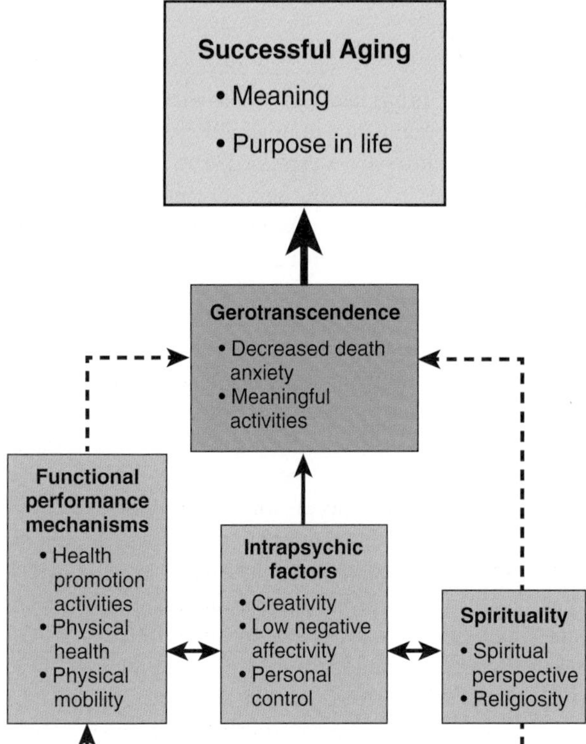

Figure 2-1 Theory of successful aging concepts and constructs. *(From Flood, M. (2006a). A mid-range theory of successful aging. J Theory Construction and Testing, 9(2), 35–39. © M. Troutman.)*

the author's extensive literature review on the phenomenon, and named accordingly.

- *Functional performance mechanisms* are one's use of conscious awareness and choice as an adaptive response to cumulative physiologic and physical losses with subsequent functional deficits occurring as a consequence of aging.
- *Intrapsychic factors* describes the innate and enduring features of an individual's character that may enhance or impair one's ability to adapt to change and to problem solve.
- *Spirituality* is the personal views and behaviors that express a sense of relatedness to something greater than oneself; the feelings, thoughts, experiences, behaviors arising from the search for the sacred. "Gerotranscendence" is a shift in metaperspective, from a materialistic and rationalistic perspective to a more mature and existential one that accompanies the process of aging (Tornstam, 2005).

The theory describes the interrelations of activity and characteristics that occur simultaneously and lead to successful aging. The foundation of the theory is physical, mental, and spiritual coping processes, which may give rise to gerotranscendence, and then lead to successful aging. The foundational coping processes of the theory exist in a cyclical fashion, relating to each other as the arrows indicate; intrapsychic factors influence the extent and success of adaptation of functional performance mechanisms. Intrapsychic factors also impact the extent and depth of spirituality in one's life. Spirituality, in turn, affects how well one can adapt functional performance mechanisms (Flood, 2006a).

Functional Performance Mechanisms

The coping process of functional performance mechanisms encompasses the ways one responds to the cumulative physiologic and functional changes that occur as a result of the passage of time (Flood, 2006a). Indicators of the functional performance mechanisms coping process are output responses of health promotion activities, physical health, and physical mobility. Each of these output responses are manifestations of the human adaptive response of functional performance mechanisms. An example of input stimuli that might initiate an output response is diagnosis of pneumonia. This input stimulus would influence the coping process of adaptation of functional performance mechanisms, producing output. Examples of output might be engaging in coughing and deep breathing (health promotion activity), stimulation of cellular immune responses (physical health), and decreased activity tolerance (physical mobility) (Flood, 2006a).

Intrapsychic Factors

The coping process intrapsychic factors describes how the person utilizes his or her inherent character traits to respond to environmental stimuli. Output responses that are indicative of intrapsychic factors include creativity, low levels of negativity, and personal control. These output responses are manifestations of the human adaptive response of intrapsychic factors. For the older adult with pneumonia, outputs of the intrapsychic factors coping process might be finding alternate ways to correspond with others while homebound (creativity); maintaining a sense of optimism and ventilating feelings of frustration, while being hopeful of speedy recovery (low levels of negative affect); and seeking out additional information about the illness to accelerate recovery (personal control) (Flood, 2006a).

Spirituality

Spirituality describes the person's views and behaviors that convey a sense of relatedness to a greater power or being (Flood, 2006a). Output responses that reflect spirituality include religiosity and spiritual perspective. Consider the case of the older adult with pneumonia; perhaps the person experiences a prolonged illness and requires hospitalization. Output responses that indicate the spirituality coping process would be personal and intercessory prayer (religiosity) and a deeper awareness of the role of spirituality in one's life (spiritual perspective) through the uncertain course of illness (Flood, 2006a). For example, the older adult might decide that the illness experience has drawn him or her closer to God, who helps him or her endure this crisis.

Interchanges occur among these foundational coping processes; output processes can impact each other, consequently, affecting the person. Considering the older adult with pneumonia, participating in health promotion activities might increase feelings of personal control. Spending time in prayer could help a person deal with frustration about this illness and the imposed limitations; effectively managed emotions can help immunity. The exchanges among the three foundational coping processes determine whether the person experiences gerotranscendence, the next adaptive process in successful aging (Flood, 2006a).

Gerotranscendence

Gerotranscendence is a more complex coping process of successful aging; whether or not someone gerotranscends depends on the foundational coping processes. Gerotranscendence is a coping process that occurs when there is a major shift in the person's worldview, where a person examines his or her place in the world and in relation to others (Tornstam, 1997). The older adult examines values held, and these may change from what they were when that person was younger. Output responses suggestive of gerotranscendence include decreased death anxiety, engagement in meaningful activities, changes in relationships, self-acceptance, and wisdom.

Gerotranscendence is a coping process that occurs when there is a major shift in the person's worldview, where a person examines his or her place in the world and in relation to others.

Roy (1997) identified the goals of the human adaptive system as survival, growth, reproduction, mastery, and personal and environmental transformation. In the theory of successful aging, survival, growth, and mastery are achieved through the integration of adaptation of functional performance mechanisms, intrapsychic factors, and spirituality. Once this integration has occurred, the older adult may gerotranscend. Through gerotranscendence, the goals of personal and environmental transformation occur. For example, an older adult who is diagnosed with cancer could rely on spirituality as a source of strength, engage in creative problem-solving and positive affirmations to manage treatment-related symptoms while promoting health through good nutrition and adequate rest. Through the integration of foundational coping processes, the individual may feel a sense of acceptance of the prognosis (decreased death anxiety), withdraw from routine social outlets, saving one's energy for spending time with close family members (engagement in meaningful activities, changes in relationships), and accept the idea of oneself as less physically able but celebrate newly found self-acceptance and wisdom (gerotranscendence).

A balanced assimilation of foundational coping processes is the initial adaptive process of successful aging. People who are more creative and have lower levels of negative affectivity and greater degrees of personal control will have more effective adaptation of functional performance mechanisms. That is to say, they will be more likely to engage in participation in health promotion activities and maintenance of physical mobility. Physical health may be influenced by intrapsychic factors—immunity and emotions, for example—and is likely to affect intrapsychic factors as well (such as how one responds psychologically to illness or accident). More creativity, less negative affectivity, and greater personal control contribute to deeper spirituality, through greater spiritual perspective and more religiosity. If one is more creative, then he or she is more receptive to new ideas and innovative problem-solving methods. Lower negative affectivity also makes one more accepting of circumstances and people, able to consider a broader range of possible outcomes to a situation, and increases the likelihood of pleasant, positive interactions with others. Greater personal control means that someone is more likely to be proactive in health promotion activities, problem solving, and disease management. A sense of spirituality contributes to one's valuation of self and sense of responsibility to appreciate and be responsible for those blessings in life such as health, relationships, and resources.

There are no set or prescribed ideal amounts or combinations of features from within the foundational coping processes. Rather, a satisfactory integration of the outputs of each foundational coping process needs to be present in order for the aging person to experience gerotranscendence, a critical step toward successful aging. Gerotranscendence is a higher-order way of thinking and being, which leads to more meaning and purpose in life, greater life satisfaction, and ultimately, successful aging (Flood, 2006a).

Related Research

Since the initial development of the theory of successful aging, it has been important to conduct research to inform and refine theory. An initial study (Flood & Scharer, 2006) examined the relationship of levels of creativity to successful aging. One challenge was finding a suitable measure for creativity. The Similes Preferences Inventory (SPI)

(Pearson & Maddi, 1966), which measures novelty of productions, was used. The proposed relationship was not supported, possibly because a number of participants had difficulty understanding and completing the 54-item instrument. However, this study brought up additional questions for future research; differences were found between Black and White older adults. Specifically, Black participants had higher creativity, life satisfaction, and purpose in life than White participants. Therefore, it became necessary to determine the feasibility of the SPI for use in older adults and whether there was racial variation in successful aging. The theory of successful aging does not specifically address race or ethnicity. However, cultural and regional influences undoubtedly impact the dimensions of physical, mental, and spiritual well-being.

A follow-up study (Flood, 2006b) examined the relationships of depression, creativity, and successful aging in middle class community-dwelling older adults. Depression moderated the relationship between creativity and successful aging, suggesting that depressive symptoms weaken the relationship between creativity and successful aging. Black older adults had significantly higher creativity levels and depressive symptoms and significantly lower purpose in life and life satisfaction than White older adults. In response to a single open-ended question on successful aging, White participants tended to emphasize a multidimensional phenomenon composed of attitude/outlook, social interaction, and self-care ability, while Black participants tended to report having their basic needs met, self-care ability, and having essential material resources (Flood, 2006b).

In a subsequent study, Troutman, Nies, Small, and Bates (2011) tested the Successful Aging Inventory (SAI), a 20-item instrument with Likert format and dichotomous format versions that reflect the conceptual domains of the mid-range theory of successful aging. Scores may range from 0 to 20 (dichotomous version) or 0 to 80 (Likert version). Higher scores indicate more successful aging. Scores on the SAI were compared with other instruments with known validity that measure underlying factors in successful aging, including life satisfaction, purpose in life, and depression, to establish psychometric properties. A sample of 200 participants who were White (n = 184 [92%]) and Black (n = 16 [8%]) residents of North Carolina completed the SAI. Principal components analysis was conducted for the Likert version using varimax rotation. Five components were retained, accounting for 62.86% of the variance. All loadings were positive. The components were named to describe the items in each: adapting and coping (20.36%), generativity and purposefulness (14.94%), gerotranscending (11.7%), religiosity (8.52%), and spirituality (7.35%). The five dimensions partially confirm the theory of successful aging (Troutman et al., in press).

Other research has been influenced by the theory of successful aging, and this work has shown support for the theory. Cozort (2008) utilized the theory of successful aging as a framework, as well as the SAI. The SAI demonstrated sound psychometric properties. McCarthy (2009) also used the theory of successful aging to frame her study, finding statistically significant relationships between the SAI and measures of related variables, thus validating the theory as well as the use of the SAI.

Further research is warranted, as theory development is an evolving process, because theory may guide research, and research can inform theory refinement. Qualitative research to explore the specific nature of racial variation in successful aging is important, as is investigation of the feasibility and effectiveness of interventions aimed at promoting successful aging.

Clinical Application

Although research on successful aging continues and questions remain, there are some areas of foci for assessment, planning, and intervention that can be targeted in the meantime. These are discussed in the following sections.

Assessment Strategies

One relatively simple component of assessment is asking older adults how they believe they are aging. This question may be met with surprise, because most people are not asked, "Tell me about how you believe you are aging. Would you say it is successful, unsuccessful, or somewhere in between?" Another important question is what things does the person feel are important at this point in life. Responses to these questions can give an indication of realistic goals that can be set based on the older adult's perceptions and expectations. Older adults' expectations regarding aging could be quantified to specifically assess the extent of importance placed on such areas as general health, sexual function, pain, urinary incontinence, and fatigue.

The Expectations Regarding Aging (ERA-38) Survey (Sarkisian, Hays, Berry, and Mangione,

2002) assesses these and other domains relevant to aging. The ERA-38 has demonstrated reliability and construct validity. The SAI (Troutman et al., in press) could be administered to evaluate the extent of an older adult's adaptation in terms of physical, mental, spiritual, and existential domains.

Physical assessment is an essential and important component in the care of the older adult, and nurses should consider age-related physiologic and physical changes. What chronic diseases are present? How effectively does the older adult manage these? What education needs, if any, are there? It may be necessary to educate an older adult about normal age-related changes as part of fostering realistic expectations of aging. Individuals who have extreme expectations (e.g., to maintain or regain the running speed they had at age 28) and demonstrate ineffective coping or poor adjustment should be referred for further evaluation by an advanced practice psychiatric nurse or a therapist. Indicators of impaired coping often include indecisiveness, self-destructive behaviors, somatic symptoms, irritability, and inappropriate use of defense mechanisms (Gulanick & Myers, 2007). Thus, it is critical to assess for the presence of symptoms such as these. Similarly, it is important to routinely assess general mental health and spiritual well-being, as these are important aspects of successful aging (Box 2-4).

Promoting Successful Aging

Functional Performance Mechanisms

Assessment findings will indicate some patient needs. For older adults in whom systems assessment reveals cardiac, respiratory, or other deviations, the nurse may need to notify the primary care provider of these findings. Patient education might also be warranted. It may also be useful to counsel the older adult on strategies to improve or maintain mobility and health. For example, education about planning activities to conserve energy and optimize oxygenation might be warranted for the older adult with chronic obstructive pulmonary disease.

BOX 2-4 Mental Health Assessment Tools

A wide variety of screening and assessment tools specific to different aspects of mental health exist. Some of these include

- Profile of Mood States (McNair, Lorr, & Droppleman, 1971)
- Positive and Negative Affect Scale (Watson, Clark, & Tellegen, 1988)
- Geriatric Depression Scale (Yesavage et al., 1983)
- Patient Health Questionnaire-9 (Pfizer, Inc., 2008)
- Centers for Epidemiologic Study Depression Scale (Radloff, 1977)
- Hamilton Anxiety Scale (Hamilton, 1959)

All of these are brief tools with sound psychometric properties that can be easily administered to older adults. If an older adult's scores on any of these tools suggest abnormality, the nurse can make referrals to a mental health professional.

Intrapsychic Factors

Nurses can encourage older adults to verbalize their feelings, perceptions, and fears and assist in setting realistic goals. Cognitive behavioral therapy from an advanced practice psychiatric nurse or other mental health professional might be warranted for older adults with feelings of limited personal control over what happens to them, or extreme negative affectivity to the extent of impaired coping and relating to others. Basic-level nurses can implement interventions such as those listed in Table 2-2. Nurses might also be instrumental in helping the older adult patient develop improved problem-solving skills.

Spirituality

Referrals to clergy or encouraging the older adult to make contact with his or her pastor, priest, rabbi, or other spiritual leader can facilitate enhanced spiritual well-being. Possible interventions targeting spirituality are identified in Table 2-2. Reading religious literature and use of prayer may also be helpful for some older adults.

Gerotranscendence

As older adults discuss their self-perceptions of aging, the nurse can use this as an opportunity to assess for indicators of gerotranscendence. What are their perceptions, fears, and/or concerns about death? Does the older adult feel that life has meaning and purpose? What activities are important or meaningful? These questions could be used to engage the older adult in initial discussions about gerotranscendence. Assuring the older adult that his or her responses are not unusual (for those who appear to be gerotranscending) and explaining gerotranscendence is an education intervention that might be well received. Wadensten and Carlsson (2007) offer specific guidelines for nursing care of older adults based on Tornstam's theory of gerotranscendence (Table 2-3).

TABLE 2-2 Nursing Interventions Classification: Intervention Descriptions for Theory of Successful Aging Dimensions

Interventions to promote effective use/well-being of intrapsychic factors	
For enhanced general coping	■ Bibliotherapy (therapeutic use of literature to enhance expression of feelings, active problem solving, coping, or insight) ■ Coping enhancement (assisting the older adults to adapt to perceived stressors, changes, or threats that interfere with meeting life demands and roles) ■ Counseling (use of interactive helping process to focus on the needs, problems, or feelings of the older adult to enhance or support coping, problem solving, and interpersonal relationships)
For enhanced creativity	■ Art therapy (facilitation of communication through drawings or other art forms) ■ Reminiscence therapy (using the recall of past evens, feelings, and thoughts via storytelling, to facilitate pleasure, quality of life, or adaptation to present circumstances)
For reducing negative affectivity	■ Animal-assisted therapy (purposeful use of animals to provide affection, attention, diversion, and relaxation) ■ Forgiveness facilitation (assisting an individual to replaces feelings of anger and resentment toward another, self or higher power, with beneficence, empathy, and humility) ■ Use of humor (facilitating the older adult to perceive, appreciate, and express what is funny, amusing, or ludicrous to establish relationships, relieve tension, release anger, facilitate learning, or cope with painful feelings) ■ Anger control assistance (facilitation of the expression of anger in an adaptive, nonviolent manner)
For increasing personal control	■ Resiliency promotion (assisting the older adult in the development, use, and strengthening of protective factors to be used in coping with environmental and societal stressors) ■ Self-efficacy enhancement (strengthening an older adult's confidence in his/her ability to perform a health behavior)
Interventions to promote spirituality	
For strengthened religiosity	■ Religious ritual enhancement (facilitating participation in religious practices) ■ Religious abuse protection support (identification of high-risk, controlling religious relationships and actions to prevent infliction of physical, sexual, or emotional harm and/or exploitation) ■ Religious addiction prevention (prevention of a self-imposed controlling religious lifestyle)
For enhanced spiritual perspective	■ Spiritual growth facilitation (facilitation of growth of an older adult's capacity to identify, connect with, and call upon the source of meaning, purpose, comfort, strength, and hope in his or her life) ■ Spiritual support (assisting the older adult to feel balance and connection with a greater power)

Source: Bulecheck, G., Butcher, H., & Dochterman, J. (2008). *Nursing interventions classification* (5th ed.). St. Louis, MO: Mosby/Elsevier.

TABLE 2-3 Suggested Gerotranscendence Nursing Interventions

Focus on the older adult as an individual.	■ Accept the possibility that behavioral signs of gerotranscendence are normal signs of aging. ■ Avoid regarding signs of gerotranscendence as undesirable and/or incorrect. ■ Avoid trying to correct older adults who show signs of gerotranscendence or change aspects of their behavior.
Reduce preoccupation with the body.	■ Choose conversation topics not focused on health and physical limitations. ■ Avoid routinely asking how the older adult feels.
Allow alternative definitions of time.	■ Respect that older people may have a different perception of time, such that the boundaries among past, present, and future are transcended. ■ Ask the older adult to talk about past "adventures." ■ Avoid routinely correcting older adults about the time; for example, when they seem to be in the past, do not always try to bring them back to the present.
Allow thoughts and conversations about death.	■ Listen when someone talks about death. Let the person speak and ask questions. Stimulate further thoughts. ■ In residential settings, inform the other residents if someone among them has died, and allow them to talk about it. ■ Do not lead the conversation away from death to other topics.
Choose topics of conversation that facilitate and further personal growth.	■ In residential or adult day care settings, ask in the morning what the older adult dreamed about instead of asking how he or she feels. If the person did dream, ask questions about the dream and what it might mean. ■ Encourage the older adult to recall and talk about childhood and earlier times, and about how the person has developed during life.
Focus on activities.	■ Allow older adults to decide for themselves whether they want to be alone or participate in activities in group settings. ■ Discuss in a group or in individual conversations the topic of growing old, and introduce older people to the theory of gerotranscendence as a possible and positive process of aging. ■ Start reminiscence therapy as a way of working with one's own life history. ■ Arrange a meditation course or encourage medication as a way to help get in touch with inherited mental structures. ■ Do not assume that participating in arranged activities is always the best alternative. ■ Do not, without reason, nag an older adult to participate in arranged activities. ■ Do not, without reason, question older adults about their desire to be alone or assume that the desire to spend a great deal of time alone as a problem.

TABLE 2-3 Suggested Gerotranscendence Nursing Interventions—cont'd

	■ Focus on organization; encourage and facilitate quiet and peaceful places and times in residential facilities. ■ Remember to plan for and organize quiet moments of rest and also to respect a person's wish to be alone in his or her room. ■ Organize so that older adults can have meals in their own room in residential care facilities, if desired. ■ Do not organize many activities in the main rooms or continuously keep the television or radio turned on in the dayroom.

Source: Wadensten, B., & Carlsson, M. (2007). The theory of gerotranscendence in practice: Guidelines for nursing, part II. *Int J Older People Nurs, 2,* 295–301.

Some interventions based on the theory of successful aging may seem obvious to the general health of older adults and not specific to the theory (such as promoting and maintaining physical health). Others are more unique and specific to the theory (such as those aimed at gerotranscendence). Some older adults will require interventions targeting only one dimension in the theory; others will need of a broader range of interventions to address multiple dimensions of successful aging. The theory is applicable to all older adults capable of self-appraisal. Thus, interventions to promote successful aging could be provided for any older adult with cognition intact to allow self-evaluation of their own aging.

Evaluating Outcomes

Nurses should assess for outcomes of each intervention/set of interventions aimed at a particular problem. Nursing outcomes can be identified according to and measured against the *Nursing Outcomes Classification* list (Moorhead, Johnson, Maas, & Swanson, 2008), which provides an index of nursing outcomes, some of which correspond with the theory of successful aging constructs.

- Outcomes relevant to functional performance mechanisms include health promotion knowledge; adaptation to physical disability, mobility, health status acceptance, compliance behavior, and health beliefs: perceived ability to perform (Moorhead et al., 2008).
- Intrapsychic factor-related outcomes consist of coping and mood equilibrium (Moorhead et al., 2008).
- Outcomes for spirituality include spiritual health and comfort status: psychospiritual (Moorhead et al., 2008).

The *Nursing Outcomes Classification* provides descriptors for each outcome that aid in determining whether the outcome has been achieved.

Outcomes for gerotranscendence interventions could be assessed by evaluating the older adult's affective and emotional response to specific interventions (i.e., those listed in Table 2-3). For example, does the older adult seem to enjoy solitude? Does he or she talk about death without fear, and as a transition, rather than an endpoint?

Gerotranscendence can also be evaluated with the Gerotranscendence Scale (Tornstam, 1994). The Gerotranscendence Scale consists of 10 items designed to tap what Tornstam (2005) calls retrospective change (p. 93), or how older adults see they have changed since age 50. The Gerotranscendence Scale uses a yes or no response scale to measure how older adults have changed since age 50. There are two dimensions for this scale, cosmic transcendence (six items) and ego transcendence (four items). Cosmic transcendence refers to the transcendence of "time, space, life, and death" (p. 81). Ego transcendence is connected to changes in the "perception of the self and relations with other people" (p. 83). For each item, there are two response choices: Yes (I do recognize myself in the statement) or No (I do not recognize myself in the statement). The Gerotranscendence Scale is brief and easily administered. It may also provide an opportunity to initiate discussions about gerotranscendence with older adults. The scale and additional information on gerotranscendence are accessible at Tornstam's website (http://www.soc.uu.se/research/gerontology/gerotrans.html).

Implications and Planning for Future Older Adults

Generally speaking, research has thus far tended to focus on understanding and describing successful aging in those who are doing well. However, it is important that we begin to examine successful aging in older adults who appear not to be doing well. These are the individuals who need intervention most. Promotion of successful aging has many positive consequences. Older adults can experience improved quality of life and physical, mental, and spiritual health, and caregivers can provide more individualized and appropriate care and, potentially, more responsible use of health care finances.

The theory of successful aging offers a framework for designing research to further understand successful aging in various groups, and to identify interventions that could be tested through clinical research. The theory also provides an organizing framework for assessment, planning, interventions, and evaluation of older adults that is individualized to the needs and situations of unique individuals and sensitive to the importance that the older adult places on various aspects of aging.

KEY POINTS

- When successful aging is defined from the reference point of the older adult, it is a possibility for most older adults.
- Shifting demographic trends, increasing diversity, and growing life expectancies require a novel and more inclusive approach to successful aging.
- Successful aging depends on the older adult's self-perception and his or her physical, mental, spiritual, and existential well-being.

CRITICAL THINKING ACTIVITIES

1. Brainstorm by writing on a sheet of paper all the things that come to mind when you think of aging and being an older adult. What kind of things did you identify? Are they positive, healthy traits? Or are they illness focused? Compare your ideas with those of a peer. What similarities are there? What differences? Why do you think you identified the characteristics that you did? What experiences have influenced your views of aging and being an older adult?
2. Identify an older adult that you know. Ask permission to conduct an interview with this person. Inquire about: Is being this age like you thought it would be? How is life different for you now, compared with when you were a young adult? What things are better? What things are worse or more difficult? How would you describe your aging? Then, think about how *you* would respond to these questions now, and when you reach older adulthood.
3. Think about your current hobbies, friends, the clothes you wear, your favorite music, and foods. Make a list of these things. Then, imagine yourself at age 70. Write down what you imagine your hobbies, friends, clothes, and so forth will be then. Do you anticipate much change over time? Why or why not? Do you look forward to aging? Dread it? Fear it?

CASE STUDY | *MR. P.*

Refer to the case study of Mr. P. earlier in the chapter. Read the following scenario and see if you can answer the questions.

After the memorial ceremony for his wife, Mr. P.'s children want to take him out to dinner. He declines, saying, "No, I would really rather go home and sit by the fireplace. Edna and I used to sit there every Sunday evening." Although they are concerned about him being alone, his children take Mr. P. home to be by himself. Mr. P. is tired from a day of activities, but he decides to get out his old photo album and reminisce. He cannot believe Edna has been gone for 1 year; sometimes it seems like she is just in the next room. Mr. P. thinks of her often. He also thinks about and misses his brother, who died 7 years ago. Mr. P. feels particularly close to

CASE STUDY | *MR. P.*—cont'd

his brother when he is outdoors in his garden because his brother used to have a garden next door to him. There was a time when he and his brother were leaders of their community, and they contributed greatly to the growth of the local library and church.

Mr. P. feels it is important to share who his brother was with his grandchildren, because they never knew what a wonderful man he was. Mr. P. finds himself concerned about his grandchildren and their growth and maturation into good citizens. He likes to try to teach them about "how life used to be" when he was their age. He primarily spends time with his family and neighbor; he prefers this close-knit support group to a senior center for socialization. Mr. P. spends the evening alone, in prayer, on this night. He skips dinner and goes to bed early.

1. Based on your awareness of developmental (and aging) theories, how would you describe Mr. P.?
2. Is he (still) aging successfully?
3. If he were referred to you as a patient, what things would be important to assess?
4. What nursing interventions might you anticipate for him?

REFERENCES

AARP. (2009). *About AARP.* Retrieved October 21, 2010, from http://www.aarp.org/about-aarp/

Adler, N., & Newman, K. (2002). Socioeconomic disparities in health: Pathways and policies. *Health Affairs, 21*(2), 60–76.

Administration on Aging. (2001). *A profile of older Americans: 2001.* Retrieved October 12, 2010, from http://www.caregiverslibrary.org/Portals/0/AOA%20Older%20American%20profile_2001.pdf

Agency for Healthcare Research and Quality and the Centers for Disease Control and Prevention. (2002). *Physical activity and older Americans: Benefits and strategies.* Retrieved October 25, 2010, from http://www.ahrq.gov/ppip/activity.htm

Arias, E. (2007). United States life tables, 2004. Table 12. Estimated life expectancy at birth in years, by race and sex: Death-registration states, 1900–28, and United States, 1929–2004. *National Vital Statistics Reports, 50*(6), 34. Retrieved October 15, 2009, from http://www.lifeexpectancy.com/articles/le_birth.pdf

Baltes, M. M., & Carstensen, L. L. (1996). The process of successful ageing. *Ageing and Society, 16,* 397–422.

Baltes, P., & Baltes, M. (1999). Psychological perspective on successful aging: The model of selective optimization with compensation. In P. Baltes & M. Baltes (Eds.), *Successful aging: Perspectives from the behavioral sciences* (pp. 1–35). New York, NY: Cambridge University Press.

Barrett, A., & Murk, P. (2006). *Life satisfaction index for the third age (LSITA): A measurement of successful aging.* Retrieved October 18, 2010, from https://scholarworks.iupui.edu/handle/1805/1160

Bearon, L. (1996). Successful aging: What does the "good life" look like? North Carolina State University. *The Forum for Family and Consumer Issues, 1*(3). Retrieved October 27, 2010, from http://ncsu.edu/ffci/publications/1996/v1-n3-1996-summer/successful-aging.php

Benner, P., & Wrubel, J. (1989). *The primacy of caring.* Menlo Park, CA: Addison-Wesley.

Bowling, A., & Dieppe, P. (2006). What is successful ageing and who should define it? *British Medical Journal, 331,* 1548–1551.

Brown, C., McGuire, F., & Voelkel, J. (2008). The link between successful aging and serious leisure. *International Journal of Aging and Human Development, 66*(1), 73–95.

Bryant, L., Corbett, K., & Kutner, J. (2001). In their own words: A model of healthy aging. *Social Science & Medicine, 53,* 927–941.

Bulecheck, G., Butcher, H., & Dochterman, J. (2008). *Nursing interventions classification* (5th ed.). St. Louis, MO: Mosby/Elsevier.

Carter, R. (2009). *Program funded to produce more college-educated geriatric nurses.* Retrieved October 18, 2010, from http://nursinghomeneglect.publishpath.com/program-funded-to-produce-more-college-educated-geriatrics-nurses

Centers for Disease Control and Prevention. (2007). *The state of aging and health in America 2007.* Retrieved October 18, 2010, from http://www.cdc.gov/aging/pdf/saha_2007.pdf

Chodzko-Zajko, W., Schwingel, A., & Park, C. (2009). Successful aging: The role of physical activity. *American Journal of Lifestyle Medicine, 3,* 20–28.

Columbia Encyclopedia. (2004). Aging. In *The Columbia encyclopedia* (6th ed.). New York, NY: Columbia University Press.

U. S. Bureau of the Census & National Institute on Aging (1993). *Racial and Ethnic Diversity of America's Elderly Population. Profiles of America's Elderly.* Retrieved March 23, 2011 from http://www.stanford.edu/group/ethnoger/index.html

Cozort, R. (2008). *Revising the gerotranscendence scale for use with older adults in the southern United States and establishing psychometric properties of the revised gerotranscendence scale.* Unpublished doctoral dissertation, University of North Carolina at Greensboro.

Crowther, M., Parker, M., Achenbaum, W. A., Larimore, W., & Koenig, H. (2002). Rowe and Kahn's model of successful aging. Spirituality: The forgotten factor. *Gerontologist, 42*(5), 613–619.

Depp, C., & Jeste, D. (2006). Definitions and predictors of successful aging: A comprehensive review of larger quantitative studies. *American Journal of Geriatric Psychiatry, 14*(1), 6–20.

Depp, C., Vahia, I., & Jeste, D. (2007). The intersection of mental health and successful aging. *Psychiatric Times, 24*(13), 20–27.

Dictionary.com. (2009). *Age.* Retrieved November 5, 2009 from http://dictionary.reference.com/browse/age

Duay, D., & Bryan, V. (2006) Senior adults' perceptions of successful aging. *Educational Gerontology, 32,* 423–445.

Erikson, E., Erikson, J., & Kivnick, H. (1986). *Vital involvement in old age.* New York, NY: Norton.

Ferri, C., James, I., & Pruchno, R. (2009). Successful aging: Definitions and subjective assessment according to older adults. *Clinical Gerontologist, 32,* 379–388.

Fisher, B. (1995). Successful aging, life satisfaction, and generativity in later life. *International Journal of Aging and Human Development, 41*(3), 239–251.

Fisher, B., & Specht, D. (1999). Successful aging and creativity in later life. *Journal of Aging Studies, 13*(4), 457–472.

Flood, M. (2002). Successful aging: A concept analysis. *Journal of Theory Construction and Testing, 6*(2), 105–108.

Flood, M. (2006a). A mid-range theory of successful aging. *Journal of Theory Construction and Testing, 9*(2), 35–39.

Flood, M. (2006b). Exploring the relationships between creativity, depression, and successful aging. *Activities, Adaptation, and Aging, 31*(1), 55–71.

Flood, M. (2008). *Developing a questionnaire to measure successful aging.* Poster presentation, Gerontological Society of America Annual Meeting. Baltimore, MD; November 24, 2008.

Flood, M., & Scharer, K. (2006). Creativity enhancement; Possibilities for successful aging. *Issues in Mental Health Nursing, 27,* 1–21.

Ford, A., Haug, M., Stange, K., Gaines, A., Noelker, L, & Jones, P. (2000). Sustained personal autonomy: A measure of successful aging. *Journal of Aging and Health, 12*(4), 470–489.

Freund, A. M. (2008). Successful aging as management of resources: The role of selection, optimization, and compensation. *Research in Human Development, 5,* 94–106.

Galbreath, J. (1995). Calista Roy. In J. B. George (Ed.), *Nursing theories: The base for professional nursing practice* (6th ed.). Prentice Hall Nursing. Upper Saddle River, NJ.

Gulanik, M., & Myers, J. (2007). *Nursing care plans: Nursing diagnosis and intervention* (5th ed.). St. Louis, MO: Mosby Elsevier.

Hamilton, M. (1959). The assessment of anxiety states by rating. *British Journal of Medical Psychology, 32,* 50–55.

Helson, H. (1964). *Adaptation level theory.* New York, NY: Harper & Row.

Heron, M., Hoyert, D. L., Murphy, S. L., et al. (2009). Death: Final data for 2006. *National Vital Statistics Reports, 57*(14), 1–136. Retrieved October 12, 2010, from http://www.cdc.gov/nchs/data/nvsr/nvsr57/nvsr57_14.pdf

Hsu, H. (2005). Gender disparity of successful aging. *Women and Health, 42*(1), 1–21.

Imperio, K. (2006). *Transcendence in successful aging: A grounded theory of older women's strategies to age successfully.* Doctoral dissertation, University of Massachusetts, Amherst.

Inui, T. (2003). The need for an integrated biopsychosocial approach to research on successful aging. *Annals of Internal Medicine, 139*(5), 391–394.

Jenerette, C., & Lauderdale, G. (2008) Successful aging with sickle cell disease: Using qualitative methods to inform theory. *Journal of Theory Construction and Testing, 12*(1), 16–24.

Kancelbaum, B. (2009). *Helping hospitals serve older patients: Nurse managers find NICHE.* Retrieved October 18, 2010, from http://www.strategiesfornursemanagers.com/ce_detail/214643.cfm

King, I. (1981). *A theory for nursing: Systems, concepts, process.* New York, NY: Delmar.

Kivett, V., Stevenson, M., & Zwane, C. (2000). Very-old rural adults: Functional status and social support. *Journal of Applied Gerontology, 19*(1), 58–75.

Knight, T., & Riccardelli, L. (2003). Successful aging: Perceptions of adults aged between 70 and 101 years. *International Journal of Aging and Human Development, 56*(3), 223–245.

Ko, K. J., Berg, C. A., Butner, J., Uchino, B. N., & Smith, T. W. (2007). Profiles of successful aging in middle-aged and older adult couples. *Psychology and Aging, 22*(4), 705–718.

Lamond, A., Depp, C., Allison, M., Langer, R., Reichstadt, J., Moore, D., . . . Jeste, D. (2008). Measurement and predictors of resilience among community-dwelling older women. *Journal of Psychiatric Research, 43*(2), 148–154.

Li, C., Wenyuan, W., Jin, H., Li, C., Wenyuan, W., Jin, H., . . . Zhang, M. (2005). Successful aging in Shanghai, China: Definition, distribution, and related factors. *International Psychogeriatrics, 18*(3), 551–563.

Litwin, H. (2005). Correlates of successful aging: Are they universal? *International Journal of Aging and Human Development, 61*(4), 313–333.

Marquez, D., Bustamante, E., Blissmer, B., & Prohaska, T. (2009). Health promotion for successful aging. *American Journal of Lifestyle Medicine, 3*(12), 12–19.

Matsubayashi, K., Ishine, M., Wada, T., & Okumiya, K. (2006). Older adults' views of "successful aging": Comparisons of older Japanese and Americans. *Journal of the American Geriatric Society, 54*(1), 184–187.

McCarthy, V. (2009). *Exploring a new view of successful aging among low-income older adults in an independent and assisted living community.* Poster presentation. Gerontological Society of American Annual Meeting, Atlanta, Georgia.

McKenna, H. P. (1997). *Nursing models and theories* (pp. 144–146). London, England: Routledge.

McNair, D. M., Lorr, M., & Droppleman, L. F. (1971). *Manual for the profile of mood states.* San Diego, CA: Educational and Industrial Testing Services.

Meleis, A. I. (1997). *Theoretical nursing: Development and progress* (3rd ed.). Philadelphia, PA: Lippincott.

Merriam-Webster. (2009). *Success.* Retrieved October 20, 2010, from http://www.merriam-webster.com/dictionary/success

Merton, R. (1968). *Social theory and social structure.* New York, NY: Free Press.

Mezey, M., & Gray-Miceli, D. (2007). *Critical thinking related to complex care of older adults.* Paper presentation, Hartford Geriatric Nursing Education Consortium. Atlanta, GA; October 3, 2007.

Moorhead, S., Johnson, M., Maas, M., & Swanson, E. (2008). *Nursing outcomes classification* (4th ed.). St. Louis, MO: Mosby.

Neugarten, B., Havighurst, R., & Tobin, S. (1961). The measurement of life satisfaction. *Journal of Gerontology, 16,* 134–143.

Nimrod, G., & Kleiber, D. (2007). Reconsidering change and continuity in later life: Toward an innovation theory of successful aging. *International Journal of Aging and Human Development, 65*(1), 1–22.

Palmore, E. (1995). Successful aging. In G. L. Maddox (Ed.). *Encyclopedia of aging: A comprehensive resource in gerontology and geriatrics* (2nd ed., pp. 914–915). New York, NY: Springer.

Pearson, P., & Maddi, S. (1966). The similes preference inventory: Development of a structured measure of the tendency toward variety. *Journal of Canadian Psychology, 30*(4), 301–308.

Pfizer, Inc. (2008). *Welcome to the patient health questionnaire (PHQ) screeners.* Retrieved October 20, 2010, from http://www.phqscreeners.com/

Phelan, E., Anderson, L., LaCroix, A., & Larson, E. (2004). Older adults' views of "successful aging." How do they compare with researchers' definitions? *Journal of the American Geriatric Society, 52,* 211–216.

Poon, L. W., Gueldner, S. H., & Sprouse, B. M. (2003). *Successful aging and adaptation with chronic diseases.* New York, NY: Springer.

Radloff, L. S. (1977). The CES-D scale: A self-report depression scale for research in the general population. *Applied Psychological Measurement, 1,* 385–401.

Reed, P. (1991). Toward a nursing theory of self-transcendence: Deductive reformulation using developmental theories. *Advances in Nursing Science, 13*(4), 64–77.

Reichstadt, J., Depp, C., Palinkas, L., Folsom, D., & Jeste, D. (2007). Building blocks of successful aging: A focus group study of older adults' perceived contributors to successful aging. *American Journal of Geriatric Psychiatry, 15*(3), 194–201.

Roos, N., & Havens, B. (1991). Predictors of successful aging: a twelve-year study of Manitoba elderly. *American Journal of Public Health, 81*(1), 63–68.

Rossen, E., Knafl, K., & Flood, M. (2008). Older women's perceptions of successful aging. *Activities, Adaptation, and Aging, 32*(2), 73–88.

Rowe, J., & Khan, R. (1987). Human aging: Usual and successful. *Science, 237,* 143–149.

Rowe, J., & Khan, R. (1998). *Successful aging.* New York, NY: Pantheon Books.

Roy, C. (1997). Future of the Roy model: Challenge to redefine adaptation. *Nursing Science Quarterly, 10,* 42–48.

Roy, C. (2010). *The Roy Adaptation Model: Assumptions.* Retrieved October 27, 2010, from http://www.bc.edu/schools/son/faculty/featured/theorist/Roy_Adaptation_Model.html

Roy, C., & Andrews, H. (1999). *The Roy Adaptation Model* (2nd ed.). Stamford, CT: Appleton & Lange.

Sarkisian, C., Hays, R., Berry, S., & Mangione, C. (2002). Development, reliability, and validity of the Expectations Regarding Aging (ERA-38) Survey. *Gerontologist, 42*(4), 534–542.

Siska, A., Truffer, C., Smith, S., Keehan, S., Cylus, J., Poisal, J. . . . (2009). Health spending projections through 2018: Recession effects add uncertainty to the outlook. *Health Affairs, 28*(2), w346–w357.

Statistics Canada. (1994). *National population health survey, 1994–1995.* Ottawa, Ontario, Canada: Author.

Strawbridge, W., Wallhagen, M., & Cohen, R. (2002). Successful aging and well-being: Self-rated compared with Rowe and Khan. *Gerontologist, 42*(6), 727–733.

Tate, R., Leedine, L., & Cuddy, E. (2003). Definition of successful aging by elderly Canadian males: The Manitoba follow-up study. *Gerontologist, 43*(5), 735–744.

Tornstam, L. (1994). Gerotranscendence: A theoretical and empirical exploration. In L. Thomas & S. A. Eisenhandler (Eds.), *Aging and the religious dimension* (pp. 203–225). Greenwood CT: Westport.

Tornstam, L. (1996). Gerotranscendence: A theory about maturing into old age. *Journal of Aging and Identity, 1*(1), 37–50.

Tornstam, L. (1997). Gerotranscendence: The contemplative dimension of aging. *Journal of Aging Studies, 11*(2), 143–154.

Tornstam, L. (2005). *Gerotranscendence: A developmental theory of positive aging.* New York, NY: Springer.

Travelbee, J. (1971). *Interpersonal aspects of nursing.* Philadelphia, PA: Davis.

Troutman, M., Nies, M.A., Small, S., & Bates, A. (2011). The development and testing of an instrument to measure successful aging. *Research in Gerontological Nursing, January 21:* 1-12. Doi: 10.3928/19404921-20110106-02.

U.S. Census Bureau. (2000). *Interim projections consistent with Census 2000.* Retrieved October 20, 2010, from http://www.census.gov/population/www/projections/popproj.html

U.S. Census Bureau. (2009). *Percent of the total population who are 65 years and over.* Retrieved October 12, 2010, from http://factfinder.census.gov/servlet/GCTTable?_bm=y&-geo_id=01000US&-ds_name=PEP_2008_EST&-_lang=en&-redoLog=false&-format=US-40S&-mt_name=PEP_2008_EST_GCTT4R_U40SC&-CONTEXT=gct

U.S. Department of Health and Human Services. (2008). *Healthy people 2010: What are its goals?* Accessed October 20, 2010, from http://www.healthypeople.gov/2010/About/goals.htm

Vaillant, G., & Mukamal, K. (2001). Successful aging. *American Journal of Psychiatry, 158*(6), 839–847.

von Bertalanffy, L. (1968). *General system theory: Foundations, development, applications.* New York, NY: Braziller.

von Faber, M., Bootsma-Van Der Wiel, A., Van Excel, E., Gussekloo, J., Lagaay, A., Van Dongen, E., . . . Westendorp, R.G.J. (2001). Successful aging in the oldest old: Who can be characterized as successfully aged? *Archives of Internal Medicine, 161*(22), 2694–2700.

Wadensten, B., & Carlsson, M. (2007). The theory of gerotranscendence in practice: Guidelines for nursing, part II. *International Journal of Older People Nursing, 2,* 295–301.

Walker, L., & Avant, K. (1995). *Strategies for theory construction in nursing* (3rd ed.). Norwalk, CT: Appleton & Lange.

Ware, J., & Sherbourne, C. (1992). The MOS 36-item short-form health survey (SF-36). Conceptual framework and item selection. *Medical Care, 30*(6), 473–483.

Watson, D., Clark, L. A., & Tellegen, A. (1988). Development and validation of brief measures of positive and negative affect: The PANAS scale. *Journal of Personality and Social Psychology, 54,* 1063–1070.

Watson, J. (1997). The theory of human caring: Retrospective and prospective. *Nursing Science Quarterly,10,* 49–52.

Webster Dictionary. (2009). *Definition of age.* Retrieved October 20, 2010, from http://www.webster-dictionary.net/definition/age

Wilmoth, J., & Longino, C. (2006). Demographic trends that will shape U.S. policy in the 21st century. *Research on Aging, 28*(3), 269–288.

Wong, P. (2000). Meaning of life and meaning of death in successful aging. In A. Tomer (Ed.), *Death attitudes and the older adult.* New York, NY: Bruner/Mazel.

Yesavage, J. A., Brink, T. L., Rose, T. L., Lum, O., Huang, V., Adey, M.B., . . . (1983). Development and validation of a geriatric depression screening scale: A preliminary report. *Journal of Psychiatric Research, 17,* 37–49.

Young, Y., Fan, M., Parrish, J., & Frick, K. (2009). Validation of a novel successful aging construct. *Journal of the American Medical Directors Association, 10*(5), 314–322.

Young, Y., Frick, K., & Phelan, E. (2009). Can successful aging and chronic illness coexist in the same individual? A multidimensional concept of successful aging. *Journal of the American Medical Directors Association, 10*(2), 87–92.

Chapter 3

Understanding Older Adults: U.S. and Global Perspectives

Alison E. Kris, RN, PhD

LEARNING OBJECTIVES

- Recognize the shifting demographics of aging in the United States.
- Understand differences in life expectancy among different people within the United States and between the United States and other countries.
- Discuss the role of obesity on life expectancy predictions.
- Describe the housing options available to older adults.
- Explain changes in educational attainment over time, and appreciate the impact of the GI Bill.

The population of older adults in the United States is increasing rapidly. The number of adults age 65 and over grew from 3 million in 1900 to 37 million in 2006, and the trend is expected to continue. Baby Boomers (people born between 1946 and 1964) will begin to turn 65 in 2011, marking the start of a dramatic rise in the population of older adults that will continue for the next several decades. The population of adults over age 65 is expected to double between 2000 and 2030. Even more dramatic will be the increase in adults over age 85. Between 2006 and 2050, the number of Americans over age 85 will grow from 5.3 million to nearly 21 million (Figs. 3-1 and 3-2). This major shift in demographics has significant implications for society as a whole, for medical care in particular, and most importantly for nursing care (Federal Interagency Forum on Aging Related Statistics, 2008).

Along with the graying of society has come the graying of the inpatient hospital unit, a trend that is expected to accelerate over the coming decades. The average age of hospitalized patients has increased dramatically over the past three decades (Fig. 3-3). By 2006, 38% of hospitalized inpatients were over age 65, and nearly a quarter of all inpatients were over age 75. This same period saw a decline in the rate of pediatric inpatient use from 13% in 1970 to 7% in 2006. The shift in inpatient utilization patterns is expected to continue as the U.S. population continues to age. Inpatient nursing care is increasingly becoming geriatric nursing care (Federal Interagency Forum on Aging Related Statistics, 2008).

As the total percentage of the population increases, so too will the population of older veterans. The historical impact of both World War II and the Korean War has already created a significant rise in the proportion of older men who are veterans. Since 1977, the proportion of older adult veterans has more than doubled from one in four to almost one in two (Horgan, Taylor & Wilensky, 1983). The number of women veterans from these wars is also on the rise. Although some older adults receive their care from the Veterans Administration (VA) health system, the overwhelming majority of veterans receive their care outside of the VA in community hospitals, clinics, and health centers.

The aging of the population will have a profound impact on the health care system. Older adults require more nursing care and more medical care than younger adults do. As people age, the

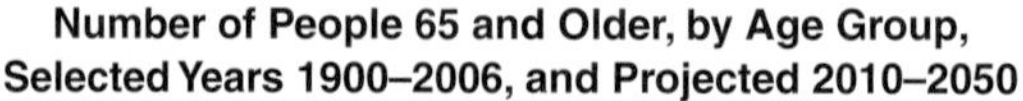

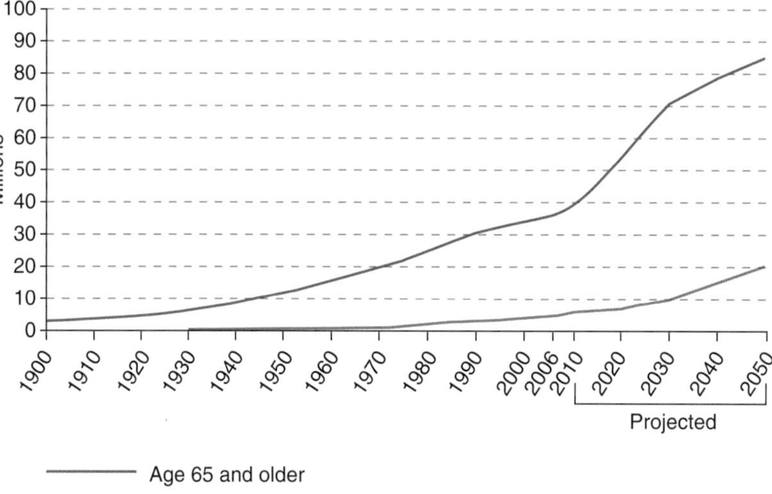

Note: Data from 2010–2050 are projections of the population.
Reference population: These data refer to the resident population.
Source: U.S. Census Bureau, Decennial Census, Population Estimates and Projections.

Figure 3-1 *(From the Federal Interagency Forum on Aging-Related Statistics. Retrieved October 20, 2010, from http://www.aoa.gov/agingstatsdotnet/Main_Site/Data/2008_Documents/Population.aspx)*

number of chronic conditions also increases, as do the number of medications used. Simply put, older adults require much more sophisticated care than younger adults due to the complex interplay of multiple chronic conditions and medications used to treat them.

Life Expectancy

Behind the graying of the population is a significant increase in life expectancy during the 20th century. In 1900, life expectancy was only 47 years for White men and 33 years for Black men. By 1950, it had risen to 67 years for White men and 61 for Black men. By 2010, estimated life expectancy had risen to 78.24 years (Central Intelligence Agency, 2010). The average was 76 years for men and 81 years for women. For those who survive to age 65, men reach an average age of 81 years and women 84 years (Centers for Disease Control and Prevention, 2008). The gap in life expectancy between Blacks and Whites remains wide, on average 6.3 years for males and 4.5 years for females (Pope, Ezzati, & Dockery, 2009). In 2005, the average life expectancy for Black men was 69.5 years; for Black women it was 76.5 years.

In 2010, the United States ranked 49th in the world in life expectancy.

In 2010, the United States ranked 49th in the world in life expectancy (Central Intelligence Agency, 2010) (Table 3-1). Reasons for the comparatively shorter life expectancy in the United States are numerous. Smoking is a major contributor to mortality from all causes, and the United States had the highest level of cigarette consumption per capita in the developed world over a 50-year period ending in the mid-1980s (Forey, Hamling, Lee, & Wald, 2002). The discrepancy in life expectancy between older men and women can be partly explained by what were once higher smoking rates among men. In addition, it is clear that air pollution is a major contributor to mortality. Residents of areas with higher levels of air pollution have lower life expectancies than those living in less polluted areas (Pope et al., 2009).

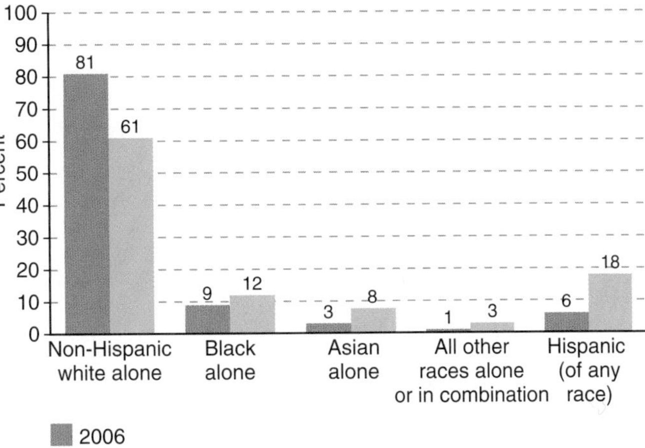

Note: The term *non-Hispanic white alone* is used to refer to people who reported being white and no other race and who are not Hispanic. The term *black alone* is used to refer to people who reported being black or African American and no other race, and the term *Asian alone* is used to refer to people who reported only Asian as their race. The use of single-race populations in this report does not imply that this is the preferred method of presenting or analyzing data. The U.S. Census Bureau uses a variety of approaches. The race group "All other races alone or in combination" includes American Indian and Alaska Native, alone; Native Hawaiian and Other Pacific Islander, alone; and all people who reported two or more races.
Reference population: These data refer to resident population.
Source: U.S. Census Bureau, Population Estimates and Projections.

Figure 3-2 *(From the Federal Interagency Forum on Aging-Related Statistics. Retrieved October 20, 2010, from http://www.aoa.gov/agingstatsdotnet/Main_Site/Data/2008_Documents/Population.aspx)*

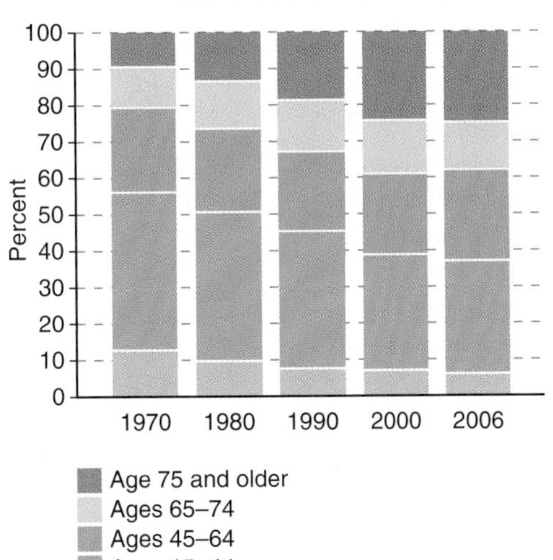

Source: CDC/NCHS, National Hospital Discharge Survey.

Figure 3-3 *(From the Centers for Disease Control and Prevention. (2008). 2006 National Hospital Discharge Survey. National Health Statistics Reports, 5, 1–20. Retrieved October 20, 2010, from http://www.cdc.gov/nchs/data/nhsr/nhsr005.pdf)*

TABLE 3-1 Life Expectancy at Birth, 2010 Estimate

RANK	COUNTRY	AGE
1	Monaco	89.78
2	Macau	84.38
3	San Marino	82.95
4	Andorra	82.36
5	Japan	82.17
6	Guernsey	82.08
7	Singapore	82.06
8	Hong Kong	81.96
9	Australia	81.72
10	Canada	81.29
11	Jersey	81.28
12	France	81.09
13	Spain	81.07
14	Sweden	80.97
15	Switzerland	80.97
16	Israel	80.86
17	Iceland	80.79
18	Anguilla	80.77
19	Bermuda	80.60
20	Cayman Islands	80.57
21	Isle of Man	80.53
22	New Zealand	80.48
23	Italy	80.33
24	Liechtenstein	80.19
25	Norway	80.08
26	Ireland	80.07
27	Jordan	79.92
28	United Kingdom	79.92
29	Greece	79.80
30	Saint Pierre and Miquelon	79.74
31	Austria	79.65
32	Malta	79.59
33	Faroe Islands	79.58
34	Netherlands	79.55
35	Luxembourg	79.48
36	Germany	79.41
37	Belgium	79.37
38	Virgin Islands	79.19
39	Finland	79.13
40	Wallis and Futuna	78.83
41	European Union	78.82
42	Korea, South	78.81
43	Puerto Rico	78.77
44	Bosnia and Herzegovina	78.66
45	Saint Helena, Ascension, and Tristan da Cunha	78.60
46	Gibraltar	78.53
47	Denmark	78.47
48	Portugal	78.38
49	United States	78.24
50	Taiwan	78.15

From Central Intelligence Agency. (2010). *The world factbook.* Retrieved October 20, 2010, from https://www.cia.gov/library/publications/the-world-factbook/rankorder/2102rank.html

Influence of Obesity

Obesity is a major contributing factor to mortality from heart disease, cancer, and diabetes. The obesity rate in the United States has been increasing for several decades, from 13% to 32% between the 1960s and 2004. It is expected to reach 41% by 2015. Among minority groups, obesity rates are even higher. For example, 80% of Black women are overweight, and 50% are obese (Wang & Beydoun, 2007). The rise in obesity may have a significant impact on overall life expectancy. Indeed, some have predicted that life expectancy may begin to decline in the near future (Olshansky et al., 2005).

High rates of obesity have a significant impact on society, on the health care system, and on nursing care. People who are obese are more likely to seek early retirement and are more likely to require disability payments (Renna & Thakur, 2010). This decreases income during the retirement years and can create gaps in income and health care coverage. Obese people are less likely to survive to age 65. When they do, total costs to the Medicare system are significantly greater (Cai, Lubitz, Flegal, & Pamuk, 2010). Finally, obesity has a significant impact on nursing care delivery. Patients who are morbidly obese require additional staff for assistance with turning, repositioning, and transfers. However, patients' weights typically are unaccounted for in staff assignments. Nurses, already at high risk for back injury, may incur even higher risk as the obesity rate rises.

Categories of Older Adults

As life expectancy rises and more people are living to older ages, society is beginning to recognize the diversity among older adults. A 65-year-old is likely to have very different life and health concerns than an 85-year-old. For this reason, the terms *older adult* or *senior citizen,* which have historically referred to all people over age 65, may prove to be too generic. Ebersole and Hess (1998) proposed several terms to help categorize the diversity of people over age 65. They include the following:

- The very young old—ages 56 to 64
- The young-old—ages 65 to 75
- The middle-old—ages 85 to 99
- The elite-old—age 100 and older

It is important to recognize that even within these subcategories of older adults, there is significant diversity in lifestyle and health status. Perhaps more importantly, there is significant variability in how older adults view themselves in terms of their age and their health status; these views may have no correlation with age.

People living beyond their 100th birthday are called *centenarians.* In recent years, the number of centenarians has grown quickly, from 37,000 in 1990 to 70,000 in 1999. This number was expected to double again over the following decade. By 2050, the number of Americans living to age 100 or more could reach 834,000 (Krach & Velkoff, 1999).

Supercentenarians are those who live beyond age 110.

There has been an equally impressive growth in the numbers of people living to even more extraordinary ages. Supercentenarians are those who live beyond age 110. More than 100 people currently living in the United States may have reached supercentenarian status. As a group, supercentenarians are in surprisingly good health. Forty-one percent need no or minimal assistance with activities of daily living. Few have cardiovascular disease, diabetes mellitus, or Parkinson's disease, and only 22% take medication for hypertension (Schoenhofen et al., 2006). Although many of the factors that contribute to exceptional longevity may be genetic, environmental factors also seem to play a significant role. Among communities with exceptional longevity, there seem to be some common themes: the importance of family and other social support networks; the consumption of large quantities of fresh, locally grown produce; and the absence of obesity and cigarette smoking (Buettner, 2005).

Geographic Distribution

About 12% of the total U.S. population is over age 65, but states vary widely in their percentage of older residents (Fig. 3-4). A number of factors contribute to the age of a population in any given state, including the birth rate, the number of young immigrants, and the number of young people moving into and out of the state for employment reasons. In addition, certain states—such as Florida, Arizona, and California—tend to attract larger than average numbers of retirees (Longino & Bradley, 2003). States that have higher than average percentages of older adults include Florida (17.4%), West Virginia (15.7%), Pennsylvania (15.3%), Maine (15.1%), Hawaii (14.8%), and Iowa (14.5%).

Rural Living

About one in five older adults lives in a rural area and thus faces special considerations and challenges. Research has demonstrated that rural elders tend to have fewer financial resources and fewer years of formal education than those living in metropolitan areas. These older adults are more likely to be in poor health and face several barriers to obtaining health care. Goins, Williams, Carter, Spencer, and Solovieva (2005) found that rural older adults identify the following barriers to obtaining quality health care: transportation difficulties, limited health care supply, lack of quality health care, social isolation, and financial constraints. Also, rural areas tend to have fewer assisted living facilities and more nursing home beds per capita. Older adults living in rural areas are more likely to live in nursing homes than their metropolitan counterparts.

Housing

More than 95% of people over age 65 live in private homes, retirement communities, or assisted living facilities rather than in institutional nursing homes. Many noninstitutional housing options are available for older adults to choose from, and it is important for nurses to understand what level of assistance each may provide to a given individual.

Noninstitutional Living

Age-Restricted Living Community

These communities allow older adults to live in houses or apartments based on age restrictions. A person typically needs to be 55 or older to qualify for residence. These facilities typically offer a range of services catering to retired adults. They often advertise clubhouses and opportunities for community

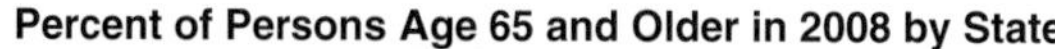

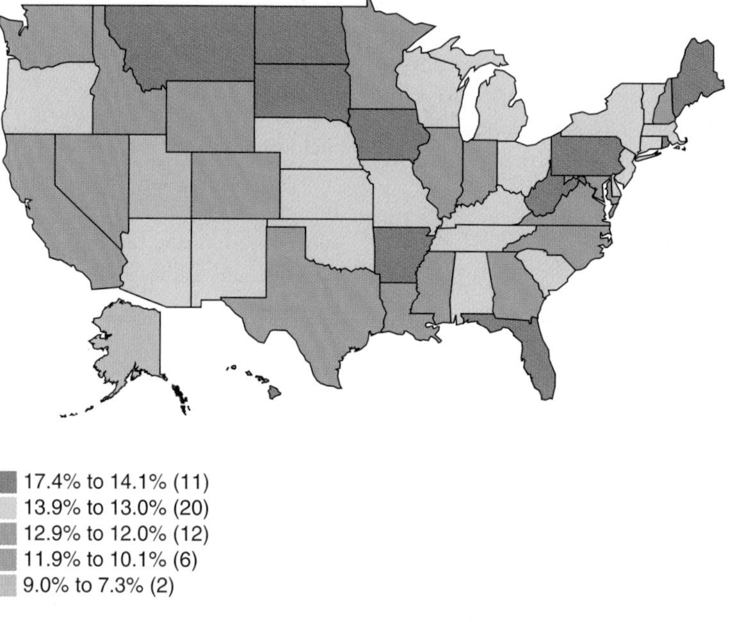

Source: 2008 Population Estimates from the U.S. Census Bureau

Figure 3-4 *(From Administration on Aging. (n.d.). A profile of older Americans: 2009. Retrieved October 20, 2010, from http://www.aoa.gov/AoAroot/Aging_Statistics/Profile/2009/docs/2009profile_508.pdf)*

and social gatherings. They cater to those in good physical and mental health who do not need assistance with their activities of daily living.

Senior-Housing Apartment Complex

This type of housing is available to seniors with demonstrated financial need. Residents live independently in their own apartments. They have their own kitchens, although many rely on the assistance of aid organizations such as Meals on Wheels to provide assistance with meals.

Assisted-Living Community

These communities cater to those who need some minimal assistance with bathing, dressing, and/or medication administration. Housing is typically in individual apartments with or without kitchens. Residents may be provided with one to three meals each day. Assisted living communities can be expensive, and many require proof of ability to pay before acceptance. The "assistance" advertised by assisted-living communities carries an additional cost, depending on the level of care required. Most assisted-living communities administer medications to most of their residents, usually through the use of unlicensed assisting personnel (Mitty, 2009).

Most assisted-living facilities administer medications to most of their residents, usually through the use of unlicensed assisting personnel.

Board and Care Home

Also known as residential care facilities for the elderly, or group homes, these are small facilities, typically homes, that provide housing and assistance to small groups of older adults. Residents may or may not share a bedroom, and a common kitchen is typically used. These facilities are not closely regulated and do not receive payment from Medicare or Medicaid. Older adults are typically charged a percentage of income (Centers for Medicare and Medicaid Services, 2009).

Life-Care or Continuing Care Retirement Community

Commonly known as CCRCs, these facilities offer different levels of care based on the resident's needs. The idea behind a CCRC is that a resident could move there in a relative state of health and stay within the same community as his or her health deteriorated and he or she needed additional assistance. Because residents of a CCRC will use the affiliated on-site nursing home, it is important for prospective buyers to consider the quality of the nursing home before moving in. These facilities typically charge a large entry fee in addition to a monthly payment (Centers for Medicare and Medicaid Services, 2009).

Institutional Living

The number of older adults living in nursing homes has declined in recent years. In 2007, about 4.4% of persons age 65 and older lived in nursing homes (Administration on Aging, 2008). However, as people age, the percentage living in nursing homes increases. Although only 1.3% of adults ages 65 to 74 currently live in a nursing home, that number climbs to 15.1% for those age 85 and over. Because nursing homes are increasingly the sites of short-term rehabilitation following hospitalization, the lifetime risk of institutionalization is higher.

About 42% of Americans age 70 and older will spend at least some time in a nursing home before they die (Murtaugh, Kemper, Spillman, & Carlson, 1997). People over age 85, women, and African-Americans are at greatest risk of nursing home placement. Most older adults living in nursing homes are women. Because women have a longer life expectancy, men often have the assistance of their wives during the final years of their lives. Unfortunately, as women age, they are more likely to be widowed and therefore do not have a spousal caregiver in their final years, increasing their risk of nursing home placement.

About 42% of Americans age 70 and older will spend at least some time in a nursing home before they die.

Nursing homes are also often called skilled nursing facilities (SNFs) or subacute rehabilitation facilities. Although the implication is that skilled nursing or rehabilitation facilities provide a higher level of care than nursing homes, there are no guidelines for the use of these terms and no regulations requiring higher levels of nurse staffing as compared with facilities using the term *nursing home* (Centers for Medicare and Medicaid Services, 2009). For decades, research has documented problems with the quality of care delivered in the nation's nursing homes.

Living Together and Alone

More than 95% of people over age 65 will have married at some point during their lives. As people age, they are more likely to be widowed, and this is particularly true of women (Fig. 3-5). However, the majority (55%) of younger older adults live with their spouses. More men (72.8%) live with their spouses than women (42%), because of the longer life expectancy of women (Fig. 3-6). About 30% of people over age 65 live alone, a number that increases with advancing age. Among women age 75 and over, for example, half live alone. Significantly smaller percentages of older adults living in noninstitutional settings live with other family members. About 6% will live with a parent, and 3.5% live with other relatives.

There are important nursing care considerations for older adults living alone. Older adults may need longer to recuperate from surgery or other acute illness, and they may need temporary placement in a nursing home before returning home. Therefore, when these patients are admitted to the hospital, discharge planning should begin upon admission to help facilitate transfer back home or to a nursing home following an acute care stay. Older adults living alone may become forgetful or may lose the ability to drive while retaining a strong desire to remain in their own homes. In these instances, community services such as Meals on Wheels and visiting nurses can be of assistance.

Older Adults Living with Domestic Partners

Domestic partnership rules and regulations vary from state to state, as do the protections they provide (Loue & Sajatovic, 2008). It is unclear as to whether same-sex domestic partners would be afforded the same rights when seeking medical care or when seeking access to long-term care facilities. Social Security survivor benefits, pensions, and 401K benefits are not extended to domestic partners. Property and inheritance rules and regulations and tax regulations differ as well. Additional legal documents, such as a durable power of attorney for health care, a will, and/or a trust may help strengthen some legal protections for same-sex couples.

Education

The educational level of older adults has been increasing for many years (Fig. 3-7). Over the past 30 years, the percentage of older adults completing high school increased substantially from 28% to 76.1%. In addition, an increasing percentage of

Martial Status of the Population Age 65 and Older, by Age Groups and Sex 2007

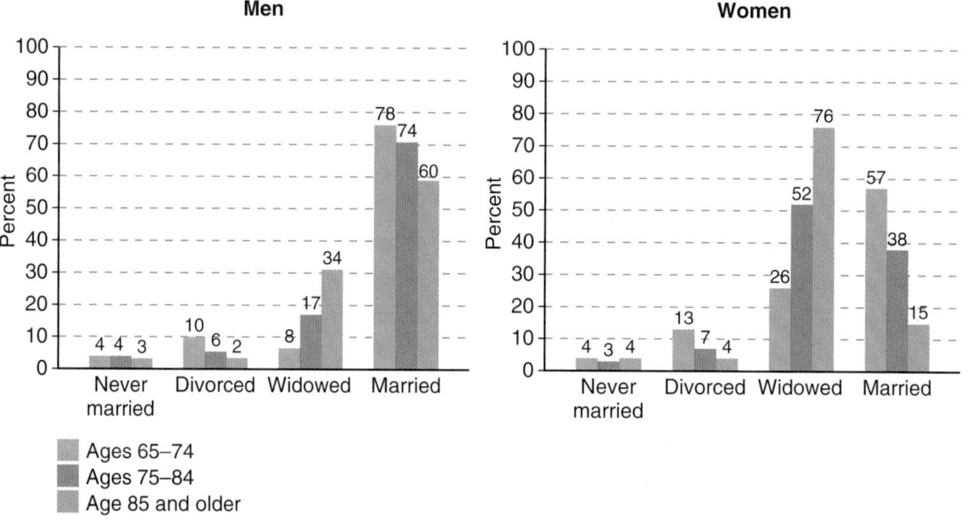

Note: Married includes married, spouse present; married, spouse absent; and separated.
Reference population: These data refer to the civilian noninstitutionalized population.
Source: U.S. Census Bureau, Current Population Survey, Annual Social and Economic Supplement.

Figure 3-5 *(From the Federal Interagency Forum on Aging-Related Statistics. Retrieved October 20, 2010, from http://www.aoa.gov/agingstatsdotnet/Main_Site/Data/2008_Documents/Population.aspx)*

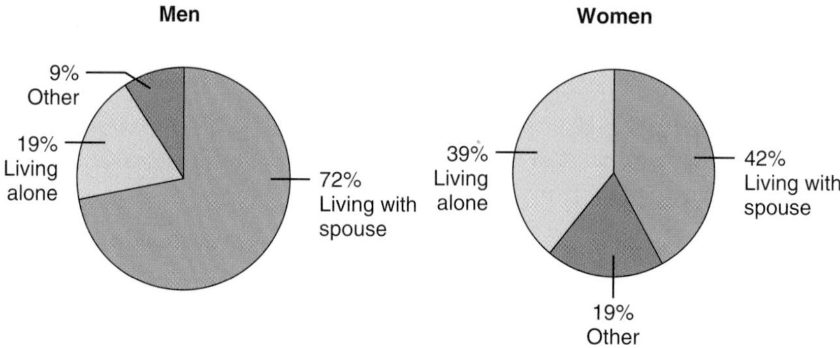

Figure 3-6 Living arrangements among those age 65 and older, 2008. (*A*) Men. (*B*) Women. *(From Administration on Aging. (n.d.). A profile of older Americans: 2009. Retrieved October 20, 2010, from http://www.aoa.gov/AoAroot/Aging_Statistics/Profile/2009/docs/2009profile_508.pdf)*

older adults have completed some form of higher education. About 20% of older adults hold bachelor's degrees or higher.

The rise in educational attainment occurred in part because of historical events, including passage of the GI Bill (U.S. Department of Veterans Affairs, 2009). The GI Bill was signed into law by Franklin Delano Roosevelt in 1944 to provide assistance to returning veterans (Fig. 3-8). In its peak year of 1947, veterans accounted for 49% of all college admissions (U.S. Department of Veterans Affairs, 2009). More than 7.8 million veterans graduated from college using benefits from the GI Bill, representing nearly half of all college graduates between 1940 and 1955 and one quarter of college graduates in the total population (Folger & Nam, 1976).

Continuing Education

Each year more than a half million people over age 60 are studying on college campuses (American Council on Education, 2007). Among people going back to school, a younger subset of older adults has been most interested in sharpening skills that could be used on the job, while an older subset of older adults studies for pleasure or to learn about new topics. Older adults should be encouraged to seek novel intellectual

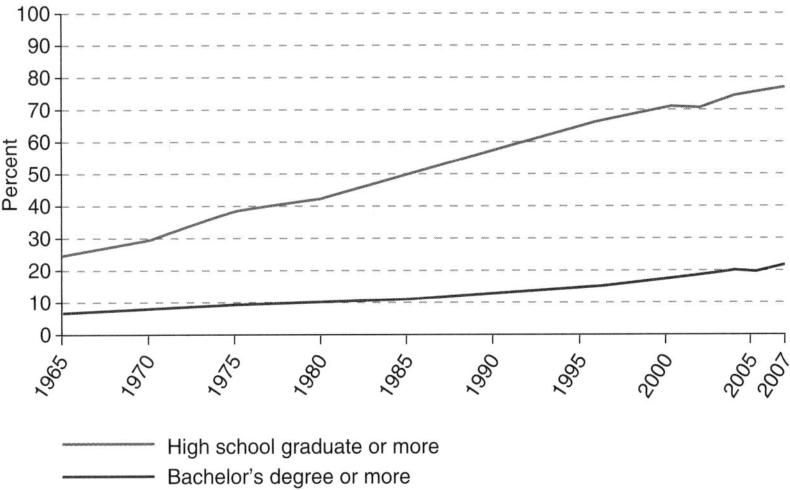

Note: A single question that asks for the highest grade or degree completed is now used to determine educational attainment. Prior to 1995, educational attainment was measured using data on years of school completed.
Reference population: These data refer to the civilian noninstitutionalized population.
Source: U.S. Census Bureau, Current Population Survey, Annual Social and Economic Supplement.

Figure 3-7 *(From the Federal Interagency Forum on Aging-Related Statistics. Retrieved October 20, 2010, from http://www.aoa.gov/agingstatsdotnet/Main_Site/Data/2008_Documents/Population.aspx)*

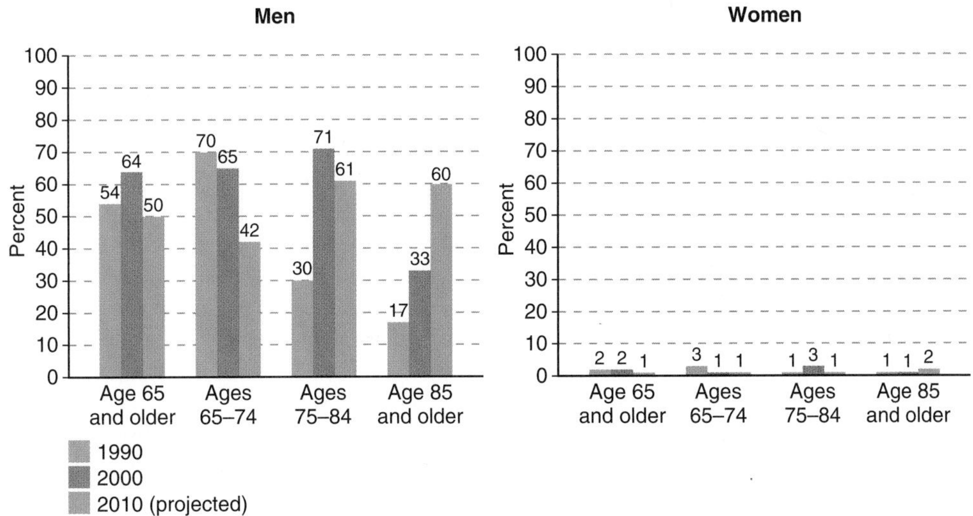

Reference population: These data refer to the resident population of the United States and Puerto Rico.
Source: U.S. Census Bureau, and Population Projections; Department of Veterans Affairs, VetPop2004.

Figure 3-8 *(From the Federal Interagency Forum on Aging-Related Statistics. Retrieved October 20, 2010, from http://www.aoa.gov/agingstatsdotnet/Main_Site/Data/2008_Documents/Population.aspx)*

challenges. There is a significant body of research demonstrating that pursuing a college education and leading an active intellectual life can help forestall the effects of Alzheimer's disease and dementia.

Occupations and Hobbies

Most people over age 65 say that they continue to work because they want to work, whereas 17% cite financial need as the main reason for working. Older adults say that they continue to work because they want to feel useful, because they want something to do, and because they want to be with others. The rate of labor force participation has increased over the past decade. About 12% of people over age 65 participated in the labor force in 1995. By 2000, the rate had increased to 13%. By 2009, 17% of the labor force was made up of people over age 65 (Pew Research Center, 2009).

PERSONAL PERSPECTIVE
Jan and Bobby Boal

When the Kaleidoscope Shop opened just inside Atlanta's perimeter, the last thing anyone would have expected is that both owners were in their late 70s. Now, a little more than 3 years later, Jan (husband) and Bobby (wife) Boal are 79 and 83, respectively, and still running their shop, which is open more than 40 hours a week. Most days, Jan and Bobby are at the shop for several hours, if not the entire day.

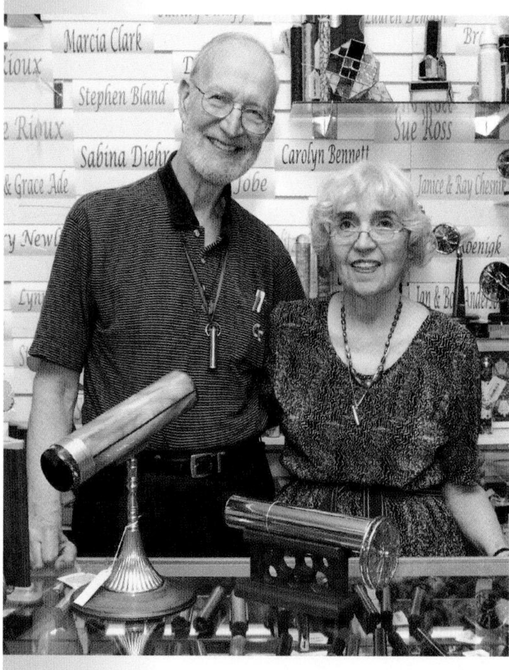

This is not the Boals' first entrepreneurial endeavor. In fact, for them, it's a downgrade. Their earlier retirement years were spent running The Veranda, a bed and breakfast in Senoia, Georgia. The Boals bought the rundown inn, renovated it, and spent 20 years as live-in owners, cooking and serving five-course breakfasts and dinners every day to the inn's guests. Before their retirement, Jan spent more than 30 years teaching at a university in downtown Atlanta while Bobby was a dedicated homemaker.

How do Jan and Bobby still continue to stay so active? It's not because they're perfectly healthy and happy. Jan has endured a Whipple surgery with a 28-day hospital recovery and then chemotherapy for hairy cell leukemia just 6 months later. Bobby has high blood pressure, is rapidly losing her hearing, has had cataract surgeries in both eyes, lost central vision in her left eye, and a few years ago had a pituitary tumor removed because it was entangling her optic nerve. Both have had their fair share of health troubles, and yet both are still active members in their church, community, and family.

"It's just something we wanted to do," Jan replied when asked how he and his wife get up every morning to run the shop. "I don't know how much longer we'll be able to keep doing it, but we're interested in people and we feel the shop is something that metro Atlanta needs. It's a beautiful art form, and people need to know about it." A passion for what they do is obviously one thing that keeps this dynamic duo running.

"We have a very active lifestyle. Our activities through our church have been very important to us. Not to mention our children and grandchildren." Jan and Bobby certainly stay active. They can be spotted taking long strolls throughout their neighborhood together. Jan still sings in the church choir, and they are very involved with their church's singles ministry. And living in Atlanta has them within 30 minutes of all three of their children and sometimes all 10 grandchildren and one great-grandchild.

Jan and Bobby are also committed to keeping their minds active. Their shop is full of challenging puzzles and games that Jan will show to his customers with a gleam of joy in his eye as he watches them struggle to figure it out. Bobby is a natural mother and homemaker to all, always eager to strike up a conversation and share some of her personal wisdom with anyone who will listen.

Maybe most importantly, they still have each other. "God gave us a great gift in each other. We are still very much in love. We joke, we laugh, we enjoy doing things together." In March 2010 they celebrated their 57th wedding anniversary, arguably more in love than they were the day they got married.

Or perhaps their health simply comes from the active responsibility they take for it. Consider Jan's actions after his Whipple surgery. "As soon as I got back to my room, I walked as much as I could. At first, it was just getting out of bed, but then I would walk around the hallway once, then twice. Four days after the surgery, I could walk a mile in the hallway. I pushed myself to walk. And I was faithful with my breathing exercises. I heartily recommend that to anyone going through a similar procedure."

Jan and Bobby have great passion for all they do, active bodies and minds, a tremendous amount of love for each other, and a sense of responsibility for their own health and wellness. They may be aging, but they are still full of life.

People over age 65 who are not working spend an increased amount of time pursuing sports and other leisure activities. Watching television accounted for about half of leisure time activity. In addition, retirees spent more time socializing and reading for personal interest than those still in the labor force. Older adults spend less time on child care and more on housework (Robinson, Godbey, & Putnam, 1997).

KEY POINTS

- As the Baby Boomers (those born between 1946 and 1964) begin to turn 65 in 2011, the United States will see dramatic increases in the number of older adults.
- A centenarian is a person who has reached age 100. A supercentenarian is a person who has reached age 110. There have been dramatic increases in the numbers of both centenarians and supercentenarians.
- More than 95% of people over age 65 do not live in nursing homes. Many alternative housing options are available for older adults.
- Women are more likely to outlive their spouses and to live alone. Consequently, they are more likely to require nursing home care.
- Older adults are concentrated in a few key states including Florida, West Virginia, Pennsylvania, and Maine. A few states draw large numbers of retirees including Florida, California, and Arizona.
- In 2010, the United States ranked 49th in overall life expectancy. A number of lifestyle factors contribute to a shortened lifespan in the United States, including smoking, lack of exercise, and obesity.
- The level of education among older adults is the highest it has ever been and continues to increase. One reason for the increases in educational attainment among older adults was the GI Bill.
- An increasing number of older adults are participating in the workforce beyond age 65.

CRITICAL THINKING ACTIVITIES

1. Go to Medicare's website and use the Nursing Home Compare research tool (http://www.medicare.gov/NHCompare/Include/DataSection/Questions/SearchCriteriaNEW.asp?version=default&browser=Firefox|3.6|WinXP&language=English&defaultstatus=0&pagelist=Home&CookiesEnabledStatus=True). How do the nursing homes in your community compare? Visit one of the nursing homes and analyze how the agency care compares with the description provided on the website.
2. We know that, in general, women are likely to outlive men. Can you think of some reasons why this might be true? What are some implications for the health care system?
3. Visit the National Geographic Website and watch the video *Secrets of Living Longer* at http://ngm.nationalgeographic.com/ngm/0511/sights_n_sounds/index.html. Write a one-page summary of the key points and your thoughts about what you learned from the video.
4. Were you surprised to discover that the United States ranks 50th in life expectancy? Aside from some of the reasons listed in the chapter, can you think of other reasons why this might be the case? Consider contributing factors.

CASE STUDY | *IDA JENNINGS*

Ida Jennings is a 93-year-old woman currently under the care of a hospice company at a local nursing home. Throughout her life Ida has lived in many different places. Initially Ida lived at home, where she cared for her spouse of more than 50 years until he died nearly 15 years ago. As Ida became older, she began to lose her vision. Her children became concerned about her ability to drive and to take care of a large house alone. Ida resisted moving out of her home for many years, despite the concerns of her children. Eventually, Ida moved to a senior housing facility. Moving proved extremely difficult for Ida. It was hard for her to let go of her possessions that she had accumulated over a lifetime. At the senior housing community, she was able to meet new friends and engage in a variety of activities. However, Ida continued to express a sense of loss about moving and giving up her home. As the years progressed, Ida became increasingly frail. Her vision became extremely poor, which made it difficult for her to take her medications accurately. In addition, Ida started to become forgetful and started to have problems with incontinence. Under pressure from her children, Ida then moved to an assisted-living community. At the assisted-living community, Ida was able to receive some assistance with her medications, and was supposed to have some assistance with activities of daily living. However, it was Rose, Ida's roommate who provided the most assistance. While at the assisted living, Ida sustained a fall, fracturing her hip. Following discharge from the hospital, Ida was placed in a nursing home for hospice care.

1. Based on what you have read in the chapter, how is Ida's case similar to other older adults?
2. Think about your own grandparents. Where do they live? Have they had to move recently? If so, what were the reasons they had to move? Has it been difficult for them to make the transition to a new home?

REFERENCES

Administration on Aging (2008). *A profile of Older Americans: 2008.* Retrieved October 22, 2010, from http://www.aoa.gov/AoARoot/Aging_Statistics/Profile/2008/docs/2008profile.pdf

American Council on Education (2007). *Framing new terrain: Older adults and higher education.* Retrieved October 22, 2010, from http://www.acenet.edu/Content/NavigationMenu/ProgramsServices/CLLL/Reinvesting/Reinvestingfinal.pdf

Buettner, D. (2005, November). New Wrinkles on Aging. *National Geographic*: 2-15.

Cai, L., Lubitz, J., Flegal, K. M., & Pamuk, E. R. (2010). The predicted effects of chronic obesity in middle age on Medicare costs and mortality. *Medical Care, 48*(6), 510–517.

Centers for Disease Control and Prevention. (2008). *Health, United States, 2008* (with Chartbook on Trends in the Health of Americans). Retrieved October 22, 2010, from http://www.cdc.gov/nchs/hus.htm

Centers for Medicare and Medicaid Services. (2009). *Types of long-term care.* Retrieved October 22, 2010, from http://www.medicare.gov/longtermcare/static/TypesOverview.asp

Central Intelligence Agency. (2010). *The world factbook.* Washington, DC: Central Intelligence Agency, 2010. https://www.cia.gov/library/publications/the-world-factbook/index.html

Ebersole, P., & Hess, P. (1998). *Toward healthy aging: Human needs and nursing response.* St. Louis, MO: Mosby.

Federal Interagency Forum on Aging Related Statistics. (2008). *Older Americans 2008: Key indicators of wellbeing.* Retrieved from http://www.aoa.gov/Agingstatsdotnet/Main_Site/Default.aspx

Folger, J., & Nam, K. (1976). *The education of the American population.* New York, NY: Amo Press.

Forey, B., Hamling, J., Lee, P., & Wald, N. (2002). *International smoking statistics: A collection of historical data from 30 economically developed countries.* London, England: Oxford University Press.

Goins, R. T., Williams, K. A., Carter, M. W., Spencer, M., & Solovieva, T. (2005). Perceived barriers to health care access among rural older adults: A qualitative study. *Journal of Rural Health, 21*(3), 206–213.

Horgan, C., Taylor, A., & Wilensky, G. (1983). Aging veterans: Will they overwhelm the VA medical care system? *Health Affairs, 2*(3), 77–86.

Longino, C. F., Jr., & Bradley, D. E. (2003). A first look at retirement migration trends in 2000. *Gerontologist, 43*(6), 904–907.

Loue, S., & Sajatovic, M. (2008). *Encyclopedia of aging and public health.* New York, NY: Springer.

Krach, C. A., & Velkoff, V. A. (1999). *U.S. Bureau of the Census, Current population reports, series P23-199RV centenarians in the United States.* U.S. Government Printing Office, Washington, DC, 1999. http://www.census.gov/prod/99pubs/p23-199.pdf

Mitty, E. (2009). Medication management in assisted living: A national survey of policies and practices. *J Am Med Dir Assoc, 10*(2), 107–114.

Murtaugh, C. M., Kemper, P., Spillman, B. C., & Carlson, B. L. (1997). The amount, distribution, and timing of lifetime nursing home use. *Med Care, 35*(3), 204–218.

Olshansky, S. J., Passaro, D. J., Hershow, R. C., Layden, J., Carnes, B. A., Brody, J., . . . Ludwig, D. S. (2005). A potential decline in life expectancy in the United States in the 21st century. *New England Journal of Medicine, 352*(11), 1138–1145.

Pew Research Center. (2009). *America's changing workforce recession turns a graying office grayer.* Retrieved from http://pewsocialtrends.org/assets/pdf/americas-changing-workforce.pdf

Pope, C. A., Ezzati, M., & Dockery, D. W. (2009). Fine-particulate air pollution and life expectancy in the United States. *New England Journal of Medicine, 360*(4), 376–386.

Renna, F., & Thakur, N. (2010). Direct and indirect effects of obesity on U.S. labor market outcomes of older working age adults. *Social Science & Medicine, 71*(2), 405–413.

Robinson, J., Godbey, G., & Putnam, R. (1997). *Time for life: The surprising way Americans use their time.* University Park, PA: Pennsylvania State University.

Schoenhofen, E. A., Wyszynski, D. F., Andersen, S., Pennington, J., Young, R., Terry, D. F., . . . (2006). Characteristics of 32 supercentenarians. *Journal of the American Geriatric Society, 54*(8), 1237–1240.

U.S. Department of Veterans Affairs. (2009). *Born of controversy: The GI Bill of Rights.* Retrieved from http://www.gibill.va.gov/GI_Bill_Info/history.htm

Wang, Y., & Beydoun, M.A. (2007). The obesity epidemic in the United States—Gender, age, socioeconomic, racial/ethnic, and geographic characteristics: A systematic review and meta-regression analysis. *Epidemiologic Reviews, 29,* 6–28.

Chapter 4

Opportunities and Challenges of Growing Old

Terry Tavella Quell, PhD, RN

LEARNING OBJECTIVES

- Consider the challenges that older adults face.
- Discuss the opportunities that come with growing older.
- Identify strategies older adults can use to optimize independence.
- Recognize ways to support older adults to keep them actively engaged.
- Explore the options for personal growth that arise upon retirement.
- Identify challenges and opportunities for older adults in the workforce.

Throughout life, each of us experiences multiple transitions. Some of these transitions open doors to new opportunities, such as the first day of elementary school, getting a driver's license, graduating from high school, landing that first real job after college, or retiring after 50 years of work. In each of these instances, changes occur that may influence the way we think about or experience the future. Other changes require adjusting to physical, social, and functional challenges that can test our coping abilities. For most people, maintaining a satisfying quality of life means having an optimal degree of independence and being socially and mentally engaged. Ensuring personal safety may require some resourceful lifestyle changes. In addition, dealing with loss and concerns about economic stability can create the need for strategies to help older adults maximize basic survival skills. As transitional periods occur, nurses can provide assessment, support, and education to help patients prepare for life changes and enhance quality of life.

Capitalizing on opportunities in the older adult's life may minimize or delay the effects of some challenges. For instance, lifestyle changes that accompany retirement and grandparenting can erase the stress of the workplace and bring new excitement to family life. New careers and ongoing educational opportunities can replace boredom with a thirst for new knowledge. Volunteerism, hobbies, and travel can renew energy and enthusiasm for daily activities. Finally, the satisfaction that comes from establishing a legacy, experiencing spiritual growth, and being seen as a purveyor of wisdom can create a sense of accomplishment and satisfaction.

Nurses can play a critical role in enhancing quality of life for older adults. Although acute care settings provide many options for patient and family education, senior centers and long-term care facilities offer ample opportunities for nurses to contribute to healthy aging by encouraging personal fulfillment.

Physical and Mental Health

Throughout life, people experience and adjust to physical changes in appearance and how the body functions. A young child who loses her front teeth learns to tackle food differently until permanent replacements emerge. Adolescents discover new interests as their bodies change during puberty. As individuals continue to age, hair begins to turn gray, skin may feel less supple, and "laugh lines" appear around the eyes. Although these developmental changes are normal, the tangible signs of aging are challenging for some people.

Throughout the aging process, physiological changes occur that may affect well-being. Bones may become more fragile, making older adults more prone to injuries such as a fractured hip. Arthritis may present a challenge to opening packages or activities that require fine motor skills such as writing or knitting. Cataracts or macular degeneration may make it difficult to read or to see at night. Such changes can adversely impact quality of life, yet they can often be minimized through prevention or treatment (Barak, Wagenaar, & Holt, 2006; Boyle, Buchman, Wilson, Bienias, & Bennett, 2007; Fagerström, Persson, Holst, & Hallberg, 2008).

Health prevention can be one of the best strategies to delay or lessen some of the most common chronic diseases of the elderly. Cardiac damage from years of untreated hypertension can lead to early myocardial infarction and stroke. Smoking increases the risk of such respiratory problems as lung cancer, emphysema, and asthma. Uncontrolled diabetes can affect kidney function, impair vision, and limit physical activities. When not treated early, the damage from these conditions can be irreversible. Further, obesity from decreased physical activity and unhealthy eating can worsen many chronic conditions that affect quality of life (Louria, 2005).

Maintaining mental health is just as important as physical health. Social and intellectual stimulation, such as keeping in touch with friends, staying abreast of current events, continuing to read newspapers, and working on crossword and jigsaw puzzles, are just a few ways to preserve brain function as we age (Barnes, 2006). Research indicates that cognitive training, physical activity, good nutrition, and social engagement are key factors in maintaining healthy brain function (Williams & Kemper, 2010). Advanced education contributes to increased mental functioning in older adults, and challenging the mind by learning a new skill or pursuing a new hobby may help maintain brain cells and stimulate cognitive processes (Robb-Nicholson, 2010).

Cognitive training, physical activity, good nutrition, and social engagement are key factors in maintaining healthy brain function.

Nurses and other health care providers can play a significant role in early detection of memory loss and cognitive deficits. Education for health providers in the assessment of older adults can lead to increased referrals for intervention and provide nurses with valuable skills for developing effective coping mechanisms for patients and families (Ballard, 2010).

Although aging and retirement are considered normal developmental stages of life, some older adults experience conditions that are not part of normal aging. The Federal Interagency Forum on Aging-Related Statistics (2008) reported that 17% of women and 11% of men age 65 and older reported depressive symptoms (Fig. 4-1). Evaluation of mood changes, decreased energy levels, disrupted sleep patterns, changes in appetite, and difficulties with concentration are important signals that should not be ignored (American Association for Geriatric Psychiatry [AAGP], 2009). Decreased self-esteem, feelings of worthlessness, and agitation can also be signs of distress that warrant evaluation (Thompsell, 2008).

Research suggests that mental disorders in older adults are underreported, in part because symptoms are disregarded as normal signs of aging, delaying diagnosis and treatment (AAGP, 2009). In addition, psychosocial histories are often overlooked during routine office visits. It is important for nurses to ask questions about retirement planning and what modifications have occurred in patients' daily lives since retirement to anticipate concerns and identify areas that need further investigation (McDaniel, 2008).

Sexual Fulfillment

In addition to physical and mental health, sexuality is another indicator of well-being that can be affected by the aging process. Physiological changes and emotional health among both men and women can present challenges and decrease sexual desire. Chronic illnesses, such as diabetes, cancer, or respiratory disease, as well a variety of medications, can affect sexuality.

Although little research exists about sexual fulfillment in the elderly, common sexual problems include decreased desire, low arousal, and orgasm difficulties (Shifren, Monz, Russo, Segreti, & Johannes, 2008). Lindau and colleagues (2007), in a study of over 3,000 adults ages 57 to 85, reported that most adults regarded sexuality

Percentage of People Age 65 and Older with Clinically Relevant Depressive Symptoms, by Sex, 1998–2004

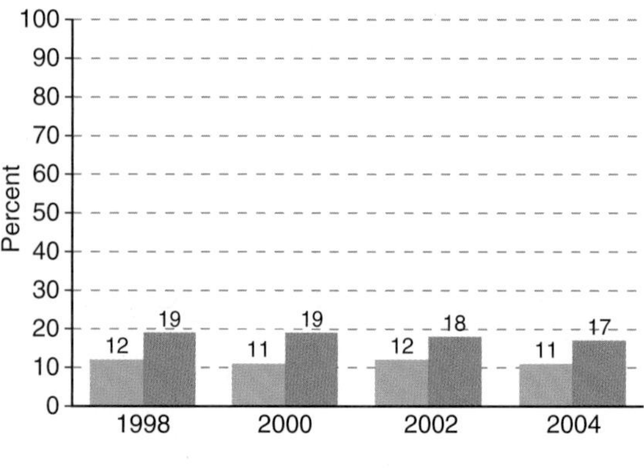

Men
Women

Note: The definition of "clinically relevant depressive symptoms" is four or more symptoms out of a list of eight depressive symptoms from an abbreviated version of the Center for Epidemiological Studies Depression Scale (CES-D) adapted by the Health and Retirement Study. The CES-D scale is a measure of depressive symptoms and is not to be used as a diagnosis of clinical depression. A detailed explanation concerning the "4 or more symptoms" cut off can be found in the following documentation, hrsonline.isr.umich.edu/docs/userg/dr-005.pdf.
Reference population: These data refer to the civilian noninstitutionalized population.
Source: Health and Retirement Study.

Figure 4-1 *(From Federal Interagency Forum on Aging-Related Statistics, 2008.)*

as important and that both men and women reported at least one sexual problem. Women reported difficulties with decreased desire, vaginal dryness, and inability to climax. Men reported concerns with erectile difficulties, with many reporting the use of medication to improve sexual function (Lindau et al., 2007).

As people age, opportunities for intimacy can change or decrease as spouses or sexual partners die. The U.S. Administration on Aging reported that among noninstitutionalized older adults, the proportion living alone increased with age, and only 30.1% of older women lived with a spouse. (See Figure 3-6 in Chapter 3.) In older adults, sexual desire is often linked to the presence of a partner, and women often marry men who are as much as a decade older (DeLamater & Sill, 2005). Thus, the loss of a partner and the accompanying grief can significantly affect well-being. For those who do have sexual partners, the decline in sexual functioning can be another loss.

Because intimacy can be difficult to discuss, sexual health is an area often avoided by health care providers (Lindau, et al., 2007). Willingness to explore one's own understanding and attitudes about sexuality and aging can make it easier for health care providers to initiate this conversation with patients (Price, 2009). Nurses can play an important role in this area by encouraging older adults to share information about their sexuality as part of an overall health assessment history.

Functional, Sensory, and Cognitive Changes

Physiological changes as we age may create functional, sensory, and cognitive changes that need to be addressed to maintain healthy well-being. The Federal Interagency Forum on Aging-Related Statistics (2008) reported that 17% of the older population had problems with sight, and 48% of men and 35% of women reported hearing difficulties. Many people find that they need glasses to read as they age, or they can no longer see well enough to drive at night. Impaired eyesight can create challenges such as difficulty in reading the daily newspaper or seeing food labels in the grocery store. Not only can this prove frustrating, but in some cases it can create safety issues, such as when directions are not followed properly with cleaning products or when street signs are misread. Carr, Flood, Steger-May, Schechtman, and Binder (2006) studied 183 adults age 75 and older living in the community. Despite a self-reported difficulty with at least one activity of daily living, 85% of the participants continued to drive. As the population over age 75 continues to rise, it will be important to consider what interventions may be necessary to help older adults maintain safe driving skills.

Nurses in all settings can assess for vision problems by asking adults to read a line or two off the television screen, a street sign, or from a consent form as a quick way to determine if there is need for concern. Vision screening, with proper referral to an ophthalmologist, is an important area of assessment in the older population to decrease the impact of limitations on activities of daily living (Fagerström et al., 2008; Spires, 2006).

The National Center for Health Statistics reports that sensory impairments affect hearing in 25% of the population between ages 70 and 79, and 17% experience problems with vision (Fig. 4-2). For people age 80 and above, these figures double (Dillon, Gu, Hoffman, & Ko, 2010). Although many people will seek out a health care provider for changing eyesight, many will ignore a problem with hearing loss. Although the myth that all elderly persons are hearing impaired is widely exaggerated, the literature has documented that age-related hearing loss is a significant concern that affects communication in older adults (Cook & Hawkins, 2006; Kochkin, 2009). With increasingly improved audiology devices, proper screening can identify new treatment options that can significantly increase quality of life (Cook & Hawkins, 2006).

Another area of concern with daily functioning is mobility. Walking and physical activity may be compromised by a number of chronic conditions including respiratory illness, cardiac disease, and neuromuscular changes. Decreasing energy levels and poor eyesight can affect activities, hinder gait, make stairs difficult to navigate, and contribute to falls in older adults. Preserving physical activity can help retain independence and maintain adequate functioning with daily activities (Boyle et al., 2007). For those with a history of falls, physical therapy and gait training can minimize the risk for another accident (Barak et al., 2006).

Finally, fine motor skills can be affected by aging. Impaired hand functioning can affect a person's ability to hold objects, open containers, or work with small tools. Even simple activities such as oral hygiene can be impaired when holding a tooth brush is compromised. In a study of 49 institutionalized older adults in Brazil, participants were scored based on motor skills and oral hygiene. Results indicated that subjects with weaker hand function had a higher level of dental plaque than those with stronger manual dexterity (Padilha, Hugo, Hilgert, & Dal Moro, 2007).

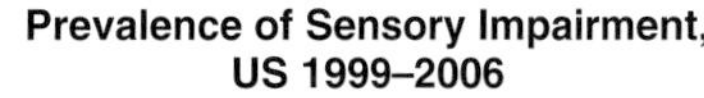

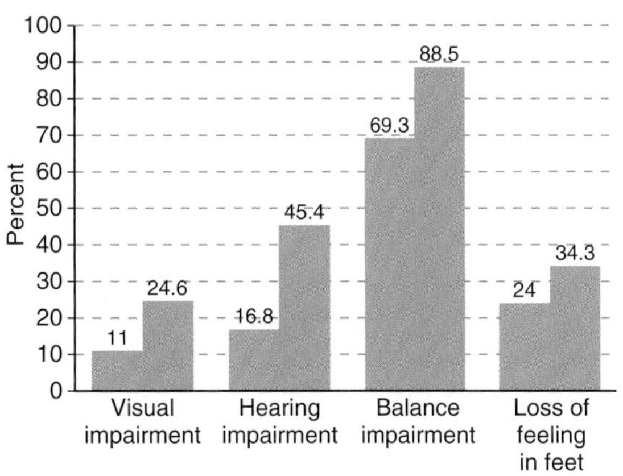

Figure 4-2 *(From CDC/NCHS, National Health and Nutrition Examination Survey; NCHS Data Brief, Number 31, April 2010.)*

Independence

For many, the biggest fear with getting old is not being able to take care of oneself. Continuing to live independently can become a challenge. The family home with several bedrooms, several baths, and additional rooms can be a lot to care for as we grow older. Even in a cozy townhouse, steep staircases, slippery polished floors, and loose throw-rugs can cause a risk of falls. Bathrooms on the second floor and washing machines in the basement can present mobility challenges and safety concerns. As families grow and members move in and out, space needs can change and may need to be modified to maintain wellness and safety in the home. Although many of us hesitate to consider the distant future, it is important that nurses consider new models to optimize independent living that foster autonomy (Sorrell, 2008).

Although many people will spend time in long-term care facilities, some will move in with family or friends and others may continue to live alone with assistance (Fig. 4-3). In a 2007 survey, the Federal Interagency Forum on Aging-Related Statistics reported that for seniors age 65 and over who were not institutionalized, 5% of men and 17% of women lived with other relatives, and 19% of older men and 39% of older women lived alone (Federal Interagency Forum on Aging-Related Statistics, 2008). Senior centers and community programs that provide transportation to doctor appointments, visits to shut-ins, and phone calls from volunteers can assist older adults in staying in their own homes while maintaining a safe environment (Redmond, 2006; Sorrell, 2008; Texas Nursing, 2006).

As older adults live longer than previous generations, caregivers—whether they are spouses,

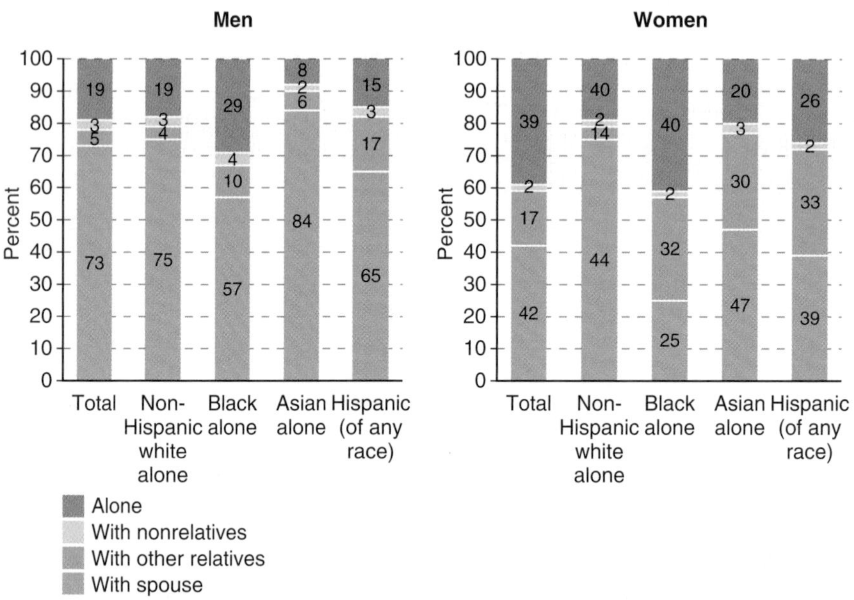

Group	Alone	With nonrelatives	With other relatives	With spouse
Men: Total	19	3	5	73
Men: Non-Hispanic white alone	19	3	4	75
Men: Black alone	29	4	10	57
Men: Asian alone	8	2	6	84
Men: Hispanic (of any race)	15	3	17	65
Women: Total	39	2	17	42
Women: Non-Hispanic white alone	40	2	14	44
Women: Black alone	40	2	32	25
Women: Asian alone	20	3	30	47
Women: Hispanic (of any race)	26	2	33	39

Note: Living with other relatives indicates no spouse present. Living with nonrelatives indicates no spouse or other relatives present. The term *non-Hispanic white alone* is used to refer to people who reported being white and no other race and who are not Hispanic. The term *black alone* is used to refer to people who reported being black or African American and no other race, and the term *Asian alone* is used to refer to people who reported only Asian as their race. The use of single-race populations in this report does not imply that this is the preferred method of presenting or analyzing data. The U.S. Census Bureau uses a variety of approaches.
Reference population: These data refer to the civilian noninstitutionalized population.
Source: U.S. Census Bureau, Current Population Survey, Annual Social and Economic Supplement.

Figure 4-3 *(From Federal Interagency Forum on Aging-Related Statistics, 2008.)*

children, or friends—may be aging themselves (Vladeck, 2005). The American Association of Geriatric Psychiatry estimates that nearly 25% of American households provide care to an older adult, and over 75% of these caretakers are female (AAGP, 2009). Programs for seniors, such as community-based adult day programs, can provide significant respite for caretakers, while contributing to engagement and maintaining quality of life for older adults (Molzahn, Gallagher, & McNulty, 2009). As the older population continues to climb, communities that are designed for retiring adults will become increasingly important to optimize independence, maintain healthy living, and provide opportunities for socialization, while offering increasing levels of care and assistance as seniors age and need more help to live independently (Brandon & Flury, 2009; Masotti, Fick, Johnson-Masotti, & MacLeod,, 2006).

Maintaining activity is an important step in preserving independence, and keeping physically active does not necessarily mean signing up for classes at the gym (Skelton & Dinan, 2007). Although some may feel that they have earned the right to hire people to cook, clean, mow the lawn, and do the gardening, these routine activities can offer physical activity, preserve cognitive functioning, and provide a sense of accomplishment. With aging, however, it may be necessary to modify some of these everyday tasks. Although dusting, vacuuming, and washing floors can be a good source of exercise, maintaining safety must be considered. For example, stepstools should be avoided to reaching high shelves, and brooms and mops should be carefully put away to avoid falls.

Routine activity also can help maintain cognitive functioning when the activity requires planning and prioritizing. Cooking a meal, for example, requires that a number of activities be prioritized so that different foods are ready to be served at the same time. In a study of 60 people ages 18 to 80, participants were asked to prepare a virtual breakfast using a touch screen monitor (Craik & Bialystok, 2006). Subjects were given the task of preparing five foods with different cooking times, all to be served at the same time. To further evaluate their ability to multitask, they were required to set four place settings around a virtual table. Results indicated that older participants checked cooking times less frequently, had more trouble switching tasks, and overall took more time to complete the activity. As we age, the ability to plan, multitask, and re-evaluate a situation can become more difficult (Craik & Bialystok, 2006). For those who are cognitively impaired, cooking may need to be simplified with a toaster oven or microwave to make preparation simpler and without the worry of a stovetop left unattended. Visits from nurses or social workers can assist in proper assessment of the home environment to maintain safety for older adults.

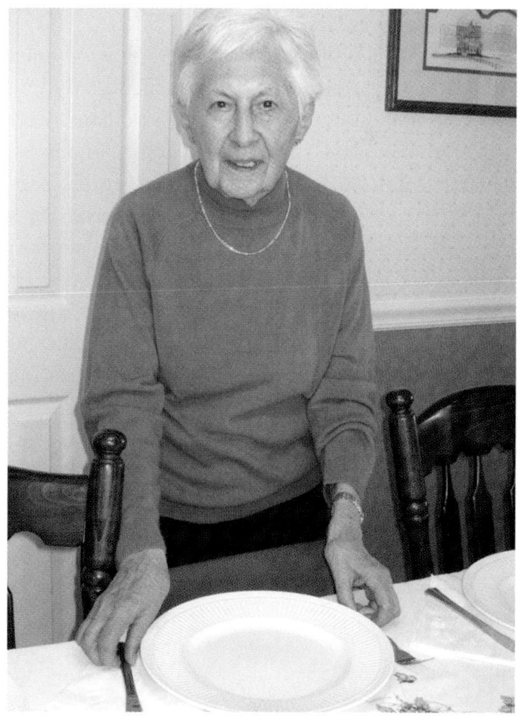

Although some consider yard work a chore, it can serve as a source of great satisfaction and accomplishment. For older adults, gardening can help improve socialization by increasing time outdoors in the neighborhood, while also maintaining physical activity. A study of 53 older adults age 58 to 86, recruited from the community, were classified as active gardeners, gardeners, and non-gardeners using the CHAMPS Physical Activity Questionnaire for Older Adults. The tool assessed the types and levels of physical activity that are meaningful and appropriate for older adults, including lighter and more vigorous activities. Results indicated that active gardeners and gardeners had significantly more hand strength than nongardeners, as well as significantly better overall health (Park, Shoemaker, & Haub, 2009). For those who grow fruits and vegetables, gardening may also encourage good nutrition and even provide cost savings to the grocery bill (Swann, 2006; Thelander, Wahlin, Olofsson, Heikkila, & Sonde, 2008).

For older adults, pets can be another method of optimizing independence. Loneliness due to loss of a partner, separation from friends, or families moving away can leave a gap in the life of an older person that can lead to depression, isolation, and decreased opportunities for communication with others (Krause-Parello, 2008; Vladeck, 2005). Krause-Parello (2008) studied 159 older women with either a cat or dog, living independently in a pet-friendly housing community. Participants were asked to complete surveys related to loneliness, general health, and pet attachment. Results supported the general health benefits of caring for a pet and indicated that pet attachment support could serve as a coping mechanism for loneliness (Krause-Parello, 2008). Especially for those who live alone, having a pet can provide companionship, elevate mood, and increase socialization (McColgan & Schofield, 2007; Prosser, Townsend, & Staiger, 2008).

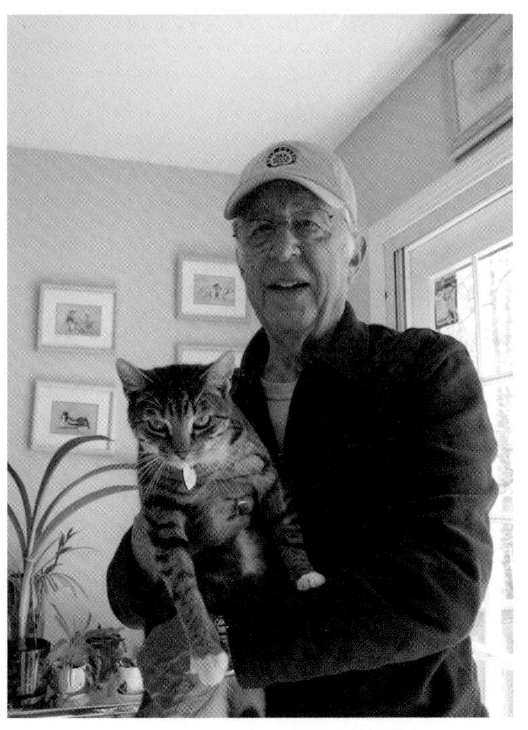

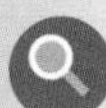

EVIDENCE FOR PRACTICE
Therapeutic Effects of Dogs

Purpose: This small research project explored the relationships that older people have with their companion animals, in particular their dogs.

Sample: Six people, three men and three women, ranging from age 22 to 70, who lived alone with dogs were interviewed in their homes with their dogs present.

Methods: The research design was qualitative and consisted of conversational interviews and observations. Semistructured interviews were tape recorded and transcribed. Field notes of the observations were written immediately following each interview to capture what could not be recorded on audiotape, including physical and verbal interactions between human and dog.

Results: Findings indicated that the participants considered their dogs to be members of the family and ranked them highly in a hierarchy of importance against other people. The animals kept them company, acted as confidants to the humans, and provided a means of emotional expression. People felt that the main advantages of having a dog were that they made them do more and acted as a social catalyst. The main disadvantage was that they missed them during periods of separation.

Implications: Dogs can play an important companionship role for older people, especially when human social circles become restricted. For some older adults, the rapport with their pet might be their most significant existing relationship. Separation from a companion animal can create distress that could worsen existing physical and mental health problems. This could have important implications for the kind of community support needed to enable older people to keep their companion animals with them either at home or in supported living accommodation.

Reference: McColgan, G., & Schofield, I. (2007). The importance of companion animal relationships in the lives of older people. *Nursing Older People, 19*(1), 21-23.

Caring for a pet, much like caring for another family member, can provide opportunity for physical activity, offer cues to eat meals, and supply a source of entertainment and companionship. Health care providers need to recognize that, for many older adults, pets can support and enhance quality of life. Risley-Curtiss (2010) surveyed 5,012 members of the National Association of Social Workers to investigate knowledge of animal-human relations, inclusion of animals in patient assessments, and history of education regarding animals in social work practice. Results indicated that 97.8% of the participants were familiar with the positive impact of animals on adults, yet only 23.2% asked questions about pets as part of their patient assessments (Risley-Curtiss, 2010).

In addition, it is important to assess concerns that can arise regarding care of pets when seniors are displaced. A hospitalized patient worrying about a hungry pet may experience additional stress that can be detrimental to both physical and mental health. Further, older adults may be reluctant to move into a retirement community or senior housing facility if unable to bring their animal companion to live with them (Krause-Parello, 2008).

Engagement

Involvement with groups and organizations can help people maintain overall health and functioning. Singing in a choir or playing an instrument in a musical ensemble can enhance communication skills and engagement with others, while providing entertainment that can enrich the mind and body. Participating in activities such as dance lessons and exercise classes at community centers can improve balance and prevent bone loss (Skelton & Dinan, 2007). Learning melodies can also enhance memory capacity and minimize cognitive decline (Sorrell & Sorrell, 2008). The Creativity and Aging Study (Cohen, 2006), conducted by the National Endowment for the Arts, compared groups of people with similar levels of health and activity to determine the impact of the fine arts on older adults. Ranging from ages 65 to 103 in three separate areas of the country, 150 people were exposed to programs run by professional artists, and data were collected at the start and at intervals of 1 and 2 years. When compared with participants in the control groups, those who experienced the cultural programs were healthier, were more involved in community activities, and had improved mental health (Cohen, 2006; Cohen et al., 2006).

Reading can stimulate the mind and help maintain communication skills, while book clubs can serve as a source of socialization with others. Reading newspapers and watching the evening news provides opportunities to keep focused on current happenings both locally and around the world. In addition, current events can be a source of conversation and encourage engagement with others (Robb-Nicholson, 2010; Williams & Kemper, 2010).

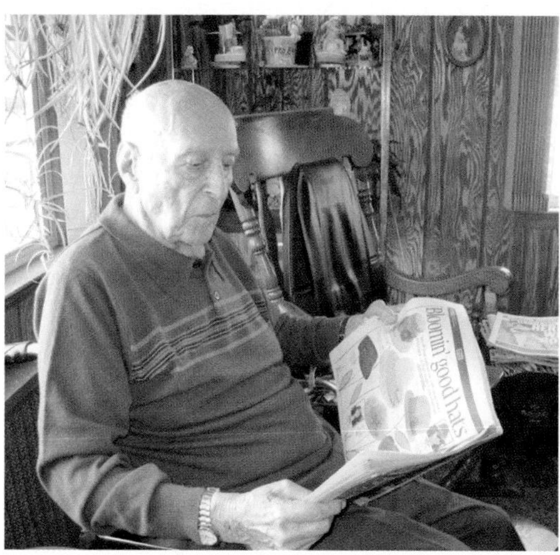

For those who have been used to going to work on a regular schedule, or having a particular daily routine, it is important to stay active and maintain friendships and connections to others. Once retired, it can be easy to lose contact with former colleagues and possibly become somewhat isolated. Once separated from one set of friends, it can be difficult to find new acquaintances that are not attached to a previous place of employment. Conversely, with decreased obligations from work, opportunities may increase for connecting with former friends and relatives. It may be easier to visit with relatives who have moved away and reconnect with old friends who were too busy to stay in touch in previous years. Staying in touch with family, friends, and colleagues can be an important factor in promoting both physical and mental health.

As longevity increases, the family structure can change significantly. Historically, aging adults raised their children, launched them into the world, then relaxed and waited for grandchildren to arrive. As older adults live longer, it is not uncommon for seniors to become caregivers for their own elderly parents at the same time that they are beginning to struggle with the aging process (Vladeck, 2005).

Concerns for safety may require that elderly relatives move in with their aging children, again making it challenging to stay connected with friends and relatives. For some extended families, more than one generation of retirees may share a household. Individuals who have been highly independent may seek out opportunities for self-fulfillment and engagement in the community; thus, the need for quality services and health care options will continue to be a challenge for the most elderly of our aging population (Brandon & Flury, 2009).

In many communities, opportunities exist for aging adults to stay involved, meet new people, and learn new activities. Senior centers provide quilting classes, computer instruction, and golf lessons. Adult day centers can provide opportunities to maintain well-being and increase interaction with others, while also providing respite for caregivers (Molzahn, Gallagher, & McNulty, 2009). Chapters of AARP provide luncheon speakers, financial planning, and legal assistance. In addition, religious and veterans organizations provide opportunities for community service, networking, and socialization.

Personal Safety

Most people are relatively independent throughout their lives. They prepare food, do laundry, clean house, run their own errands. This makes many older adults reluctant to ask for help, even if they have relatives and friends who are willing to help out. Unaccustomed to giving up power and control, some will try to manage on their own rather than admit to being needy or vulnerable. Nurses can often help families identify strategies to provide independence while maintaining the need for a secure environment.

For older adults, cognitive and physical functioning can be affected in ways that present a number of hazards. Unsteady hands, or miscalculating the heat of a bowl of soup, can lead to painful burns. Polished hardwood floors and loose throw rugs can lead to nasty spills, and trying to reach the top cabinet shelf with an unsteady chair or stepstool can lead to severe bruises and broken bones. Switching to easier food preparation, removal of loose floor rugs, and rearranging cabinets for easier access can all decrease the risk of accidents.

Fears of giving up independence, or not wanting to wait to get things done, can prevent older adults from asking for assistance when needed. For many, the apprehension about safety and the risk of falling can be very anxiety producing. Even taking a bath or shower can become a significant source of worry (Molzahn, Gallagher, & McNulty, 2009). Providing opportunities for daily interaction with others and establishing a system for a daily check-in with an older person may be a good way to help maintain independence while providing a measure of safety.

Assessment of the living situation, environmental conditions, and available social supports must be incorporated into all health care visits for older adults.

Many communities have programs developed by schools and churches in which students or volunteers make daily calls to older adults who live alone. Adult day centers provide opportunities for interaction, recreation, and inclusion (Molzahn, Gallagher, & McNulty, 2009). Parish nurse programs, many of which have been in existence for over 30 years, can be good avenues to contact older adults through an already established community organization. Opportunities for meeting other members of the community while providing health screening and teaching can assist the elderly in maintaining health and wellness (Redmond, 2006). Safety alert bracelets that can be activated in case of an emergency can provide immediate assistance as needed. Assessment of the living situation, environmental conditions, and available social supports must be incorporated into all health care visits for older adults.

Loss

Although some people experience the loss of a young friend or relative to illness or injury, it is not a common occurrence. Often, the loss is both sudden and unexpected, and this may make individuals question their own mortality. For many, the first significant death in life is a grandparent or elderly aunt or uncle. Although these losses can hit hard, most people understand that people do not live forever and expect to lose loved ones as they age.

Life expectancy rates in the United States are lower than some other industrialized nations worldwide (Federal Interagency Forum on Aging-Related Statistics, 2008) (Fig. 4-4). In the past century, life expectancy has increased by 30 years, and a child born in 2006 is now predicted to live to almost 80 years old (Administration on Aging, 2008).

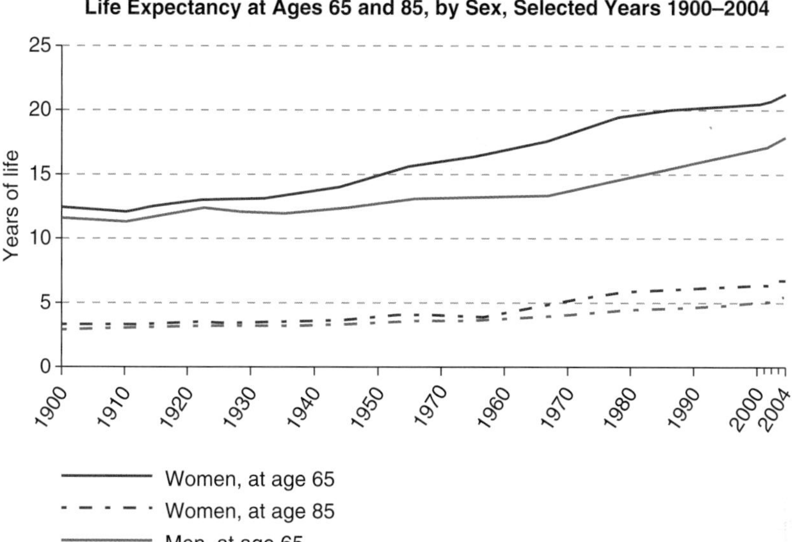

Figure 4-4 *(From Federal Interagency Forum on Aging-Related Statistics. (2008). Older Americans 2008: Key indicators of well-being. Washington, DC: U.S. Government Printing Office.)*

As we age, it becomes more and more common to lose loved ones. As older adults begin to lose friends one at a time, their circle of peers begins to grow smaller, and as the numbers decrease, it becomes more and more inevitable that soon everyone in the group will leave this world. Perhaps the most difficult loss is the death of a spouse. In 2007, the U.S. Census Bureau reported that 13% of men and 42% of women age 65 and above were widowed (Administration on Aging, 2008). Especially for those who have been together for a long time, a spouse can be a life partner that they are with for a longer time period than they were alone.

For many health care providers, loss is a difficult subject to discuss. Often people do not know what to say, so they avoid the topic. As loss occurs at many levels, the risk for social isolation increases, often compounding the process of grieving (Vladeck, 2005). The need for continued support after the death of a family member is critical because depression, loss of appetite, and sleep disorders can be highly common in family members who have cared for dying relatives (Holtslander, 2008). Strategies to assist older adults with the grief process, such as bereavement counseling, and widows' and widowers' groups can facilitate coping with loss and reduce the risk of isolation during this transitional period.

Economic Stability

Ensuring finances for the retirement years can be a challenge. Too often, people put off saving for the future and find that they are unable to maintain their lifestyle in later years. Overall, older adults are more prosperous than in any other generation (Federal Interagency Forum on Aging-Related Statistics, 2008). However, the U.S. Department of Health and Human Services reported that almost 10% of elderly persons were below the national poverty level in 2007 (Administration on Aging, 2008).

Seniors are especially vulnerable to the overall economic climate because they may no longer be employed and need to support themselves with retirement accounts, Social Security, and interest from investments (Beard, 2009) (Fig. 4-5).

As the average life span increases, there are many concerns that older adults will outlive their financial resources (Louria, 2005). For many

Sources of Income for Married Couples and Nonmarried People Who are Age 65 and Older, by Income Quintile, 2006

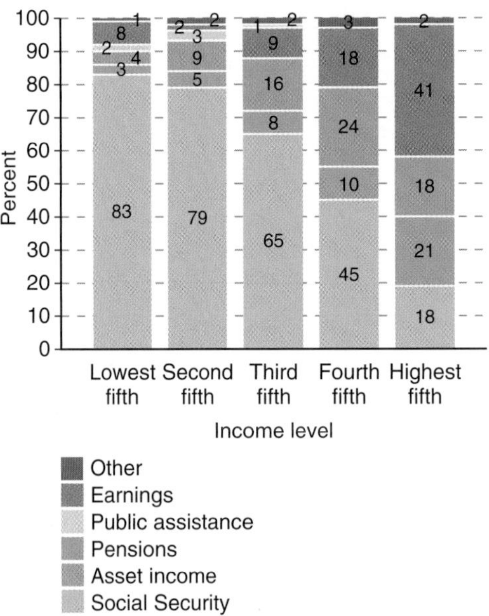

Note: A married couple is considered age 65 and older if the husband is age 65 or older or the husband is younger than age 55 and the wife is age 65 or older. The definition of "other" includes, but is not limited to, unemployment compensation, worker's compensation, alimony, child support, and personal contributions. Quintile limits are $11,519 for the lowest quintile, $18,622 for the second quintile, $28,911 for the third quintile, $50,064 for the fourth quintile, and open-ended for the highest quintile.
Reference population: These data refer to the civilian noninstitutionalized population.
Source: U.S. Census Bureau, Current Population Survey, Annual Social and Economic Supplement, 2007.

Figure 4-5 *(From Administration on Aging. (2008). A profile of older Americans: 2008. U.S. Department of Health and Human Services. Washington, D. C. Retrieved from http://www.mowaa.org/Document.Doc?id=69)*

years, the U.S. government identified the retirement age as 65; however, the age has been extended as far as 67 for those born after 1959 (Social Security Online, 2009). In 2007, the median income for older men was $24,323, while older women had an income of only $14,021 (Administration on Aging, 2008). With a limited income, it may be difficult for some seniors to continue to afford their previous lifestyle.

Although participation rates in the labor force declined steadily for older men and women from 1900 to 2002, increasing numbers of seniors are now staying in the workforce (Administration on Aging, 2008). In 2007, 16% of Americans age 65 and older were actively working or seeking employment (Fig. 4-6). As many Americans live longer than ever before, keeping individuals in the workplace for a longer period of time may be something that should be encouraged. However, many current employment practices make this difficult to achieve. The Organization for Economic Cooperation and Development proposed three key issues that discourage older adults in the workplace: Current retirement systems that penalize older adults from working while earning pensions, employer attitudes toward older workers, and lack of training in current technology are all barriers for older workers who want to remain in the job market (Gurria, 2008).

For Americans reaching age 65, the average life expectancy is an additional 19 years (Administration on Aging, 2008). Thus, retiring at age 62 or 65

Labor Force Participation Rates of the Population Age 55 and Older, by Age Group, Annual Averages, 1963–2006

Men

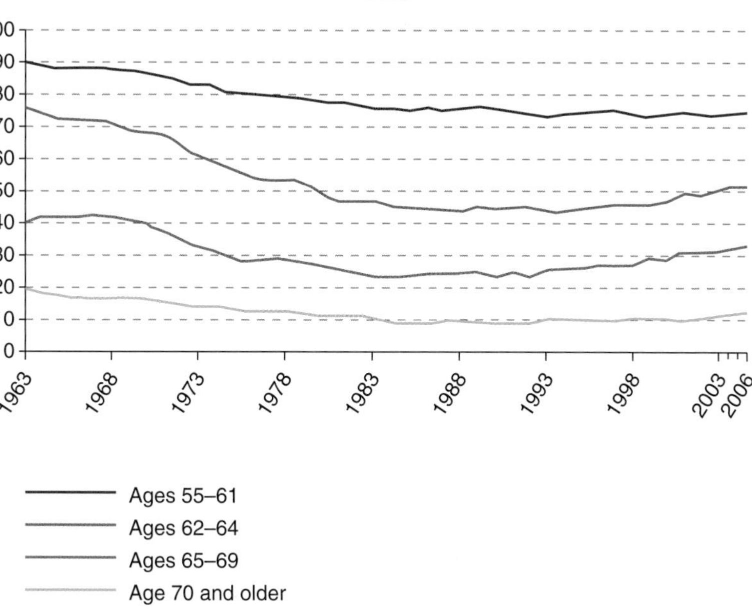

Note: Data for 1994 and later years are not strictly comparable with data for 1993 and earlier years due to a redesign of the survey and methodology of the Current Population Survey. Beginning in 2000, data incorporate population controls from Census 2000.
Reference population: These data refer to the civilian noninstitutionalized population.
Source: Bureau of Labor Statistics, Current Population Survey.

Labor Force Participation Rates of the Population Age 55 and Older, by Age Group, Annual Averages, 1963–2006

Women

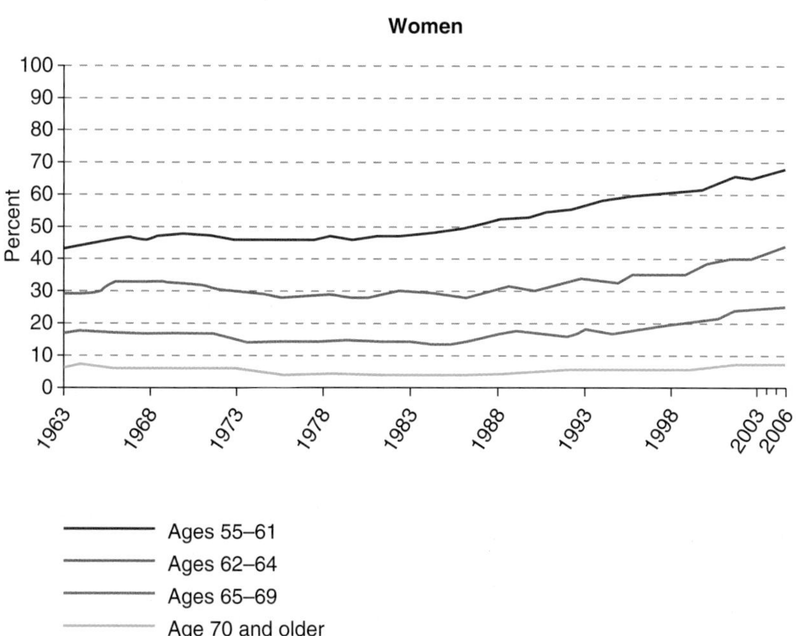

Figure 4-6 *(From Administration on Aging. (2008). A profile of older Americans: 2008. U.S. Department of Health and Human Services. Washington, D. C. Retrieved from http://www.mowaa.org/Document.Doc?id=69)*

may no longer be the norm. Proper financial planning and smart investing in earlier years can help ensure enough money to live, travel, and enjoy life in later years. Health insurance for older adults is also a concern because for many, insurance is tied to employment. Although Medicare will cover many health care expenses in our later years, often the elderly must choose between paying for expensive medication and buying food at the grocery store.

Paying for housing may also be a concern. For those who have lived in their home for many decades, property values may have climbed, with taxes that outpace income. Not wanting to leave their familiar surroundings, or not being in a position to move somewhere cheaper, often older adults find themselves unable to maintain the costs of a home. Reduced utility rates for seniors, tax benefits for veterans, and reverse mortgages can all be explored to help ease this burden. Nurses and health care providers can be a valuable resource in negotiating community programs that can assist older adults with these concerns.

While dealing with financial concerns, maintaining health, optimizing independence, and staying engaged with the outside world are real challenges for the aging adult, early identification of risks related to environmental stressors and social support systems can help minimize losses. By identifying potential concerns and creating new opportunities, the effect of some hardships can be minimized or delayed.

Opportunities

Retirement

The transition to retirement can be a life-changing milestone where many might say that they are closing one chapter of their lives and beginning anew. For some, this new found freedom from the day-to-day work routine brings wonderful opportunities. They now have time to do all the things they have been putting off, such as volunteering, playing golf, and traveling. For others, retirement can be a very stressful life event. Facing the challenges of loneliness, worrying about having enough money, and staying healthy can create additional burdens and overwhelm coping skills (McDaniel, 2008). Ideally, the challenges of aging can be minimized by increasing opportunities for new adventures.

PERSONAL PERSPECTIVE

Challenges and Opportunities of Aging

At age 82, Bill, a handsome and fit retired engineer, speaks frankly and thoughtfully about aging, both the challenges and opportunities. "One of the most apparent things I've found," he says, "is my memory isn't nearly as good as it should be. Where I once could store a lot of data—I wouldn't even bother with notes—now I find that I forget an appointment unless I write it down. Last year I forgot to pay my taxes. That's startling. It's so unlike me. But then I say, 'maybe it was unlike me then, but maybe it's what I am now.' I don't want to dwell on that, but I do find myself making more notes than I did before, and my notes aren't as cryptic as they once were. Now I will put everything down because I won't remember what I thought about two months ago." Although Bill admits that this change is a hard one for him to accept, he nonetheless does so without adding onto himself the destructive burden of self-judgment.

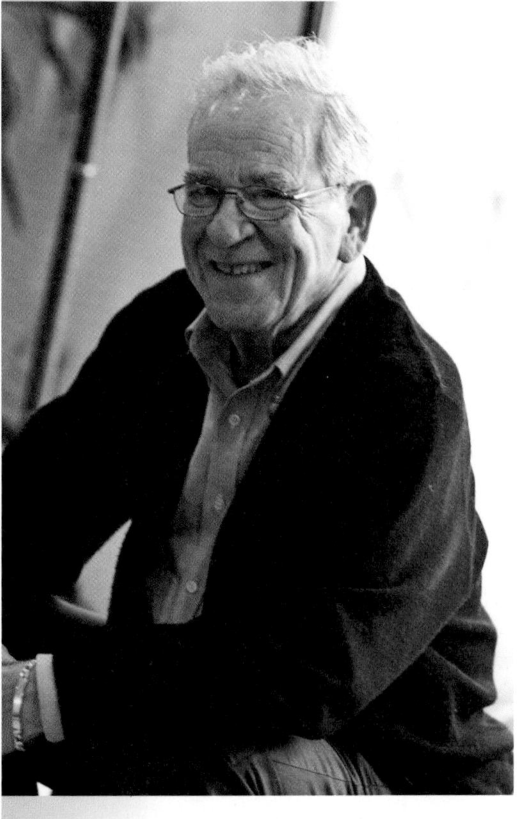

Perhaps the greatest challenge of aging is loss. Bill spoke openly about the dark days after his wife died, describing the months after the funeral as "empty, frightening, bewildering, and confusing," with "long empty days and nights, that were overpowering" for him. "Time is a problem," he says. However, "if you keep yourself busy, then time isn't a problem." His desire to find a light at the end of this dark tunnel allowed him to see the unbounded stretch of time as an opportunity to explore new interests. Bill says, "I have always, since I was maybe fourteen years old, wanted to play the trombone, as silly as that may seem. And one day I remembered that I never fulfilled that wish. Now I have all the time in the world, so I bought a trombone and took ten or twelve lessons and bought some books to get me off and running. It's a challenge, but it's okay. It's something I always wanted to do even though I forgot about it for 50 years because I was busy with life in general." Now, though the nature of "life in general" has been re-defined, Bill has found that the extra time afforded during the elder years is not the enemy.

About Bill Bill Marullo, a widowed father of three, is in close touch with all three of his children and finds great joy in his six grandchildren. A navy veteran of World War II, Bill returned to the States and joined the Coast Guard after the war. After his military service, he had a long career as an electrical design engineer. When his dear wife Marie passed away after 54 years of marriage, Bill turned to community work to help him combat the feelings of loneliness and isolation, and he remains a committed Catholic, attending church regularly. Today, he is a valued volunteer at a local hospital where he works in both the thrift shop and the mail room. Bill recently took up the trombone, made a new close friendship, and befriended a cat named Max.

Lorri Danzig, MS, CSL

Grandparenting

One of the most exciting experiences of aging is seeing children begin families of their own. There is nothing that can be compared to giving new life as a child is born. Those who have been lucky enough to experience this joy know the happiness and the heartbreak that can occur as children grow up and follow in their parents' footsteps or walk in another direction.

Parents will often say that, regardless of age, their children are always a part of them, and the days of worrying never end. With newborns, parents express concern about babies getting proper nutrition and sleeping through the night. Parents of toddlers baby-proof their houses to minimize the dangers of choking on small objects and getting a shock from electrical outlets. During the elementary and middle school years, parents worry about their child's academic ability and fitting in with peers. And even when the children are out of the house and on their own, the concern for their well-being still persists.

Grandchildren can bring mixed blessings. For many, the experience of becoming a grandparent means all the fun of having a little one yet the ability to send that child home with parents at the end of the day. Some grandparents carry dozens of photos, while others give their grandchildren gifts. Others may try to provide all the opportunities that they were unable to give their own children. No longer the sole provider of discipline, some grandparents feel that occasionally bending the rules should be allowed.

For others, grandchildren can be a challenge. The makeup of American families has changed. The U.S. Census Bureau reported that in 2000, 3.6% of U.S. households were identified as having grandparents in the home. Of those, 42% reported having primary responsibility for their grandchildren younger than age 18 (Simmons & Dye, 2003).

A grandchild may be a burden for some older adults, another child to raise, when they thought they were done with little ones (Ebert & Alemán, 2008). If economic times are difficult, grandchildren can bring more mouths to feed when budgets are already stretched. Although grandparents may love the little ones, they may not want to trade the stress of a full-time job for a new position as babysitter. For those adults who are serving as surrogate grandparents, the roles of parents and grandparents can be confused, leading to anger, frustration, and issues of responsibility for authority (Ebert & Alemán, 2008).

New Careers

As people age, they grow in different ways depending upon how their lives evolve. Some will spend their whole life in the same job or with the same company, enjoying the stability of working in one place for many years. Others may move around until they find a good fit with their personal goals.

Recent statistics indicate that the average American holds more than 10 jobs from ages 18 to 42 (U.S. Department of Labor, 2008).

For some, early retirement creates an opportunity to seek out a long-held passion. For example, a 50-year-old police officer, knowing she can retire after 25 years of working in law enforcement, might decide to return to nursing school as a second career.

For others, second careers will emerge that stem from individual interests. For example, a 58-year-old construction worker, knowing he has 30 years in with the union, can retire with a full pension. With 60% of his salary as his pension income, he can take a part-time position as a gardener, thus being able to combine his work and his favorite hobby. Examples like these illustrate the new wave of Baby Boomers who are changing the face of retirement as we know it. These older adults, born shortly after World War II, are healthier and better educated than their predecessors and are likely to pursue personal fulfillment through a second career (Brandon & Flury, 2009; Leach, Philipson, Beggs, & Money, 2008).

As longevity for older adults continues to extend to an average of 15 or more years after retirement (Federal Interagency Forum on Aging-Related Statistics, 2008), increasing numbers of people will choose to pursue second careers. Whether looking to fulfill a lifetime dream, pick up a few dollars while pursuing a much-loved pastime, or supplement pensions due to continued financial need, older Americans may look to put off a total break from the world of work (Leach et al., 2008).

As longevity continues to extend to an average of 15 or more years after retirement, increasing numbers of people will choose to pursue second careers, hobbies, continuing education, and volunteering.

As increasing numbers of older adults choose to stay employed after age 65; it will be important for employers to create workplaces that are conducive to employing older adults. From 2010 to 2030, the population of Americans who are age 65 and older is predicted to increase from 12% to 20% (AAGP, 2009; Vladeck, 2005). With the present generation of Baby Boomers now beginning to retire, and significantly fewer workers available to take their places, the ability to maintain the current workforce level may not be possible.

As older adults stay healthier and have less physically demanding jobs, incentives could help retain these individuals in the workforce. Creative strategies to reduce financial penalties for working while receiving retirement benefits and changing attitudes toward older workers can provide diversity and celebrate the expertise that comes with years of experience. Innovative methods of modifying the workplace to be more considerate of physical and cognitive limitations, and increased efforts to maintain and improve technological skills of aging employees, can keep more older adults in the workforce and foster healthy and productive lives (Gurria, 2008; Vladeck, 2005; Wolf, 2009).

Ongoing Education

For some aging people, the free time that comes when children marry or move out, or when they retire from a full-time job, can be frightening. Financial concerns, illness, and loss of social supports can lead to additional stress and strain coping responses (McDaniel, 2008). Knowing that they no longer have children or job duties to worry about can leave individuals with a sense of restlessness and nothing to do. This time, however, presents opportunities to grow and learn in different ways. As Baby Boomers begin to retire in record numbers, the need for lifelong learning and personal fulfillment will become exceedingly important (Wilson et al., 2006). Golf lessons at the local high school, quilting classes at the senior center, and cake decorating at the nearby arts and crafts store provide opportunities to learn new skills, meet new friends, and gain satisfaction from accomplishing a new goal.

Although these types of personal growth activities may be designed for adult learners, educational needs may also include new knowledge needed for a changing work environment, whether in a current position or in transferring to a new career (Gurria, 2008; Vladeck, 2005, Wolf, 2009). Opportunities for personal and professional development will need to be supported in the learning environment through creative strategies designed to address the needs of older adults. For those returning to the classroom after many years, current teaching methods may include technology such as PowerPoint lectures, downloaded class documents, and discussions in chat rooms. Especially for older adults seeking education through traditional classroom settings with young adults, teaching methods must be enhanced and modified to address the challenges of seniors who bring life experience to the discussion but may need additional support with new methods of instruction (Earle & Myrick, 2009; Wolf, 2009).

Hobbies

Ask anyone what they would do with a few extra hours a week, and there is a good chance that they would start a new hobby. One person might say she always wanted to learn quilting. Another might say, "One of these days I'm going to find time to play golf." Although these goals may seem ambitious, the free time afforded by retirement gives many people the opportunity to focus on new projects with renewed energy, changing the face of retirement as we have known it.

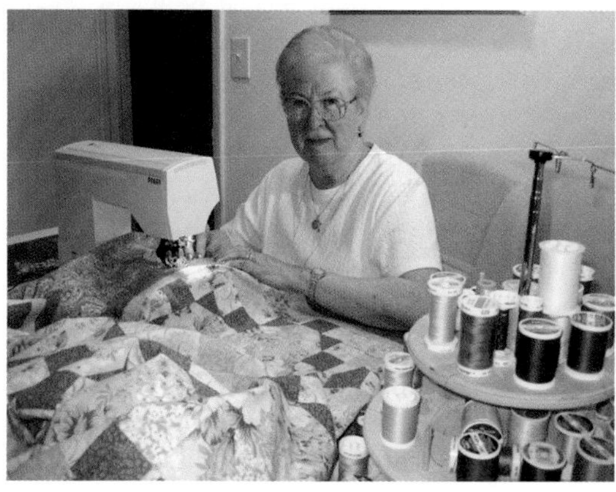

Many retirees have high expectations for their quality of life in their older years (Leach et al., 2008). The prospect of freedom from a set daily routine, where seniors can pursue different lifestyles and explore new activities in their leisure time, creates many opportunities for social engagement and contributions to the community.

Volunteering

Many people have a desire to volunteer for all types of organizations, but a full-time job and family responsibilities provide little free time. As situations change through the life stages, volunteering may once again be something that can bring great rewards.

The 2005 White House Conference on Aging identified five resolutions specifically related to civic and social engagement. Implementation strategies moving forward emphasized continued support for Senior Corps programs and national strategies to decrease barriers, promote meaningful volunteer activities, and encourage volunteerism in the workplace (O'Neill, 2006). As a group, older adults are a valuable resource for giving back to their communities.

Volunteering comes in many forms. Regardless of one's previous career, the possibilities are endless to share talents and skills with others. Data comparing volunteerism from 1995 to 2005 indicated that those in the first cohort of Baby Boomers, born from 1946 to 1955, volunteered more often than those born in previous years. Considering the numbers of older adults who will soon be retiring, the outlook for an increasing cadre of senior volunteers seems positive (Einolf, 2009). Recognizing the need to keep seniors involved in their communities, the 2006 Older Americans Act (H.B. 6197) reauthorized five additional years of community programs for older adults and called for the development of a comprehensive strategic plan for supporting older adults in civic engagement (O'Neill, 2006). As longevity of the American population increases, the role of older adults in promoting and creating new strategies for productive contributions to the community will become increasingly important (Rozario, 2007).

Travel

Some are lucky enough to get the opportunity to travel while they are young. Spending summers with grandparents or vacations with relatives at the beach can spark warm childhood memories. Frequent moves due to family business or the armed services can also bring people around the world. Once responsibilities end for working every day, caring for young children, or paying for college, the opportunity to travel for more than an overnight trip may become a possibility. Indeed, many seniors have become "snowbirds" who head south to warmer climates in the cold months. With increased longevity, health, and prosperity, it is becoming more likely to see older adults traveling for extended periods of time, once work is over and children have left the home (Leach et al., 2008).

Establishing a Legacy

As people age, they begin to realize that they will not live forever. For many, making a mark on the world or leaving something that will be remembered after they are gone is an important part of aging. The ability to impact the lives of others can be a goal that lives from one generation to the next (Hunter, 2008).

Often people feel that they want to be remembered for something they have accomplished. Sometimes, it is by providing service that brings honor and prestige while helping the community. Sometimes, it might be through establishing a philanthropic foundation. Whether passing on financial resources, donating collections of historical value, or building a successful business from the ground up, the desire to give part of ourselves to future generations is a meaningful way to contribute to society in our older years (Hunter, 2008).

For some, preserving family history may be the legacy that they wish to bestow upon future generations. Tracing family roots, building family trees, and creating albums filled with memorabilia can close the gap between generations. Classes on memoir writing, scrapbooking, and quilting are offered at many senior centers and community facilities to assist in preserving the past (Matthiessen, 2010). The ability to connect with our ancestors and leave a memento of our lives can be a lasting gift to future generations.

Spiritual Growth

The experience of religion and spiritual practices changes over time. As young children, we learn the cultural and spiritual values of our family, but as we move into young adulthood, sometimes these values become less important to us. Although some continue to practice their beliefs throughout life, for some, the hectic pace of life gets in the way. As we age, we often find that we have more time to consider our spiritual side. Spirituality can be an effective coping mechanism for the challenges of aging. Often, it provides a foundation for a positive viewpoint in the face of adversity. For many who seek a connection to their inner being, there is less fear of death, decreased stress, and a more positive attitude toward life challenges (Atchley, 2008).

As societal gathering places through the years, community services have often been provided in places of worship (Ellor, 2008). In the early 2000s, the White House Office of Faith-Based and Community Initiatives was founded to help support the work of congregations of all denominations to fill gaps in community services (Ellor, 2008).

Of particular interest to many health care providers is the practice of parish nursing that has been in existence since the 1970s (Redmond, 2006). Programs across the country, serving many religions and faiths, offer the opportunity for health care services and teaching provided in a faith-based setting. The ability to stay connected to spiritual practices and one's community of faith can be a source of great strength as we age.

Offering Wisdom

Throughout the history of many cultures, the elders were revered and turned to for advice and counsel. Although that is not always the perception in current times, some say that we learn from our elders' mistakes and gain strength from their wisdom. Although technology sometimes outpaces us as a source of knowledge, 60 or 70 years of making mistakes and learning from them is something we cannot deny. As we age, we continue to gather experience and hone our skills, thus increasing our expertise as we move on in years.

Conclusion

Maintaining physical and mental health in today's world is critical as the profile of aging Americans begins to change. The Federal Interagency Forum on Aging-Related Statistics (2008) reports that the older population is expected to grow to 71.5 million Americans, representing almost 20% of the U.S. population by 2030. The country is now beginning to see the changing characteristics depicted by the Baby Boom generation, born between 1946 and 1964. These seniors are more educated, are more culturally diverse, and have the highest rate of participation in the workforce in American history (Administration on Aging, 2008; Texas Nursing, 2006). In addition, the healthier status of today's older adults is a frequent topic in the literature. Although many older Americans have chronic health conditions, they are more physically fit and experience fewer functional limitations than their predecessors (Federal Interagency Forum on Aging-Related Statistics, 2008). Opportunities for second careers, ongoing education, travel, and healthy engagement in the community provide a new perspective on the future for retired adults. This changing profile of older Americans will require a health care work force that is more multilingual, increasingly culturally competent, better trained in geriatric best practices, and more creative in care delivery (Health Resources and Services Administration, 2006).

KEY POINTS

- By capitalizing on opportunities for older adults, the effect of some challenges can be minimized or delayed.

- Physiological changes and emotional health among both men and women can present challenges and decrease sexual desire.
- Because intimacy can be difficult to discuss, sexual health is an area that is often overlooked by health care providers caring for older adults.
- Physiological changes as we age may create functional, sensory, and cognitive changes that need to be addressed to maintain healthy well-being.
- For many, the biggest fear with getting old is not being able to take care of oneself, and living independently can become a challenge.
- As older adults live longer than previous generations, caregivers, whether they are spouses, children, or friends, may be aging themselves.
- Maintaining physical activity can preserve independence, and routine tasks such as cleaning and gardening can help preserve cognitive function and provide a sense of accomplishment.
- When individuals are cognitively impaired, tasks such as cooking may need to be simplified to provide a safe environment.
- Health care providers need to recognize that for many older adults, pets can provide companionship, elevate mood, and increase socialization.
- Involvement with groups and organizations can help people maintain overall health and functioning.
- Staying in touch with family, friends, and colleagues can be an important factor in promoting both physical and mental health.
- As adults live longer, it is not uncommon for seniors to become caregivers for their own elderly parents at the same time that they are beginning to struggle with the aging process.
- Community programs such as adult day centers can provide opportunities to maintain well-being and increase interaction with others, while also providing respite for caregivers.
- Fears of giving up independence can prevent older adults from asking for assistance when needed.
- Assessment of the living situation, environmental conditions, and available social supports must be incorporated into all health care visits for older adults.
- For many health care providers, loss is a difficult subject to discuss. Strategies to assist older adults with the grief process, such as bereavement counseling and widow's and widower's groups, can facilitate coping with loss.
- As the average life span increases, many older adults are concerned about outliving their financial resources.
- The transition to retirement can be a life-changing milestone, both an opportunity and a stressful challenge.
- For older adults serving as surrogate grandparents, the roles of parents and grandparents can be confused, leading to anger, frustration, and issues of responsibility for authority.
- As longevity for older adults continues to extend well past retirement, increasing numbers of people will chose to pursue second careers.
- Opportunities for personal and professional development will need to be supported in the learning environment through creative strategies designed to address the needs of older adults.
- The prospect of freedom from a set daily routine, where seniors can pursue different lifestyles and explore new activities in their leisure time, creates many opportunities for social engagement and contributions to the community.
- For many individuals, making a mark on the world, or leaving a legacy, is an important part of aging.
- As we age, we often find that we have more time to consider our spiritual side.
- Parish nurse programs, many of which have been in existence for over 30 years, can be good avenues to contact older adults through an already established community organization.

CRITICAL THINKING ACTIVITIES

1. Consider an older adult who is experiencing vision changes and has trouble reading the small print in the newspaper. Identify ways to assist this patient in taking six daily medications that come in individually labeled pill containers.
2. Think about one of your favorite high school teachers who may be approaching retirement age. What activities could you suggest that would keep him or her actively engaged in the senior years?
3. Call your local health department, or visit their website. Identify community resources for older adults that you can share with your patients.
4. Imagine yourself when you are approaching retirement. What legacy would you like to leave for your grandchildren, younger relatives, or community?
5. Reflect on your vision for older adults. If you could change one thing about the health care system, what would that be?

CASE STUDY | *MR. FRANK*

Mr. Frank, a 79-year-old music teacher, retired 10 years ago. Since leaving his full-time job, he has been teaching piano lessons at students' homes and maintaining his backyard garden. He was recently discharged after a below-the-knee amputation related to complications of diabetes and decreased perfusion. He currently lives with his elderly sister in the home where they both grew up.

When you arrive at his home, he is sleeping on the couch because his bedroom is on the second floor and he is afraid to climb the stairs. Although he has been fitted with a prosthetic leg and crutches, he has already fallen once trying to get up to his bedroom, and a second time trying to get to the bathroom, which is also on the second floor. His sister is concerned that he may fall again and that he seems to be "down in the dumps."

Before his surgery, Mr. Frank walked to the corner coffee shop every day to visit with friends and buy the daily newspaper. He has not seen his friends in several weeks, and misses reading the sports section now that it is baseball season. He frequently talks about his 15-year old dog, who died about 6 months ago.

1. What strategies should be considered to help maintain a safe home environment for Mr. Frank and his sister?
2. Identify opportunities for keeping Mr. Frank actively engaged while he is recuperating from his surgery.
3. Consider interventions to support the losses that Mr. Frank has recently experienced.
4. Describe the challenges that Mr. Frank's sister will be facing as a caregiver for her brother.

REFERENCES

Administration on Aging. (2008). *A profile of older Americans: 2008.* U.S. Department of Health and Human Services. Washington, DC. Retrieved March 27, 2011, from http://www.mowaa.org/Document.Doc?id=69

American Association for Geriatric Psychiatry (AAGP). (2009). *Geriatrics and mental health–The facts.* Retrieved November 3, 2010, from http://www.aagpgpa.org/prof/facts_mh.asp

Atchley, R. C. (2008). Spirituality, meaning, and the experience of aging. *Generations, 32*(2), 12-16.

Ballard, J. (2010). Forgetfulness and older adults: Concept analysis. *Journal of Advanced Nursing, 66*(6), 1409-1419.

Barak, Y., Wagenaar, R. C., & Holt, K. G. (2006). Gait characteristics of elderly people with a history of falls: A dynamic approach. *Physical Therapy, 86*(11), 1501-1510.

Barnes, I. (2006). Preventative maintenance for the brain. *Canadian Nursing Home,* 17(3), 15-17.

Beard, J. (2009, August 4). The financial crisis and the health of older people. *The Journal: AARP International,* 66.

Boyle, P. A., Buchman, A. S., Wilson, R. S., Bienias, J. L., & Bennett, D. A. (2007). Physical activity is associated with incident disability in community-based older persons. *Journal of the American Geriatrics Society, 55*(2), 195-201.

Brandon, B., & Flury, E. (2009). Aging with choice: Coping with a changing marketplace. *Long-Term Living, 58*(1), 14-18.

Carr, D. B., Flood, K. L., Steger-May, K., Schechtman, K. B., & Binder, E. F. (2006). Characteristics of frail older adult drivers. *Journal of the American Geriatrics Society, 54*(7), 1126-1129.

Cohen, G. D. (2006). *The creativity and aging study.* National Endowment for the Arts, Washington, DC. Retrieved November 3, 2010, from http://www.nea.gov/resources/accessibility/CnA-Rep4-30-06.pdf

Cohen, G. D., Perlstein, S., Chapline, J., Kelly, J., Firth, K. M., & Simmens, S. (2006). The impact of professionally conducted cultural programs on the physical health, mental health, and social functioning of older adults. *Gerontologist, 46*(6), 726-734.

Cook, J. A., & Hawkins, D. B. (2006). Hearing loss and hearing aid treatment options. *Mayo Clinic Proceedings, 81*(2), 234-237.

Craik, F. I., & Bialystok, E. (2006). Planning and task management in older adults: Cooking breakfast. *Memory and Cognition, 34*(6), 1236-1249.

DeLamater, J. D., & Sill, M. (2005). Sexual desire in later life. *Journal of Sex Research, 42*(2), 138-149.

Dillon, C. F., Gu, Q., Hoffman, H., & Ko, C. W. (2010). Vision, hearing, balance, and sensory impairment in Americans aged 70 years and over: United States, 1999-2006. NCHS Data Brief, no. 31. Hyattsville, MD: National Center for Health Statistics.

Earle, V., & Myrick, F. (2009). Nursing pedagogy and the intergenerational discourse. *Journal of Nursing Education, 48*(11), 624-630.

Ebert, L. A., & Alemán, M. W. (2008). Taking the grand out of grandparent: Dialectical tensions in grandparent perceptions of surrogate parenting. *Journal of Social and Personal Relationships, 25*(4), 671-695.

Einolf, C. J. (2009). Will the boomers volunteer during retirement? Comparing the baby boom, silent, and long civic cohorts. *Nonprofit and Voluntary Sector Quarterly, 38*(2), 181-199.

Ellor, J. W. (2008). The role of "faith-based" social services programs for older people. *Generations, 32*(2), 60-64.

Fagerström, C., Persson, H., Holst, G., & Hallberg, I. R. (2008). Determinants of feeling hindered by health problems in daily living at 60 years and above. *Scandinavian Journal of Caring Sciences, 22*(3), 410-421.

Federal Interagency Forum on Aging-Related Statistics. (2008). *Older Americans 2008: Key indicators of well-being.* Federal Interagency Forum on Aging-Related Statistics. Washington, DC: U.S. Government Printing Office.

Gurria, A. (2008). Living longer, working longer. AARP International. Retrieved March 27, 2011, from http://www.aarpinternational.org/resourcelibrary/resourcelibrary_show.htm?doc_id=727357

Health Resources and Services Administration (HRSA). (2006). *The impact of the aging population on the health workforce in the United States: Summary of key findings.* National Center for Health Workforce Analysis of the Bureau of Health Professions. Health Resources and Services Administration, Washington, DC. Grant number U79HP00001. Retrieved March 27, 2011, from http://www.albany.edu/news/pdf_files/impact_of_aging_excerpt.pdf

Holtslander, L. F. (2008). Caring for bereaved family caregivers: Analyzing the context of care. *Clinical Journal of Oncology Nursing, 12*(3), 501-506.

Hunter, E. G. (2008). Beyond death: Inheriting the past and giving to the future, transmitting the legacy of one's self. *OMEGA: Journal of Death and Dying, 56*(4), 313-329.

Kochkin, S. (2009). MarkeTrak VIII: 25-Year trends in the hearing health market. *The Hearing Review, 16*(11), 12-31.

Krause-Parello, C. A. (2008). The mediating effect of pet attachment support between loneliness and general health in older females living in the community. *Journal of Community Health Nursing, 25*(1), 1-14.

Leach, R., Philipson, C. Beggs, S., & Money, A. (2008). Sociological perspectives on the baby boomers: An exploration of social change. *Quality in Aging, 9*(4), 19-26.

Lindau, S. T., Schumm, P., Laumann, E. O., Levinson,W., O'Muircheartaigh, C. A., & Waite, L. J. (2007). A study of sexuality and health among older adults in the United States. *New England Journal of Medicine, 357*(8), 762-774.

Louria, D. B. (2005). Extraordinary longevity: Individual and societal issues. *Journal of the American Geriatrics Society, 53*(9), 317-319.

Masotti, P. J., Fick, R., Johnson-Masotti, A., & MacLeod, S. (2006).Community matters in healthy aging. Healthy naturally occurring retirement communities: A low-cost approach to facilitating healthy aging. *American Journal of Public Health, 96*(7), 1164-1170.

Matthiessen, C. (2010). *How to help an older adult create a lasting legacy.* Retrieved November 3, 2010, from http://www.caring.com/articles/lasting-legacy

McDaniel, J. G. (2008). "Normal" adult development and aging can also be stressful: Considering the case of retirement. *Journal of Gerontological Nursing, 34*(12), 3-4.

McColgan, G., & Schofield, I. (2007). The importance of companion animal relationships in the lives of older people. *Nursing Older People, 19*(1), 21-3.

Molzahn, A. E., Gallagher, E., & McNulty, V. (2009).Quality of life associated with adult day centers. *Journal of Gerontological Nursing, 35*(8), 37-46.

O'Neill, G. (2006). Civic engagement on the agenda at the 2005 White House Conference on Aging. *Generations, 30*(4), 95-100.

Padilha, D. M., Hugo, F. N., Hilgert, J. B., & Dal Moro, R. G. (2007). Hand function and oral hygiene in older institutionalized Brazilians. *Journal of the American Geriatrics Society, 55*(9), 1333-1338.

Park, S., Shoemaker, C. A., & Haub, M. D. (2009). Physical and psychological health conditions of older adults classified as gardeners or nongardeners. *Horticultural Science, 44*(1), 206-210.

Price, B. (2009). Exploring attitudes towards older people's sexuality. *Nursing Older People, 21*(6), 32-39.

Prosser, L., Townsend, M., & Staiger, P. (2008). Older people's relationships with companion animals: A pilot study. *Nursing Older People, 20*(3), 29-32.

Redmond, G. M. (2006). Developing programs for older adults in a faith community. *Journal of Psychosocial Nursing & Mental Health Services, 44*(11), 15-18.

Risley-Curtiss, C. (2010). Social work practitioners and the human-companion animal bond: A national study. *Social Work, 55*(1), 38-46.

Robb-Nicholson, C. (2010). Preserving and improving memory as we age. *Harvard Women's Health Watch, 17*(6), 1-3.

Rozario, P. A. (2007). Volunteering among current cohorts of older adults and baby boomers. *Generations, 30*(4), 31-36.

Shifren, J. L., Monz, B. U., Russo, P. A., Segreti, A., & Johannes, C. B. (2008). Sexual problems and distress in United States women: Prevalence and correlates. *Obstetrics & Gynecology, 112*(5), 970-978.

Simmons, T., & Dye, J. L. (2003). *Grandparents living with grandchildren: 2000.* U.S. Census Bureau. U.S. Department of Commerce, Washington DC. Retrieved March 27, 2011, from http://www.census.gov/prod/2003pubs/c2kbr-31.pdf

Skelton, D., & Dinan, S. (2007). Explaining about the benefits of active ageing. *Working With Older People, 11*(4), 10-14.

Social Security Online. (2009). *Retirement age: The full r etirement age is increasing.* Social Security Administration, Baltimore, MD. Retrieved March 27, 2011, from http://www.socialsecurity.gov/pubs/ageincrease.htm

Sorrell, J. M. (2008). As good as it gets? Rethinking old age. *Journal of Psychosocial Nursing and Mental Health Service, 46*(5), 21-25.

Sorrell, J. A., & Sorrell, J. M. (2008). Aging matters: Music as a healing art for older adults. *Journal of Psychosocial Nursing and Mental Health Service, 46*(3), 21-24.

Spires, R. A. (2006). How you can help when older eyes fail. *RN, 69*(2), 38-44.

Swann, J. (2006). Making gardening activities easier to manage. *Nursing & Residential Care, 8*(5), 215-218.

Texas Nursing. (2006). Aging population is redefining health care delivery. *Texas Nursing, 80*(6), 6-7, 12.

Thelander, V. B., Wahlin, T. R., Olofsson, L., Heikkila, K. A., & Sonde, L. (2008). Gardening activities for nursing home residents with dementia. *Advances in Physiotherapy, 10,* 53-56.

Thompsell, A. (2008). Recognizing depression in older adults in care homes. *Nursing & Residential Care, 10*(2), 95-97.

U.S. Department of Labor. (2008). *Number of jobs held, labor market activity, and earnings growth among the youngest baby boomers: Results from a longitudinal survey summary.* U.S. Department of Labor, Washington, DC. Retrieved from http://www.bls.gov/news.release/nlsoy.nr0.htm

Vladeck, B. C. (2005). Economic and policy implications of improving longevity. *Journal of the American Geriatrics Society, 53*(9), 304-307.

Williams, K. N., & Kemper, S. (2010). Interventions to reduce cognitive decline in aging. *Journal of Psychosocial Nursing and Mental Health Service, 48*(5), 42-51.

Wilson, L. B., Harlow-Rosentraub, K., Manning, T., Simson, S., & Steele, J. (2006). Civic engagement and lifelong learning. *Generations, 30*(4), 90-94.

Wolf, M. A. (2009). Older adult women learners in transition. *New Directions for Adult and Continuing Education, 122,* 53-62.

Chapter 5

An Evidence-Based Team Approach to Optimal Wellness

Jean W. Lange, PhD, RN, FAAN and Debbie Tolson, RGN, PhD, BSc, MSc

LEARNING OBJECTIVES

- Describe the environments in which health professionals deliver care to older adults.
- Identify sources of evidence-based, best practice guidelines.
- Discuss the nurse's role as a member of an interprofessional team.
- Explain how global and national population trends have impacted health care.
- Discuss the rationale for interprofessional teamwork.
- Identify international and national health care priorities for older adults.
- Compare the roles, educational requirements, and credentialing process of other health care professionals who participate on geriatric teams.
- Discuss how the Caledonian Development Model contributes to the development of evidence-based teamwork.

Environments of Care

Nurses care for older adults in community, residential, and inpatient settings. In your public health course, you may participate in a blood pressure screening or immunization clinic at a senior housing center or outpatient clinic. You may visit a recently discharged diabetic patient in his or her home to monitor healing of an amputated foot. Your hospital experiences will take you to inpatient medical and surgical units where older adults account for more hospital stays than any other age group and comprise more than 35% of the patients you will care for (Nagamine, Jiang, & Merrill, 2006). You may go to residential settings such as senior housing, assisted living, or skilled nursing facilities to learn interviewing, assessment, and interpersonal communication skills.

Nurses collaborate with other health professionals to care for older adults in a variety of residential settings as well as in hospital, rehabilitative, and outpatient environments (Table 5-1). In recent years, housing options for older adults have expanded to meet the needs and preferences of this growing population. Although most older adults live independently, they may transition to settings where care is more accessible as their circumstances change or an illness requires more specialized care (Figure 5-1). For example, maintaining a private residence can be a significant burden that motivates an older adult to seek less demanding accommodations. Older adults typically seek alternative living arrangements for reasons of safety, socialization, proximity to family members, or the need for services such as transportation, meal preparation, or assistance with personal care.

Living at Home

A variety of short- and long-term options provide incremental levels of service depending on an older adult's needs. Seventy percent of Americans over age 65 choose to remain in privately owned, single-family homes (Fig. 5-2) (Administration on Aging, 2008). The phrase *aging in place* is often used to describe this increasing trend. Community-based home-care services such as meal delivery and home health caregivers can support an older person's decision to remain at home.

TABLE 5-1 Environments of Care

Community settings	Independent living (senior housing, private homes) Community clinics Health care provider offices Adult day care centers
Residential settings	
Short term	Mental health rehabilitation centers (psychiatric, substance abuse) Convalescent/physical rehabilitation centers
Long term	Skilled nursing facilities Assisted-living centers
Inpatient settings	Hospitals Veterans Administration Medical Centers

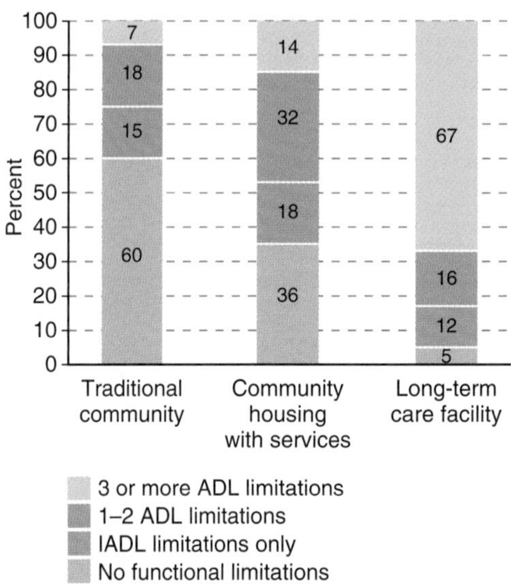

Note: Community housing refers to retirement communities or apartments, senior housing, continued care retirement facilities, assisted living facilities, housecleaning, laundry service, or help with medications. Respondents in settings were asked about the availability of services but not whether they used the services. Long-term care facility refers to a licensed, multi-bed facility certified by Medicare or Medicaid that offers personal care (activities of daily living [ADLs] or instrumental ADLs [IADLs]) or 24-hour supervision.
Source: Centers for Medicare and Medicaid Services, Medicare Current Beneficiary Survey.

Figure 5-1 *(Reprinted from Federal Interagency Forum on Aging-Related Statistics. (2008) Older Americans 2008: Key indicators of well-being. Washington, DC: U.S. Government Printing Office. Retrieved December 3, 2010, from http://www.agingstats.gov/agingstatsdotnet/Main_Site/Data/2010_Documents/Docs/OA_2010.pdf)*

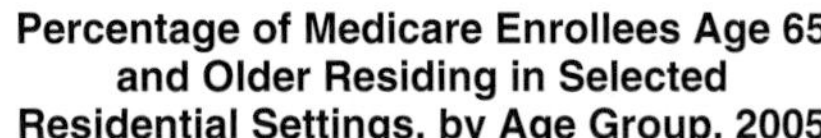

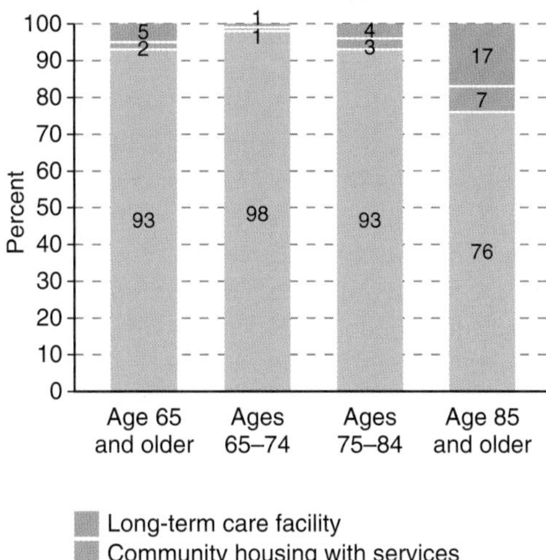

Note: Community housing refers to retirement communities or apartments, senior housing, continued care retirement facilities, assisted living facilities, housecleaning, laundry service, or help with medications. Respondents in settings were asked about the availability of services but not whether they used the services. Long-term care facility refers to a licensed, multi-bed facility certified by Medicare or Medicaid that offers personal care (activities of daily living [ADLs] or instrumental ADLs [IADLs]) or 24-hour supervision. Source: Centers for Medicare and Medicaid Services, Medicare Current Beneficiary Survey.

Figure 5-2 *(Reprinted from Federal Interagency Forum on Aging-Related Statistics. Older Americans 2010: Key indicators of well-being. Washington, DC: U.S. Government Printing Office. Retrieved March 22, 2011, from http://www.agingstats.gov/agingstatsdotnet/Main_Site/Data/2010_Documents/Docs/OA_2010.pdf)*

Housing Communities Designed for Independent Living

Senior or elderly housing offers independent living in a retirement community that reduces the burden of private home maintenance. Independent senior housing communities may also provide opportunities for socialization through planned activities, access to public transportation, and meal or housekeeping services. Residents who need additional assistance with daily tasks such as bathing or dressing can access outside services to supplement those provided by the housing community. Senior housing may be owned or rented. Government subsidized housing provides an option for older adults with lower incomes.

Continuing care retirement communities (commonly called CCRCs, life care communities, or active-adult communities) typically target younger, active adults who are at or above a minimum age (usually between ages 55 and 65). They often include an array of recreational facilities, such as swimming pools, tennis courts, and fitness centers. Residents of continuing care retirement communities usually must sign a contract and include the option to transition into affiliated or on-site assisted living or skilled nursing care facilities if necessary.

Community Options for Adults With Care Needs

Assisted-living centers (also called adult care facilities, adult residential care, or enhanced living) may be owned or rented. Living quarters may be in private units or rented rooms that generally include additional service options, such as assistance with personal care, medication supervision, group meals, laundry, and on site health care personnel trained to handle emergencies or adverse events. Group homes (adult homes) where residents share common areas but have private bedrooms offer similar services. State regulations mandate the level of skilled care that can be provided at assisted-living sites; however, regular care of a licensed nurse is generally not an option in assisted-living settings.

If a person's care needs exceed the state guidelines for assisted living, the older adult must seek alternative care, typically in the home of a relative who assumes a caregiver role, or in a facility where 24-hour nursing care is provided. Less than 5% of people over age 65 reside in skilled nursing facilities; however, this percentage increases to 25% to 30% of those 85 years of age and older (Administration on Aging, 2008). Many skilled nursing facilities (commonly known as SNFs, also called nursing homes or long-term care facilities) provide short-term and long-term services. Short-term services include physical, occupational, and speech rehabilitation and convalescence after hospitalization. Long-term services provide custodial care to residents on a permanent basis. Skilled nursing facilities also may have specialty units designed to safely care for patients with dementia in a "least restrictive" environment or for patients with more advanced care needs, such as ventilator dependence or hospice. Nurses and other health professionals help older adults maintain an optimal quality of life across all environments of care.

The Value of Collaborative Care

During the course of our lives, most of us seek health care from a variety of professionals. You may have started seeing a dentist or hygienist during childhood, attended peer luncheon sessions led by your school psychologist, recall visits to a pediatrician for immunizations, or seen a surgeon to remove an inflamed appendix. Perhaps you played sports and received training by an exercise physiologist or had an injury requiring physical therapy during your recovery. A multitude of health care professionals contribute in unique ways to the physical, social, financial, and psychological aspects of our well-being throughout our lives. Often, we are not aware of the services some disciplines can provide until we find ourselves in need or another provider makes a referral.

Whose responsibility is it to recognize and address these needs? Is this a realistic expectation of a nurse? Do we have sufficient knowledge about our patients to recognize that an unmet need requires the help of another discipline? Do we have the authority to make a referral that may help to improve the health outcomes of a particular patient?

Nurses have a central role in patient care and, in this role, have an opportunity to understand the patient's health in the broader context in which he or she lives. Nurses gather information from patients about many aspects of their lives, such as diet and exercise patterns, living and work environments, spiritual concerns, relationships, financial resources, physical and psychological health, cultural beliefs and values, hobbies, and language preferences. Knowing where patients live, their health-related beliefs and practices, and what resources are available to them gives the nurse insight about whether a newly released but expensive medication is affordable for that patient. Understanding that a patient who comes to the clinic to check his cholesterol level just lost his wife of 45 years may suggest to you that this person could have psychosocial, as well as physical, needs. Clearly, nurses view patients from a broad or holistic perspective and gather information that may reveal patient needs that go beyond physical complaints.

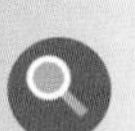

EVIDENCE FOR PRACTICE
Multidisciplinary Case Management

Purpose: To evaluate the effect of a multidisciplinary case management model used in a rural primary health care practice on hospital admission rates among vulnerable older adults.

Sample: Fifty-nine patients aged 75 and over were identified as meeting the criteria for vulnerability (two or more emergency room visits or hospital admissions; high need for social services; caregiver dependent; history of falling; poorly controlled chronic condition). Patients' mean age was 84 and ranged from 57 to 99 years old.

Methods: Researchers met with 34 practice partners to describe the study and elicit participation. A checklist, reviewed during regular team meetings, documented actions and progress of each vulnerable patient in the study. Team members included physicians, community psychiatric nurses, social workers, pharmacists, physiotherapists, nurses, and case managers.

Results: Sixteen of 34 practice teams agreed to participate. During the first year, 17 emergency admissions were avoided in 13 of the participants by team interventions such as additional social support, home rehabilitation post falls, and improved monitoring of diabetes. During the 3-year period, 17 participants (29%) died, 11 were transferred to long-term care, and 39 (66%) were admitted to the hospital (4 of these twice and 7 more than twice).

Implications: The team meeting/checklist approach reduced emergency room visits and facilitated team member understanding about the availability of services provided by other disciplines. Partnerships with an administratively designated champion were able to hold team meetings more consistently. Barriers to implementation included allocating time for meetings at the expense of seeing additional patients, lack of administrative support, difficulty coordinating meeting times among team members, and lack of participation by some of the primary care physicians.

Reference: Graffy, J., Grande, M., & Campbell, J. (2008). Case management for elderly patients at risk of hospital admission: A team approach. *Primary Health Care Research & Development, 9,* 7-13.

The Nurses' Role on Interprofessional Teams

Nurses have the knowledge needed to recognize unmet needs. Now, what is the role of nurses in addressing those needs? The International Council of Nurses proclaims in *The ICN Code of Ethics for Nurses* (2006) that working in cooperative relationships with other disciplines is a primary responsibility of the nurse. The Social Policy Statement of the American Nurses Association (ANA) further states that registered nurses not only cooperate with other disciplines but also hold a leadership role in organizing, delivering, and advocating for beneficial patient care (ANA, 2003). Both of these documents define on international and national levels what the public can expect of a nurse, including what we do in the context of our relationship with society at large and our obligation to the recipients of our care. The beneficial impact that a coordinated team approach can have on patient outcomes is also recognized outside of the nursing discipline. The World Health Organization (WHO), a global leader in defining international priorities for health care, submits that coordinating referral systems, community networks, and resources is not only necessary but foundational to the effective management of disease (WHO, 2007a).

Clearly, nurses must collaborate with other health disciplines to deliver the quality of care promised by our profession. A nurse who suspects that a patient is not eating or taking his medications because of depression has an obligation to share this knowledge with other members of the health care team and to recommend appropriate referrals. In this case, one or more disciplines might be appropriate, such as a dietitian, pharmacist, mental health professional, and physician. Adequately addressing patients' needs often involves teaming with an array of professionals such as social workers, physical therapists, physician specialists, podiatrists, and home-care providers. Collaboration also involves communicating with allied health professionals (e.g., nursing assistants, technicians) and nonmedical healers with whom the patient may consult, as well as with the patient and his or her significant others.

The Consequences of Fragmented Care

Unfortunately, the current U.S. system has failed to coordinate its health care services in a way that produces cost-effective, quality outcomes. At the end of a comprehensive study, the Institute of Medicine (2000) concluded that U.S. health care is fragmented and poorly organized. They reported that "the delivery of care often is overly complex and uncoordinated, requiring unnecessary steps and patient 'handoffs' that slow down care and de-crease rather than improve safety" (Institute of Medicine, 2001, p. 1). This lack of coordination increases health care costs and contributes to poorer patient outcomes by wasting resources and creating gaps in coverage, as well as loss of information. One reason cited for this inefficiency is that our current health care system "fails to build on the strengths of all health professionals involved to ensure that care is appropriate, timely, and safe" (Institute of Medicine, 2001, p.1). The consequences of fragmented care include an estimated 44,000 to 98,000 deaths in the United States annually from medical errors (Institute of Medicine, 2000; Thomas et al., 2000; Thomas et al., 1999), failure to provide care according to established standards (Institute of Medicine, 2003c; McGlynn et al., 2003), and longer hospital stays that cost more than $2 billion each year (Institute of Medicine, 2000, 2003a; Bates et al., 1997) (Table 5-2).

To remedy the problem, the Institute of Medicine (2003b) challenged health professionals to change current practice from multidisciplinary professionals working in isolation of one another to collaborating together on interprofessional teams. Interprofessional teams define patient-centered goals and make collective decisions about treatment. The patient and significant others are members of this team and must have a central voice in determining the treatment plan. The Institute of Medicine predicted that working collaboratively in patient-centered teams would improve communication and care coordination, reduce complications, and lead to safer care and better patient outcomes (Barnsteiner, Disch, Hall, Mayer, & Moore, 2007). In support of this prediction, numerous studies have documented the positive results that occur when health professionals use a collaborative care model. The positive outcomes realized in some of these studies are listed in Table 5-3 and illustrated in the United Kingdom Model of Interprofessional Teamwork discussed later in this chapter.

TABLE 5-2 Adverse Patient Outcomes Resulting from Fragmented and Uncoordinated Care

Institute of Medicine, 2000 Thomas et al., 1999 Thomas et al., 2000	Between 44,000 and 98,000 Americans die from medical errors annually.
McGlynn et al., 2003	Only 55% of patients in a recent random sample of adults received recommended care, with little difference found between care recommended for prevention, treatment of acute episodes, or treatment of chronic conditions.
Bates et al., 1997 Institute of Medicine, 2000	Medication-related errors for hospitalized patients cost roughly $2 billion annually.
Institute of Medicine, 2002 Institute of Medicine, 2003a	41 million uninsured Americans have consistently worse clinical outcomes than the insured and are at increased risk for dying.
Balas, 2001 Institute of Medicine, 2003b	The lag between discovery of more effective forms of treatment and their incorporation into routine patient care averages 17 years.
Chassin, 1997 Institute of Medicine, 2003a	18,000 Americans die each year from myocardial infarction because they did not receive preventive medications, although they were eligible for them.
Centers for Disease Control and Prevention, 1999 Institute of Medicine, 2000	Medical errors kill more people per year than breast cancer, AIDS, or motor vehicle accidents.
Clark et al., 2000 Institute of Medicine, 2003c Legorreta, Liu, Zaher, & Jatulis, 2000 McBride, Schrott, Plane, Underbakke, & Brown, 1998 Ni, Nauman, & Hershberger, 1998 Perez-Stable & Fuentes-Afflick, 1998 Samsa et al., 2000 Young, Klap, Sherbourne, & Wells, 2001	More than 50% of patients with diabetes, hypertension, tobacco addiction, hyperlipidemia, congestive heart failure, asthma, depression, or chronic atrial fibrillation are currently managed inadequately.

Reprinted with permission from Institute of Medicine. (2006). *The chasm in quality: Select indicators from recent reports.* Washington, DC: The National Academies Press, National Academy of Sciences.

TABLE 5-3 Evidence of Benefits of Teamwork on Patient Outcomes

Graffy, Grande, & Campbell, 2008	A multidisciplinary case management approach including identification of high-risk elderly clinic patients reduced hospitalization rates among 973 British participants, and improved coordination of services and communication among team members.
Masanori, Jun, Toshio, & Yoshinori, 2007	Rehospitalization rates among Japanese older adults with heart failure were significantly lower using a multidisciplinary management model versus traditional care. Readmission rates were 21% in 100 days in the team-managed group ($n = 66$) versus 41% in the traditional care group ($n = 112$; $p < .01$). In 30 days, readmission rates were 1.5% for the team-care group versus 17% in the traditional care group ($p < .05$).
Krishnan, Nash, Baker, Fowler, & Rayman, 2007	After introduction of a multidisciplinary foot team, incidence of amputations among more than 11,000 diabetic patients declined by 70% to 82% over an 11-year period.
Lingard et al., 2008	After implementation of checklist-guided preoperative team debriefing meetings among Canadian surgical staff, the number of communication failures per procedure declined by nearly 400%. Unanticipated problems were identified or resolved in more than 33% of 172 case observations.
von Renteln-Kruse & Krause, 2007	After instituting a team-based fall-prevention program including assessment; risk alert; supervision and transfer assistance; patient, caregiver, and staff education; and use of sensory and mobility aids when appropriate, the fall rate of inpatients over age 80 ($n = 2{,}982$) decreased by nearly half compared the rate before the fall program began ($n = 4{,}272$).
Harari, Martin, Buttery, O'Neill, & Hopper, 2007	Conducting a multidisciplinary comprehensive geriatric screening to assess newly hospitalized patients over age 70 resulted in better identification and management of common problems, such as fall risk, delirium, chronic pain, constipation, and urinary incontinence. In-hospital transfers of high-risk patients to specialized units decreased the average length of stay 4 days. Outpatient referrals for follow-up after discharge more than doubled.
Darroch, 2007	Multidisciplinary Community Older People's Team assessments facilitated comprehensive problem identification and rapid intervention among home-dwelling adults over age 65, reducing hospitalization and unnecessary admission to long-term care. Dietary intervention with 25 at-risk participants averaging age 82 resulted in weight gain and improved risk scores in more than half of the sample.
Cummings, 2009	Treatment of 69 community-dwelling older adults with severe mental disorders by a specialized interprofessional geriatric mental health team resulted in decreased symptoms of depression and inpatient psychiatric hospitalization. Participant life satisfaction also increased significantly after 6 months of treatment.

Nursing Standards of Care

To accomplish the necessary transformation of the U.S. health care system, the Institute of Medicine's Committee on Quality of Health Care in America advised that change begin by educating students to "work in interprofessional teams that cooperate, collaborate, communicate, and integrate care that is continuous and reliable" (Institute of Medicine, 2000). The American Association of Colleges of Nursing (AACN, 2008) underscored nursing's critical role on health care teams in its document, *The Essentials of Baccalaureate Nursing Education.* The nine essentials will be used by schools of nursing across the country to shape curricula. The document explains the key position of the nurse as "the human link between the patient and the complex health care environment" and emphasizes that "future [nurse] clinicians [must] deliver patient centered care as members of an interprofessional team" (p. 22).

A second document, *Recommended Baccalaureate Competencies and Curricular Guidelines for the Nursing Care of Older Adults,* holds educators as well as practicing nurses accountable for having the necessary information and skills to competently and collaboratively care for older adults (AACN & John A. Hartford Foundation Institute for Geriatric Nursing, 2010) (Table 5-4).

Bridging the Evidence-to-Practice Gap

Keeping up to date about best practices in the care of older adults enables nurses to proactively plan care that can reduce patients' risk for developing diseases, complications, and injuries (AACN, 2008). Nursing knowledge provides a foundation for decision making that directly impacts patients' recovery. The National Quality Forum (NQF) and the ANA identified numerous patient outcomes that are affected by the quality of nursing care received. Many of these outcomes reflect problems more common among older adults such as falls, pressure ulcers, use of restraints, infections acquired as a result of hospitalization (nosocomial infections), urinary catheter-associated bladder infections, and ventilator-associated pneumonias (Kurtzman & Corrigan, 2007). Using current evidence to guide practice involves collaborating with other members of the health team and the patient to produce the best possible result.

Research provides the evidence to support changes in practice. Keeping abreast of new information in gerontology, however, can be a challenge because our graying population has led to a proliferation of aging research. Historically, the application of new knowledge to practice has taken far too long, in part because nurses do not feel that they have the time to keep abreast of new developments in the literature or that they lack the confidence to competently interpret research reports (Melnyk, Fineout-Overholt, Feinstein, Sadler, & Green-Hernandez, 2008). The consequence of not keeping abreast of new developments means that nurses risk applying yesterday's solutions to today's problems. In recognition of the need to expedite translation of new evidence into practice, foundations such as the John A. Hartford Institute for Geriatric Nursing (http://hartfordign.org/) and federally funded Geriatric Education Centers (http://www.pogoe.org) have attempted to bridge this gap by providing free online access to excellent resources about the latest evidence in caring for older adults. ConsultGeriRN (http://consultgerirn.org/), sponsored by the Hartford Institute for Geriatric Nursing, provides current information regarding common topics in aging. The Nurses Improving Care for Healthsystem Elders (http://www.nicheprogram.org/) is a model for hospital care developed by the Hartford Institute for Geriatric Nursing that provides the necessary resources for nurses to achieve patient-centered care for older adults.

Original studies related to aging research are published in numerous journals such as *Geriatric Nursing* and the *Journal of Gerontological Nursing.* A list of more than 140 journals dedicated to aging topics can be found on the website of the University of North Carolina's Institute on Aging (http://www.uncioa.org/agelib/journalslist.asp). Other credible resources that review the literature about a wide variety of health care topics include the Cochrane Library, the National Guideline Clearinghouse, the Agency for Healthcare Research and Quality, and the Joanna Briggs Institute. Nursing journals such as *Evidence-Based Nursing, Worldviews on Evidence-Based Nursing,* and *Online Journal of Knowledge Synthesis for Nursing* also publish reviews on a wide variety of health care topics.

Over the past three decades, a growing body of knowledge surrounding the unique needs of older adults has led to geriatric nursing as a specialty area with its own scope of practice and performance standards (ANA, 2001). Nurses can become certified in geriatric nursing by successfully completing an examination through the American Nurses

TABLE 5-4 Gerontological Nursing Competency Statements

1	Incorporate professional attitudes, values, and expectations about physical and mental aging in the provision of patient-centered care for older adults and their families.
2	Assess barriers for older adults in receiving, understanding, and giving of information.
3	Use valid and reliable assessment tools to guide nursing practice for older adults.
4	Assess the living environment as it relates to functional, physical, cognitive, psychological, and social needs of older adults.
5	Intervene to assist older adults and their support network to achieve personal goals, based on the analysis of the living environment and availability of community resources.
6	Identify actual or potential mistreatment (physical, mental, or financial abuse, and/or self-neglect) in older adults and refer appropriately.
7	Implement strategies and use online guidelines to prevent and/or identify and manage geriatric syndromes.
8	Recognize and respect the variations of care, the increased complexity, and the increased use of health care resources inherent in caring for older adults.
9	Recognize the complex interaction of acute and chronic comorbid physical and mental conditions and associated treatments common to older adults.
10	Compare models of care that promote safe, quality physical and mental health care for older adults such as PACE, NICHE, Guided Care, Culture Change, and Transitional Care Models.
11	Facilitate ethical, noncoercive decision making by older adults and/or families/caregivers for maintaining everyday living, receiving treatment, initiating advance directives, and implementing end-of-life care.
12	Promote adherence to the evidence-based practice of providing restraint-free care (both physical and chemical restraints).
13	Integrate leadership and communication techniques that foster discussion and reflection on the extent to which diversity (among nurses, nurse assistive personnel, therapists, physicians, and patients) has the potential to impact the care of older adults.
14	Facilitate safe and effective transitions across levels of care, including acute, community-based, and long-term care (e.g., home, assisted living, hospice, nursing homes) for older adults and their families.
15	Plan patient-centered care with consideration for mental and physical health and well-being of informal and formal caregivers of older adults.
16	Advocate for timely and appropriate palliative and hospice care for older adults with physical and cognitive impairments.
17	Implement and monitor strategies to prevent risk and promote quality and safety (e.g., falls, medication mismanagement, pressure ulcers) in the nursing care of older adults with physical and cognitive needs.
18	Utilize resources/programs to promote functional, physical, and mental wellness in older adults.
19	Integrate relevant theories and concepts included in a liberal education into the delivery of patient-centered care for older adults.

From American Association of Colleges of Nursing & The Hartford Institute for Geriatric Nursing at New York University. (2010). *Recommended baccalaureate competencies and curricular guidelines for the nursing care of older adults.* Retrieved January 10, 2011, from http://www.aacn.nche.edu/education/pdf/AACN_Gerocompetencies.pdf

Credentialing Center. Certification is available at basic and advanced practice levels.

The Nurse as Coordinator of Care

Future nurses will likely spend a great deal of their time serving on gerontology-focused teams because, with advances in technology and treatment options, individuals with chronic diseases are living longer. Older adult are also the fastest growing segment of our population (He, Sengupta, Velkoff, & DeBarros, 2005). In fact, the number of adults living past age 85 is expected to double by the year 2030 and account for about 20 percent of U.S. residents (Federal Interagency Forum on Age-Related Statistics, 2008). Our aging population challenges nurses to better understand how to promote wellness, maximize independence, and help individuals successfully manage coexisting health problems (comorbidities). Most older people have at least one chronic condition, and many have multiple conditions (Administration on Aging, 2008). It is not surprising, therefore that people over age 65 tend to have more health care needs and spend, on average, nearly four times as many days in the hospital as do younger people (Nagamine, Jiang, & Merrill, 2006). Complex needs often require the coordination of several disciplines.

The value of nursing involvement in coordinating team efforts is well recognized (Institute of Medicine, 2003b). Nursing's contributions include a holistic patient perspective and expertise in interpersonal communication, translating evidence into practice, quality improvement approaches, and informatics (AACN, 2008). Realizing nursing's capacity to positively influence care outcomes, Robert Woods Johnson funded the Quality and Safety Education for Nurses (QSEN) initiative. The goal of the project is "to address the challenge of preparing future nurses with the knowledge, skills and attitudes necessary to continuously improve the quality and safety of the health care systems in which they work in six key areas: patient-centered care, teamwork and collaboration, evidence-based practice, quality improvement, informatics, and safety (QSEN, 2010). This initiative provides resources for nurse educators and students to learn how to provide patient-centered care and to be effective collaborators on the health care team (Cronenwett et al., 2007).

Roles of Interprofessional Team Members

Effective team collaboration requires understanding the roles and potential contributions of other team members. Knowing who does what helps nurses decide when another discipline can help to address a patient's needs. For example, let's suppose that your 85-year-old patient, Mrs. Altman, was admitted for repair of a hip fracture. During surgery, Mrs. Altman had a stroke (cerebrovascular accident). As a result, she requires help with feeding, bathing, and dressing herself. Before this hospitalization, Mrs. Altman lived alone. The initial treatment plan is to send Mrs. Altman to a rehabilitation center, but the patient is not expected to fully regain her previous level of functioning. The family is unable to assume her care, and they ask you to help them find a place where their mother can go after she leaves the rehabilitation center. Questions about needed services, patient and family resources, care options, and patient and family preferences all need to be answered.

How do you determine who is best qualified to assist you in responding to the family's request? Looking at Table 5-5, with what disciplines would you choose to collaborate? You would probably want to invite several individuals to a team meeting, including the physician who is her medical provider, a social worker who can inform the family about placement options, a case manager who can explain what services are covered through the patient's insurance plan, and perhaps an elder law attorney who can help the family explore financing long-term care costs beyond what Mrs. Altman's insurance will cover. Interprofessional teams work collaboratively to address complex problems that require the varied expertise of several disciplines. Effective teamwork depends on the ability of members to "establish shared and explicit goals, and work collaboratively to define and treat patient problems" (Drinka & Clark, 2000, p. 7).

Geriatric team members typically include

- The primary care provider (physician or nurse practitioner)
- Nurse
- Social worker
- Case manager
- Psychologist
- Pharmacist

Additional members may include a physical therapist, an occupational therapist, a dietitian, a dentist, and a chiropractor, as well as an elder law specialist, community advocate, and spiritual leader (Long & Wilson, 2001). The patient and significant others are key members of all patient-centered

TABLE 5-5 Interprofessional Scope of Practice, Education, and Licensure

DISCIPLINE	PRACTICE ROLES/SKILLS	EDUCATION/TRAINING	LICENSURE/CREDENTIALS
Nurse	LVN uses basic nursing skills as dictated by the facility and under the supervision of an RN	1 year of training	Exam required for licensing CEUs required in some states
	RN (AD, BS, or higher) has increased scope of practice, including planning for optimal functioning, coordination of care, teaching, and direct and indirect patient care	*RN with AD*—2 years of training, usually in a community college *RN with BS degree*—4 years in college	Must pass national licensure exam CEUs required annually in some states
Nurse Practitioner (NP)	Health assessment, health promotion, histories and physicals in outpatient and acute/home/long-term care settings Orders, conducts, and interprets lab and diagnostic tests Prescribes medications, teaching and counseling	Masters degree with a defined specialty area such as gerontology (GPN) or a post-master's certificate program	RN licensure required National certification exam in desired specialty area (e.g., gerontology, family practice)
Physician	Diagnoses and treats diseases and injuries Provides preventive care Does routine checkups Prescribes drugs Performs some surgery	Medical school (4 years) Additional 3 to 7 years of graduate medical education	State licensure and exam required for MD degree Possible exam required for specialty areas CEU requirements
Geriatrician	Physician with special training in diagnosis, treatment, and prevention of disorders in older people Recognizes aging as a normal process and not a disease	Medical school Residency training in family medicine and internal medicine 1-year fellowship program in geriatric medicine	Physician licensure required Completion of fellowship training program and/or exam for Certificate of Added Qualifications in Geriatric Medicine (CAQ) Recertification by examination required every 6 years

Continued

TABLE 5-5 Interprofessional Scope of Practice, Education, and Licensure—cont'd

DISCIPLINE	PRACTICE ROLES/SKILLS	EDUCATION/TRAINING	LICENSURE/CREDENTIALS
Physician Assistant (PA)	Practices medicine under supervision of licensed physician Exercises autonomy in medical decision making Provides a broad range of diagnostic and therapeutic services Practice is centered on patient care	Specially designed 2-year PA program located at medical colleges and universities Most have bachelor's degree and more than 4 years' health care experience before entering PA program	State licensure or registration Certification by national association (NCCPA) Recertification every 6 years by examination 100 CEUs every 2 years
Social worker	Assesses individual and family psychosocial functioning Provides care to help enhance or restore capacities, possibly including locating services or providing counseling	4-year college degree (for BSW), 2 years of graduate work (for MSW), and doctoral degree (PhD)	LMSW for master's level LSW for BS level SWA (social work associate) for combination of education and experience ACP signifies licensure for independent clinical practice 15 hours continuing education required every year
Case manager	Typically works for a hospital or third-party payor Collaborates with other disciplines to determine need for services and monitor their delivery in a cost-effective manner	Nurses, social workers, and sometimes occupational therapists function in this role	See requirements for each discipline
Psychologist	Assesses, treats, and manages mental disorders Does psychotherapy with individuals, groups, and families	5 years graduate training beyond undergraduate work Most coursework includes gerontology and clinical experience	PhD, EdD, and PsyD are degrees awarded State licensure American Psychological Association has ethics codes, as do most states
Psychiatrist	Treats mental, emotional, and behavioral symptoms	Medical school and residency specializing in psychiatry Residency, including both general residency and 2 to 3 years in specialty area (e.g., geriatrics, pediatrics)	State exam to practice medicine Board of Psychiatry and Neurology offers exam for diplomate in psychiatry

TABLE 5-5 Interprofessional Scope of Practice, Education, and Licensure—cont'd

DISCIPLINE	PRACTICE ROLES/SKILLS	EDUCATION/TRAINING	LICENSURE/CREDENTIALS
Pharmacist	Devises and revises medication therapy to achieve optimal regimen for patient's medical and therapeutic needs Provides information resource for patient and medical team	B.S. 5-year program or doctorate degree (PharmD)	National exam (NABPLEX) given every quarter Board certifications in specialties available (pharmacotherapy, nuclear pharmacy, nutrition, psychiatry and oncology in near future) Annual CEUs required from 10 to 15 hours
Speech-language pathologist	Assesses and treats full range of speech, language, and swallowing disorders Functions in ambulatory or inpatient clinical settings Provides individual or group therapy to maximize functional communication and swallowing ability	Masters degree Completion of 9-month CFY post-MA/MS required to practice nationwide	CCC in speech language pathology awarded by American Speech Language Hearing Association after completion of national exam (NESPA) and CFY State licensure required in 45 states Annual CEUs required
Audiologist	Identifies, assesses, and manages auditory and balance disorders Provides audiological rehabilitation with selection, fitting, and management of devices	Masters degree Completion of 9-month CFY post-MA/MS required to practice nationwide	CCC in audiology awarded by American Speech Language Hearing Association after completion of national exam (NESPA) and CFY State licensure required in 47 states
Occupational therapist (OT)	Uses therapeutic goal-directed activities to evaluate, prevent, or correct physical, mental, or emotional dysfunction or to maximize function in the life of the individual	BS or MS in occupational therapy with minimum of 6 months field work For OT assistant, an AD or OT assistant certificate with minimum of 2 months field work	For OTR or COTA, national certification exam required 36 PDUs required every 3 years
Physical therapist	Evaluates, examines, and uses exercises, rehabilitative procedures, massage,	Entry-level graduate degree (master's or doctorate) in physical therapy	For PT or PTA state exam required CEU requirements vary state by state

Continued

TABLE 5-5 Interprofessional Scope of Practice, Education, and Licensure—cont'd

DISCIPLINE	PRACTICE ROLES/SKILLS	EDUCATION/TRAINING	LICENSURE/CREDENTIALS
	manipulations, and physical agents including, but not limited to, mechanical devices, heat, cold, air, light, water, electricity, and sound in the aid of diagnosis or treatment		
Chaplain	Provide visits and ministry to patients and family	Masters degree in theology Minimum of 1 year of clinical supervision, if fully certified Can work in some settings without being fully certified	Most but not all chaplains are ordained ministers Certification is through Chaplaincy Board of Certification (BCC), but credentials not normally used CEU requirement 50 hours per year
Dietitian	Evaluates nutritional status Works with family members and medical team to determine appropriate nutrition goals	BS in food and nutrition, plus experience to be eligible for exam MS degree available	For RD, must pass the national exam of the American Dietetic Association For LD, same exam is required but processing of paperwork and fees is different CEUs required for LD (6 clock hours/year) and RD (75 clock hours/year every 5 years)
Elder law attorney	Represents legal concerns of older adults, including guardianship, conservatorship, retirement, estate planning/disposition, financing long-term care, preparing advance directives, and benefits issues (e.g., Social Security, Medicare/Medicaid, Veterans)	Bachelor's degree followed by a graduate degree in law (JD) with a concentration in elder law	State license to practice law earned by passing the bar exam For Elder Law Attorney Certification (CELA) available through the National Elder Law Foundation, requires exam, at least 5 years experience with emphasis on elder law cases, 45 related CEUs in previous 3 years

AD, associate degree; BCC, board-certified chaplain; BS, bachelor of science; CCC, certificate of clinical competence; CEU, continuing education unit; CFY, clinical fellowship year; COTA, certified occupational therapy assistant; LD, licensed dietitian; LVN, licensed vocational nurse; MA, master of arts; MS, master of science; NP, nurse practitioner; OT, occupational therapist; OTR, occupational therapist registered; PA, physician assistant; PT, licensed physical therapist; PTA, licensed physical therapist assistant; PDU, professional development unit; RD, registered dietitian; RN, registered nurse.

Reprinted with permission from Long, D. M., & Wilson, N. L. (Eds.). (2001) *Houston geriatric interdisciplinary team training curriculum.* Houston, TX: Baylor College of Medicine's Huffington Center on Aging.

teams and should participate in all health care decisions. Advocating for the inclusion of other disciplines to address complex health challenges can improve patient outcomes and the quality of care received. Two interprofessional organizations that provide excellent resources and networking opportunities are the Gerontological Society of America and the Association for Gerontology in Higher Education.

Geriatric Team Models

Geriatric team models combine the expertise of several disciplines who work collaboratively to improve the care outcomes of older adults. Most use a team approach headed by a physician specializing in the care of older adults (geriatrician). Teams meet regularly to review and update the treatment plan for each patient. Team members typically include disciplines such as nursing, medicine, social work, dietetics, pharmacy, and rehabilitation. The goals are generally to minimize complications, reduce hospital length of stay or readmissions, and ease transitions between care settings, such as hospital to home, convalescence, or long-term care. Higher-risk patients typically are targeted for follow-up by the team. High-risk patients can include those who are frail, have cognitive impairment, or were admitted from residential settings such as assisted living or skilled nursing facilities (Amador, Reed & Lehman, 2007). Geriatric teams function in acute, rehabilitative, outpatient, and long-term care settings. Some common geriatric team models include the Acute Care for Elders units designed to improve hospital care for older adults and Geriatric Assessment Teams or Geriatric Evaluation and Management Teams that conduct detailed psychological, physical, and social assessments in outpatient or inpatient settings. The Geriatric Education Centers has published a curriculum entitled "Geriatric Interdisciplinary Team Training (GITT)." The program focuses on learning to work with other disciplines as a team and to apply a team approach to the care of older adults.

A Model of Evidence-Informed Gerontological Practice

The Caledonian Development Model of Interprofessional Practice in the United Kingdom is one example of a team approach to improve geriatric care. The Caledonian Model is an improvement model to help professionals work in teams to change, improve, and develop their practice (Tolson, Booth, & Lowndes, 2008; Tolson, Schofield, Booth, Kelly, & James, 2006). The model capitalizes on a special type of group known as a community of practice (CoP). Members of the CoP are recruited from one or several organizations (e.g., National Health System, hospital ward, day hospital, or independent sector care home). CoP members may include nurses, patients and their families, therapists, dietitians, physicians, and other individuals connected to a team's goal. CoP members collaborate and pool their expertise on an improvement project designed to advance a selected goal of care (e.g., the promotion of oral health among older adults in a government subsidized senior housing community). The focus of CoPs is to identify common problems experienced by the many patients each team serves and to review the research evidence and suggest strate gies to manage these problems in ways that improve practice. An expert practitioner acts as the CoP's clinical/practice advisor; for example, in a project focused on nutritional aspects, a dietitian would act as the clinical expert or in a project to maximize oral health, a dental practitioner would serve as the expert. Patients who are admitted to clinical areas where CoP teams are using this improvement approach benefit from more evidence-informed care.

Although project goals vary for each CoP, all involve learning activities undertaken within the development college (collaborative Internet-based learning place) (Andrew, Tolson, & Ferguson, 2008). The group learns by sharing and comparing how they work locally with others and by understanding how closely their team's practice resembles either national care guidelines or a consensus view of best practice. Such participatory models encourage individuals to bring their own practice know-how and experience into the learning community and to see learning as an exchange among members where ideas are tested in practice.

The basic framework of the Caledonian Model is illustrated in Figure 5-3. The figure depicts the process used to create and implement national best practice statements that address a patient concern and are designed to improve patient outcomes. Best practice statements incorporate a blend of evidence-based systematic reviews, practice experience, and patient preferences for care (Booth, Tolson, Hotchkiss, & Schofield, 2007). This framework was applied to a project designed to maximize communication among health professionals working with

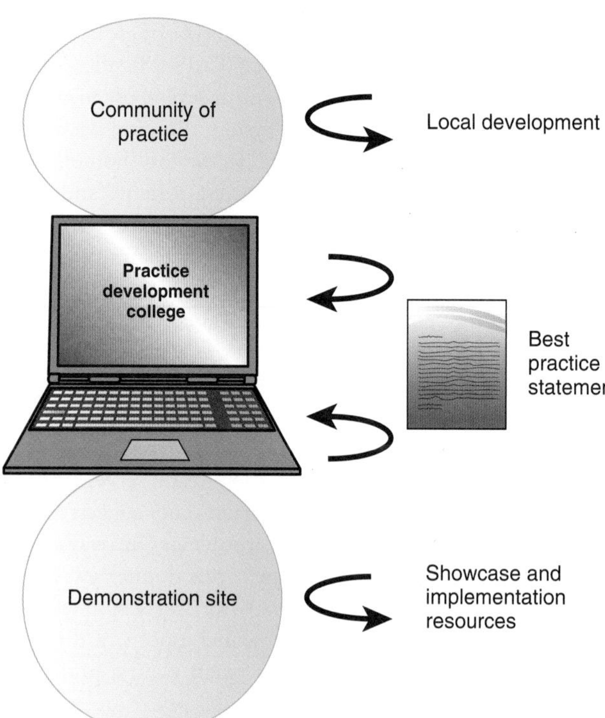

Figure 5-3 Overview of the Caledonian Model.

older adults who have difficulty hearing (NHS Quality Improvement Scotland, 2005a). Key stakeholders were nurses who led the project and patients, families, audiologists, and physicians. Each stakeholder gave input into the best practice statement designed to improve the communication environment and the auditory rehabilitation process.

Working on a CoP team involves developing an appreciation for how to optimize the various expert contributions of different team members and creating shared resources such as templates for interdisciplinary care documentation. Each CoP is supported by a practice development facilitator who helps the team to identify and learn the skills needed to achieve the desired goal. The facilitator also helps the team create an action plan to manage the change process. CoPs interact with facilitators and one another through an Internet-based college. CoPs also occasionally meet in real-time to share implementation strategies. The team also supports its members through the process of championing changes designed to meet their goal. In a way, the CoP becomes a sophisticated and energized development team with a shared agenda that they facilitate in their respective workplaces.

The following example illustrates one practice change accomplished by a CoP at a long-term care facility. Nurses at this facility wanted to improve the fluid intake of frail residents, some of whom suffered from dementia. The nurse CoP member brought this challenge to the team. When the residents were asked for input, several commented that they would drink more if they had "control of the tea pot." They proposed that individual pots be served on demand to give residents a choice about the timing and strength of the tea rather than the current practice where tea was served at set times from a large community pot. The nurse identified that to implement this new procedure, finding a low-cost, light, unbreakable insulated teapot would be essential for the safety of those who wanted this independence. The nurse was doubtful that such a vessel existed or that such a change could be safely introduced. A fellow CoP member from another region was able to source a supplier, share her approach to its successful introduction, and demonstrate through static accident reports that these were considered safe where she worked. She was also able to share information that convinced the catering manager that this change would not be onerous in terms of staff time or his budget. Thus a team approach accomplished a cost-effective change in this agency with the potential to improve the quality of life for residents, as well as to increase their fluid intake.

Improved Teamwork Using the Caledonian Model

The Caledonian Model has significantly improved practice in the United Kingdom. To illustrate its impact, we share the experience of a Rehabilitation and Assessment Directorate (RAD) in a large Scottish Health Board. Health Boards are regional governing bodies in the United Kingdom responsible for administering all National Health Services (NHS) services in accordance with national policy. NHS services are offered to citizens at no charge. The Health Boards control their regional budgets and are accountable for the quality of all NHS services in their region.

A RAD manages health services across the region, including inpatient, outpatient, and preventive services (such as falls prevention); rehabilitative and palliative care; and community services. Each RAD aspires to achieve an integrated and holistic approach to assessment, rehabilitation, and enablement through multiprofessional teams whose primary focus is to work with older adults and those with chronic conditions. The RAD within the Scottish Health Board covers a large geographic area with about 1,000 health professionals. Most of these are nurses without bachelor degrees (68%) who lack the skill to appraise research evidence. Concerns about variations in care standards led the Scottish RAD team to build their 2007 improvement plan around the Caledonian Development Framework. This multiprofessional project was nurse-led and undertaken in partnership with Glasgow Caledonian University. The focus of the project was to implement a best practice statement on promoting movement and physical activity with older people (NHS Quality Improvement Scotland, 2005b).

Initial barriers to recruiting volunteers for a CoP included staff complaints of being too busy, lack of confidence with Internet use, and their ability to work online in the virtual practice development college. Nonnursing disciplines hesitated to adopt what was seen as a nursing model. As work among CoP members progressed, it became apparent that disciplines communicated differently and had contrasting views on the nature of evidence. For example, nurses were more willing to embrace qualitative forms of evidence that accommodated the older person's perspectives than several therapists who valued scientific objectivity and provider preferences over those of patients. Over time, however, therapists seemed to take their cue from nurses about when to limit exercises if a patient seemed reluctant to continue. Initially, the tendency of physiotherapists to protect their role in promoting movement and activity limited patient progress. As teamwork progressed, however, movement and activity became the domain of all providers such that every patient movement (e.g., during transfers, repositioning, or hygiene care) was viewed as an opportunity for therapeutic intervention. Nursing leadership was instrumental in delineating a multiprofessional care pathway and in shaping shared documentation (McAloon, Reid, & Tolson, 2005).

Integrating Evidence into Practice Guidelines

After 1 year, there were measureable improvements from this team approach with respect to assessing, evaluating, and planning patient care. Patients expressed that care was more consistent and tailored to their preferences. Consequently, patients were more engaged in their rehabilitation plans. Better recognition of factors contributing to fall risk led to proactive planning. For one man, this meant minimizing the risk of falling on the stairs in his home by installing a chair lift. These changes represent a new valuing of shared practice among CoP members fueled by a learned respect for each member's contributions (Nolan, Davis, Brown, Keady, & Nolan, 2004).

Lessons Learned from the Caledonian Model Integration Project

At the start of the project, it was assumed that different disciplines would understand one another's roles and expertise; however, this was not the case. Discipline-specific ways of doing and talking hindered progress. It was therefore essential to spend time exploring professional role boundaries, teasing out staff thoughts about respective roles in relation to promoting movement and activity, and finding a common language. A key lesson learned by managers was that progress often means changing practices that are culturally embedded into the health care system, so sustained change takes time. Quick fixes that lack adequate evidence are not likely to lead to improved outcomes (Pipe, 2007).

For RAD practitioners there have been many lessons and discoveries about how they can work better together. Nurses often find it hard to describe the specific contribution they make to care. The RAD improvement project highlighted the leadership role of nursing as critical to interprofessional, evidence-informed care. Members of this project became vested in this evidence-informed team model of practice. When budget cuts threatened the next phase of development, the multiprofessional team rallied to publicize its benefits and successfully procured funding for a second phase (Pearson, Wiechula, Lockwood, & Court, 2005).

KEY POINTS

- Nurses and other health professionals care for older adults in a variety of residential settings, as well as in hospital, rehabilitative, and outpatient environments.
- Most older adults live independently (age in place) but may seek alternative living arrangements for reasons of safety, socialization, proximity to family members, or the need for services such as transportation, meal preparation, or assistance with personal care.
- Senior housing communities, assisted-living centers, and skilled nursing facilities provide incremental levels of service depending on an older adult's needs.
- Nurses' holistic perspective on patient care provides a foundation for identifying problems that require the expertise of other disciplines.
- Key documents published by The International Council of Nursing, the American Association of Colleges of Nursing, and the American Nurses Association assert that working in cooperative relationships with other disciplines is a primary responsibility of nurses.
- Adequately addressing patients' needs often involves teaming with an array of health disciplines, allied health workers, and nonmedical healers, as well as with the patient and significant others.
- According to the Institute of Medicine, the lack of coordinated health care in the United States has resulted in poorer patient outcomes, wasted resources, and increasing costs. Working in collaborative and patient-centered interprofessional teams is necessary to transform the current system. Change must begin by educating students using a team model of care.
- Nursing knowledge provides a foundation for decision making that directly impacts patient outcomes.
- Two resources dedicated to helping professionals keep abreast of gerontological best care practices include the John A. Hartford Institute for Geriatric Nursing and the Geriatric Education Centers.
- Basic and advanced certification in geriatric nursing is available through the American Nurses Credentialing Center.
- Because nurses will spend time caring for older adults, nurses must understand how to promote wellness, maximize independence, and help individuals successfully manage coexisting health problems (comorbidities).
- The Robert Woods Johnson Quality and Safety Education for Nurses initiative provides resources for nurse educators and students to learn how to provide patient-centered care and to be effective collaborators on the health care team.
- Understanding the roles of other team members is essential for effective teamwork, which depends on the ability of members to define common goals and treatment plans.
- Geriatric team members include a variety of disciplines such as the primary care provider, nurse, social worker, case manager, psychologist, pharmacist, physical or occupational therapist, dietitian, dentist, chiropractor, and the patient and significant others. Disciplines such as elder law specialists, community advocates, or spiritual leaders also may be beneficial in addressing patients' health-related needs.
- The Gerontological Society of America and the Association for Gerontology in Higher Education are interprofessional organizations that provide interdisciplinary resources.
- Geriatric team models work collaboratively to minimize complications, reduce hospital length of stay or readmission rates, and facilitate transitions between care settings. Team models include the Acute Care for Elders units, Geriatric Assessment Teams, or Geriatric Evaluation and Management Teams.
- The goal of the Geriatric Education Centers' Geriatric Interdisciplinary Team Training curriculum is to help disciplines learn to apply a team approach to the care of older adults.

CRITICAL THINKING ACTIVITIES

1. Arrange to participate in interprofessional grand rounds or team meetings.
2. Design a patient simulation experience where students represent different disciplines.
3. Arrange for student clinical placements across a range of care environments focusing on older adults (e.g., outpatient clinics with a geriatric assessment team, hospital units functioning under a geriatric team model, assisted living, adult day care, rehabilitation and convalescent centers, visiting nurse home care agencies, long-term care).
4. Create student projects that require collaboration with other disciplines.
5. Assign students to shadow a member of another discipline that participates on a geriatric assessment team.
6. Invite members of a geriatric assessment team to participate in a panel discussion during class about the roles of each member in managing selected patient situations.
7. Imagine that your elderly patient recently moved to the long-term care facility where you work. You have concerns that the patient is not adjusting well and decide to arrange a meeting with the various disciplines involved in the patient's care. What disciplines might you involve?

CASE STUDY | *JESSIE MacDONALD*

Jessie MacDonald was admitted to the assessment ward via the emergency department. She was found on the floor by her son during his weekly visit. Jessie was mildly hypothermic on admission, dehydrated, and badly bruised. It was not clear how long she had lain on the floor or why she had fallen, because Jessie had no recollection of the event. Her neighbors reported having seen Jessie in her garden earlier that day, so it was likely less than a few hours. A nonspecific medical diagnosis of "an unexplained fall resulting in minor injury" was made.

Following administration of intravenous fluids, the physicians recommended home discharge as soon as possible. Jessie concurred with this, stating that there was nothing wrong with her and that it was "just one of those silly accidents that happen." The nurse responsible for Jessie's care disagreed, however, and was concerned by Jessie's poor performance on the Get Up and Go test.

By explaining to Jessie that she seemed to be at higher than average risk of falling and persuading her that it might be possible to work with her to reduce the risk of further falls, Jessie's discharged was delayed. Through evidence-informed decision making and in partnership with Jessie, it was agreed that the physiotherapist would complete a more thorough assessment on the ward and that a home visit would be undertaken with the occupational therapist. Jessie was discharged home 5 days after admission, following home modifications to enhance Jessie's safety (e.g., removal of hazardous rugs and rearrangement of furniture). Jessie also reluctantly accepted a walking aid. Jessie continues to visit the day hospital for further investigation of her postural hypotension and goes to a supervised gym to improve her mobility.

1. Dignity and respect are important dimensions of health care for older people. What strategies did the nurse used to promote a sense of dignity and respect throughout Jessie's experience of hospital care?
2. How might Jessie's son have been involved in assessing her immediate and future care needs?
3. What risks did the staff perceive in Jessie's home environment? What other issues should be considered in terms of her safety at home?
4. Fear of falling can lead to self-imposed restrictions on mobility and participation. How will staff know if this is an issue for Jessie in the longer term?

REFERENCES

Administration on Aging. (2008). *A profile of older Americans: 2008.* Washington, DC: Author.

Amador, L. F., Reed, D., & Lehman, C. A. (2007). The acute care for elders unit: Taking the rehabilitation model into the hospital setting. *Rehabilitation Nursing, 32*(3), 126-132.

American Association of Colleges of Nursing (AACN). (2008). *Essentials of baccalaureate nursing education.* Washington, DC: Author.

American Association of Colleges of Nursing & The Hartford Institute for Geriatric Nursing at New York University. (2010). *Recommended baccalaureate competencies and curricular guidelines for the nursing care of older adults.* Retrieved January 10, 2011, from http://www.aacn.nche.edu/education/pdf/AACN_Gerocompetencies.pdf

American Nurses Association (ANA). (2001). *ANA gerontological nursing scope and standards of gerontological nursing practice* (2nd ed.). Silver Spring, MD: Author.

American Nurses Association (ANA). (2003). *Nursing's social policy statement* (2nd ed.). Silver Spring, MD: Author.

Andrew, N., Tolson, D., & Ferguson, D. (2008). Building on Wenger: Communities of practice in nursing. *Nurse Education Today, 28*(2), 246-252.

Balas, E. A. (2001). Information systems can prevent errors and improve quality [Comment]. *Journal of the American Medical Informatics Association, 8*(4), 398-399.

Barnsteiner, J., Disch, J., Hall, H., Mayer, D., & Moore, S. (2007). Interprofessional education: It can't be left to chance. *Nursing Outlook, 55,* 144-150.

Bates, D. W., Spell, N., Cullen, D. J., et al. (1997). The costs of adverse drug events in hospitalized patients. Adverse drug events prevention study group. *JAMA, 277*(4), 307-311.

Booth, J., Tolson, D., Hotchkiss, R., & Schofield. I. (2007). Using action research to construct national evidence-based nursing care guidance for gerontological nursing. *Journal of Clinical Nursing, 16,* 945-953.

Centers for Disease Control and Prevention (National Center for Health Statistics). (1999). *Births and deaths: Preliminary data for* 1998. *National Vital Statistics Reports.* Washington, DC: U.S. Department of Health and Human Services.

Chassin, M. R. (1997). Assessing strategies for quality improvement. *Health Aff (Millwood), 16*(3), 151-161.

Clark, C. M., Fradkin, J. E., Hiss, R. G., Lorenz, R. A., Vinicor, F., & Warren-Boulton, E. (2000). Promoting early diagnosis and treatment of type 2 diabetes: The national diabetes education program. *Journal of the American Medical Association, 284*(3), 363-365.

Cronenwett, L., Sherwood, G., Barnsteiner J., Disch, J., Johnson, J., Mitchell, P., . . . (2007). Quality and safety education for nurses. *Nursing Outlook, 55*(3), 122-131.

Cummings, S. M. (2009). Treating older persons with severe mental illness in the community: Impact of an interdisciplinary geriatric mental health team. *Journal of Gerontological Social Work, 52*(1), 17-31.

Darroch, K. (2007). An audit to measure the outcome of nutritional intervention 3 months post-discharge from the Community Older People's Team. In Selected abstracts from the British Dietetic Association Conference (p. 372). *Journal of Human Nutrition and Dietetics, 20*(4), 362-387.

Drinka, T., & Clark, P. (2000). *Health care teamwork: Interdisciplinary practice and teaching.* Westport, CT: Auburn House.

Graffy, J., Grande, M., & Campbell, J. (2008). Case management for elderly patients at risk of hospital admission: A team approach. *Primary Health Care Research & Development, 9,* 7-13.

Federal Interagency Forum on Aging-Related Statistics. (2008). *Older Americans 2008: Key indicators of well-being.* Washington, DC: U.S. Government Printing Office.

Harari, D., Martin, D., Buttery, A., O'Neill, S., & Hopper, A. (2007). The older persons' assessment and liaison team 'OPAL': Evaluation of comprehensive geriatric assessment in acute medical inpatients. *Age and Ageing, 36,* 670-675.

He, W., Sengupta, M., Velkoff, V., & DeBarros, K. (2005). *65+ in the United States: 2005.* Washington, DC: U.S. Government Printing Office.

Institute of Medicine. (2000). In L. T. Kohn, J. M. Corrigan, & M. S. Donaldson (Eds.), *To err is human: Building a safer health system.* Washington, DC: The National Academies Press.

Institute of Medicine. (2001). *Crossing the quality chasm: A new health system for the 21st century.* Washington, DC: The National Academies Press.

Institute of Medicine. (2002). *Care without coverage: Too little, too late.* Washington, DC: The National Academies Press.

Institute of Medicine. (2003a). In J. M. Corrigan, A. Greiner, & S. M. Erickson (Eds.), *Fostering rapid advances in health care: Learning from system demonstrations.* Washington, DC: The National Academies Press.

Institute of Medicine. (2003b). In A. C. Greiner & E. Knebel (Eds.), *Health professions education: A bridge to quality.* Washington, DC: The National Academies Press.

Institute of Medicine. (2003c). In K. Adams & J. M. Corrigan (Eds.), *Priority areas for national action: Transforming health care Quality.* Washington, DC: The National Academies Press.

International Council of Nurses. (2006). *The ICN code of ethics for nurses.* Geneva, Switzerland: Author.

Krishnan, S., Nash, F., Baker, N., Fowler, D., & Rayman, G. (2007). Reduction in diabetic amputations over eleven years in a defined UK population-benefits of multidisciplinary team working and prospective audit. *Diabetes Care, 31,* 99-101.

Kurtzman, E. T., & Corrigan, J. M. (2007). Measuring the contribution of nursing to quality, patient safety, and health care outcomes. *Policy, Politics & Nursing Practice, 8*(1), 20-36.

Legorreta, A. P., Liu, X., Zaher, C. A., & Jatulis, D. E. (2000). Variation in managing asthma: Experience at the medical group level in California. *American Journal of Managed Care, 6*(4), 445-453.

Lingard, L., Regehr, G., Orser, B., Reznick, R., Baker, G. R., Doran, D., . . . Whyte, S. (2008). Evaluation of a preoperative checklist and team briefing among surgeons, nurses, and anesthesiologists to reduce failures in communication. *Archives of Surgery, 143*(1), 12-17.

Long, D. M., & Wilson, N. L. (Eds.). (2001) *Houston geriatric interdisciplinary team training curriculum.* Houston, TX: Baylor College of Medicine's Huffington Center on Aging.

Masanori, N., Jun, T., Toshio, O., & Yoshinori, D. (2007). Multidisciplinary team approach for elderly patients with chronic heart failure. *Circulation Journal: Official Journal of the Japanese Circulation Society, Supplement I, 71,* 60.

McAloon, M., Reid, W., & Tolson, D. (2005). An overview of the development of a generic integrated care pathway in a department of medicine for the elderly. *Journal of Integrated Care Pathways, 9,* 1-7.

McBride, P., Schrott, H. G., Plane, M. B., Underbakke, G., & Brown, R. L. (1998). Primary care practice adherence to National Cholesterol Education Program guidelines for patients with coronary heart disease. *Archives of Internal Medicine, 158*(11), 1238-1244.

McGlynn, E. A., Asch, S. M., Adams, J. Keesey, J., Hicks, J., DeCristofaro, A., . . . (2003). The quality of health care delivered to adults in the United States [Comment]. *New England Journal of Medicine, 348*(26), 2635-2645.

Melnyk, B. M., Fineout-Overholt, E., Feinstein, N. F., Sadler, L. S., & Green-Hernandez, C. (2008). Nurse practitioner educators' perceived knowledge, beliefs, and teaching strategies regarding evidence-based practice: Implications for accelerating the integration of evidence-based practice into graduate programs. *Journal of Professional Nursing, 24,* 7-13.

Nagamine, M., Jiang, H. J., & Merrill, C. T. (2006). *Trends in elderly hospitalizations, 1997–2004. HCUP Statistical Brief #14.* Rockville, MD: Agency for Health Care Research and Quality. Retrieved November 5, 2010, from http://www.hcup-us.ahrq.gov/reports/statbriefs/sb14.pdf

NHS Quality Improvement Scotland. (2005a) *Maximising communication with older people who have hearing disability.* Edinburgh, Scotland: Author. Retrieved December 3, 2010, from http://www.nhshealthquality.org/nhsqis/2776.html

NHS Quality Improvement Scotland. (2005b) *Working with dependent older people towards promoting movement and physical activity.* Edinburgh, Scotland: Author. Retrieved December 3, 2010, from http://www.nhshealthquality.org/nhsqis/2727.html

Ni, H., Nauman, D. J., & Hershberger, R. E. (1998). Managed care and outcomes of hospitalization among elderly patients with congestive heart failure. *Archives of Internal Medicine, 158*(11), 1231-1236.

Nolan, M. R., Davis, S., Brown, J., Keady, J., & Nolan, J. (2004). Beyond 'person-centred' care: A new vision for gerontological nursing. *International Journal of Older People Nursing, 13*(3a), 45-53.

Pearson, A., Wiechula, R., Lockwood, C., & Court, A. (2005). The JBI model of evidence based health care. *International Journal of Evidence based Health Care, 3*(8), 207-216.

Perez-Stable, E. J., & Fuentes-Afflick, E. (1998). Role of clinicians in cigarette smoking prevention. *Western Journal of Medicine, 169*(1), 23-29.

Pipe, T. B. (2007). Optimising nursing care by integrating theory-driven evidence based practice. *Journal of Nursing Care Quarterly, 22*(3), 234-238.

Quality and Safety Education for Nurses (QSEN). (2010). *Quality and safety competencies.* Retrieved December 3, 2010, from http://www.qsen.org/competencies.php

Samsa, G. P., Matchar, D. B., Goldstein, L. B., Bonito, A. J., Lux, L. J., Witter, D. M., . . . (2000). Quality of anticoagulation management among patients with atrial fibrillation: Results of a review of medical records from 2 communities. *Archives of Internal Medicine, 160*(7), 967-973.

Thomas, E. J., Studdert, D. M., Burstin, H. R., Orav, E. J., Zeena, T., Williams, E. J., . . . Brennan, T. A. (2000). Incidence and types of adverse events and negligent care in Utah and Colorado [Comment]. *Medical Care, 38*(3), 261-271.

Thomas, E. J., Studdert, D. M., Newhouse, J. P., Zbar, B. I. W., Howard, K. M., Williams, E. J., . . . (1999). Costs of medical injuries in Utah and Colorado. *Inquiry, 36*(3), 255-264.

Tolson, D., Booth, J., & Lowndes, A. (2008). Achieving evidence based practice: Impact of the Caledonian development model. *Journal of Nursing Management, 16,* 682-691.

Tolson, D., Schofield, I., Booth, J., Kelly, T. B., & James, L. (2006). Constructing a new approach to developing evidence based practice with nurses and older people. *World Views on Evidence Based Nursing, 3*(2), 62-72.

von Renteln-Kruse, W., & Krause, T. (2007). Incidence of in-hospital falls in geriatric patients before and after the introduction of an interdisciplinary team–based fall-prevention intervention. *Journal of the American Geriatrics Society, 55,* 2068-2074.

World Health Organization (WHO). (2007). *Age-friendly primary health care centres toolkit.* Geneva, Switzerland: Author. Retrieved December 3, 2010, from http://www.who.int/ageing/publications/upcoming_publications/en/index.html

Young, A. S., Klap, R., Sherbourne, C. D., & Wells, K. B. (2001). The quality of care for depressive and anxiety disorders in the United States. *Archives of General Psychiatry, 58*(1), 55-61.

Chapter 6

Engaging Older Adults as Partners in Their Care

Philip A. Greiner, DNSc, RN

LEARNING OBJECTIVES

- Recognize the prevailing theories of behavioral change at the individual level.
- Discuss relevant environmental factors that influence behavioral change at the individual level.
- Use theory, facts about the environment, and evidence to suggest potential policy changes that can support behavioral change.
- Examine the patient-as-partner approach to care delivery and the effect of this approach on the structure of health-related services.
- Present an argument for preventive health services for the older adult population as an issue of social justice.
- Reflect on personal behaviors and clinical practice with older adults to better understand the need for institutional change in older adult services.

One of the goals for this chapter is for the reader to better understand the roles that older adults can play in health-related activities. A second goal is to have the reader grasp the impact that the immediate and larger environment can have in determining the options available for older adults in any given society. To meet either of these goals, it is helpful to have an understanding of the terms used in this chapter and how those terms are applied.

Influences on the Older Adult

What do we mean when we say *older adults?* Traditionally, age 65 has been the point at which we identify a person as an older adult, in part because this age is when the person qualifies for full Medicare coverage and Social Security benefits. However, there is growing recognition that behaviors developed and maintained through one's lifecourse set the stage for how a person ages. In 1996, the World Health Organization issued guidelines for promoting physical activity among older adults. The guidelines concluded that people age 50 and older were the most appropriate target for increasing physical activity. Subsequently, the *National Blueprint: Increasing Physical Activity Among Adults Aged 50 and Older* (Chodzko-Zajko, 2001) highlighted the need for midlife physical activity as the basis for extending the years of active independent living as one ages. More recently, the National Institute on Aging has taken a lifecourse approach to research on aging, recognizing that there are multiple factors throughout life that may influence how a person ages (National Institute on Aging, 2009). The term *older adult,* then, refers to a point in the lifecourse when a person reaches an age determined as the point that society designates as the beginning of old age, but it is an individual's lifecourse that influences how the person ages and what health-related services may be needed. It is more helpful to examine aging as a process that proceeds over a lifetime, to recognize that not all people survive to become older adults, and to note that people enter older adulthood with varying social, physical, and cognitive abilities.

Health care is often viewed as the interaction between a care provider and a patient. Although this approach helps the provider understand an individual person, it is also important to understand how this patient's experience fits with other people in similar situations. Data collected on groups of people can be organized in several ways. Often, data are organized into cohorts based on age. By examining cohort data, it is possible to see which behaviors occur most often and fall within an expected range and which behaviors occur less often and outside the expected range. Cohorts can then be compared to see how behaviors change over time. They also can be compared internally by such variables as sex, race, income, and education.

An example of this phenomenon is the recognition about 15 years ago of the wide variability among older adults based on their age. (See Chapter 3 for more information.) One way to categorize the range of older adults is as the newer old and the oldest-old. The oldest-old cohort includes people age 85 and older (Suzman, Willis, & Manton, 1996). This is the most rapidly growing cohort of older adults. People in the oldest-old cohort are also called hearty survivors (Olshansky & Carnes, 2001) or sometimes the elite old (see Chapter 3) because they have successfully outlived others in their age cohort. In general, women tend to outlive men, and White women and men tend to outlive their fellow citizens who are Black or Hispanic.

The new old, those ages 65 to 70, represent the cohort of people leading up to the Baby Boom generation. The Baby Boom cohort (those born between 1946 and 1964) includes about 78 million people—the largest cohort of older adults American society has ever faced. This pending increase in the older adult population comes with dramatic changes in lifestyle and activities compared with the World War II generation. As a result, there is a recognition that older adult services will need to change dramatically to match the behaviors and meet the needs of this new older adult cohort.

In addition to age itself, the place where a person lives and works plays an important role in determining social and health outcomes (Robert Wood Johnson Foundation, 2009). For example, senior housing for low-income older adults may be located in inner city areas where it is unsafe to walk alone, lighting is poor, and sidewalks are broken or uneven. As a result, these older adults may limit walking and other physical activities, which may contribute to weight gain and decreasing flexibility, balance, and mobility. In contrast, older adults who can afford to live in a life-care community have an environment that promotes walking and other physical activities, is well-lit and safe, and boasts well-maintained walking paths. These older adults are more likely to be active and to retain or improve their physical abilities.

People with higher levels of education and income tend to live longer, healthier lives than do people with lower levels of education and income. This relationship is not just for high education/income as compared with low education/income. Rather, this relationship holds across all levels of education and income and is referred to as a *social gradient* (Wilkinson & Marmot, 2003).

Location also influences what choices are available. Older adults living in a rural setting may have no public transportation, limited food options, and a single source of health care as compared with older adults living in an affluent suburb where there is a well-funded infrastructure offering multiple options in each of these areas. These attributes of place and socioeconomic status add a social justice component to behavior change that cannot be ignored at the level of the provider-patient relationship.

In summary, becoming an older adult is influenced by a person's lifecourse, the cohort into which that person was born, the relative education and income of that person in society, and the place in which the person lives and works. These external environmental factors are referred to as *social determinants* of health (Wilkinson & Marmot, 2003). These social determinants represent the cutting edge of health research, including aging research. They relate directly to individual contributions to health outcomes, which include those behaviors that a person can change and attributes that a person cannot change. Attributes that a person cannot change are things like one's race or genetic makeup. Behaviors that a person can change include one's diet, exercise, and tobacco use. These personal choices, however, are shaped by the place where that person lives, the company he or she keeps, the type of work he or she does, his or her income and education, and the resources available and policies in the community and larger environment. It is insufficient to suggest that a person change behavior without also addressing the social, cultural, economic, and educational resources available. Working for change at these higher levels involves social justice activities, including patient and community advocacy, community capacity building, and professional involvement in social change through setting policy and standards. The social determinants of health serve as the underpinnings of the current *Healthy People 2010* framework and for the *Healthy People 2020* framework and specific objectives currently under development (Box 6-1).

Engagement and Partnership

What do we mean by *engagement* and *partnership?* Both of these terms relate to health care interactions that move the patient from being a passive recipient of care, with the provider as the knowledgeable expert, to becoming an active participant in the care process as promoted in *Healthy People 2010* (Calkins, Boult, Wagner, et al., 1999; U.S. Department of Health and Human Services, 2000).

Engagement refers to the process the provider uses to enlist the patient's involvement in the health care process. Engagement also implies commitment to an ongoing relationship between provider and patient.

Partnership refers to the equal status and power of those involved in the care process, but specifically between patient and provider. The goal is to have a meaningful partnership wherein each partner is engaged in the process of improving the patient's health status. Core work in this area of health care reform comes from the Chronic Care Model (Improving Chronic Illness Care, 2009), supported by the Robert Wood Johnson Foundation. This patient-centered approach places the patient in a partnership relationship, equal to that of others in the partnership. Others in the partnership become resources that the patient can draw on when needed. The goals of this patient-as-partner process are (1) that the various providers gain a better understanding of the context in which the patient lives and functions and (2) that the patient assumes more responsibility and accountability for his or her health.

Engagement, then, represents the initial and ongoing phases of establishing the provider-patient relationship and the partnership. This process requires continual work on the part of each partner to develop and enrich the partnership. The patient's contribution to this process is a commitment to work on health and lifestyle behaviors that are legitimately under his or her control. Through the partnership process, a plan is developed. It establishes short-term and long-term goals toward which each of the partners contributes their efforts. Each meeting is used to identify progress toward these goals and possible barriers that could limit or preclude such progress. The plan of care and related goals are modified based on this continual input and evaluation by the provider, patient, and others involved in the patient's care. National care standards can be used to benchmark the patient's progress toward meeting specific goals, while local knowledge is needed to deal with identified barriers. Local knowledge can come from the patient but should also come from the provider becoming knowledgeable about and involved in the community. This patient-as-partner approach has important implications for how providers work with patients to encourage behavior change. It is also an example of grassroots social justice activities in that it promotes an equal partnership among the people involved and values the lived experiences of the patient.

Through the partnership process, a plan is developed that establishes short-term and long-term goals toward which each of the partners contributes their efforts.

BOX 6-1 Healthy People 2020 Goals

The *Healthy People 2020* overarching goals include

- Attaining high quality, longer lives free of preventable disease, disability, injury, and premature death
- Achieving health equity, eliminating disparities, and improving the health of all groups
- Creating social and physical environments that promote good health for all
- Promoting quality of life, healthy development, and healthy behaviors across all life stages (U.S. Department of Health and Human Services, 2010)

Source: U.S. Department of Health and Human Services. (2010). Healthy people 2020 framework. Retrieved November 27, 2010, from http://healthypeople.gov/2020/

Health Promotion for Older Adults?

People younger than 65 and even some who are older than 65 may question the need for health-promoting behavior change in the older adult population. After all, the primary focus of behavior change is for people to adopt healthy lifestyles early in life to increase life expectancy and the quality of life (U.S. Department of Health and Human Services, 2000). However, these same goals apply to older adults, especially with the increasing longevity within the older adult population. Take, for example, the role of exercise and nutrition on the risk of hypertension and stroke. In older adults, micro infarcts (small infarcts 1 cm in diameter or smaller) can cause cognitive and physical changes from which the person may not recover. Multiple small strokes like these can cause cumulative damage that is similar to or worse than the decline seen in Alzheimer's disease. Stroke prevention in older adults is critical to prevent these small infarcts and to maintain an acceptable quality of life. Therefore, exercise and nutrition to lower hypertension should continue as a clinical goal throughout the lifecourse for older adults (Greiner, Snowdon, & Greiner, 1999).

Individual Approaches to Behavior Change

The tendency is to view health care interactions from a provider-patient perspective, perhaps because that relationship has the most immediate relevance to both providers and patients. It is within this interaction that patients have the opportunity to discuss personal concerns and goals, and providers can offer recommendations about areas for health improvement. The relevance of these concerns, goals, and areas for health improvement is often based on changing the patient's behavior. Although there are many theories related to behavioral change, an overview of four key theories will provide a basis for understanding how these theories may be used in clinical practice. The four theories include the Health Belief Model (Janz & Becker, 1984), Self-Efficacy Theory (Bandura, 1977), the Health Promotion Model (Pender, Murdaugh, & Parsons, 2006), and the Stages of Change Theory (Velicer, Prochaska, Fava, Norman, & Redding, 1998).

Health Belief Model

The Health Belief Model (Janz & Becker, 1984) is one of the oldest models from social psychology, having been developed in the 1950s. The model aims to explain current behavior and predict future action based on five important components: perceived threat, perceived benefits, perceived barriers, cues to action, and other variables.

- Perceived threat contains two interrelated components: perceived susceptibility (the sense of the risk of getting the health problem) and perceived severity (the sense of how serious the threat of illness or health consequences are as compared to inaction). If people believe that they are healthy and seldom exposed to a health risk, they perceive a lesser threat and are less likely to change their behavior.
- Perceived benefits relate to the person's sense that a recommended action will be effective. People are more likely to change their behavior if the perceived benefits are high.
- Perceived barriers refers to factors that can have a negative effect on changing the behavior. Barriers can be physical, psychological, social, and/or financial. People are more likely to change a behavior if there are few barriers or barriers are easily overcome.
- Cues to action are motivating factors that cause a person to change behavior. People are more likely to change a behavior if something has happened to make action more acceptable at this moment in time.
- Other variables might include environmental factors that affect the person's decisions to indirectly contribute to behavioral change. People are more likely to change behavior if their friends and family are adopting similar changes.

These five components make up the classic Health Belief Model. By assessing each of the five parts, the provider can work with the patient to determine ways to increase the chances of successful behavioral change. For example, if an 80-year-old man is considering the need for Pneumovax vaccination to decrease his risk of pneumonia, an assessment is first made of his concerns about pneumonia. The provider may determine the extent of his understanding of the risk of pneumonia for older adults, the possible consequences of developing pneumonia, and the risk of death from pneumonia. The provider also can provide evidence of the success of Pneumovax in preventing pneumonia. Possible barriers to receiving the Pneumovax may be the patient's fear of injections, concern about vaccination side effects, and the potential cost of the medication. The patient also can suggest factors that might make behavior change more acceptable to him, such low-cost or free vaccination services. By using a patient-as-partner approach, the provider and patient can identify best options, set realistic goals, and establish a timeframe for receiving the Pneumovax injection. Public health officials can further reduce barriers by making the

Pneumovax vaccine available at influenza clinics where accessibility and peer pressure may increase the possibility of the patient receiving the Pneumovax.

Self-Efficacy Theory

The Self-Efficacy Theory (Bandura, 1977) represents an expansion of the Health Belief Model. In fact, current depictions of the Health Belief Model include self-efficacy as a sixth component (Rosenstock, Strecher, & Becker, 1994). Bandura proposed Self-Efficacy Theory as a solution to a growing division in his field that focused on cognitive processes on the one hand and successful performance on the other hand as measures of human behavior. Self-efficacy is a cognitive process learned from the consequences of previous responses. If a behavioral response worked well in the past, and the person sees that such behavioral responses have also worked for others, that person experiences an increase in self-efficacy. Self-efficacy is the person's sense that he or she can behave differently to achieve a given outcome. The more strongly a person believes that he or she can effect a change in behavior, the more likely it is that behavior change will occur. Bandura also stated that self-efficacy varied by the magnitude or difficulty of the task, the generality of one's sense of mastery, and the strength of one's expectations of efficacy.

The sense of efficacy can be enhanced through successful performance experiences, the observed successful performance experiences of others, verbal persuasion by others or oneself, and emotional arousal. The concept of self-efficacy has gained acceptance as a driving factor in behavioral change but is also viewed as a component part in newer versions of the Health Belief Model.

In applying the Self-Efficacy Theory, the provider would need to determine the patient's sense of self-efficacy in relation to the desired behavior change. If an older adult woman has never participated in formal exercise activities, her perceived self-efficacy in this area may be low. However, most people have had successful experiences walking. This woman may be willing to start a tailored walking program as a pathway to increased exercise. Goals, therefore, are set low so that she can gain a sense of mastery by successfully reaching several goals. She might start with the goals of purchasing appropriate walking shoes and completing a walk from her apartment to a nearby park and back. Having attained these goals, she could be asked to complete this walk three times a week for the next month. By this time, her confidence in her ability to walk for exercise will be increased, along with her endurance. She should find that each walk becomes easier to do and that these benefits make doing other activities easier as well. The next set of goals may be to find a walking buddy or group with which to continue walking, while also increasing either the distance walked or the pace of that walk. It is important for the provider and patient to anticipate setbacks due to weather or pain and to develop possible solutions to these problems. Other resources in the community should also be identified so that the patient has additional sources of support for this new behavior.

Health Promotion Model

The Health Promotion Model (Pender, Murdaugh, & Parsons, 2006) focuses on three general areas: individual characteristics and experiences, behavior-specific cognitions and affect, and behavioral outcomes. Each of these general areas has component parts.

- Individual characteristics and experiences are made up of prior related behavior and biological, psychological, and sociocultural personal factors. These characteristics and experiences set the stage for behavior change.
- Behavior-specific cognitions and affect are made up of aspects drawn from the Health Belief Model. These include perceived benefits of action, perceived barriers to action, perceived self-efficacy, activity-related affect, interpersonal influences, and situational influences.
- Each of these aspects contributes to the expected behavioral outcome through a commitment to a plan of change, immediate competing demands and preferences, and health-promoting behavior.

The Health Promotion Model is more complex than the previously mentioned models, in part because it incorporates and expands both of those models and includes expectancy-value theory and social cognitive theory (Pender, Murdaugh, & Parsons, 2006). This model combines personal decision making with interpersonal and situational factors that influence personal action.

Application of this model involves more complexity but allows both the provider and the patient to focus on specific concerns and benefits. For example, an older adult woman living in a large extended-family home wants to quit smoking. She has used tobacco products for 38 years, but recently realized that she is addicted to nicotine through reading a popular magazine. Her previous attempts to quit smoking where halfhearted, but she now finds that few of her contacts at social events will tolerate smoking. Her health care provider gave her printed material to review before their scheduled appointment, so she understands the many health benefits of smoking cessation. She believes that she is in control of her life, has the support of her family and friends in making this change, and recognizes the social benefits of being smoke-free. She feels ready to commit to changing her behavior, sees few competing demands in her life, and perceives multiple preferences for her to quit. An assessment of each of these aspects indicates that her chance of successfully reaching the desired behavioral outcome is high.

Stages of Change Theory

This theory presents five components in a cyclical process of stages that varies for each individual (Velicer, Prochaska, Fava, Norman, & Redding, 1998). The stages include precontemplation, contemplation, preparation for action, action, and maintenance.

- Precontemplation is when the person has recognized a problem but is not ready to change the behavior. It is believed that the person in this stage needs more information and a broader sense of the general environment to understand the need for change.
- The contemplation stage is reached when the person recognizes the problem and gives serious consideration to the need for change. The person reevaluates his or her previous perspective.
- The preparation for action stage occurs when the person begins to think that behavior change is possible in the immediate future. This stage is somewhat related to self-efficacy but is situation specific.
- In the action stage, the person has consistently engaged in behavior change for less than 6 months. In this stage, rewards, support from others, and avoidance of triggering situations are helpful in continuation of the change.
- Finally, the maintenance stage is reached, when the person has successfully continued the behavior change for 6 months or more.

The entire process is viewed as cyclical because factors that support the behavior change can shift and the person can revert to prior behavior patterns.

An application of this theoretical approach to older adults can be seen in attempts to reduce risky sexual behavior in those aged 60 and older. This age cohort may have avoided or ignored much of the HIV/AIDS education since the late 1980s by being in a monogamous relationship for most of that time yet find themselves now divorced or widowed. Being new to dating and not accustomed to using barrier protection against exchange of body fluids, these older adults are at risk of sexually transmitted infections, including HIV/AIDS. A health care provider can use the Stages of Change Theory to determine which stage the patient may be in with regard to sexual activity. A patient in the precontemplation or contemplation stage should be given information about the risk and encouraged to ask for further information before resuming sexual activities. Those in the preparation for action stage need more of the provider's time and involvement to review possible barrier methods and to assess the patient's willingness to change behavior.

Broader social issues may need to be addressed before individual change can occur.

Each of these four theories can be used with individuals. Some of these theories, such as Self-Efficacy Theory, give little consideration to the environment in which people act. Others, such as the Health Promotion Model, provide indirect pathways for environmental influences of personal decisions about behavior. There is, however, growing evidence and recognition that individual change can be limited by an unsupportive environment or enhanced through community-level change (Institute of Medicine, 2003). That is, individual models alone may be insufficient to explain why some people are unable or unwilling to make changes in health-related behavior. To imply that people are not compliant with treatment is to blame them for a situation in which they may be victimized by greater societal issues. These broader social issues may need to be addressed before individual change can occur.

Community Approaches to Behavior Change

Several models are currently being applied at the community level. The two models of community-level theory included here have been used widely and incorporated into both large- and small-scale community interventions. They are the PRECEDE-PROCEED Model (Green & Kreuter, 2005) and the Ecological Model (Institute of Medicine, 2003).

PRECEDE-PROCEED Model

The PRECEDE-PROCEED Model (Green & Kreuter, 1999) consists of six phases: social assessment and situational analysis, epidemiological assessment, educational and ecological assessment, intervention alignment, administrative and policy assessment, and evaluation. These phases are presented as a linear, stepwise process, although each phase informs and provides feedback for prior and future phases.

- Social assessment and situation analysis consists of gathering data on community assets and capacity within the community from those people living in the community. Assessment is done through a variety of methods designed to involve various stakeholders, leaders, followers, and residents. This phase provides information from various perspectives on the current state of the community.
- The epidemiological assessment is completed by a thorough review of available epidemiological data, an assessment of risk factors and health concerns, factors that link individual health to ecological facts, and identifying behavioral factors amenable to change in this community. Communities vary on the types and amount of data that are routinely collected and the quality of those data. This phase provides hard facts to link to the social assessment.
- The educational and ecological assessment contains predisposing factors (awareness, knowledge, beliefs, attitudes, values, self-efficacy, behavioral intent, and existing skills) and enabling factors (health care environment, other environmental conditions that affect health-related behavior, new skills, and reinforcing factors). These factors are similar to those seen in the individual models of behavior change but are now assessed at the population level as well. Combined with the other assessment phases, it is possible to construct an asset map, as well as areas of strength and areas for further development.
- The intervention alignment refers to a process of identifying methods and setting priorities within and among categories. The goal is to reach agreement among participants on what to address and how best to address the identified areas for further development. This phase is also used to specify assets that exist in the community that might be useful in addressing priority goals.
- The administrative and policy assessment determines the resources available to make the changes, the values, attitudes, and beliefs of the staff, political will, and the other attributes of the agencies needed to effect the changes. It can also help to identify key people to assist in community change.
- Evaluation refers to the multiple methods available and the data to be used to determine outcomes of the proposed changes. Evaluation includes an assessment of goal attainment and the processes used to reach those goals. It also includes areas for continued work and analyzes the problems that may have been encountered along the way.

The PRECEDE-PROCEED Model has been used successfully in a wide variety of situations, including worksite and school settings. For example, the model could be used to examine the types of activities that older adults have available to them in their communities. A task force could be organized to interview older adults and agency representatives on existing activities and current levels of participation in those activities, desired activities, and potential sites for those activities; gather data on the health benefits of a broad range of activities; establish a list of available sites for activities, agencies with which to coordinate activities, and social and environmental considerations related to those activities; decide on the best activities for older adults in this community, given the resources; and establish the methods to put those activities in place. After several months of operation, an evaluation of activity participation and attendance could be gathered, along with additional suggestions for improving activity use.

Ecological Model

The Ecological Model (Institute of Medicine, 2003) has evolved from work in multiple fields in the area of social ecology (Dahlberg & Krug, 2002; Krieger, 2001). Social ecology, as it relates to health behavior, explores the relationship between people and their environment on a broad scale. The model as presented here was incorporated into several Institute of Medicine publications (Gebbie, Rosenstock, & Hernandez, 2003; Institute of Medicine, 2003). This model highlights the social determinants of health (Wilkinson & Marmot, 2003) that directly and indirectly influence health-related behaviors. It uses a lifecourse approach to examine individual behaviors within the context of social, family, and community networks; living and working conditions; and broad social, economic, cultural, health, and environmental conditions and policies at the global, national, state, and local levels. Because of the social and contextual approach used in this model, it is an excellent choice from a social justice perspective. Each level provides opportunities for change that can directly or indirectly enhance the health and well-being of individuals.

- The social, family, and community networks layer represents the social and peer groups within which people function on a daily basis. These networks can influence individual decision making and may support or block individual behavior change. They can also define acceptable and unacceptable behavior within the neighborhood, workplace, church, and larger community.
- The living and working conditions layer refers to the immediate environmental factors in which the person must function. These include such things as the air, water, transportation, and food options; opportunities for nutrition, health care, education, and exercise; and possible environmental exposures to harmful substances.
- The broad social, economic, cultural, health, and environmental conditions and policies at the global, national, state, and local levels layer addresses the multiple ecosocial influences on health and behavior. It is at this level where consideration is given to factors that facilitate or limit access to care providers, promote or negatively affect health outcomes, encourage or discourage behaviors that are risky, and foster or curtail social action to improve society.

KEY POINTS

- Old age is defined by age as well as other societal considerations.
- One's lifecourse is important as it reflects a more comprehensive explanation of the various factors that contribute to the aging process than age alone.
- Health promotion is a vital component of disease prevention and health maintenance for adults of any age.
- Individual behavior change is influenced by a variety of factors, some of which are outside the control of the individual.
- Self-efficacy is an important addition to our understanding of why people differ in their ability to make behavior change.
- Individual behavior change can be facilitated or hindered by factors that occur at levels above that of the individual. Population-level change models help to explain these higher-level concerns and suggest points of intervention to support change at the individual level.
- Social justice is an important concept for both individual-and community-level behavior change. The patient-as-partner approach and the ecological model can be combined to provide care that is more socially just.

CRITICAL THINKING ACTIVITIES

1. Visit a senior housing residence in your neighborhood. Evaluate the neighborhood. Does it appear safe and well lit at night? Are grocery stores, pharmacies, and other resources nearby? How does the community support its older adults? Is there a senior center, public transportation, library, or churches that might provide important services?
2. Using the PRECEDE-PROCEED Model as a guide, what additional information would you want to assess in the previously described neighborhood?
3. Arrange an interview with a staff member of the local Area Agency on Aging to learn what services they provide.
4. Consider the following situation. You are caring for a diabetic patient who is not well controlled with oral hypoglycemic medication and will need to learn how to inject insulin. The patient has a history of fainting whenever he has blood drawn and tells you he has a fear of needles. Using the Health Belief Model and Self-Efficacy Theory as a framework, how might you strategize your teaching? This patient would be in which Stage of Change?

CASE STUDY | *HARRIET AND SMOKING CESSATION*

This chapter's case study demonstrates the usefulness of the Ecological Model and its interaction with individual-focused interventions, and it also draws together information from other models discussed in the chapter. The case study is presented in segments that a lifecourse as well as an episodic perspective of factors involved in the case. It provides a perspective of the social changes that allow individual behavior changes to succeed, while also examining some of the processes involved in individual change. For these reasons, this case study is longer than others in this book.

Smoking is one of the most harmful behaviors in which a person can engage. It affects every major organ system, and second-hand smoke harms those around the smoker (U.S. Department of Health and Human Services, 2004). Smoking is also one of the most difficult behaviors to change because of the addictive nature of nicotine and because of the social cues that support smoking behavior. It usually takes several attempts before a smoker can become smoke free (U.S. Department of Health and Human Services, 1998). Smoking is a social phenomenon that is linked to other behaviors, like eating and drinking. The decision to smoke is influenced by depictions of smoking and tobacco products in movies, on television, and in advertisements.

Brief Health and Social History

Harriet is a 78-year-old white female who worked most of her life in a factory in a northeastern "rust-belt" city. Because she was a line worker assembling parts that went into small appliances, she had no pension benefits or retirement plan contributions. She earned just enough to pay for her monthly living expenses, with a small amount left over for small luxuries. As a result, she now lives in senior housing, which means that her rent is subsidized by state and federal funds because her income is low and she has no other financial assets to draw upon. She lives on a fixed income of $620 monthly from Social Security and receives Medicare/Medicaid combined benefits to partly cover her health care costs. Her ever-increasing health care copayments are a concern to her because she is on a fixed income. She has little money in her budget to pay for extras, so cigarettes are for her a substitute for entertainment, cable television, and dinners out. She has smoked for more than 50 years, starting in high school and continuing through her working years. All of her friends and coworkers smoked as well. For much of Harriett's adult life, people smoked wherever she went. Her motivation to quit smoking now comes from the recent deaths of close friends from smoking-related causes and the need to conserve her money. Cigarettes cost her about $40/week or $160/month—one-quarter of her monthly income.

Clinical Management

Harriet went to the local Community Health Center to see her nurse practitioner. During that visit, Harriet asked about ways to stop smoking. Her practitioner used the five A's (Ask, Advise, Assess, Assist, Arrange) approach to cessation counseling and found Harriet receptive to quitting (*Helping Smokers Quit,* 2009). The nurse practitioner provided assistance and information on various methods of smoking cessation. She also explained that this behavior change could take several attempts to be successful.

After further assessment of her current health, choice of cessation methods, and ability to adhere to the plan, Harriet left the Community Health Center with a plan for support, a follow-up appointment, and enough resources at her disposal to "kick the habit." She selected nicotine patches in a decreasing dosage so she could control the expected withdrawal symptoms. She also had nicotine gum to supplement the patches, if needed. Harriet joined a telephone support group, run by a registered nurse and open to others trying to quit smoking, so she had someone to call if she felt unable to manage on her own. She could also call the nurse practitioner if these approaches did not seem to be helping.

CASE STUDY | *HARRIET AND SMOKING CESSATION*—cont'd

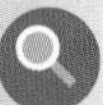

EVIDENCE FOR PRACTICE
Approach to Smoking Cessation

Harriet's nurse practitioner used an evidence-based approach to smoking cessation that was specifically designed for primary care clinicians and published as a clinical practice guideline by the U.S. Department of Health and Human Services.

Sample: The updated 2008 guideline includes the results of almost 9,000 research articles published between 1975 and 1999.

Methods: Members of a multiagency governmental and nonprofit public health consortium conducted extensive literature searches to develop updated recommendations for effective clinical treatments for nicotine addiction.

Results: Based on literature review, peer review, and public comment, the 2008 guideline reveals substantial progress in the rate at which smokers are advised to quit smoking and in the intensity and success of smoking cessation interventions. It provides 10 key recommendations aimed at maintaining and increasing the rate at which clinicians advise patients to quit smoking and at making sure patients have access to effective treatments.

Implications: The 2008 guideline contains many resources and strategies for helping patients quit smoking. One such strategy is the 5 A's (like on p..104) approach, which includes these steps:

- Ask about tobacco use.
- Advise the patient to quit.
- Assess the patient's willingness to try quitting.
- Assist the patient in the attempt to quit.
- Arrange for follow-up.

Evidence suggests that using all 5 A's yields better results than using only some of them.

Reference: Fiore, M., Jaén, C., Baker, T., et al. (2008). *Treating Tobacco Use and Dependence: 2008 Update. Clinical Practice Guideline.* Rockville, MD: U.S. Department of Health and Human Services. Public Health Service. Retrieved November 27, 2010, from http://www.surgeongeneral.gov/tobacco/treating_tobacco_use08.pdf

Societal Change to Support Cessation

There were other changes, however, that contributed to both Harriet's decision to quit smoking and to her provider's ability to help her quit smoking. When Harriet was younger, almost all of her family, friends, and coworkers smoked. Everywhere she went people smoked, including hotels, movie theaters, restaurants, bars, and stores. Her doctor even smoked during her periodic visits! The tobacco industry had incredible influence within state and federal government, lobbying for farm subsidies for growing tobacco, tax credits for manufacturing facilities, and contracts to distribute tobacco products on government sites. The tobacco industry also hired psychologists to better understand consumer behavior and to develop marketing methods to reach people who were less likely to smoke. They provided free tobacco products to the armed forces during World War II, gave away free samples on street corners and in restaurants, and created new products that appealed to women and African-Americans (Glantz et al., 1998). By 1964, the Advisory Committee to the Surgeon General issued its landmark report titled *Smoking and Health* (U.S. Department of Health, Education, and Welfare, 1964). In response to the

Continued

CASE STUDY | *HARRIET AND SMOKING CESSATION*—cont'd

many people who stopped smoking as a result of this report, the tobacco industry increased sales and marketing efforts.

As Harriet got older, she had friends who became ill with respiratory diseases, friends who died because of smoking-related illnesses such as heart disease and hypertension, and friends who quit smoking. As her age cohort shrank in size due to death, Harriet became more aware of the decrease in smoking around her.

From the 1980s until more recently, laws were enacted to establish smoke-free worksites, buses, public spaces, and restaurants. She now had to leave the building in most places if she needed to smoke. Taxes on cigarette purchases continued to rise on a regular basis, making them an increasing percentage of her monthly expenditures, and her nurse practitioner constantly provided her with new information on the harmful effects that smoking could have on her health. At first Harriet just ignored the information. After all, she was well over 65 years old! Surely quitting smoking would not benefit her at this point.

Harriet noticed that she became short of breath walking up the stairs in her apartment building. She also had a persistent cough that got worse if she had the slightest cold. Once, she developed pneumonia that required hospitalization in part because of the damage that smoking caused in her lungs. While in the hospital, she was not allowed to smoke due to the oxygen therapy she received and the risk of fire and explosion the oxygen presented. Several of the registered nurses talked with her about quitting smoking and described the damage to her lungs from this behavior. That hospitalization was the only other time that she had stopped smoking. As soon as she returned home from the hospital, the cigarettes were there and, with little else to keep her occupied during the day, she was soon smoking just as much as before her pneumonia episode and hospitalization.

Now, however, she was ready to quit smoking. In addition to the mutually developed treatment plan, she also agreed to two positive incentives. First, she was placing $50 each month into a savings account to be used for entertainment. Going out with other older adults was her personal reward for stopping smoking. Second, the Medicare Health Maintenance Organization (HMO) she belonged to reduced her copayments if she successfully stopped smoking. This change made even more of her monthly income available to pay bills. This HMO also provided a telephone resource nurse whom she could call with any questions. All of these changes she believed would motivate her to quit and stay smoke-free.

Bumpy Road to Recovery

Harriet found that all the motivation and supports were not enough, at first. Within days, she was smoking again. She had not used the telephone support group or the HMO resource nurse because she felt as though she had let everyone down. A follow-up telephone call from her nurse practitioner, however, was just what she needed. After a good cry and chat about what went wrong, Harriet was willing to try again. Her nurse practitioner had suggested that Harriet try hypnosis as an adjunct to her other methods and recommended a nontraditional health specialist near her apartment building. Although the hypnosis session cost her some money out-of-pocket, she found that she was now able to get through breakfast and the mid-afternoon without needing to smoke. At her next scheduled visit with the nurse practitioner a month later, Harriet was smoke free for 2 weeks.

At this point, her nurse practitioner suggested that Harriet begin walking after breakfast and in the mid-afternoon. Her thinking was that, because these seemed to be the most difficult periods of Harriet's day, supplanting a positive behavior for the negative one might help Harriet. In addition, the walking should help increase Harriet's endurance and decrease her shortness of breath. After some additional discussion, Harriet agreed to try this plan. Again, Harriet had some difficulty implementing this additional change. First it rained. Then a friend stopped by

CASE STUDY | *HARRIET AND SMOKING CESSATION*—cont'd

just as she was getting ready to go out, so she stayed in and talked instead. But 2 weeks later she went out for a walk. She started slowly, as her nurse practitioner suggested, but soon was walking over 1 mile every day. Two weeks after that, she had increased her pace and distance. She did call the HMO resource nurse for suggestions on better shoes for walking and on nutritional changes she could make to keep from gaining weight. Harriet was now smoke free for 2 months and was actually feeling better physically. She noticed that she only felt short of breath when climbing more than one flight of stairs and seldom when just walking. She also noticed that she felt stronger, more able to do things like cleaning her apartment, than she had in the months prior to these behavior changes. As a treat, she took the bus to the mall, bought herself lunch at a restaurant, and purchased some walking shoes to replace the older shoes she had been wearing. All of these changes reinforced that it had been a good decision to stop smoking.

Unexpected Benefits

The next visit Harriet made to the nurse practitioner was for her yearly visit. She was surprised to find that she had lost 20 pounds! Part of her weight loss was clearly due to the amount of walking she was doing—almost 2 miles each day. Her second surprise was that her blood pressure, which had always been higher than normal, was now below normal. Her weight loss and increased exercise combined to lower her blood pressure, and the nurse practitioner took her off her antihypertensive medication. The nurse practitioner also suggested some higher protein foods that Harriet might try to further build up her muscle mass. Plus, she added some exercises to strengthen muscles not affected by walking. These additional exercises would address upper body strength and balance. The nurse practitioner praised Harriet for her success at making such difficult life changes and reminded her how far she had come in a relatively short time. The nurse practitioner also suggested that Harriet explore an indoor walking group that met at the local mall because colder weather was coming and she wanted Harriet to continue these activities.

1. What parts of the models of individual behavior change would explain why people do not change behavior when presented with information alone?
2. Using the Ecological Model of Health, which factors in her lifecourse fit into the living and working conditions and encouraged her smoking behavior?
3. What social and environmental factors made it easier for Harriet to quit smoking at this point in her life?
4. At what points did various nurses interact with Harriet? Why might have some nurses been more effective than others?

REFERENCES

Bandura, A. (1977). Self-efficacy: Toward a unifying theory of behavioral change. *Psychological Review, 84*(2), 191-215.

Calkins, E., Boult, C., Wagner, E., & Pacala, J. (1999). *New ways to care for older people: Building systems based on evidence.* New York: Springer.

Chodzko-Zajko, W. (2001). The national blueprint: Increasing physical activity among adults age 50 and older. *Journal of Aging and Physical Activity, 9*(Suppl.).

Dahlberg, L., & Krug, E. (2002). Violence: A global public health problem. In E. Krug, L. Dahlberg, J. Mercy, A. Zwi, & R. Lozano (Eds.), *World report on violence and health.* (pp. 1–19). Geneva, Switzerland: World Health Organization.

Federal Interagency Forum on Age-Related Statistics. (2008). *Older Americans 2008: Key indicators of well-being.* Washington, DC: U.S. Government Printing Office.

Fiore, M., Jaén, C., Baker, T., Bailey, W. C., Benowitz, N. L., Curry, S. J., . . . Wewers, M. E. (2008). *Treating tobacco use and dependence: 2008 update.* Clinical Practice Guideline. Rockville, MD: U.S. Department of Health and Human Services. Public Health Service.

Fishbein, M., Middlestadt, S., & Hitchcock, P. (1991). Using information to change STD related behaviors: An analysis based on the theory of reasoned action. In J. Wasserheit, S. Aral, & K. Holmes (Eds.), *Research issues in human behavior and sexually transmitted diseases in the AIDS era.* (pp. 243–257). Washington, DC: American Society for Microbiology.

Gebbie, K., Rosenstock, D., & Hernandez, L. (2003). *Who will keep the public healthy?: Educating public health professionals for the 21st Century.* Washington, DC: National Academies Press.

Glantz, S., Slade, J., Bero, L., Hanauer, P., & Barnes, L. (1998). *The cigarette papers.* Berkeley: University of California Press.

Green, L., & Kreuter, M. (2005). *Health program planning: An educational and ecological approach* (4th ed.). Boston: McGraw Hill.

Greiner, P., Snowdon, D., & Greiner, L. (1999). Self-rated function, self-rated health, and postmortem evidence of brain infarcts: Findings from the nun study. *Journal of Gerontology: Social Sciences, 54B*(4), S219-S222.

Helping smokers quit: A guide for clinicians. (2008, May). Agency for Healthcare Research and Quality. Rockville, MD. Retrieved November 26, 2010, from http://www.ahrq.gov/clinic/tobacco/clinhlpsmksqt.htm

Improving Chronic Illness Care. (2009). *The chronic care model.* Retrieved November 27, 2010, from http://www.improvingchroniccare.org/index.php?p=The_Chronic_Care_Model&s=2

Institute of Medicine. (2003). *The future of the public's health in the 21st century.* Washington, D.C.: The National Academies Press.

Janz, N., & Becker, M. (1984). The health belief model: A decade later. *Health Education Quarterly, 11*(1),1-47.

Krieger, N. (2001). Theories for social epidemiology in the 21st century: An ecosocial perspective. *International Journal of Epidemiology, 30,* 668-677.

National Institute on Aging. (2009). *DBSR review committee report.* Retrieved November 27, 2010, from http://www.nia.nih.gov/ResearchInformation/ExtramuralPrograms/BehavioralAndSocialResearch/

Olshansky, S., & Carnes, B. (2001). *The quest for immortality,* New York: Norton.

Pender, N., Murdaugh, C., & Parsons, M. (2006). *Health promotion in nursing practice* (5th ed.). Upper Saddle River, NJ: Pearson.

Rosenstock I., Strecher, V., & Becker, M. (1994).The Health Belief Model and HIV risk behavior change. In R.J. DiClemente, and J.L.Peterson (Eds.), Preventing AIDS: Theories and Methods of Behavioral Interventions (pp. 5-24). New York: Plenum Press.

Robert Wood Johnson Foundation. (2009). *Commission to build a healthier America.* Retrieved November 26, 2010, from http://www.commissiononhealth.org/

Suzman, R., Willis, D., & Manton, K. (1996). *The oldest old.* Oxford, UK: Oxford University Press.

U.S. Department of Health and Human Services. (1998). *The health consequences of smoking. Nicotine addiction: A report of the Surgeon General.* Washington, DC: U.S. Government Printing Office.

U.S. Department of Health and Human Services. (2000). *Healthy people 2010: Understanding and improving health* (2nd ed.). Washington, DC: U.S. Government Printing Office.

U.S. Department of Health and Human Services. (2004). *The health consequences of smoking: A report of the Surgeon General.* Washington, DC: U.S. Government Printing Office.

U.S. Department of Health and Human Services. (2010). *Healthy people 2020 framework.* Retrieved November 27, 2010, from http://healthypeople.gov/2020/

U.S. Department of Health, Education, and Welfare. (1964). *Smoking and health.* Washington, DC: U.S. Government Printing Office.

Velicer, W., Prochaska, J., Fava, J., Norman, G., & Redding, C. (1998) Smoking cessation and stress management: Applications of the transtheoretical model of behavior change. *Homeostasis, 38,* 216-233.

Wilkinson, R., & Marmot, M. (2003). *Social determinants of health: The solid facts* (2nd ed.). Copenhagen, Denmark: World Health Organization.

Unit II

Optimizing Physical Health and Functioning

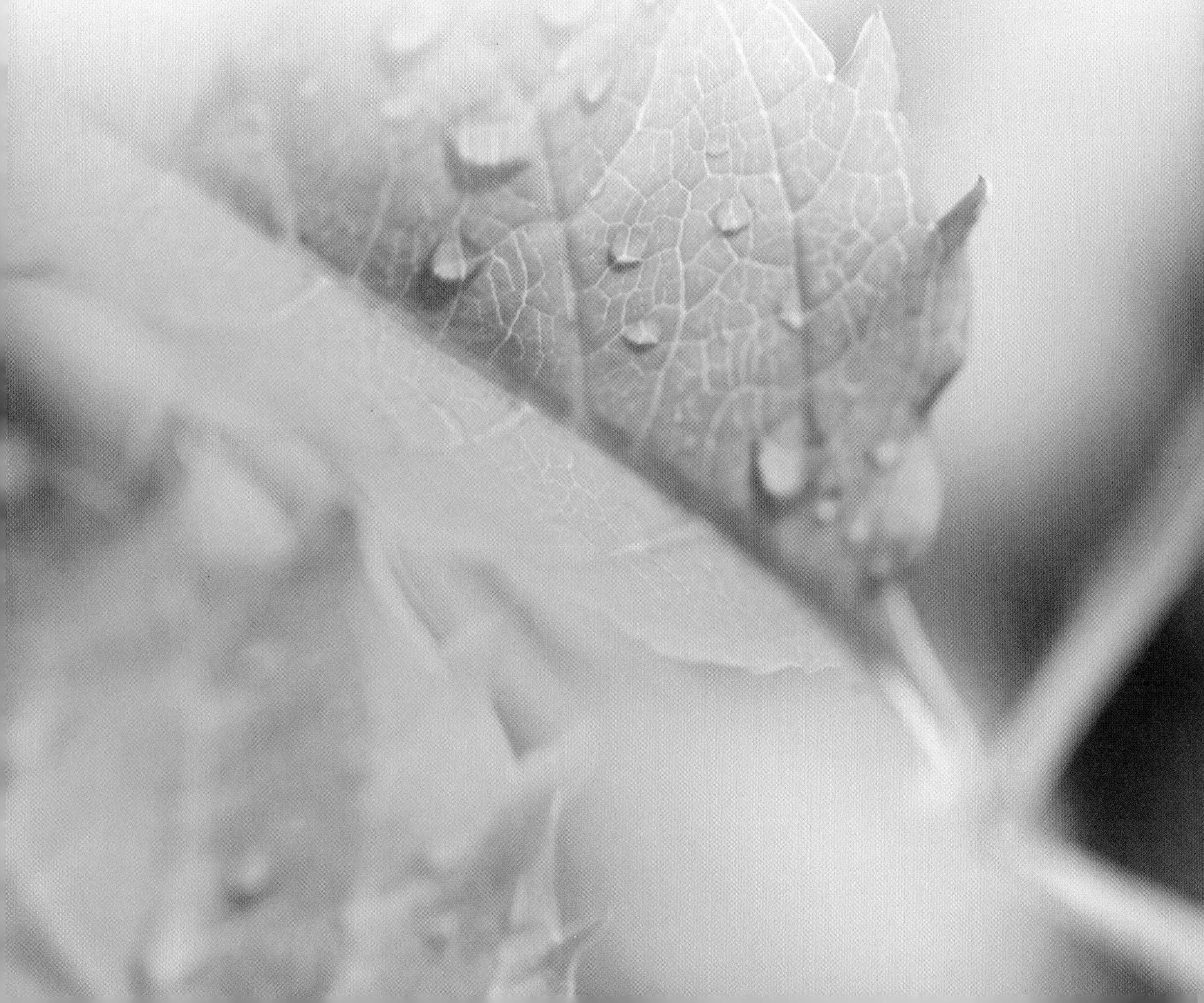

Chapter 7

Health Priorities for the Older Adult

Kathryn A. Blair, PhD, FNP-BC, FAANP

LEARNING OBJECTIVES

- Review the 2020 health care priorities for older adults.
- Explain the role of prevention and early identification of disease in the older adult as a means to promote healthy aging.
- Outline the role of the nurse in meeting the health care priorities for older adults.
- Detail the role of exercise and adequate nutrition in both the physical and mental health of the aging individual.
- Identify appropriate screening for older adults.

Health care providers play an important role in the process of guiding older adults toward healthy aging, a process that should integrate health maintenance and disease prevention. As early as 1979, the U.S. Surgeon General proposed national goals to reduce premature deaths and to maintain the independence of older adults. The document containing these national goals was called *Healthy People: The Surgeon General's Report on Health Promotion and Disease Prevention* (U.S. Department of Health, Education, and Welfare, 1979). Since that time, the nation's prevention goals have been updated in *Healthy People 2000, Healthy People 2010,* and the currently *Healthy People 2020* (U.S. Department of Health & Human Services, n.d.). The purpose of the *Healthy People* documents was and is to design a template that promotes health, prevents illness, reduces disability, and lowers the rate of premature deaths. Table 7-1 lists goals and indicators from *Healthy People 2010.*Delete this table Box 7-1 lists objectives for older adults as in *Healthy People 2020.*

To review *Healthy People 2020* in its entirety is beyond the scope of this chapter; however, the chapter provides an overview of some of the components of healthy aging as laid out in *Healthy People.* Topics to be introduced include health promotion, patient education, access to care, physical activity, nutrition, fall prevention, smoking cessation, immunizations, mental health, and preventive screening in the older adult. An in-depth analysis of these issues appears in subsequent chapters.

Health Promotion

Since the beginning of the 20th century, nurses have assumed responsibility for improving health across the life span through prevention and health promotion strategies (Wilhelmsson & Lindberg, 2007). Nurse-led interventions (patient education, care coordination, and health promotion) have resulted in better physical functioning and reduced health care costs for older adults (Meng, Wamsley, Eggert, & Van Nosttrand, 2007; Ozminkowski et al., 2006).

Indeed, the health of the nation is dependent on reducing the occurrence and the need to manage chronic diseases. Recent estimates indicate that 40% of premature deaths annually are caused by chronic diseases linked to preventable or modifiable behaviors (Zoorob & Morelli, 2008). The elderly have the greatest risk for developing or having multiple chronic diseases that may interfere with optimal physical and mental functioning (DeJonge, Taler, & Boling, 2009).

About 40% of premature deaths are caused by chronic diseases linked to preventable or modifiable behaviors.

TABLE 7-1 *Healthy People 2010:* Goals, Indicators, and Focus Areas

Goals	Increase quality and years of healthy life Eliminate health disparities
Leading indicators	Physical activity Overweight and obesity Tobacco use Substance abuse Responsible sexual behavior Mental health Injury and violence Environmental quality Immunization Access to health care
Focus areas	Access to quality health services Arthritis, osteoporosis, and chronic back conditions Cancer Chronic kidney disease Diabetes Disability and secondary conditions Educational and community-based programs Environmental health Family planning Food safety Health communication Heart disease and stroke HIV Immunization and infectious diseases Injury and violence prevention Maternal, infant, and child health Medical product safety Mental health and mental disorders Nutrition and overweight Occupational safety and health Oral health Physical activity and fitness Public health infrastructure Respiratory disease Sexually transmitted diseases Substance abuse Tobacco use Vision and hearing

From http://healthypeople.gov/2020/

BOX 7-1 Objectives from *Healthy People 2020* for Older Adults

- Reduce the proportion of older adults who have moderate to severe functional limitations.
- Reduce the proportion of unpaid caregivers of older adults who report an unmet need for caregiver support services. (Developmental)
- Increase the proportion of older adults with one or more chronic health conditions who report confidence in managing their conditions. (Developmental)
- Reduce the proportion of noninstitutionalized older adults with disabilities who have an unmet need for long-term services and supports. (Developmental)
- Reduce the rate of pressure ulcer–related hospitalizations among older adults.
- Increase the proportion of the health care workforce with geriatric certification.
- Increase the number of States and Tribes that publicly report elder maltreatment and neglect.
- Increase the proportion of older adults with reduced physical or cognitive function who engage in light, moderate, or vigorous leisure-time physical activities.
- Reduce the rate of emergency department visits due to falls among older adults.

From U.S. Department of Health & Human Services. (2009). Healthy People 2020 Public Meetings: 2009 Draft Objectives. Retrieved November 10, 2010, from http://healthypeople.gov/2020

Health promotion is an interdisciplinary and multidimensional process that encompasses prevention, screening, and disease management. Its components include risk assessment, health education, and addressing such topics as physical activity, nutrition, stress management, smoking cessation, and immunizations. Although the full benefits of health promotion are realized through lifetime behaviors, data suggest health promotion activities have a positive effect even when started later in life (Nelson et al., 2007). In fact, even frail older adults can profit from health promotion (Markle-Reid et al., 2006).

Patient Education

The foundation of health promotion and prevention is effective patient education. This requires that the nurse be familiar with basic principles of adult learning as they apply to the older adult (Polzien, 2006). These principles include the following:

- Adult learners want to be partners in the educational offering instead of being passive recipients.
- Adult learners will filter information through their value system.
- Adult learners will use life experiences to integrate concepts.
- Adult learners are self-directed.

Before an educational program can be designed and teaching can begin, the patient should be assessed for readiness to learn, current knowledge, and ability to change. A simple assessment should address the following questions.

- Is the older adult motivated to learn?
- Does the older adult have the ability to learn, or is there a sensory or cognitive barrier?
- What is the older adult's attitude about the benefits of change?
- Does the older adult have the skills and support systems needed for change to occur?

Nurses should then individualize each educational session to meet the patient's needs and learning style (Box 7-2). When planning educational offerings, nurses must appreciate that intelligence does not decline with age, but processing and comprehension of information may require more time for the older adult (Thomas, 2007). Additional considerations would include making sure that visual aides are large enough for the elderly to see and that audio presentations are slow enough and loud enough for the older adult to hear and process (Mauk, 2006). Finally, make sure to include written material if the patient is literate and allow time for questions.

BOX 7-2 Understanding Learning Styles

Some people are auditory learners, meaning that they learn best by hearing educational materials spoken aloud. Other people are visual learners, meaning that they learn best by reading. Finally, some people are kinetic learners, meaning that they learn best through active engagement in a task that fosters learning. Because most adult learners have a mixed style of learning, health educators should try to incorporate elements of all three learning styles for each patient.

Access to Care

For elders to participate in health promotion and disease prevention, they must be able to access the health care delivery system. Organizational barriers for older adults and particularly for minorities include not knowing how to make appointments, lack of referral for services needed, waiting lists, language barriers, transportation problems, and conflicting treatment options.

Policy at the state level can also serve as a barrier to care for older adults. A recent study found that more than 70% of eligible older adults were not enrolled in supplemental Medicaid (Ungaro & Federman, 2009). Even older adults with dual Medicare and Medicaid, especially low-income African Americans, were less likely to receive preventive care, follow-up care, and medical testing (Niefeld & Kasper, 2005).

Another consideration that impacts access to care is provider density, or the number of health care providers per capita in a community or region (Pathman, Ricketts, & Konrad, 2006). Access to care is especially difficult for rural-dwelling older adults because often the supply of health care providers is very limited. When the community has no provider, older adults may choose not to seek health care rather than travel long distances to the closest source.

If nurses are to be effective in promoting health and successful aging, they must serve as change agents to improve access to care for older adults. One way to facilitate this change is through political activism at the local and state levels by participating in professional nursing organizations. Other ways to help older adults access care include becoming familiar with volunteer and local agencies that provide services for older adults and developing relationships with local health care providers.

If nurses are to be effective in promoting health and successful aging, they must serve as change agents to improve access to care for older adults.

Physical Activity

Increasing exercise is a national health priority, especially for older adults. The physical benefits of exercise are well known and include increased muscle strength, flexibility, and improved balance, and yet less than one third of older adults participate in regular physical activity (Hildebrand & Neufel, 2009). Not only does increased activity (physical, leisure, or both) confer physical benefits but psychological benefits as well. Older adults who remain active have less depression, anxiety, and loneliness (Lampinen, Heikkinen, Kauppinen, & Heikkinen, 2006).

FOCUS ON SAFETY
Starting and Exercise Program

The focus of increased activity among older adults should be on balance, aerobic activity of moderate intensity, and flexibility exercises (Nelson et al., 2007). When instituting an exercise program, activity should increase in a stepwise approach, starting with reducing sedentary behaviors and gradually increasing muscle strength (Nelson et al., 2007).

As with any health promotion activity, motivating and sustaining the behavior can be problematic. One successful strategy may be incorporating a group or neighborhood approach, rather than focusing on the individual participant (Jancey, 2008). Another consideration to facilitate participation is to be realistic about the types of activities expected of the older adult.

Nutrition

Poor nutrition is a major contributor to the four leading causes of premature death: coronary heart disease, cancer, stroke, and diabetes (Chahbazi & Grow, 2008). As part of normal aging, older adults may experience a variety of changes associated with alterations in nutrition. For example, many older adults have reduced lean body mass and increased fat mass, which in turn increases the risk of insulin resistance and obesity. In addition, access to food for older adults may be problematic, especially when transportation is a problem.

Some older adults develop a condition called anorexia of aging. This is a physiologic reduction in appetite that has been associated with impaired immune function, altered cognitive function, poor wound healing, and reduced bone mass (Chapman, 2006). Its etiology may be associated with a reduced energy expenditure, but other contributing factors include living alone, being depressed, having poor dentition, and having a reduced sense of smell and taste.

In contrast to those who develop anorexia of aging, some older adults struggle with obesity. Current predictions suggest that the prevalence of obesity will increase to 5.4% of the aging population (Harrington & Lee-Chiong, 2009). Being overweight does not necessarily indicate adequate nutrition and confers an increased risk of diabetes, hypertension, cardiovascular disease, and arthritis.

Basic dietary education guidelines should include the need to limit fat consumption to 25% to 30% of total caloric intake, increase fiber intake to 30 grams for men and 21 grams for women over age 50, and reduce salt intake to about 2,300 mg daily for those without heart disease (Shewmacke & Huntington, 2009). Any nutritional program also should examine strategies to address vitamin and mineral deficiencies, which may occur whether an older adult is underweight or overweight. Commonly deficient vitamins and minerals include vitamin D, calcium, vitamin B_{12}, and folate (Shewmacke & Huntington, 2009).

Finally, the psychosocial component of nutrition should not be ignored. Older adults who eat with others may have a greater overall intake (Krondl, Coleman, & Lau, 2008).

Fall Prevention

Recent statistics indicate that 5.8 million adults age 65 and older reported falling, with 1.8 million older adults sustaining an injury that needed medical intervention (Stevens, Mack, Paulozzi, & Ballesteros, 2008). Unintentional injuries, such as hip fracture after falling, are the fifth leading cause of death in older adults (Moylan & Binder, 2007). Risk factors for falling include muscle weakness, gait and balance problems, polypharmacy, vision problems, and orthostatic hypotension. All of these are modifiable risks that can be addressed by nurses.

Unintentional injuries, such as hip fracture after falling, are the fifth leading cause of death in older adults.

Nurses can begin by recognizing conditions that may increase the risk for falling in the healthy older adult. For example, a neurologic disorder (e.g., vestibular disorders), musculoskeletal disorder (e.g., osteoarthritis or kyphosis), sleep disorder, depression, or substance abuse (e.g., alcohol) may all be risk factors. Environmental hazards also should be evaluated as well, by assessing the older adult's home for such risks as cluttered, damaged, or slippery floors and inadequate lighting.

Two simple balance tests that nurses can perform to assess older adults are the Romberg and Get Up and Go (GUG) test (American Academy of Neurology, n.d.). The Romberg test is performed by having the older adult stand with eyes closed; it allows assessment of cerebellar function, which is responsible for balance. The GUG test is performed by having the older adult rise from a chair and walk a designated distance and then return to the chair. This test evaluates gait and balance.

Evidence suggests that a decline in cognitive function increases the risk for falls (McMichael, VanderBilt, Lavery, Rodriguez, & Ganguly, 2008). A tool commonly used to assess cognitive function is the Mini Mental State Examination (MMSE). It allows evaluation of cognitive function by assessing orientation, attention, calculation, recall, language, and motor skills. (To see a copy, go to http://www.nmaging.state.nm.us/pdf_files/Mini_Mental_Status_Exam.pdf)

For older adults at risk of falling, nurses can develop specific interventions that could include exercises to improve balance, leg strength, and gait. Evidence strongly supports the notion that performing such exercises reduces falls (Yokoya, Demura, & Sato, 2008). Another strategy to reduce falls involves modifying the environment by removing such hazards as throw rugs and employing assistive devices such as handrails and raised toilet seats (Rubenstein & Josephson, 2006).

Smoking Cessation

The medical consequences of smoking are well documented and include an increased risk for cancer, stroke, cardiovascular disease, peripheral vascular disease, chronic obstructive pulmonary disease, and reduced brain function (Crane, 2007; Flicker, 2010). Unfortunately, discussions of smoking cessation are relatively uncommon between older adults and health care providers because both patient and provider may feel that there would be little benefit. However, evidence points strongly to the contrary. Smoking cessation in older adults can reduce the risks and reduce comorbid conditions (Whitson, Helfin, & Burchett, 2006).

Numerous strategies exist to aid in smoking cessation, including nicotine replacement, external support systems, and drug interventions. Nurses can facilitate the transition from smoker to nonsmoker by serving as a support system. Nurses can also educate older adults about the risks of smoking and the benefits of smoking cessation.

To help older adults stop smoking, nurses must be aware of the characteristics of people who are likely to quit. These include living with someone, having mobility problems, being a nondrinker, and having smoked for a shorter duration. People who are more likely to stop smoking include women and those (both male and female) with a recent cancer diagnosis (Abdullah et al., 2006). About 35% to 45% of patients who stop smoking will relapse (Whitson, Heflin, & Burchett, 2006); therefore, nurses should be vigilant and continue to ask about smoking at each encounter with a patient.

Immunizations

Immune senescence and the increased presence of comorbid conditions (such as diabetes and obesity) make older adults particularly vulnerable to the adverse effects of infectious diseases. Immunization is a proven prevention strategy in the total care of healthy older adults and yet is often forgotten, avoided, or unavailable. High (2007) reported that immunization rates among older adults lag behind national goals despite evidence that an annual influenza vaccination is cost-effective for those age 65 and older as measured by quality-adjusted life years (Maciosek, Solberg, Coffield, Edwards, & Goodman, 2006). Two common barriers to older adults receiving vaccinations are access and fear. Many elders fear that immunization will cause the disease it is designed to prevent.

Immunizations that nurses should address with older adults include the pneumococcal vaccine, annual influenza vaccine, zoster vaccine, and tetanus boosters. Nurses can educate older adults about the safety of vaccines and recommend appropriate immunizations at each encounter. To improve access to immunization, nurses can set up immunization clinics at the local senior center.

Mental Health

Sustaining mental well-being and recognizing mental health issues are priorities when caring for the aging population. Older adults are at increased risk for mental health issues because of their significant life losses (health, partners, jobs, etc.) and medication side effects. However, many older adults avoid seeking mental health care because of the stigma of mental illness, the perceived cost of care, or the sense that mental and emotional issues should not be talked about.

Nurses are responsible for addressing the whole person, including not just physical health but also mental and spiritual health. This means explaining to the older adult that mental health and well-being does not mean simply the absence of a diagnosable mental illness but continued growth, development, and fulfillment throughout the lifespan.

Nurses can help older adults avoid social isolation by identifying community resources. Nurses can highlight older adults' strengths rather than their weaknesses. At community and state levels, nurses can help formulate public health programs to assess and address the mental health issues of the aging population.

Prevention and Screening

Prevention of diseases and their complications is a major health goal when caring for older adults. Prevention efforts may be primary, secondary, or tertiary (Box 7-3). The value of primary prevention is clear, but role of secondary prevention is less clear for older adults who have reached their 70s and beyond.

The mainstay of any prevention model is screening, and guidelines are available for many diseases. Table 7-2 lists screening and counseling resources from the U.S. Preventive Services Task Force.

Cancer is a common focus of screening efforts, and although age is a risk factor for cancer, there are no specific guidelines for cancer screening in older adults. However, data suggest that the more comorbid conditions a person has, the less effective cancer screening becomes, especially in terms of cost-benefit (Terret, Castel-Kramer, Albrand, & Droz, 2009).

BOX 7-3 Types of Prevention

- Primary prevention focuses on behaviors that reduce the risk of chronic disease, such as maintaining a normal weight to reduce the risk of diabetes or having recommended vaccinations to prevent infectious disease.
- Secondary prevention focuses on screening for disease in its earliest stages, before it is evident. An example is mammography used to screen for breast cancer.
- Tertiary prevention focuses on treating and managing disease as effectively as possible to reduce the risk of complications. An example is treating hypertension to reduce the risk of myocardial infarction and stroke.

TABLE 7-2 Resources for Health Screening and Counseling

The U.S. Preventive Services Task Force provides the following resources, available on the Internet, for primary care screening and counseling.

SCREENING TOPIC	INTERNET RESOURCE
Coronary heart disease	http://www.uspreventiveservicestaskforce.org/uspstf/uspsacad.htm
Coronary heart disease, nontraditional risk factors	http://www.uspreventiveservicestaskforce.org/uspstf/uspscoronaryhd.htm
High blood pressure	http://www.uspreventiveservicestaskforce.org/uspstf/uspshype.htm
Lipid disorders	http://www.uspreventiveservicestaskforce.org/uspstf/uspschol.htm
Diabetes type 2	http://www.uspreventiveservicestaskforce.org/uspstf/uspsdiab.htm
Breast cancer	http://www.uspreventiveservicestaskforce.org/uspstf/uspsbrca.htm
Colorectal cancer	http://www.uspreventiveservicestaskforce.org/uspstf/uspscolo.htm
Cervical cancer	http://www.uspreventiveservicestaskforce.org/uspstf/uspscerv.htm
Ovarian cancer	http://www.uspreventiveservicestaskforce.org/uspstf/uspsovar.htm
Prostate cancer	http://www.uspreventiveservicestaskforce.org/uspstf/uspsprca.htm
Visual acuity	http://www.uspreventiveservicestaskforce.org/uspstf/uspsviseld.htm
Obesity	http://www.uspreventiveservicestaskforce.org/uspstf/uspsobes.htm
COUNSELING TOPIC	**INTERNET RESOURCE**
Tobacco use	http://www.uspreventiveservicestaskforce.org/uspstf/uspstbac2.htm
Diet	http://www.uspreventiveservicestaskforce.org/uspstf/uspsdiet.htm
Exercise	http://www.uspreventiveservicestaskforce.org/uspstf/uspsphys.htm

EVIDENCE FOR PRACTICE
Cancer Screening in Older Women

Purpose: The authors hypothesized that cancer screening for older women regardless of health status would not be a priority for health care providers, and preventive services such as immunizations and exercise counseling would be underutilized.

Sample: Data were gathered from the 2005 National Health Interview Survey. The final sample included 4,683 women age 65 and older. The sample was categorized into five age groups: those ages 65 to 69, those ages 70 to 74, those ages 75 to 79, those ages 80 to 84, and those age 85 and older.

Methods: Data extracted from the survey included cancer screening (mammography, colon cancer screening, and Pap smears), immunizations (pneumococcus and influenza), and exercise counseling. Additional data regarding health status and sociodemographic variables (age, race/ethnicity, education, income, insurance, and geographic location) were also included in the analysis.

Results: Among patients included in the study, 30% were ages 65 to 69, almost 24% were ages 70 to 74, about 20% were ages 75 to 79, and 10% were age 85 years or older. About 80% were non-Hispanic white. About 21% of subjects reported above-average health, 58% reported average health, and 20% reported below-average health.

Age was a predictor for cancer screening. The older the age of the woman, the less likely she would be screening for cancer except for those women who reported below-average health. Only 33.7% of older women received exercise counseling. In general, immunizations increased with age until age 85.

Implications: Many older women are not receiving age-appropriate cancer screening and health promotion services, including exercise counseling.

Reference: Schonberg, M., Leveille, S., & Marcantonio, E. (2008). Preventive health care among older women: Missed opportunities and poor targeting. *Am J Med, 121*, 974-981.

As with cancer, the risks for cardiovascular events increase with age. Research reports that risk factors for cardiovascular disease—such as diabetes, hypertension, and dyslipidemia—are not treated aggressively or appropriately in older adults (Andrawes, Bussey, & Belmin, 2005; Selvin, Coresh, & Brancati, 2006).

In summary, successful aging is dependent on disease prevention and health promotion. The health care priorities for older adults focus on such topics as access to care, patient education, physical activity, a healthy diet, smoking cessation, age-appropriate screening, and immunizations. Although the value of health promotion is clear, there is less clarity about appropriate screening recommendations. As with any intervention, decisions regarding care should not be based on age but on life expectancy and quality of life.

KEY POINTS

- *Healthy People 2010* is a guide that can be used for health priorities for older adults.
- Older adults can benefit from health promotions activities.
- Nurses are important members of the health promotion team.
- Patient education must be tailored for the older adults' learning style and sensory deficits.
- The concept of empowerment can facilitate learning and health maintenance in the older adult.
- Improved access to care is a necessity for older adults to maintain health.
- Increasing activity has numerous health benefits such as increased bone and muscle strength, improved balance, increased flexibility, and improved mental health.
- Anorexia of aging is associated with poor nutrition in older adults.
- Overweight and obesity can be as problematic for older adults as undernutrition.
- Smoking cessation has benefits for older adults and should be included in health promotion activities.
- Older adults are vulnerable for infectious disease and should have routine immunizations.
- Mental health issues in older adults should be incorporated into health promotion and maintenance.
- Screening and treatment for cardiovascular risks should be addressed in the care of older adults.
- Cancer screening in older adults should be individualized and is dependent on preexisting conditions.

CRITICAL THINKING ACTIVITIES

1. Interview an older adult in a nursing home and one in assisted living regarding health promoting behaviors. They should be the same age and gender. Compare and contrast the two. What are the differences and what are the similarities?
2. In your hometown, identify community resources that facilitate healthy aging.
3. Examine the older adult's perceived barriers for exercise and adequate nutrition.
4. Propose solutions to the previously mentioned barriers on an individual and community level.
5. Examine the proposed *Healthy People 2020* and identify any gaps in terms of health promotion and health care needs of the aging adult.

CASE STUDY | *MRS. GRANT*

Mrs. Grant is a 69-year-old widow who asks you what can she do to get healthy. She is slightly overweight and has hypertension, arthritis, and chronic obstructive pulmonary disease (COPD). She moved to the area recently, so she has few friends and lives alone. She lives in a quiet neighborhood but is afraid to go out at night. She still drives but does not drive at night. Her home is close to a local supermarket and several fast food restaurants. She says she finds it hard to cook for one, so she goes to a fast food restaurant for her main meal each day. She does very little exercise because of her arthritis and COPD. She continues to smoke even though she knows this habit is contributing to her COPD.

1. How would you prioritize Mrs. Grant's health care needs?
2. How would you address her lack of exercise and diet?
3. What strategies might you use to encourage smoking cessation?
4. How would you help Mrs. Grant become engaged in social networking?

REFERENCES

Abdullah, A., Ho, L., Kwan, Y., Cheung, W., McGhee, S., & Chan, W. (2006). Promoting smoking cessation among the elderly: What are the predictors of intention to quit and successful quitting. *Journal of Aging and Health, 18*(4), 552-564.

American Academy of Neurology. (n.d.) *Get up and go test.* Retrieved November 10, 2010, from http://www.aan.com/practice/guideline/uploads/273.pdf

Andrawes, A., Bussey, C., & Belmin, J. (2005). Prevention of cardiovascular events in elderly. *Drugs and Aging, 22,* 859-876.

Chahbazi, J., & Grow, S. (2008).Common foods and farming methods thought to promote health what the data show. *Primary Care: Clinics in Office Practice, 35,* 769-788.

Chapman, I. (2006). Nutritional disorders in the elderly. *Medical Clinics of North America, 90,* 887-907.

Crane, R. (2007). The most addictive drug, the most deadly substance: Smoking cessation tactics for a busy clinician. *Primary Care: Clinics in Office Medicine, 37,* 117-135.

DeJonge, K., Taler, G., & Boling, P. (2009). Independence at home: Community-based care for older adults with severe chronic illness. *Clinics in Geriatric Medicine, 25,* 159-169.

Flicker, L. (2010). Cardiovascular risk factors, cerebrovascular disease burden and health brain aging. *Clinics in Geriatric Medicine, 26,* 17-27.

Harrington, J., & Lee-Chiong, T. (2009). Obesity and aging. *Clinics in Chest Medicine, 30,* 609-614.

High, K. (2007). Immunizations in older adults. *Clinics in Geriatric Medicine, 23,* 669-685.

Hildebrand, M., & Neufeld, P. (2009). Recruiting older adults into a physical activity promotion program: *Active Living Every Day* offered in a naturally occurring retirement community. *Gerontologist, 49,* 702-710.

Jancey, J. (2008). A physical activity program to mobilize older people: A practical and sustainable approach. *Gerontologist, 48,* 251-257.

Krondl, M., Coleman, P., & Lau, D. (2008). Helping older adults meet nutritional challenges. *Journal of Nutrition for the Elderly, 27,* 205-220.

Lampinen, P., Heikkinen, R., Kauppinen, M., & Heikkinen, E. (2006). Activity as a predictor of mental well-being among older adults. *Aging and Mental Health, 10,* 454-466.

Maciosek, M., Solberg, L., Coffield, A., Edwards, N., & Goodman, M. (2006). Influenza vaccine: Health impact and cost effectiveness among adults aged 50-64 and 65 and older. *American Journal of Preventive Medicine, 31,* 72-79.

Markle-Reid, M., Weir, R., Browne, G., Roberts, J., Gafni, A., & Henderson, S. (2006). Health promotion for frail elderly home care clients. *Journal of Advanced Nursing, 54,* 380-395.

Mauk, K. (2006). Reaching and teaching older adults. *Nursing, 36,* 17.

McMichael, K., VanderBilt, J., Lavery, L., Rodriguez, E., & Ganguly, M. (2008). Simple balance and mobility tests can assess fall risk when cognition is impaired. *Geriatric Nursing, 29,* 311-323.

Meng, H., Wamsley, B., Eggert, G., & Van Nostrand, J. (2007). Impact of a health promotion nurse intervention on disability and health care costs among elderly adults with heart conditions. *Journal of Rural Health, 23,* 322-331.

Moylan, K., & Binder, E. (2007). Falls in older adults: Risk assessment, management and prevention. *American Journal of Medicine, 120,* 493-497.

Nelson, M., Rejeski, W., Blair, S., Duncan, P., Judge, J., King, A., . . . (2007). Physical activity and public health in older adults: Recommendations from the American College of Sports Medicine and the American Heart Association. *Circulation, 116,* 1094-1105.

Niefeld, M., & Kasper, J. (2005). Access to ambulatory medical and long-term care services among elderly Medicare and Medicaid beneficiaries: Organizational, financial, and geographic barriers. *Medial Care Research and Review, 62,* 300-319.

Ozminkowski, R., Goetzel, R., Wang, F., Gibson, T., Shechter, D., Musich, S., . . . (2006). The savings gained from participation in health promotion programs for Medicare beneficiaries. *Journal of Occupational and Environmental Medicine, 48,* 1125-1132.

Pathman, D., Ricketts, T., & Konrad, T. (2006). How adults' access outpatient physician services relates to the local supply of primary care physicians in rural southeast. *Health Services Research, 41,* 79-102.

Polzien, C. (2006). The ABC's of teaching older adults: Implications for hoe care and hospice. *Home Healthcare Nurse, 24,* 487-489.

Rubenstein, L., & Josephson, K. (2006). Falls and their prevention in elderly people: What does the evidence show? *Medical Clinics of North America, 80,* 807-824.

Schonberg, M., Leveille, S., & Marcantonio, E. (2008). Preventive health care among older women: Missed opportunities and poor targeting. *American Journal of Medicine, 121,* 974-981.

Selvin, E., Coresh, J., & Brancati, F. (2006). The burden and treatment of diabetes in elderly individuals in the U.S. *Diabetes Care, 29,* 2415-2419.

Shewmacke, R., & Huntington, M. (2009). Nutritional treatment for obesity. *Primary Care: Clinics in Office Medicine, 36,* 357-377.

Stevens, J., Mack, K., Paulozzi, L. & Ballesteros, M. (2008). Self-reported falls and fall-related injuries among person aged > or = 65 years: United States, 2006. *Journal of Safety Research, 39,* 345-349.

Terret, C., Castel-Kremer, E., Albrand, G., & Droz, J. (2009). Effects of comorbidity on screening and early diagnosis of cancer in elderly persons. *Lancet, 10,* 80-86.

Thomas, C. (2007). Bulletin boards: A teaching strategy for older adult audiences. *Journal of Gerontological Nursing, 33,* 45-52.

Ungaro, R., & Federman, A. (2009). Restrictiveness of eligibility determination and Medicaid enrollment by low-income seniors. *Journal of Aging and Social Policy, 21,* 338-351.

U.S. Department of Health and Human Services. (n.d.). Healthy people: What is its history? Retrieved November 12, 2010, from http://www.healthypeople.gov/

U.S. Department of Health, Education, and Welfare. (1979). *Healthy people: The surgeon general's report on health promotion and disease prevention.* Retrieved November 12, 2010, from http://profiles.nlm.nih.gov/NN/B/B/G/K/_/nnbbgk.pdf

Wihelmsson, S., & Lindberg, M. (2007). Prevention and health promotion and evidence-based fields of nursing: A literature review. *International Journal of Nursing, 13,* 254-265.

Whitson, H., Heflin, M., & Burchett, B. (2006). Patterns and predictors of smoking cessation in an elderly cohort. *Journal of the American Geriatrics Society, 54,* 466-471.

Yokoya, T., Demura, S., & Sato, S. (2008). Three-year follow-up of the fall risk and physical function characteristics of elderly participating in a community exercise class. *Journal of Physiological Anthropology, 28,* 55-62.

Zoorob, R., & Morelli, V. (2008). Disease prevention and wellness in the twenty-first century. *Primary Care: Clinics in Office Practice, 35,* 663-667.

Chapter 8

Challenges to Physical Health

Alison Kris, RN, PhD, Sally Gerard, RN, DNP, and Susan Fisher, APRN, EdD

LEARNING OBJECTIVES

- Describe what an atypical presentation is, and how an older adult may present with an atypical presentation.
- Synopsize diseases prevalent in older adults, and discuss how they may present differently in older adults.
- Discuss lifestyle modifications, including changes in diet and physical activity, that may be helpful in treating or preventing these common conditions.
- Understand the ways in which these conditions are treated, the goals of drug therapy, and any important cautions associated with drug use.

Causes of death have been associated with the economic well-being of nations. In countries with a lower average income, the cause of death among older adults may be more likely to be from an infectious disease or acute illness, while older adults in more developed countries are more likely to die from the complications of chronic disease (Table 8-1A, Table 8-1B).

Learning to live with the consequences or morbidities of chronic disease can be a challenge. Diagnosing chronic disease also may present challenges because, in the older adult, these conditions may present differently than in younger people. Changes in condition, including diminished appetite or a decline in functional status, may indicate a significant underlying medical condition. In addition, older adults may have decreased subjective perception of signs and symptoms, such as a blunted pain response. Physiological changes, such as leukocytosis, may be diminished or absent. Dementia, cognitive impairment, or other conditions that impair communication may make it difficult to obtain an accurate history.

The absence of cardinal symptoms of disease combined with the presence of novel yet subtle signs and symptoms in an older adult may cause a person to present in an unusual way. This is called an *atypical* presentation. Atypical presentations are most common in people over age 85, those with multiple comorbidities and multiple medications, and those with impaired cognitive status (http://consultgerirn.org/topics/atypical_presentation/want_to_know_more). Common conditions associated with atypical presentations include infections, falls, urinary incontinence, myocardial infarction (MI), and congestive heart failure. Other conditions that may present in an atypical manner include silent malignancy, silent acute abdomen, depression, and thyroid disease.

The older adult may have an atypical presentation, including absence of cardinal symptoms of disease and presence of novel yet subtle signs and symptoms.

Infections

In older adults, infections often appear quite different than they do in children. For young people, hallmarks of infection include a high fever, swollen lymph nodes, and an elevated white blood cell count. In older adults, all of these signs may be diminished or absent. When evaluating fever in an older adult, it is important to note the deviation from baseline rather than the number itself because older adults often have baseline temperatures below 98.6°F. Instead of the more common signs and

TABLE 8-1A Top 10 Causes of Death by Country Income

CAUSE OF DEATH	HIGH-INCOME COUNTRY		MIDDLE-INCOME COUNTRY		LOW-INCOME COUNTRY	
	%	RANK	%	RANK	%	RANK
Coronary heart disease	16.3	1	13.9	2	9.4	2
Stroke and other cerebrovascular diseases	9.3	2	14.2	1	5.6	5
Cancer of trachea, bronchus, lung	5.9	3	2.9	5		
Lower respiratory infection	3.8	4	3.8	4	11.2	1
Chronic obstructive pulmonary disease	3.5	5	7.4	3	3.6	6
Alzheimer's disease and other dementias	3.4	6				
Cancer of colon or rectum	3.3	7				
Diabetes mellitus	2.8	8	2.1	10		
Breast cancer	2.0	9				
Cancer of stomach	1.8	10	2.2	8		
Road traffic accidents			2.8	6		
Hypertensive heart disease			2.5	7		
Tuberculosis			2.2	9	3.5	7
Diarrheal diseases					6.9	3
HIV/AIDS					5.7	4
Neonatal infections					3.4	8
Malaria					3.3	9
Prematurity and low birth weight					3.2	10

From World Health Organization. (2009). *World health statistics.* Retrieved December 12, 2010, from http://www.who.int/whosis/whostat/EN_WHS09_Full.pdf

TABLE 8-1B Top 10 Causes of Death Worldwide

CAUSE OF DEATH	PERCENTAGE OF DEATHS
Coronary heart disease	12.2
Stroke and other cerebrovascular diseases	9.7
Lower respiratory infections	7.1
Chronic obstructive pulmonary disease	5.1
Diarrheal diseases	3.7
HIV/AIDS	3.5
Tuberculosis	2.5
Trachea, bronchus, lung cancers	2.3
Road traffic accidents	2.2
Prematurity and low birth weight	2.0

From World Health Organization. (2009). *World health statistics.* Retrieved December 12, 2010, from http://www.who.int/whosis/whostat/EN_WHS09_Full.pdf

symptoms, older adults with new onset of infection may present with an acute change in mental status. In fact, delirium may occur in 50% of older adults with infection. Decreased oral intake, leading to weight loss and dehydration, should be evaluated as a potential sign of an underlying infection. Acute changes in functional status and falls may also mask infection. Changes in respiratory status, such as an increase in respiratory rate or a decrease in oxygenation, can indicate a respiratory infection. The hypoxia that can accompany changes in respiratory status can result in confusion in older adults. For subtle changes to be noticed, it is important to carry out detailed assessments on a regular basis, and for the results of those assessments to be accurately recorded.

Falls

Falls are common in older adults and are a leading cause of disability and death (Box 8-1). They also may indicate underlying disease. In fact, in about 10% of cases, the fall may be the only symptom of an underlying acute illness (Tinetti, Speechley, & Ginter, 1988). Therefore, whenever an older adult falls, the cause of the fall should be ascertained. Never assume that it is normal for an older adult to fall. A variety of acute and chronic conditions can increase the risk of falls among older adults.

- By far the greatest risk factor for future falls is a history of falls.
- The risk of falling is more than doubled in persons with cognitive impairment when compared with older adults who are not cognitively impaired (Tinetti, Speechley, & Ginter, 1988).
- Older adults living in nursing homes fall about three times more often than those living in the community (Rubenstein & Josephson, 2002).
- People over age 75 who fall are at increased risk of admission to nursing homes, have an increased risk of fracture, and have increased mortality (CDC, 2010b).
- Some chronic conditions, such as diabetes and severe atherosclerosis, can impair sensation in the lower extremities. Impaired sensation can make it difficult to ensure proper footing, increasing the risk of falls.
- Many drugs can increase fall risk. Drugs given to reduce blood pressure can lead to orthostatic hypotension. This drop in blood pressure upon standing can cause dizziness, leading to a fall.

BOX 8-1 Facts about Falls

- More than one third of adults age 65 and older fall each year.
- Falls are more serious in older people and are a leading cause of injury and death.
- In 2009, more than 2 million older adults were treated in emergency departments after falling, 581,000 of whom were hospitalized.
- Some 20% to 30% of older adults who fall sustain moderate to severe injuries.
- In 2007, more than 80% of deaths from falling were among those age 65 or older, and 18,000 older adults died from injuries sustained in a fall.
- Almost half of older adults who die after a fall do so because they sustained a traumatic brain injury.

From Centers for Disease Control and Prevention. (2010b). Falls among older adults: An overview. Atlanta, GA: Author. Retrieved December 12, 2010, from http://www.cdc.gov/homeandrecreationalsafety/falls/adultfalls.html

Assessing an Older Adult after a Fall

Evaluate the patient's environment after a fall. Make sure lighting is adequate, particularly near steps and stairways. Check if stairways have sturdy and functioning handrails on both sides of the stairway, if possible. Reduce the number of throw rugs, and make sure the ones in use are secure. Because a significant number of falls that happen at home occur in the bathroom, careful attention should be paid to this space. Install grab bars in showers and near toilets and nonslip surfaces on shower floors. The Centers for Disease Control and Prevention offers a toolkit to aid in assessing home safety at http://www.cdc.gov/Ncipc/pub-res/toolkit/CheckListForSafety.htm.

A good physical exam following a fall should move from head to toe, looking for new changes or opportunities to improve safety. Changes in vision are important to address. Cataracts create a haze that can impair the ability to judge subtle variations in floor surfaces, while macular degeneration can create dark spots in the center of the visual field. Stroke or transient ischemic attack may lead to unilateral weakness, contributing to a fall. Gross motor strength can be assessed, noting differences in strength from one side to the other.

It can be difficult for older adults to find properly fitted footwear. Older people who have conditions such as congestive heart failure may experience significant fluctuations in foot size based on time of day and compliance with the drug regimen. Shoes with laces can present challenges for older adults who have limited range of motion or reduced manual dexterity because of arthritis. Velcro footwear that has some stretch and that can be easily adjusted throughout the day may be of benefit.

Polypharmacy, or the use of multiple interacting drugs, can increase fall risk. In an older adult who has recently fallen, gather a list of drugs from all prescribing physicians. Try to determine if the drugs are being taken as prescribed. Older adults with even mild cognitive impairment are at risk for either omitting important drugs or taking more than the prescribed dosages. Drugs that impede blood clotting should be taken at night to prevent serious bleeding complications after a fall. Over-the-counter products, such as nonsteroidal anti-inflammatory drugs (NSAIDs), can increase the risk of gastrointestinal bleeding, which can lead to a fall.

In a long-term care facility, patients who are cognitively impaired are at increased risk of falling, as are residents who have had a previous fall. People in long-term care may incorrectly assume that the use of physical restraints will prevent falls. However, this is not true (Capezuti, Strumpf, Evans, Grisso, & Maislin, 1998; Neufeld et al., 1999; Tinetti, Liu, & Ginter, 1992). In fact, residents who are physically restrained are at increased risk of serious complications from a fall (Neufeld et al., 1999).

Falls also may be an atypical indicator of other diseases or conditions. Vitamin deficiencies, such as a vitamin B_{12} deficiency common in older adults, can increase fall risk. Parkinson's disease can cause gait changes leading to an increased risk of falls. In addition, depression and hypothyroidism also increase fall risk. For patients with conditions that cause lower extremity pain, such as osteoarthritis, falls can indicate a worsening of the condition, or may be an indication of poorly controlled pain (Riefkohl et al., 2007).

Urinary Incontinence

Urinary incontinence is defined as the involuntary loss of urine. Although many older adults and even some practitioners may think urinary incontinence is a normal part of aging, it is not. Therefore, if an older adult experiences a new onset of urinary incontinence, efforts should be undertaken to understand the cause and treat the condition.

Although many older adults and even some practitioners may think urinary incontinence is a normal part of aging, it is not.

There are several types of urinary incontinence including stress, urge, overflow, and functional incontinence. Stress incontinence is the most common type of urinary incontinence. It occurs when pressure is increased in the abdominal cavity by such activities as coughing, sneezing, or lifting a heavy object. Stress incontinence is also common in younger women during pregnancy. Urge incontinence refers to an abrupt onset of an intense urge to urinate, followed by an uncontrollable loss of urine. Urge incontinence can occur when there are changes in the frontal lobe of the brain that inhibit urination. Overflow incontinence is common in men with benign prostatic hypertrophy or prostate cancer. The enlarged prostate obstructs the flow of urine from the bladder, causing the bladder to overfill and eventually overflow. Functional incontinence refers to incontinence due to a non-bladder–related cause, such as if a person cannot get to a bathroom in a timely fashion because of osteoarthritis or some other cause. Pay careful attention to the patient's choice of clothing. It may be helpful for the person to wear pants that are easily removed in situations when movement or hand strength is limited. The use of urinary catheters to manage urinary incontinence should be avoided. Urinary catheters irritate the lining of the bladder and increase the risk of infection. Urinary catheters are the leading cause of institutionally acquired urinary tract infection (UTI).

For older adults with new-onset urinary incontinence, precipitating factors should be assessed. UTIs often present in an atypical manner in older adults. They increase urinary frequency, resulting in incontinence. In fact, bladder infections are the most common cause of transient incontinence in older adults. UTIs can go undiagnosed in older adults because there may be an absence of dysuria (painful urination) because of the blunted pain response that can accompany aging. In addition, there may be an absence of leukocytosis in older adults experiencing UTIs. Because of the difficulty in diagnosing UTI early, particularly in older adults who cannot communicate, the UTI may progress to a more serious condition called urosepsis.

In addition, several types and classes of drugs can create problems with incontinence. Diuretics are commonly prescribed to older adults with hypertension and congestive heart failure. These drugs can significantly increase urine output and are a common cause of incontinence. As a result, the older adults may skip doses of a prescribed diuretic, which could lead to an exacerbation of hypertension and heart failure. Older adults hospitalized for exacerbations of heart failure should be assessed for their ability to comply with a prescribed diuretic regimen.

Cardiovascular Disease

Overall, cardiovascular disease is the leading cause of death in the United States, accounting for more than 27% of all deaths nationwide. Cardiovascular disease is also the leading cause of death for people over 60 (Heron et al., 2009). The term *cardiovascular disease* includes numerous diseases and conditions, including MI, stroke, hypertension, peripheral artery disease, and heart failure (Fig. 8-1). Each of these diseases is caused, in part, by diseased blood vessels, which interrupt the flow of oxygenated blood to vital organs.

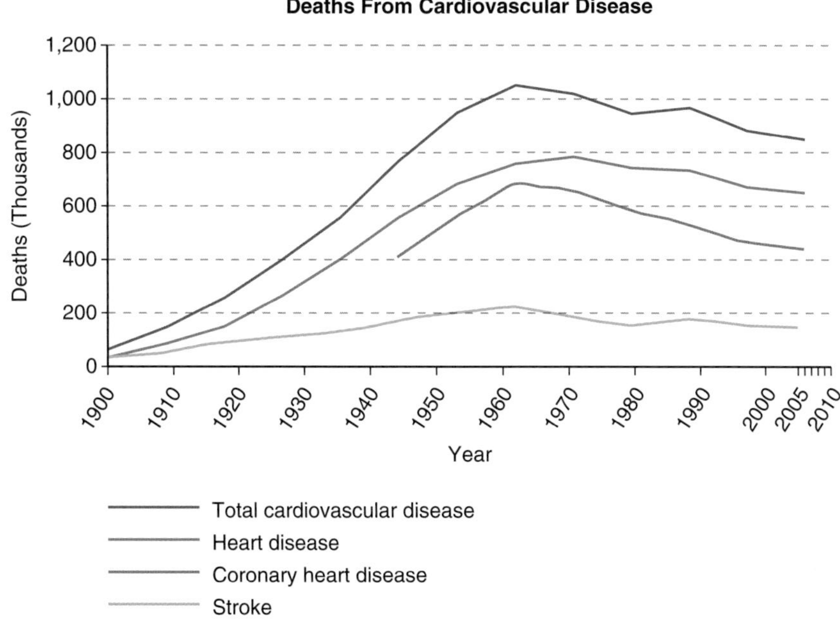

Figure 8-1 Deaths from cardiovascular disease in the United States from 1900 to 2006. (Data for 2006 are preliminary.) *(From National Heart, Lung, and Blood Institute. (2008). Fact book fiscal year 2008. Washington, DC: U.S. Department of Health and Human Services, p. 35. Retrieved December 12, 2010, from http://www.nhlbi.nih.gov/about/factbook-08/FactBookFinal.pdf)*

Many factors have been associated with an increased risk of cardiovascular disease. Hypertension, high cholesterol (especially high low-density lipoprotein [LDL]), smoking, and obesity all cause damage to the vascular system increasing the incidence of cardiovascular diseases. To reduce risk, blood pressure should be maintained below 120 systolic and below 80 diastolic. Cholesterol levels should be regularly assessed. LDL levels greater than 160 mg/dL are associated with increased risk, while increases in high-density lipoprotein (HDL) levels have a protective effect. Ideally, HDL levels should be above 40 mg/dL for men and above 50 mg/dL for women, with higher levels conveying greater protective benefit. High triglyceride levels also pose a risk for cardiovascular disease and are associated with lifestyle factors such as obesity and inactivity. Ideally, triglyceride levels should be maintained less than 150 mg/dL (American Heart Association, 2010).

Although cardiovascular diseases are more common with age, they are not an inevitable consequence of aging. In fact, many of the causes of cardiovascular disease are entirely preventable. The major causes of cardiovascular disease include smoking, poor diet leading to obesity, and lack of physical activity. It is thought that these modifiable risk factors account for about 80% of coronary heart disease and cerebrovascular disease. Moderate exercise has demonstrated to significantly reduce the risk of developing cardiovascular disease. Diet plays a major role in the development of cardiovascular disease. Diets that aid in preventing the development of cardiovascular disease include those that are rich in fruits, vegetables, and fiber and low in sodium and saturated fat.

Myocardial Infarction

Although heart disease occurs with great frequency in both men and women, many people, both young and old, do not realize the degree to which heart disease affects women. Stereotypical images of a young male grabbing his chest and dropping to the floor in a dramatic fashion are often quite different from the picture witnessed by many health care professionals. In fact, more women than men die from heart disease every year. It is important to note that heart disease is the number one killer of women over age 25. In addition, although 1 in 29 women will die of breast cancer, about 1 in 2 women will die of heart disease (Lloyd-Jones et al., 2009).

Although 1 in 29 women will die of breast cancer, about 1 in 2 women will die of heart disease.

In an MI, the blood supply to the heart is interrupted, typically because a blood vessel has become occluded. The lack of blood supply to the heart muscle is of major significance. Without blood supplying the heart, there is no oxygen being delivered to the heart either. Without oxygen, the cells in the heart muscle begin to die. As an increasing number of cardiac muscle cells begin to die off, the heart muscle begins to weaken. The electrical signals that generate the heart beat have difficulty passing through the incapacitated cardiac muscle tissue and dysrhythmias can occur.

In younger people, the interruption in blood supply to the heart and the consequent damage can be painful. However, many older adults do not experience MI with the classic symptom of crushing chest pain. Older patients may instead experience what feels like indigestion or abdominal discomfort, nausea or vomiting, and shortness of breath. Other atypical symptoms of MI include upper back pain, pain between the shoulder blades, and jaw pain in the absence of chest pain. Older adults are less likely to experience chest pain or pain in the arm and shoulder than younger patients, and the presentation of MI becomes less and less typical with increasing age (Hwang, Park, Shin, & Jeong, 2009). Syncope, stroke, and acute confusion are more likely to be the sole presenting symptoms of MI as people age.

Syncope, stroke, and acute confusion are more likely to be the sole presenting symptoms of MI as people age.

In addition, we know that there are gender differences in the presentation of MI. Although men are more likely to experience more classic symptoms, women are more likely to experience symptoms that are more diffuse such as fatigue or weakness, or flulike symptoms. The atypical presentation often found in women may be a reason why women delay seeking treatment for MI and may be a factor in the increased mortality following MI in women.

Absence of symptoms associated with MIs may be particularly pronounced in older adults with diabetes (DeVon, Penckofer, & Larimer, 2008). Diabetics tend to have impaired pain sensation peripherally and are also less likely to perceive pain associated with MI. Complicating matters is the fact that atypical signs and symptoms of MI such as sweating, fatigue, dizziness, and shaking can be mistakenly attributed to blood glucose variability. Older adults, particularly older adults with diabetes, require careful monitoring for subtle signs and symptoms that may indicate an underlying disease. In patients with an acute MI, early diagnosis is critical, so treatment can start as soon as possible to halt the progression of irreversible cardiac damage.

Congestive Heart Failure

Congestive heart failure is a condition in which the heart is unable to pump enough blood to meet physiological needs. Heart failure occurs most commonly in older adults because of a combination of the normal changes of aging (see Chapter 9), as well as the increased prevalence of conditions that underlie the disease. Heart failure typically results from several other common health problems, including hypertension and coronary artery disease. The heart muscle must pump blood out to the periphery with each systolic beat. In a person with high blood pressure, the heart must pump against the increased pressure. Eventually, this increased workload causes the left ventricle to enlarge and stiffen. The enlarged, thickened, and stiff left ventricle becomes unable to fill adequately with blood, and hence the heart is not able to pump out enough blood to meet physiological needs. Other conditions such as MI and myocarditis weaken cardiac muscle and prevent the heart from being able to pump blood with enough force to allow for adequate circulatory function. Conditions that affect the heart rhythm, causing it to beat too quickly or in a disorganized way, also prevent the heart from being able to get enough blood circulating to and from the periphery, leading to heart failure.

There are a variety of symptoms associated with heart failure. The inability of the heart to send oxygen and nutrient-rich blood to the body leads to fatigue and muscle weakness. Kidney failure is common in heart failure because poor perfusion makes the kidneys less able to filter blood efficiently. The kidney failure associated with heart failure may lead to higher than normal levels of blood urea nitrogen and creatinine in the blood. In addition, the renal failure associated with heart failure may result in decreases in hemoglobin and hematocrit. In addition, when the kidneys are poorly perfused, or when there is underlying renal damage, the kidneys become unable to remove excess fluid from the bloodstream. This causes the body to retain excess fluid, putting additional strain on the heart, which needs to pump the excess blood volume.

Heart failure may present in an atypical manner in older adults. For many, heart failure may come on gradually and may manifest as a set of seemingly unrelated symptoms. Increases in fatigue and shortness of breath may be the consequence of fluid retention. When fluid is retained in the legs as a result of heart failure, the legs may feel heavy and may become more difficult to move, increasing the risk of falls. An older adult with heart failure may be able to rise in the morning and walk to a chair without any difficulty. However, once seated for several hours, excess fluid may begin to accumulate in the legs, making it more difficult to walk as the day progresses. Some older adults may experience confusion if the brain is not being well perfused.

Lifestyle modification may prove helpful, particularly in the early stages of the disease. Patients who are overweight should be encouraged to lose weight, which will reduce excess burden on the heart. In addition, patients with mild to moderate heart failure should exercise regularly to stay as fit as possible. Excess sodium should be avoided because it may lead to fluid retention, again increasing the workload on the heart.

It is important for those with heart failure to monitor their weight closely. Fluid retention can quickly worsen symptoms and can further damage an already weakened heart. Often, patients with heart failure will take several different drugs in several different drug classes to manage the condition. The goals of drug management are to:

- Help the heart beat more forcefully and efficiently
- Reduce blood pressure (thereby reducing cardiac workload)
- Remove excess water (to help prevent fluid overload)

Because people with heart failure often have other underlying health problems—such as arteriosclerosis—for which they may also take medicine, the list of drugs may be long and polypharmacy is a concern. Many of the drugs used to manage heart failure can have significant and unpleasant side effects such as incontinence, dizziness, and fatigue. Fluctuations in levels of certain drugs can lead to unsafe drops in blood pressure and heart rate. In addition, managing the multiple drugs prescribed for patients with heart failure can prove to be a cognitive challenge as well as a financial burden. If an older adult begins to experience frequent exacerbations of heart failure, it may be important to investigate if drugs are being taken as prescribed.

Cancer

A cancer diagnosis is often seen as a threat to one's sense of well-being and loss of independence, but in the elderly it can be a devastating threat to one's life. It can lead to a complex array of issues associated with the disease itself, as well as comorbid conditions, and treatment side effects. Cancer patients over 70 years have at least three comorbid conditions (e.g., metabolic disorders, cardiopulmonary disease, and obesity) and these conditions can influence cancer detection, the clinical presentation of the disease, and treatment outcomes, especially survival and quality of life (Extermann, 2007; Extermann, Overcash, Lyman, Parr, & Balducci, 1998; Hurria et al., 2009).

More than 60% of patients diagnosed with cancer are over age 65 (Kagan, 2008), and the incidence of cancer in this population is 11 times higher than that of younger people (Yancik & Ries, 2000). The lifetime risk of developing cancer is higher in men than in women (559.6 per 100,000 versus 420.1 per 100,000) (Edwards et al., 2002). The risk of a person age 45 developing cancer during the next 10 years is 1 in 24, whereas a person age 65 has a 1 in 6 risk of being diagnosed with cancer by age 75 (Hayat, Howlader, Reichman, & Edwards, 2007).

About half of the malignancies that occur in older adults include lung and bronchus, breast, colorectal, and prostate cancers (Jemal et al., 2009). Lung cancer is the most common cancer in both men and women older than age 60, accounting for about 28% of all cancer deaths in this age group (Jemal et al., 2009). In women ages 60 to 79, the second- and third-ranked fatal cancers in women are breast cancer and colorectal cancer; in men, they are colorectal and prostate cancer (Jemal et al., 2003). The lifetime incidence of breast cancer in women is similar to that of prostate cancer in men (28.8 per 100,000 and 33.9 per 100,000), respectively (Edwards et al., 2002). The incidence of certain other cancers has shown a dramatic increase in older adults since 1970, including non-Hodgkin's lymphoma (Balducci & Ballester, 1996), non-melanoma skin cancer (Glass & Hoover, 1989), and brain cancer (Flowers, 2000). The incidence of lymphoma in particular has nearly doubled since 1970, for no known reason (Jemal et al., 2009).

Although the reasons for these increases are unclear, age-related molecular changes plus longer exposure to carcinogens are thought to make the older person more susceptible (Balducci & Extermann, 2000a). The incidence of most cancers increases with age up to age 85 and then begins to level off after age 95. Cancer as a cause of death in this age group becomes less likely as other chronic diseases become more prevalent (Extermann, 2007; Saltzein, Behling, & Baergen, 1998).

Cancer Screening in Older Adults

As the population ages, cancer incidence, prevalence, and mortality will also increase. The aim of cancer screening is to detect early cancers in asymptomatic and high-risk individuals when it is most curable (Mahon, 2005; Terret, Castel-Kremer, Albrand, & Droz, 2009). The usefulness of a screening program is based on characteristics of the disease and the attributes of the screening test (Table 8-2). When screening patients age 65 and older, consideration should be given to the effectiveness of the test, potential risks and benefits, and cost (Sheinfield-Gorin, Gauthier, Hay, Miles, & Wardle, 2008).

How do patient preferences/family preferences influence the decision-making process? Beliefs and values about screening, the relationship with their health care provider, cognitive status, lack of education about screening, varied perceptions about cancer risk, and diminished lack of social and financial support can influence a person's decision to participate in screening (Resnick & McLesky, 2008). If screening is considered, a discussion of the risk and benefits of the test must occur between the provider and the patient. False-positive results require additional testing to rule out cancer. Also, testing may cause unnecessary stress, morbidity, and even mortality without significantly prolonging life (Walter, Bertenthal, Lindquist, & Konety, 2006; Walter, Eng, & Covinsky 2001; Walter, Lindquist, & Covinsky, 2004).

One area where nurses can be helpful with screening decisions is in educating older adults about symptoms that would be suggestive of a

TABLE 8-2 Screening Test Requirements

Disease characteristics	Common enough to justify efforts to detect High prevalence in preclinical state Mortality and morbidity are high Presymptomatic treatment improves outcomes Effective treatment available
Screening test attributes	Acceptable sensitivity and specificity Ease of administration Cost effective Safe Acceptable to patient

From Sheinfield-Gorin, S., Gauthier, J., Hay, J., Miles, A., & Wardle, J. (2008). Cancer screening and aging: Research barriers and opportunities. *Cancer, 113* (Suppl. 12), 3493–3504.

cancer. These early signs might be things like new onset of fatigue, weight loss, changes in bowel habits, and unexplained lumps. Early recognition of symptoms suggestive of a cancer is critical in this population. In older adults, early warning signs of cancer may be incorrectly attributed to "just getting old." For example, an elderly patient may attribute his persistent constipation to "old age" rather than suspecting a colon cancer; or an older woman with pain may think that it may be "arthritis" rather than a bone metastasis from a malignancy. Both patients and health care providers can be prone to make incorrect assumptions in this area.

Current evidence suggests that older individuals do not delay appreciably in seeking medical help once having noted a symptom that appears to be related to cancer. However, health care professionals may be guilty of delaying further diagnostic work-up in elderly patients (Cohen, 2007). Failure to recognize new symptoms in older individuals may be due in part to the multiple comorbidities, age, and overall health status. Discovery of a new symptom in a previously very active 80-year-old may be approached differently than in someone with severe congestive heart failure, diabetes, and pulmonary failure.

Treatment of the Older Adult with Cancer

Cancer is a disease of aging, and the biological changes associated with aging impact the treatment of cancer (Ershler & Longo, 1997). Age bias often influences treatment decisions, despite the fact that each person's physiological aging is different (Westin & Longo, 2004). Older patients, when appropriately selected, can benefit from cancer regimens similar to that offered to younger patients (Balducci & Beghe, 2001). Although misconceptions and fears exist about the older patient's tolerance, safety, and feasibility of undergoing cancer treatment, several authors have found that they appear to tolerate treatment-associated toxicities reasonably well (Balducci, 2009; Bouchardy, Rapiti, Blagojevic, Vlastos, & Vlastos, 2007; Kemeny, 2004; Monson, Litvak, & Bold, 2003; Townsley, Selby, & Siu, 2005).

Many older adults may see the prospect of treating their cancer as a choice to extend life at the expense of physical functioning and independence.

Many older adults see the prospect of treating their cancer as problematic (Trask, Blank, & Jacobsen, 2008). Loss of independence is a common fear of older patients in their decision to proceed with treatment. Other coexisting factors such availability of financial and economic resources, family support, and perceived life expectancy may affect their ability to choose what may be in their best interest (Given & Given, 2008).

In an attempt to address some of these concerns, several geriatric oncologists suggest that patient selection should be based on life expectancy, comorbidity, and functional status using a comprehensive geriatric assessment tool rather than a standard medical evaluation for making treatment choices aimed at cure or palliative treatment (Balducci & Beghe, 2000; Burdett-Radoux & Muss, 2006; Extermann, 2007; Muss, Biganzoli,

Sargent, & Aapro, 2007; Repetto, 2003; Terret, Zuliam, Naiem, & Albrand, 2007). In oncology, functional status is measured by two brief scales (e.g., Karnofsky performance score and the Eastern Cooperative Group (ECOG score) that are somewhat predictive for treatment tolerance. Neither scale evaluates a patient's activities of daily living or the impact of functional decline on psychological status (Hurria et al., 2009). Instead, the Comprehensive Geriatric Assessment (CGA, Box 8-2) is a multidisciplinary tool that examines several components of aging, including functional status, that can be somewhat predictive of survival, tolerance to chemotherapy, and postoperative morbidity and mortality (Balducci 2003a; Extermann et al., 2005; Extermann & Hurria, 2007; Hurria, 2007; Kumar, Soares, Balducci, & Djulbegovic, 2007; National Comprehensive Cancer Network, 2010; Terret, Zuliam, Naiem, & Albrand, 2007). Although the CGA is not standardized or widely used in oncology practice, the benefits appear to lead to more appropriate patient selection and outcomes. Identification of reversible conditions that may interfere with treatment, estimates of life expectancy, predictions of treatment tolerance, and availability of family support can assist in the development and implementation of a comprehensive therapeutic plan (Given & Given, 2008). It also establishes a common language in which to communicate information rather than relying on chronological age as a basis for decision making (Carrera, Balducci, & Extermann, 2005).

BOX 8-2 Elements of a Comprehensive Geriatric Assessment

- Mental status
- Functional status
  - Activities of daily living
  - Instrumental activities of daily living
- Comorbid conditions (e.g., cardiovascular disease, anemia, depression)
- Social support
- Cognitive status
- Emotional status/depression
- Presence of geriatric syndromes (e.g., dementia, falls, neglect and abuse)
- Socioeconomic conditions
- Nutrition
- Polypharmacy

From Balducci, L. (2007). Aging, frailty, and chemotherapy. Cancer Control, 14, 7–12.

Surgery

Surgery remains an important first step in treatment of cancer, especially if the goal is to achieve a cure. It is also an effective intervention in the case of advanced disease to provide palliative relief of an obstruction or pressure from a tumor. Most diagnoses of cancer will require an initial surgical procedure either to confirm the presence of a cancer or to excise solid tumors such as breast, colorectal, gastric, or pancreatic. Although surgery is the most frequently used treatment modality, it has been viewed as a prohibitive risk in the elderly in terms of morbidity and mortality. However, this fact is not supported in the literature because the elderly have benefited from these surgical interventions (Audisio, Zbar, & Jaklitsch, 2007; Kemeny, 2004).

Radiation

Radiation therapy plays an important role in the multimodality approach to treatment of commonly occurring cancers in the elderly such as lung, lymphoma, colorectal, breast, head and neck, prostate, and malignant gliomas. Radiotherapy uses high-energy particles or waves, such as x-rays, gamma rays, electrons, and protons, to destroy or damage cancer cells. The primary aim of radiation is to provide local control of disease by delivering a precisely measured dose of irradiation to a defined tumor volume with as little as possible damage to surrounding tissue (Gosselin-Acomb, 2005). The main effects are seen at the cellular level where damage to either DNA or RNA is evident in tissues, organs, and/or the entire body depending on the extent of the treatment field.

About 60% of cancer patients receive radiation therapy for cure or control at some time during the course of their disease (Casey, Zachariah, & Balducci, 2003; Iwamoto, 2001). Depending on the stage of disease, patients can be treated for curative or palliative intent with special attention given to survival and quality of life. If the goal of treatment is palliative in nature, then radiation therapy can be effective in the management of symptoms associated with progressive or advanced disease (e.g., pain, pathological fractures due to bone metastasis). Elderly patients do not appear to experience increased radiation toxicity to normal tissues; rather, functional status appears to be a better indicator of treatment tolerance (Zachariah & Balducci, 2000).

However, one distinct disadvantage of radiotherapy, especially for older adults, is the long duration of therapy and the resulting fatigue. Treatment with curative intent can last 6 to 7 weeks, usually 5 days a week, and palliative treatment occurs daily for 2 to 4 weeks. Cancer-related fatigue is one of the most distressing symptoms of cancer treatment and may have profound effects on functional status and quality of life. Because physiological reserves diminished with age, older adults often experience protracted delays in recovery after treatment (Zachariah & Balducci, 2000).

Acute side effects of radiotherapy tend to be site specific (i.e., toxicities of the skin, mucous membranes, and gastrointestinal tract) depending on the area included in the treatment field. Acute symptoms include nausea, vomiting, dyspnea, esophagitis, weakness, weight loss, and change in functional status (Zachariah & Balducci, 2000). The limited knowledge about the experience of radiation for the older adults provides opportunities for further research in the area of interventions and management of the side effects of radiation therapy.

Chemotherapy/Biotherapy

Chemotherapy/biotherapy is a major foundation of cancer treatment for many solid and hematological tumors. It is associated with varying degrees of toxicity in the elderly (Wedding, Röhrig, Klippstein, Pientka, & Hoffken, 2007). Failure to include older adults in chemotherapy clinical trials exposes them to increasing drug toxicities because the standard doses are largely derived from data in younger patient cohorts. Lack of safety and efficacy at standard doses does not allow for the age-related changes in physiology and can lead to poorer outcomes in the older person (Dale, 2003; Hurria, 2007). The progressive decline in functional reserve associated with aging, the presence of comorbid disease, and the high prevalence of polypharmacy contribute to morbidity and mortality in the elderly receiving chemotherapy (Extermann, 2007; Extermann, Overcash, Lyman, Parr, & Balducci,1998; Schwartz, 2006; Townsley, Selby, & Siu, 2005.

Numerous pharmacokinetic and pharmacodynamic changes occur as part of the progressive physiological decline caused by aging and must be considered in patients receiving chemotherapy (Balducci, 2009). Changes in the pharmacokinetic parameters can influence how drugs are absorbed, distributed, metabolized, and excreted (Balducci & Extermann, 2000b; Wasil & Lichtman, 2005). Cancer therapies can cause side effects and when used in combination, whether with drugs or other treatments, more side effects can occur.

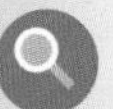

EVIDENCE FOR PRACTICE
Testing Cancer Treatments

Purpose: To accurately determine the number of patients over age 65 who are exclusively enrolled in randomized clinical trials. Additional variables of the study looked at type of intervention (i.e., cure or palliative), morbidity and mortality outcomes associated with treatment of elderly patients compared with younger patients, the methodological value of the clinical trial, and evidence of age bias in the published results.

Method: All completed Phase III randomized clinical trials conducted by five National Cancer Institute Cooperative Groups (NCI-COG) were reviewed from 1955 to 2000. Using enrollment criteria of age 65 or older, data were obtained on a proportion of participants older than 65.

Results: Of the 345 studies enrolling 122,186 patients, only one clinical trial exclusively enrolled older patients (0.29%). Stratification by age 65 or older was evident in only 6.3% ($n = 22$), and 5% of the trials ($n = 17$) excluded patients aged 70 or older. One trial evaluating the role of tamoxifen versus placebo for women with stage II breast cancer exclusively enrolled older patients. Tamoxifen is one of the safest drugs used in cancer treatment; this fact limited generalization about cytotoxic effect of chemotherapy. Only 15 trials had a population of greater than 40% patients over age 65 that showed a comparable survival benefit from experimental treatments. Favorable outcomes from 4% ($n = 15$) of trials using experimental versus standard treatment showed similar treatment-related morbidity and mortality in both arms of the study. Ninety-six percent of the studies reviewed (331 of 345 trials) showed no age bias in published results.

Implications: The study clearly recognized that despite the number of elderly patients being treated for cancer, there are inadequate data as to the efficacy and tolerance of these cytotoxic therapies. Persistent underrepresentation of older adults in these trials weakens the evidence base to guide treatment therapy. Although the older adults enrolled these clinical trials did not suffer more toxicity with experimental treatments, physician perception persists regarding treatment benefit/tolerance in the older patients in clinical trials. This fear contributes to produce underrepresentation in clinical trials, yet this study demonstrated that age is not an independent risk factor for toxicity. With the pervasive rise in incidence and prevalence as the population ages, the need to treat older patients adequately should be based on reliable evidence and this can only occur if they are included in clinical trials.

Reference: Kumar, A., Soares, L. P., Balducci, L., & Djulbegovic, B. (2007). Treatment tolerance and efficacy in geriatric oncology: A systemic review of phase III randomized trials conducted by five National Cancer Institute–sponsored cooperative groups. *J Clin Oncol, 25,* 1272–1276.

Complications of chemotherapy are a direct result of the cytotoxic effect on rapidly dividing cells of the bone marrow, gastrointestinal tract, skin, and hair. Myelotoxicity, especially neutropenia, is one of the most serious complications of chemotherapy and older individuals appear to be at increased risk because of reduction in hematopoietic reserves. Elderly patients tend to experience neutropenia within the first few cycles of treatment and are more likely to be hospitalized due to life-threatening infectious complications (Balducci, 2003b). A growing body of evidence supports the use of standard therapy in older patients without significant comorbidities and good functional status, but little is known as to how to treat less "fit" elderly patients. When nonstandard doses are used in this population to reduce toxicities, treatment outcomes are poorer (Burdette-Radoux & Muss, 2006).

Although the evidence is sparse, older patients with careful selection appear to tolerate and respond well to chemotherapy (Balducci, 2007; Balducci & Corcoran, 2000; Burdette-Radoux & Muss, 2006; Hood, 2002; Wasil & Lichtman, 2005). Older patients with breast, colorectal, and non–small cell lung cancer have demonstrated a benefit from adjuvant therapies provided their life expectancy is greater than 5 years (Balducci, 2009; Burdett-Radoux & Muss, 2006; Muss, Biganzoli, Sargent, & Aapro, 2007; Repetto, 2003). Lack of data on efficacy of chemotherapy in older patients and the tendency of treatment selection to be based on chronological age versus physiological age may correlate with undertreatment and poor outcomes (Dale, 2003).

With the increased use of biotherapy and molecular targeted therapy as a treatment modality, limited data are available regarding tolerance in the older patient. Many of the molecular targeted agents are oral, and little is known about the bioavailability and efficacy in the older patient. A recent study found that older patients seem to tolerate these therapies either alone or in combination with chemotherapy as well as younger patients (Townsley et al., 2006). Although research shows that older patients seem to tolerate molecular targeted therapy as well as younger patients, issues of adherence, malnutrition, and cost may be a deterrent in this population. Further research is required to address the efficacy and toxicities of cancer therapies in older adults to include less than "fit" patients in clinical trials to provide evidence-based data. Additional strategies focusing on survival and quality of life will need to be developed for management of this unique population.

Diabetes

As the population of older Americans increases, so does the growth of diabetes mellitus. Diabetes is a major health concern for all age groups including older adults. One of the most dramatic aspects of diabetes is the rapid rise in the number of Americans who have developed diabetes and the possible predictions for the future. Currently, there are 23.6 million Americans or 7.8% of the population who have diabetes (American Diabetes Association, 2010b). This is an increase of 45% in the past 20 years. If current trends continue, 1 in 3 Americans will develop diabetes at some point, and they will lose an average of 10 to 15 years of their lifespan (CDC, 2010a).

When we look specifically at older Americans, the statistics are even more dramatic. For Americans age 65 and older the prevalence of diabetes is as high as 12% with expectations that that number will grow to almost 20% by the year 2020 (Selvin, Coresh, & Brancati, 2006). Almost 50% of all people diagnosed are age 60 or older (Engelgau, Murphy, Narayan, & Vinicor, 2006). Implications of the growth of diabetes in this age group are vast, ranging from interference in quality of life, full or partial disability, frequent hospitalizations, and the increased demand for health care services. The associated health care costs related to treating this chronic, incurable disease are also quite dramatic.

There are a variety of types of diabetes mellitus present in both younger and older adults. All types are characterized by high levels of blood glucose due to some type of defect in the body's use of insulin. Two common types of diabetes are type 1 diabetes and type 2 diabetes. Although both types are diagnosed by high blood glucose, they are quite different in their etiology. Type 1 diabetes accounts for approximately 5% to 10% of diabetes cases and usually develops early in life (Banion & Valentine, 2006). Although the cause of type 1 diabetes is not certain, it involves an autoimmune response in which the body's immune system attacks and kills insulin-producing beta cells in the pancreas (NIDDK, 2010). This lack of insulin production triggers dramatic symptoms and requires rapid intervention. These individuals will require some form of supplemental insulin for the rest of their lives. Because of improvements in the treatment of type I diabetes, these patients once termed "juvenile diabetics" are now living to older ages.

Type 2 diabetes accounts for 90% to 95% of all cases of diagnosed diabetes (CDC, 2007) and is the diabetes that affects large numbers of older adults. The risks for type 2 diabetes include older age, obesity, a family history of diabetes, a personal history of gestational diabetes, impaired glucose metabolism, physical inactivity, and race/ethnicity (CDC, 2007). This more common form of diabetes is characterized by the body's inability to use insulin properly. For a variety of reasons, some known and some unknown, the body either fails to produce enough insulin or the cells become resistant to insulin. In the latter case, the body produces more insulin in an attempt to overcome the resistance. Over time, this increased production causes the beta cells to burn out and insulin production is impaired (Donath et al., 2005). This impairment eventually leads to hyperglycemia. Because the mechanism of insulin impairment occurs over time, the onset of diabetes and its associated symptoms are more gradual and often undiagnosed for years.

Typical and Atypical Presentations

The insidious nature of diabetes is that very often people have no symptoms of elevated blood glucose in type 2 diabetes. Statistical data related to type 2 diabetes often include estimates of undiagnosed cases. For example, of the current estimate of over 23 million people with diabetes in America, the American Diabetes Association (2010b) estimates that almost 6 million of those are currently undiagnosed. For this reason, diabetes is a common focus of community health promotion events, screening at-risk senior populations.

Classic symptoms of diabetes in both younger and older adults are the 3 Ps: polyuria (frequency of urination), polydipsia (increased thirst), and polyphagia (increased hunger) (Table 8-3). Other symptoms associated with the elevated blood glucose of diabetes include unusual weight loss, frequent infections, blurred vision, and slow healing of wounds. Because of the variety of symptoms, the diagnosis of diabetes varies and may be quite unexpected for some people.

In older adults, the subtle signs of diabetes may be missed. Patients experiencing polyuria may misinterpret this as a urinary infection or some other urinary dysfunction (Gray-Miceli & McDonald, 2007). Gradual weight loss can be associated with cancer in

TABLE 8-3 Symptoms of Diabetes Mellitus

Type 1 or type 2 Diabetes	Frequent urination Unusual thirst Extreme hunger Unusual weight loss Extreme fatigue Irritability
Type 2 Diabetes	Frequent infections Blurred vision Cuts and bruises that are slow to heal Tingling or numbness in the hands or feet Recurring skin, gum, or bladder infections

American Diabetes Association. (2010a). *Diabetes basics: Symptoms.* Retrieved December 12, 2010, from http://www.diabetes.org/diabetes-basics/symptoms/

the mind of the individual and cause great anxiety. A nonhealing skin condition or infection may send a person to a dermatologist, which may eventually lead to a diagnosis of diabetes. In addition, because older adults may have a blunted thirst sensation, they may be missing one of the three Ps. Therefore, the presentation of diabetes in an older adult may differ from that in younger people. Specifically, an older adult may present with dehydration, confusion, delirium, and decreased visual acuity (Jett, 2008).

The formal diagnosis of diabetes is evaluated through laboratory testing of glucose levels and is the same for both younger and older adults. A normal blood glucose level is below 100 mg/dL after an 8-hour fast (American Diabetes Association, 2010c). Diabetes is diagnosed if the patient has:

- A blood glucose level of 126 mg/dL or higher after an 8-hour fast
- A blood glucose level of 200 mg/dL or higher 2 hours after drinking 75 grams of glucose dissolved in water (a glucose tolerance test)
- A blood glucose level of 200 mg/dL or higher at any random time of the day and the presence of diabetes symptoms (NIDDK, 2010)

There is also a growing group of people with prediabetes. For these people, blood glucose levels exceed 100 mg/dL but are not high enough for a diagnosis of diabetes (NIDDK, 2010). This glucose finding indicates a risk to develop diabetes and allows the opportunity to implement strategies to reduce the likelihood of disease onset.

Hemoglobin A1C is another measure of glucose control and helps patients and practitioners understand how well blood glucose levels are controlled over time. Ideally, hemoglobin A1C levels should fall below 7% to avoid long-term complications from diabetes. However, for some older adults, tight glucose control may be difficult or impractical to achieve. In these patients higher hemoglobin A1C levels are acceptable, particularly in those with a shortened a life expectancy and in those with other advanced comorbidities. In these patients, blood glucose control should attempt to minimize the risk of hypoglycemic episodes. For patients nearing the end of life, blood glucose rarely needs to be monitored and only requires treatment if episodes of hyperglycemia interfere with patient comfort (Joslin Diabetes Center, 2007).

Risk factors for the development of type 2 diabetes are varied, but the incidence of onset increases with age (Box 8-3). The age-related risk for diabetes starts at 45 years old and increases in combination with other risk factors such as racial/ethnic groups, family history, and those previously identified to have prediabetes (http://www.diabetes.org). These risk factors should be identified, although they cannot be altered. Risk factors that can be altered include weight and a sedentary lifestyle. Health care members should review risk factors with older adults to identify opportunities to reduce the risk of diabetes through lifestyle modifications.

BOX 8-3 Risk Factors for Type 2 Diabetes

- Age 45 or older
- Impaired glucose tolerance or impaired fasting glucose
- Family history of diabetes
- Overweight or obese
- Sedentary lifestyle or lack of regular exercise
- Low high-density lipoprotein cholesterol level, high triglyceride level, high blood pressure
- Racial/ethnic groups: non-Hispanic Blacks, Hispanic/Latin Americans, Asian Americans, American Indians, and Alaska Natives
- History of gestational diabetes or having a baby weighing 9 lb or more at birth

From American Diabetes Association. (2009a). Diabetes basics: Who is at greater risk for type 2 diabetes? Retrieved December 12, 2010, from http://www.diabetes.org/diabetes-basics/prevention/risk-factors

Once diabetes is diagnosed, the management of blood glucose is crucial to patient outcomes and the ability to minimize complications. Altering patterns of diet and exercise in a population with long-standing habits presents a unique set of challenges. It is imperative for this population to understand that the adoption of healthy lifestyle changes can have multiple positive outcomes on their health. When a person with a chronic illness assumes self-management responsibilities, the person gains the opportunity to better control the disease and retain the highest possible quality of life (Anderson, Funnell, & Tang, 2006).

Successful self-management of a chronic illness can be a difficult challenge to the older adult. The importance of establishing the support of health care practitioners cannot be underestimated in diabetes care. Diabetes self-management education is available in various forms and often incorporates physicians, nurses, dietitians, and social workers. Unfortunately, many people with diabetes are not offered, or do not seek out, these opportunities for diabetes support. Research shows that up to 54% of people with type 2 diabetes are above target levels for glycemic control (Leeman, 2007). This inability to control glucose levels often relates to insufficient knowledge.

Elements of diabetes management involve proper nutrition, exercise, drug treatment, blood glucose testing, and other health promotion activities (Table 8-4). Nutrition issues can be problematic for all age groups. Nationally, our consumption of processed foods and excess calories has caused a variety of health concerns including increased obesity rates. Dietary habits are developed over a lifetime for older adults and can be difficult to alter. For older Americans dietary habits can be significantly influenced by finances, living conditions, loss of a significant other, or physiological changes in metabolism and appetite.

Understanding the concepts of food and its impact on blood glucose is a cornerstone of diabetes management. Nutrition counseling with trained professionals is referred to as medical nutrition therapy. No longer rigid or based on many calculations, medical nutrition therapy seeks small, incremental changes to benefit overall health (Freeman & Franz, 2006), and it may be effective for glycemic control. Additionally, nutritional emphasis on saturated fat and cholesterol supports cardiac health in this at-risk population.

Physical activity is a desired behavior in all age groups and has multiple benefits for older adults with diabetes. About 30% of adults ages 65 to 74 and 40% of those age 75 or older pursue no leisure-time physical activity (Agency for Healthcare Research and Quality, 2002). Physical activity can help maintain or lose weight, lower blood glucose levels, improve the body's use of insulin, and promote cardiac and psychological health along with other benefits (Mullooly, 2006). In older adults, even a small amount of exercise can improve health and help maintain optimal mobility, muscle strength, and circulation (Agency for Healthcare Research and Quality, 2002). National standards for diabetes care recommend 150 minutes per week of moderately intense aerobic physical activity in addition to resistance training three times weekly if there are no medical contraindications (American Diabetes Association, 2008).

Although nutrition and physical activity are indicated for all persons with diabetes, many will

TABLE 8-4 Summary of Standards of Care in Diabetes

TEST/EXAM	FREQUENCY
Self-monitoring of blood glucose	As needed for treatment goals (type 2 diabetes) More often when using insulin
A1C (3-month average of blood glucose)	Twice yearly if at goal Four times yearly if not at goal Goal: At or below 7%
Weight	Each regular diabetes visit
Blood pressure	Each regular diabetes visit Goal: Systolic less than 130 mm Hg; Diastolic less than 80 mm Hg
Lipids (cholesterol profile)	Yearly (less if normal)
Microalbumin (protein in urine)	Yearly
Dilated eye exam	Yearly
Comprehensive foot exam	Yearly (more often if high risk)
Medical nutrition therapy	As needed to meet treatment goals
Physical activity plan	As needed to meet treatment goals Goal: 150 minutes moderate activity weekly; resistance training 3 times weekly
Immunizations	Flu annually Pneumonia at least once
Dental care	At least twice yearly

American Diabetes Association. (2009b). Executive summary: Standards of medical care in diabetes. *Diabetes Care, 32,* S1–S21.

also require drug treatment to support glycemic control. As mentioned previously, those persons with type 1 diabetes need to administer insulin to themselves for the rest of their life due to the body's inability to produce endogenous insulin. Type 2 diabetes has a variety of drugs available for glycemic control that may include oral products or insulin.

Non-insulin drugs for treating diabetes come in a variety of categories. Older adults may take one type of drug or several drugs with different mechanisms of action. Collaboration with all members of the health care team is especially important when multiple practitioners are prescribing drugs for a patient with diabetes. Often, older adults take multiple drugs for multiple health issues and the effects of diabetes drugs should be considered in light of the patient's complete drug regimen from all prescribers. For example, an older adult could easily have a primary care physician, cardiologist, and endocrinologist, all prescribing drugs. For this at-risk population, older adults should be encouraged to keep an updated list of drugs and should ask prescribers about the possible effect on blood glucose or other interactions when new drugs are ordered.

Older adults with type 2 diabetes may also use insulin to control blood glucose either alone or, commonly, with oral drugs. Because of the progressive nature of diabetes, there is an ongoing need for medication changes that could include the use of insulin (Gray-Miceli & McDonald, 2007). This addition of insulin is usually recommended when oral therapy alone does not produce recommended glycemic goals. Like oral drugs, there are a number of choices of insulin and the ways it can be incorporated into a plan of glucose management. Because it is only available as an injection, many older adults resist the initiation of insulin to their regimen or refuse to start it for a variety of reasons (Johnson & Dang, 2006). Fears of self-injections, progression of the disease, or other issues may be overcome with patient support and education. Although very effective in controlling blood glucose, when used correctly, insulin is considered a high-risk drug and requires proper training and education to avoid unwanted outcomes.

Self-monitoring of blood glucose is a component of self-care to help manage diabetes. Information gained through self-monitoring reflects how food, physical activity, drugs, and stress are affecting the patient's blood glucose level (Kulkarni, 2006). Also, being able to quickly check the blood glucose level helps to support the patient's target goals and detect and prevent dangerous fluctuations in blood glucose. Self-monitoring is indicated for all older adults who take diabetes medication, and especially those who use insulin. Barriers caused by physical status, cognition, or dexterity may necessitate assistance from a family member, caretaker, or home health resource to test blood glucose (Kulkarni, 2006).

Exacerbations and Complications

Complications of diabetes can be classified as acute and chronic in nature. The ultimate goal of blood glucose management is to stay "average," not too high and not too low, thus minimizing the acute and chronic complications. Hypoglycemia (low blood glucose) is a significant consideration in all age groups, especially older adults (Box 8-4). Slowed counter-regulation of hormones, erratic food intake, certain drugs, and slowed intestinal absorption put older adults at higher risk for hypoglycemia (Spollett, 2006). The actual glucose level that produces hypoglycemia varies by individual. With severe hypoglycemia, persons are impaired to the point that they cannot help themselves to correct the problem due to an altered mental state (Banion & Valentine, 2006). The most important

BOX 8-4 Hypoglycemia Symptoms and Treatments

Possible Symptoms of Hypoglycemia

- Shaking
- Sweating
- Dizziness
- Anxiety
- Trouble concentrating
- Lack of coordination

Sources of 15 to 20 Grams Carbohydrate

- 4 ounces juice
- 4 ounces regular soda
- Glucose tablets (according to label instructions)
- 3 to 4 hard candies, chewed
- 1 cup lowfat or nonfat milk
- 2 tablespoons raisins

Treatment may be followed in 15 minutes by repeat test of blood glucose level. Keep in mind that severe hypoglycemia causes more severe symptoms and may prevent the affected person from taking self-treatment.

From Steil, C. F. (2006). Pharmacologic therapies for glucose management. In C. Mensing (Ed.), The art and science of diabetes self-management education: A desk reference for healthcare professionals (pp. 321–355). Chicago: American Association of Diabetes Educators.

issues with hypoglycemia are to recognize the condition, treat it as early as possible, and investigate what caused the episode so that it can be prevented in the future.

Hyperglycemia is above-normal blood glucose (Arnold & Trence, 2006). Elevated blood glucose can occur before the diagnosis of diabetes and transiently throughout the long-term management of diabetes. Many factors can contribute to hyperglycemia, such as ingestion of excessive carbohydrates, lack of exercise, inadequate adherence to the drug regimen, and stress. Severe hyperglycemia can cause dehydration and electrolyte imbalance leading to hospitalization and possible death.

Chronic complications of diabetes are characterized as macrovascular and microvascular. This terminology refers to larger blood vessels (macrovascular) and smaller, more delicate, vessels (microvascular). The reason for these disorders of the vasculature has to do with the long-term effects of glucose on the blood vessels. The physiological effects of excess glucose increase the formation of plaque, clots, and inflammation (Lorber, 2006). This alteration in small and large blood vessels manifests in a variety of ways in older adults.

Macrovascular complications include coronary artery disease, cerebrovascular disease, and peripheral vascular disease. People with diabetes are two to four times more likely to have a stroke, an MI, and sudden death, and 65% of deaths in diabetes are due to coronary artery disease (Lorber, 2006). For these reasons proper diabetes management must include a heart-healthy approach to life. Fortunately, those who incorporate the suggested nutrition and exercise practices for diabetes are simultaneously helping reduce their risk of heart disease and other macrovascular complications.

Although macrovascular disease is the leading cause of death in diabetes, complications make a significant impact on the quality of life. Microvascular complications can affect varied areas of the body and involve the delicate microscopic vessels. Microvascular complications of the eyes, kidneys, and nerves are most commonly discussed. Diabetes is the leading cause of blindness, chronic renal failure, and loss of lower extremities due to the destruction of these vessels (American Diabetes Association, 2010b). These types of disabilities can lead to loss of independence or require a change in living situations for older adults.

In addition to the traditional complications of diabetes, there are also exacerbations of glucose control that can be caused by common short-term illnesses such as influenza or a gastric virus. Because stress, both physical and psychological, can raise blood glucose due to the hormonal response of the body, certain situations can cause significant blood glucose problems (Ruggiero, Wagner, & de Groot, 2006. These factors can lead to the unpredictable fluctuations in blood glucose. In older adults and the frail elderly, this can require hospitalization.

In summary, the successful management of diabetes requires the older adult to be knowledgeable on a variety of related topics. Some older adults are very active and motivated to adapt healthy lifestyle patterns that support glycemic control, and some may suffer from a variety of other illnesses that makes care more difficult (Spollett, 2006). The educational support of these people should reflect individual needs related to any deficits they may have (Gray-Miceli & McDonald, 2007) Using a team of health care providers to teach and support the multiple aspects of diabetes care is optimal for success. Priorities of care may change over the patient's lifespan and as the diabetes evolves. Nurses have countless opportunities to support older adults in the challenges of maintaining health and preventing complications in the spectrum of diabetes.

Using a team of health care providers to teach and support the multiple aspects of diabetes care is optimal for success.

Osteoarthritis

Osteoarthritis (also called degenerative arthritis or degenerative joint disease) is the most common form of arthritis, and a large majority of older adults will experience some degree of osteoarthritis during their lifetime. The most common sites of arthritis are the knees, hips, and hands. People who engage in repetitive activities that stress the joints, such as athletes, are at increased risk of osteoarthritis, and these individuals may experience osteoarthritis at a younger age, particularly if there is a history of joint injury. Weight is a significant factor in the development of osteoarthritis in the knees. According to Vrezas, Elsner, Bolm-Audorff, Abolmaali, and Seidler (2010), people who are overweight or obese are about 10 times more likely to develop osteoarthritis in their knees as compared with people who were not overweight. Weight and repetitive use causes the cartilage between the joints to break down more quickly, leading to the development of painful arthritis. In addition, there is an effect of gender and genetics (Spector & MacGregor, 2004). Women are more likely to develop osteoarthritis, and the risk of developing the disease is higher when there is a family history present.

The pain of osteoarthritis may vary throughout the course of the disease. Patients may initially have joint stiffness after a period of rest (in the morning) that dissipates with use. Later in the course of the disease, joints become painful with use and activity may become limited. There may be atrophy of the muscles surrounding the joints secondary to disuse.

Lifestyle modifications may be helpful, particularly early in the disease. Patients with osteoarthritis in the knees and hips should be counseled to lose weight. Non-weight-bearing exercises, such as swimming, have demonstrated some efficacy in reducing some of the painful symptoms of osteoarthritis. Using cold packs, taking oral glucosamine, and using topical rubs containing capsaicin have shown to be of modest benefit in treating osteoarthritis. Ultrasound has been determined to be ineffective in the treatment of pain from osteoarthritis.

Drugs and Other Treatments

Acetaminophen is often among the first drugs used in osteoarthritis because it has an established record of safety. NSAIDs such as ibuprofen and naproxen are more effective than acetaminophen but may raise the risk of certain side effects, including gastrointestinal bleeding. Newer anti-inflammatory drugs called COX-2 inhibitors are effective in relieving the pain of osteoarthritis but have raised concerns about cardiovascular side effects, including MI and stroke. In addition to oral drugs, some drugs may be injected directly into the joint. Corticosteroids can reduce pain and inflammation for short periods. Adding cushioning fluid back into the joint can help decrease friction between bones and hence reduce pain. This method, termed viscosupplementation, tends to reduce pain for longer periods than injected corticosteroids and can delay (but not prevent) the need for joint replacement.

When these interventions fail, joint replacement is an option. Currently, the most common sites of joint replacement are the hips and knees. Following joint replacement surgery, patients usually stay in the hospital for 2 to 3 days before being discharged to home or to a nursing home to receive physical therapy. Physical therapy following joint replacement surgery may last several weeks, as the muscles and tendons are retrained around the new joint. Most patients experience a significant reduction in symptoms following joint replacement. Complications, although uncommon, can be significant. Infection following joint replacement is perhaps the most common and significant complication. Older adults, in particular, are at increased risk of complications related to disorientation and disuse during hospitalization. A combination of drugs, physiological stress, and a change in environment can bring about delirium in a person who may have been cognitively intact. These patients will require assistance with ambulation after surgery and have an increased risk of falls.

Osteoporosis

Osteoporosis refers to a reduction in bone strength and density that can increase the risk of fracture. It is literally the presence of "porous bone" that appears almost spongelike upon examination. This reduction in bone strength increases the risk of fractures among older adults. The most common osteoporotic fracture is a compression fracture of the spine, followed by fractures to the hip and wrist. There are several different types, forms, and causes of osteoporosis. Among women between ages 51 and 75, the most common type of osteoporosis is referred to as type 1 osteoporosis. It results mainly from the loss of estrogen following menopause. Type 2 osteoporosis tends to occur after age 70 in both men and women and is thought to result from reduced vitamin D synthesis, resistance to vitamin D activity, or both. Older women may experience a combination of types 1 and 2 (Merck Manuals Online Medical Library, 2010). Osteoporosis also may occur as a result of disuse; disuse osteoporosis can occur in either sex at any age.

Osteoporosis is typically a disease without any symptoms; therefore, an older adult can experience bone loss for years without diagnosis or treatment. These individuals may present with a broken bone following a minor fall or injury. These fractures can be a cause of bone pain, particularly in those who are unable to communicate that they have fallen. In addition, younger patients who have been taking steroids for long periods may be at increased risk of osteoporosis.

Women are at significantly greater risk of osteoporosis than are men. About 80% of older adults affected by osteoporosis are women. Although people of all ethnicities may develop osteoporosis, those at increased risk are Caucasians, Asians, and Hispanics. In addition, people who are small and thin, those with a family history of osteoporosis, those who are inactive, and those who smoke are at increased risk.

Musculoskeletal changes in osteoporosis can increase the risk of falls. Kyphosis or kyphoscoliosis refers to an increased curvature of the spine. These kyphotic changes are often the result of vertebral compression fractures from osteoporosis. Kyphosis increases the risk of falls as the center of gravity moves forward over the toes.

The most common test to check for osteoporosis is the dual energy x-ray absorptiometry (DEXA) scan. This text is recommended for all women over age 65. It shows changes in bone density and allows diagnosis of osteopenia (slightly reduced bone density) and osteoporosis (significantly reduced bone density).

Increasing the intake of calcium, through the use of supplements or through dietary modification, can help to strengthen bone. Foods that are high in calcium include milk, cheese, yogurt, collard greens, and sardines. Because estrogen is essential for calcium to be absorbed and deposited in bone, increasing the intake of dietary calcium alone is often insufficient to rebuild bone in postmenopausal women. Although supplemental estrogen used to be given together with calcium to treat osteoporosis, it is now understood that the risks associated with the long-term use of supplemental estrogen (heart disease and cancer) outweigh the benefit. In addition to the use of prescribed drugs and supplements, weight-bearing exercise helps build bone density. The stress of exercise stimulates the bones to grow and remineralize. Activities proven to help prevent bone loss include walking, hiking, dancing, and weight-lifting.

Bisphosphonates have become the main drugs used to treat osteoporosis. They work by inhibiting the activity of osteoclasts. Osteoclasts work to break down bone, and drugs that prevent their activity will allow the osteoblasts (cells that work to build up bone) to gain ground. These drugs therefore help prevent bone loss and, in some cases, will help to build up and strengthen existing bone. In older adults, it is important to note that these drugs can be extremely irritating to the gastroesophageal tract. Therefore, they should be taken with a full glass of water, and the patient should remain upright for 30 minutes. Nurses working in hospitals and long-term care facilities need to assess patients for their ability to tolerate liquids and to remain sitting up before giving these drugs.

Chronic Obstructive Pulmonary Disease

Chronic obstructive pulmonary disease (COPD) is a condition that impairs the movement of air through the lungs. It is the fourth leading cause of death in the United States. Smoking is the major cause of COPD, and roughly 80% to 90% of deaths from COPD are attributable to smoking (U.S. Department of Health and Human Services, 2004). Although men have traditionally been most affected by COPD, the rates of disease are increasing in women as a result of changes in trends in cigarette smoking.

The disease is composed of two different, yet interrelated conditions: chronic bronchitis and emphysema. In chronic bronchitis, airways are inflamed and excessive amounts of mucus are formed. The lungs lose the ability to recoil with expiration, and the air gets trapped in the collapsed lung tissue. Most patients with COPD have varying degrees of both chronic bronchitis and emphysema.

COPD is a progressive disease, and although drug treatments and lifestyle changes can help improve some of the symptoms, the underlying damage to lung tissue cannot be reversed (Merck Manuals Online Medical Library, 2010; Wise & Tashkin, 2007).

Over time, patients with COPD can develop signs and symptoms of the disease. Shortness of breath with exertion is the cardinal symptom. Dyspnea worsens progressively throughout the course of the disease, often leading to oxygen dependency. The inability of the lungs to fully retract with expiration leads to enlargement of the lung tissue. The presence of enlarged, nonfunctioning lung tissue causes outward pressure on the rib cage, leading to the development of a characteristic barrel chest. The hypoxia associated with COPD results in pale lips and fingernail beds. Clubbing is often seen in the fingers.

Nutrition

People with COPD often have difficulty meeting nutritional needs (Odencrants, Ehnfors, & Ehrenberg, 2008). There are significant stressors increasing metabolic demands, including increased work of breathing. In addition, it is thought that the pathophysiology of the disease itself combined with the use of steroids contributes to muscle wasting (Schols & Gosker, 2009). There are several ways patients with COPD may alter their diets to boost their nutritional intake (Box 8-5).

BOX 8-5 Nutritional Goals for Patients with COPD

- Maintain a healthy body weight.
- Drink 48 to 64 ounces or more of noncaffeinated fluid daily to help keep secretions thin. Patients who need fluid restriction should check with their health care provider about how much fluid to consume.
- Consume about 25 to 30 grams of fiber daily by eating high-fiber foods, such as vegetables, legumes, whole-grain foods, and fresh fruit.
- Limit sodium consumption.
- Avoid eating too much or eating foods that cause bloating, which can make breathing more difficult.
- Eat highly nutritious foods rather than foods that sap energy without giving energy in return.
- Try eating higher calorie foods earlier in the meal.
- To minimize shortness of breath while eating, clear the airways at least 1 hour before eating, eat slowly, eat foods that are easy to chew, eat five or six smaller meals daily, eat sitting up, and avoid drinking fluids until after eating.
- To minimize the effects of tiredness late in the day, eat food that are easy to prepare, ask for help with meal preparation, investigate a meal delivery program, eat the main meal early in the day, and rest before eating.

From Cleveland Clinic Foundation. (1995–2009). Nutritional guidelines for people with COPD. Cleveland, OH: Author. Retrieved December 12, 2010, from http://my.clevelandclinic.org/disorders/chronic_obstructive_pulmonary_disease_copd/hic_nutritional_guidelines_for_people_with_copd.aspx

Physical Activity

Older adults living with COPD should be encouraged to remain physically active. Research has demonstrated that a variety of exercise training programs, including the use of yoga, can help reduce feelings of breathlessness in this patient population (Carrieri-Kohlman et al., 2005; Donesky-Cuenco, Nguyen, Paul, & Carrieri-Kohlman, 2009). In addition, physical activity can help prevent or alleviate some of the comorbidities commonly associated with COPD including depression, osteoporosis, and diabetes. Nurses can support patients in efforts to remain physically active by ensuring patients have access to portable oxygen devices when needed and by encouraging patients to develop techniques to manage breathlessness while exercising.

Drug Treatment

The goals of drug use in patients with COPD are to reduce inflammation and open airways to improve the movement of air through the lungs. Bronchodilators help open the airways as wide as possible, while inhaled corticosteroids work to reduce inflammation. Patients with COPD may be on combinations of different drugs to help alleviate dyspnea and to allow patients to be more active. The drugs used to treat COPD are not curative and do not alter the course of the disease.

Many of the drugs used to treat COPD in older adults are administered through the use of multidose inhalers (commonly known as MDIs). In order for these drugs to work effectively, they must be inhaled as deeply as possible into the lung tissue. Coordinating the timing of drug release from the MDI with inspiration can prove difficult for some patients (Allen, Jain, Ragab, & Malik, 2003; Board & Allen, 2006). When possible, nurses should observe their patients using their MDIs to help ensure proper technique. For patients who have trouble using an MDI, nebulizer treatments may provide a more effective means of administering the prescribed drug.

Exacerbations and Complications

Patients with COPD may experience exacerbations throughout the course of the disease. As the disease progresses, exacerbations may become increasingly frequent. Older adults are more likely to require hospitalization due to exacerbations of COPD (American Lung Association, 2010). The course of treatment for an older adult with COPD typically requires the use of corticosteroids to reduce inflammation and the administration of oxygen therapy.

During periods of acute exacerbation, patients may be taught to breathe using a "pursed-lip breathing" technique. Breathing through pursed lips has been reported to alleviate sensations of breathlessness in these patients. Many patients will sit upright and lean forward over an overbed table in bed, or tripod their hands on their knees while in a wheelchair. These positions can also help ease feelings of dyspnea. For some older adults with otherwise limited mobility, sitting upright to alleviate sensations of dyspnea can increase the risk of pressure ulcers. Patients who need to sit upright for extended periods should be encouraged to change positions frequently and use pressure-relieving devices.

Older adults with COPD are also at increased risk from other pulmonary diseases and infections. Nurses should ensure that these patients receive vaccinations for seasonal flu and pneumococcal pneumonia. Pneumonia in those with COPD is a potentially life-threatening complication because the already limited gas exchange becomes further impaired. Airway-opening drugs may be used with antibiotic therapy and sometimes with ventilator support.

Comorbid Conditions

Patients with COPD often present with other comorbid conditions associated with the treatments for COPD and the underlying disease process. In particular, the use of steroids is associated with diabetes, depression, and osteoporosis. These comorbid conditions may be overlooked in patients with COPD and may present in an unusual way, in absence of other risk factors.

For many patients, feeling short of breath goes hand in hand with feelings of anxiety. Drugs and other interventions that improve oxygenation also help reduce the anxiety that dyspnea can cause. The physical limitations of breathlessness, including decreases in the ability to perform basic activities of daily living, can also be associated with depression.

End-of-Life Care

At the end of life, drugs to alleviate dyspnea and anxiety should be given without regard to their effects on oxygenation. Pulse oximetry is not a particularly useful tool for patients dying of COPD. Instead, symptom management should be provided with the ultimate goal of alleviating the sensations of dyspnea, anxiety, and pain. Although oxygen is a useful tool, it is rarely an adequate intervention when used alone at the end of life. Sublingual opiates in combination with antianxiety drugs should be titrated in response to frequent nursing assessments. Adjuvant therapies to alleviate feelings of breathlessness and anxiety such as the use of fans, fresh air, and massage should also be used.

Maintaining Health in Chronic Illness

Although many of the conditions covered in this chapter are experienced by large numbers of older adults, they do not necessarily have to have a negative impact on quality of life. Recognition of the differences between normal and pathological changes associated with aging is an important step in detecting an underlying disease early so that it can be effectively treated or managed. The knowledge that subtle changes in weight, cognition, and affect can signal underlying disease should inform the way a patient history is taken. When patients are found to have one or more chronic diseases, nurses play a key role in assisting older adults to maintain function while managing underlying illness.

PERSONAL PERSPECTIVE

Facing the Challenges of Decline

Agnes, a retired social worker and onetime world traveler, lights up when she talks about her long career and days of community involvement. But today, it is not just retirement that has radically changed the rhythm of her life. At 84, she walks with difficulty and finds her thinking is not as sharp as it used to be. "Now that I'm older," she reflects, "I feel that opportunities are limited due to physical problems and even mental problems. I used to have access to a car to get out and go wherever I wanted to go, and now it's more difficult. I have to see if it's worth going on a bus trip, or ask someone to drive me, or ask myself if I am physically strong enough and determined enough to walk where I want to go."

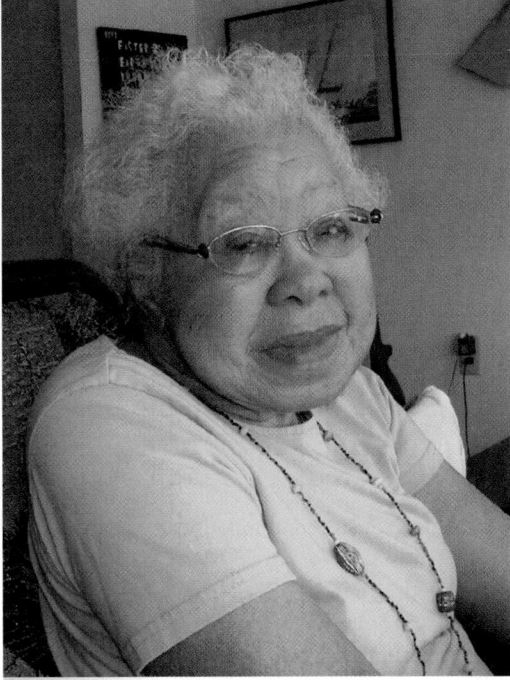

As if to emphasize the point, Agnes leans into her walker and, with slow, measured steps, crosses the room to the window overlooking the busy New Haven streets below. "You know," she says somewhat wistfully, "we live directly south of Yale and there are a lot of things I would like to visit. I used to always go to the museums and the lectures at the law school. Now I find I have to stop and think how I'm going to get there, and how I'm going to get back, and it's not worth it. I don't have the mental energy to plan for it."

Agnes speaks of the challenges of her own physical decline matter of factly and without a trace of self-pity: "If your knees hurt and your hips hurt and your back hurts, sometimes you wonder if it's easier to just sit down and do nothing. But I think that's a dangerous attitude, so you have to combat the physical problems. No difficulty is too great for you to overcome or surmount and so you have to look for the kind of help you need," counsels Agnes, a model of determination and grace.

About Agnes Agnes Timpson began a career as a medical technologist but soon discovered that she'd rather work with people, so she changed course. For many years, she was a social worker at Fellowship House, an agency that helps people with mental illnesses live independently in the community. However, her career always came second. Her first priority was her family. Widowed after 59 years of marriage, she is blessed with six children and eight grandchildren. Agnes served on the Board of Governors for the Connecticut Department of Higher Education. She still remains active in the Alpha Kappa Alpha sorority of black professional women and in two national associations focused on leadership, education, and training, with a dedication to helping young people stay in school. Agnes is an avid reader who finds great enjoyment in perusing the shelves of her local library.

Lorri B. Danzig, MS, CSL

KEY POINTS

- In older adults, common diseases may present differently due to physiological changes associated with aging.
- Common conditions associated with atypical presentations include infections, falls, urinary incontinence, MI, and heart failure.
- In older adults, hallmarks of infection such as fever, swollen lymph nodes, and leukocytosis may be diminished or absent.
- Falls should not be considered a normal part of aging. When an older adult has a fall, an underlying cause should be investigated.
- Urinary incontinence is not a normal part of aging. In older adults with new onset, precipitating factors should be assessed.
- Heart disease is the number one killer of women over age 25.
- Older adults with MI may not experience "crushing chest pain." Instead, they may experience upper back pain, pain between the shoulder pain, indigestion, or abdominal discomfort.
- Congestive heart failure is a condition in which the heart is unable to pump enough blood to meet physiological demands.
- Kidney failure is often associated with heart failure, as the kidneys become poorly perfused and unable to function properly. If the kidneys are unable to remove sufficient amounts of fluid, excess fluid can be retained, leading to exacerbations of heart failure.
- Cancer and its treatment can compromise an individual's already declining functional reserve and can impact diminishing social and financial resources.
- Age is the single most important risk factor in the elderly for the development of cancer.
- Patients with cancer have at least three comorbid conditions that can influence cancer detection, clinical presentation, and treatment outcomes.
- Medical decision making related to cancer treatment, barriers to cancer screening, undertreatment, and issues of quality of life present complex problems in the elderly population.
- More than 60% of patients diagnosed with cancer are over age 65. The average age of developing cancer is 68 for men and 65 for women.
- People age 75 years and older are expected to triple the rate of cancer cases over the next 30 years.
- Cancer treatments are major physiological stressors and successful outcomes depend on an individual's functional reserve to tolerate those stressors.
- Age bias influences treatment decisions despite the fact that physiological aging is different for each person.
- With the advances made in the management of other comorbid diseases, many elderly patients can live well beyond their diagnosis of cancer, thus making adjuvant therapy a viable option.
- Older patients with a diagnosis of cancer need to be evaluated on life expectancy, comorbidity, and functional status rather than chronological age.
- Elderly patients with cancer are at risk for undertreatment, inappropriate treatment, or both when chronological age is used as a basis for decision making.
- Uncertainty exists as to how to best assess the older person with cancer's ability to tolerate treatment and will require closer collaboration between oncologists and gerontologists to determine the most effective tools.

- Comorbid illness increases with age and can influence an individual's tolerance to cancer therapy.
- Research has shown that the elderly with careful assessment can tolerate surgery, radiation therapy, and chemotherapy/biotherapy.
- Informal caregivers, usually family members, are largely responsible for providing care to elderly patients undergoing cancer treatment.
- Prolonged caregiving can exhaust the resources of the caregiver and place him or her at risk for physiological, psychological, and economic issues.
- Type 2 diabetes is a common disease with increased incidence in older adults.
- Type 2 diabetes is increasing nationally due to the aging population and increased incidence of obesity.
- Type 2 diabetes is often undiagnosed for years because there may be no symptoms.
- Once a diagnosis is made, a comprehensive patient assessment should be done to determine current health status and goals for care.
- Management of blood glucoses to avoid hypoglycemia and hyperglycemia is the goal.
- Establishing a team of health care members to support knowledge of diabetes management is preferred.
- Management involves proper nutrition, exercise, self-monitoring of blood glucose, and, for many, drug treatment.
- The goal for care is to avoid short-term and long-term complications that can interfere with the quality of life for older adults or cause death.
- Nurses have countless opportunities to teach older adults with diabetes skills for health living with diabetes.
- Arthritis is a condition marked by painful deterioration of the cartilage surrounding the joints and the growth of bony prominences at the ends of bones.
- Osteoarthritis is an extremely common condition affecting 80% of older adults.
- Non-weight-bearing exercises such as swimming have demonstrated some efficacy in reducing some of the painful symptoms of osteoarthritis.
- Joint replacement is an option for patients with severe osteoarthritis. The most common sites of replacement are knees and hips.
- Osteoporosis is a reduction in bone strength and density. This reduction in bone strength increases the risk of fracture in older adults.
- Interventions for patients with osteoporosis include engaging in weight-bearing exercises, nutritional supplementation with calcium and vitamin D, and the administration of drugs that inhibit the action of osteoclasts.
- COPD impairs air movement through the lungs and is the fourth leading cause of death in the United States.
- The overwhelming majority of COPD cases stem from exposure to cigarette smoke.
- COPD is a progressive disease. Symptoms can be managed with lifestyle interventions and drug therapy.
- For patients with COPD at the end of life, high-quality symptom management should be provided with the ultimate goal of alleviating the sensations of dyspnea, anxiety, and pain.

CRITICAL THINKING ACTIVITIES

1. Describe what you envision your health status will be at 75 years of age in terms of comorbid illnesses, functional status, and comorbidity. What types of comorbidities do you feel that you might be at risk for? Is there anything that you can do to prevent them later in life?
2. Talk to some older adults whom you know and ask them what they know about screening for cancer. Find out what screening tests they have had in the past. Find out who referred them.
3. Look up the side effects of the following drug regimen (rituximab, cyclophosphamide, doxorubicin, vincristine, and prednisone). Your patient is 78 years old and has both diabetes and heart disease. What are the possible toxicities related to this treatment?
4. Think about what would happen if your elderly parent who provides babysitting for your children while you worked suddenly developed cancer. Treatment entails daily transportation to radiation therapy for the next 6 to 8 weeks. How will this impact you and your family? Identify what issues will arise. How will you manage this? Do you need to find additional services? How would you go about doing this?
5. To show changes in acid base balance, a simple demonstration using bromthymol blue, a color-sensitive pH indicator, may be conducted. To a clear glass of water, add a few drops of bromthymol blue. The water will now be blue. Next, using a straw, exhale to blow air bubbles through the solution. The color of the water will change to yellow, indicating that it is now acidic, from the CO_2 that has just been added to it. Next add some sodium bicarbonate to the glass, and

note the color change. Discuss pH changes that may occur in people with COPD, sometimes also called CO_2 retainers, and how the buffer system works. More advanced students might be asked to discuss specific laboratory value changes that occur in patients with COPD.

6. To demonstrate the relationship of atherosclerosis to blood pressure, an example of a garden hose may be used. What happens when you put your thumb over the end of a running garden hose? Even with a small occlusion, the pressure increases dramatically. This is similar to what happens when atherosclerotic plaques form in the arteries. They partially occlude the blood flow, increasing blood pressure in the system.
7. Imagine yourself diagnosed with a chronic disease like diabetes. After examining your own coping skills, think how you would react to this type of news. How successful would you be in changing your diet, exercising, monitoring blood glucose, taking prescribed drugs, and having regular check-ups?

CASE STUDY | *MR. BERBER*

Mr. Berber is a 75-year-old retired high school principle who up to 6 months ago lived in his own home. His wife died 5 years ago after a long illness with colon cancer. He recently decided to move in with his only son, who is unmarried. Mr. Berber has become increasingly more forgetful over the past year and has recently been diagnosed with mild dementia. Despite his comorbid conditions, ischemic heart disease, hyperlipidemia, and diabetes, he played golf twice a week. Lately, his son, a sales manager, has noticed his father having some constipation that is unrelieved with over-the-counter drugs. Mr. B. has never had a colorectal or prostate screening, even though his primary health care provider has requested him to do so over the years. Mr. Berber's son is concerned about leaving his father alone when he is on business trips, which occur about twice a month, for several days.

1. What is your assessment of Mr. Berber's functional status and mental status? How do they influence screening and treatment decisions?
2. Would it be appropriate to screen Mr. Berber for colon cancer and prostate cancers? What are the associated risks for this patient if he should be diagnosed with cancer?
3. What factors may have influenced his decision in the past not to undergo screening exams?
4. What is the probability of Berber's son becoming a caregiver for his father? How will this impact him? What are the primary issues he will have to address regarding his father?

CASE STUDY | *MARCIA GOMEZ*

Marcia Gallagher is a 63-year-old woman who works as a nursing assistant and lives with her husband. She has two grown children whom she sees frequently, and she especially enjoys visiting with her grandchildren. She has been in relatively good health, although she is slightly overweight and does not exercise regularly. Because she has not been having any significant problems, she has not seen her physician for a few years.

For some time now, Marcia has been having difficulty with her vision when she is at work. She attributes this to getting older and plans to have an eye exam sometime in the future. On a recent visit Marcia has difficulty reading a book to her grandchildren and decides it is time to see the eye doctor to get a prescription for glasses like many people she knows who are her age. During the eye exam, the doctor asks her if anyone in her family has type 2 diabetes. She shares that she thinks her father had an issue with "sugar."

Marcia is shocked when the doctor refers her back to her primary health provider for a full checkup because he suspects she has diabetes. When she visits her physician, she finds that her blood glucose is 328 mg/dL. The doctor initially discusses lifestyle management of type 2

CASE STUDY | *MARCIA GOMEZ*—cont'd

diabetes and prescribes a drug. He shares with her that her vision may improve as her blood glucose returns to normal. He advises that she should have a full eye exam yearly now that she knows she has diabetes. The physician also shares that it is likely that her blood glucose has been elevated for months or years due to the results of her A1C test. Marcia leaves the doctor's office shocked and upset about the news of this chronic illness.

1. Considering what you have learned about the symptoms of type 2 diabetes, is Marcia's story unusual and why?
2. What types of lifestyle changes can Marcia adopt to maximize her health now that she has diabetes?
3. What resources will support Marcia in her new challenge to manage this progressive chronic condition?

CASE STUDY | *MRS. ROSSI*

Mrs. Rossi is an 89-year-old woman with end-stage COPD. She currently resides in a nursing home in a large metropolitan city. Her husband died many years ago, and her children live far away. Mrs. Rossi prefers to be out of bed in her wheelchair. She often sits forward in her wheelchair leaning over the over bed tray because this is the position in which she can breathe most easily. Usually she wears oxygen, 2 L via nasal cannula.

One day you notice Mrs. Rossi lying flat on her back in bed. Her lips are blue and she says, "help ... I'm suffocating ... I feel like I can't get any air." You see the nasal cannula has slipped away from her nose and is dangling from the side of the bed.

Her drugs are albuterol/Atrovent via nebulizer bid.; morphine 2 mg every 6 hr, PRN, for pain; lorazepam 5 mg every 12 hr, PRN, for anxiety.

1. Which interventions would you plan for Mrs. Rossi?
2. How would you prioritize these interventions and why?
3. What information would you want to communicate to the nursing assistants caring for Mrs. Rossi? What should be communicated to her family and to her physician?

REFERENCES

Agency for Healthcare Research and Quality. (2002). *Physical activity and older Americans.* Washington, DC: U.S. Department of Health and Human Services. Retrieved December 12, 2010, from http://www.ahrq.gov/ppip/activity.htm

Allen, S. C., Jain, M., Ragab, S., & Malik, N. (2003). Acquisition and short-term retention of inhaler techniques require intact executive function in elderly subjects. *Age and Ageing, 32*(3), 299–302.

American Diabetes Association. (2008). Standards of medical care in diabetes—2008. *Diabetes Care, 31*(Suppl. 1), S12–S54.

American Diabetes Association. (2009a). *Diabetes basics: Who is at greater risk for type 2 diabetes?* Retrieved December 12, 2010, from http://www.diabetes.org/diabetes-basics/prevention/risk-factors

American Diabetes Association. (2009b). Executive summary: Standards of medical care in diabetes. *Diabetes Care, 32,* S1–S21.

American Diabetes Association. (2010a). *Diabetes basics: Symptoms.* Retrieved December 12, 2010, from http://www.diabetes.org/diabetes-basics/symptoms/

American Diabetes Association. (2010b). *Diabetes statistics.* Alexandria, VA: Author. Retrieved December 12, 2010, from http://www.diabetes.org/diabetes-basics/diabetes-statistics/?utm_source=WWW&utm_medium=DropDownDB&utm_content=Statistics&utm_campaign=CON

American Diabetes Association. (2010c). *Prediabetes FAQs.* Alexandria, VA: Author. Retrieved December 12, 2010, from http://www.diabetes.org/diabetes-basics/prevention/pre-diabetes/pre-diabetes-faqs.html

American Heart Association. (2010). *What your cholesterol levels mean.* Retrieved December 12, 2010, from http://www.heart.org/HEARTORG/Conditions/What-Your-Cholesterol-Levels-Mean_UCM_305562_Article.jsp

American Lung Association. (2010). *Trends in COPD (chronic bronchitis and emphysema): Morbidity and mortality.* Washington, DC: Author. Retrieved December 3, 2010, from http://www.lungusa.org/finding-cures/our-research/trend-reports/copd-trend-report.pdf

Anderson, B., Funnell, M., & Tang, T. (2006). Self management of health. In C. Mensing (Ed.), *The art and science of diabetes self-management education* (pp. 43–58). Chicago: American Association of Diabetes Educators.

Arnold, M. S., & Trence, D. L. (2006). Hyperglycemia. In C. Mensing (Ed.), *The art and science of diabetes self-management education* (pp. 163–186). Chicago: American Association of Diabetes Educators.

Audisio, R. A., Zbar, A. P., & Jaklitch, M. T. (2007). Surgical management of oncogeriatric patients. *Journal of Clinical Oncology, 25,* 1924–1929.

Balducci, L. (2003a). New paradigms for treating elderly patients with cancer: The Comprehensive Geriatric Assessment and guidelines for supportive care. *Journal of Supportive Oncology, 1*(S), 30–37.

Balducci, L. (2003b). Myelosuppression and its consequences in elderly patients with cancer. *Oncology, 17,* 27–32.

Balducci, L. (2007). Aging, frailty, and chemotherapy. *Cancer Control, 14,* 7–12.

Balducci, L. (2009). Pharmacology of antineoplastic medications in older cancer patients. Retrieved December 12, 2010, from http://www.cancernetwork.com/display/article/10165/99583

Balducci, L., & Ballester, O. F. (1996). Non-Hodgkin's lymphoma in the elderly. *Cancer Control, 3,* 5–14.

Balducci, L., & Beghe, C. (2000). The application of the principles of geriatric to the management of the older person with cancer. *Critical Reviewws in Oncology/Hematology, 35,* 147–154.

Balducci, L., & Beghe, B. (2001). Cancer and age in the USA. *Critical Reviews in Oncology/Hematology, 37,* 137–145.

Balducci, L., & Corcoran, M. B. (2000). Antineoplastic chemotherapy of the older cancer patient. *Hematology/Oncology Clinics of North America, 14,* 193–211.

Balducci, L., & Extermann, M. (2000a), Cancer and aging—An evolving panorama. *Hematology/Oncology Clinics of North America, 14,* 1–16.

Balducci, L., & Extermann, M. (2000b). Management of cancer in the older person: A practical approach. *Oncologist, 5,* 224–237.

Banion, C., & Valentine, V. (2006). Type 1 diabetes throughout the life span. In C. Mensing (Ed.), *The art and science of diabetes self-management education* (pp. 187–213). Chicago: American Association of Diabetes Educators.

Board, M., & Allen, S. C. (2006). A simple drawing test to identify patients who are unlikely to be able to learn to use an inhaler. *International Journal of Clinical Practice, 60*(5), 510–513.

Bouchardy, C., Rapiti, E., Blagojevic, S., Vlastos, A., & Vlastos, G. (2007). Older female cancer patients: Importance, causes, and consequences of undertreatment. *Journal of Clinical Oncology, 25,* 1858–1869.

Burdette-Radoux, S., & Muss, H. B. (2006). Adjuvant chemotherapy in the elderly: Whom to treat, what regimen? *Oncologist, 11,* 234–242.

Capezuti, E., Strumpf, N. E., Evans, L. K., Grisso, J. A., & Maislin, G. (1998). The relationship between physical restraint removal and falls and injuries among nursing home residents. *Journals of Gerontology, Series A, Biological Sciences and Medical Sciences, 53*(1), M47–M52.

Carrera, I., Balducci, L., & Extermann, M. (2005). Cancer in the older person. *Cancer Treatment Review, 31,* 380–402.

Carrieri-Kohlman, V., Nguyen, H. Q., Donesky-Cuenco, D., Demir-Deviren, S., Neuhaus, J., & Stulbarg, M. S. (2005). Impact of brief or extended exercise training on the benefit of a dyspnea self-management program in COPD. *Journal of Cardiopulmonary Rehabilitation, 25*(5), 275–284.

Casey, I., Zachariah, B., & Balducci, L. (2003. Radiation therapy of older persons. In J. Overcash & L. Balducci (Eds.), *The older cancer patient* (pp. 131–143). New York: Springer.

Centers for Disease Control and Prevention. (CDC, 2007). *National diabetes fact sheet.* Atlanta, GA: Author. Retrieved December 12, 2010, from http://www.cdc.gov/diabetes/pubs/pdf/ndfs_2007.pdf

Centers for Disease Control and Prevention. (CDC, 2010a). *Diabetes.* Atlanta, GA: Author. Retrieved December 12, 2010, from http://www.cdc.gov/chronicdisease/resources/publications/AAG/ddt.htm

Centers for Disease Control and Prevention. (CDC, 2010b). *Falls among older adults: An overview.* Atlanta, GA: Author. Retrieved December 12, 2010, from http://www.cdc.gov/homeandrecreationalsafety/falls/adultfalls.html

Cleveland Clinic Foundation. (1995–2009). *Nutritional guidelines for people with COPD.* Cleveland, OH: Author. Retrieved December 12, 2010, from http://my.clevelandclinic.org/disorders/chronic_obstructive_pulmonary_disease_copd/hic_nutritional_guidelines_for_people_with_copd.aspx

Cohen, H. J. (2007). The cancer aging interface: A research agenda. *Journal of Clinical Oncology, 25,* 1945–1948.

Dale, D. C. (2003). Poor prognosis in elder patient with cancer: The role of bias and undertreatment. *Journal of Supportive Oncology, 1,* 11–17.

DeVon, H. A., Penckofer, S., & Larimer, K. (2008). The association of diabetes and older age with the absence of chest pain during acute coronary syndromes. *Western Journal of Nursing Research, 30*(1), 130–144.

Donath, M. Y., Ehses, J. A., Maedler, K., et al. (2005). Mechanisms of beta-cell death in type 2 diabetes. *Diabetes, 54*(Suppl. 2), S108–S113.

Donesky-Cuenco, D., Nguyen, H.Q., Paul, S., & Carrieri-Kohlman, V. (2009). Yoga therapy decreases dyspnea-related distress and improves functional performance in people with chronic obstructive pulmonary disease: A pilot study. *Journal of Alternative and Complementary Medicine, 15*(3), 225–234.

Edwards, B. K., Howe, H. L., Ries, L. A. G., Thun, M. J., Rosenberg, H. M., Yancik, R., . . . Feigal, E. G. (2002). Annual report to the nation on the status of cancer, 1973-1999, featuring implications of age and aging on the U.S. cancer burden. *Cancer, 94,* 2766–2792.

Engelgau, M., Murphy, D., Narayan, K., & Vinicor, F. (2006). Diabetes and the public health perspective. In C. Mensing (Ed.), *The art and science of diabetes self-management education* (pp. 7–19). Chicago: American Association of Diabetes Educators.

Ershler, W. B., & Longo, D. L. (1997). Aging and cancer: Issues of basic and clinical science. *Journal of the National Cancer Institute, 89,* 1489–1497.

Extermann, M. (2007). The interaction between comorbidity and cancer. *Cancer Control, 14,* 13-22.

Extermann, M., Aapro, M., Bernabei, R., Cohen, H. J., Droz J. P., Lichtman, S., . . . Topinkova, E. (2005). Use of comprehensive geriatric assessment in older cancer patients: Recommendations from the Task Force on CGA of the International Society of Geriatric Oncology. *Critical Reviews in Oncology/Hematology, 55,* 241–252.

Extermann, M., & Hurria, A. (2007). Comprehensive geriatric assessment for older patients with cancer. *Journal of Clinical Oncology, 25,* 1824–1831.

Extermann, M., Overcash, J., Lyman, G.H., Parr, J., & Balducci, L. (1998). Comorbidity and functional status are independent in older cancer patients. *Journal of Clinical Oncology, 16,* 1582–1587.

Flowers, A. (2000). Brain tumors in the older person. *Cancer Control, 7,* 523–538.

Freeman, J., & Franz, M. (2006). Medical nutrition therapy. In C. Mensing (Ed.), *The art and science of diabetes self-management education* (pp. 279–295). Chicago: American Association of Diabetes Educators.

Given, B., & Given C. W. (2008). Older adults and cancer treatment. *Cancer, 113*(12), 3505–3511.

Glass, A. G., & Hoover, R. N. (1989). The emerging epidemic of melanoma and squamous cell skin cancer. *Journal of the American Medical Association, 262,* 2097–2100.

Gosselin-Acomb, T. K. (2005). Principles of radiation therapy. In C. Henke-Yarbro, M. Hansen Frogge, & M. Goodman (Eds.), *Cancer nursing: Principle and practice* (6th ed., pp. 229–249). Sudbury, MA: Jones & Bartlett Learning.

Gray-Miceli, D., & McDonald, K. (2007). *Assessment and management of type 2 diabetes in older adults with complex care needs.* White paper presented at Geriatric Nursing Education Consortium Faculty Development Institute, June, 2007, Portland, OR.

Hayat, M. J., Howlader, N., Reichman, M. E., & Edwards, B. K. (2007). Cancer statistics, trends, and multiple primary cancer analyses from the Surveillance, Epidemiology, and End Results (SEER) Program [Electronic version]. *Oncologist, 12,* 20–37.

Heron, M., Hoyert, D., Murphy, S., Xu, J., Kochanek, K. & Tejada-Vera, B. (2009). Deaths: Final data for 2006. *National Vital Statistics Reports, 57*(14). Hyattsville, MD: National Center for Health Statistics.

Hood, L. E. (2002). Chemotherapy in the elderly: Supportive measures for chemotherapy-induced myelotoxicity. *Clinical Journal of Oncology Nursing, 7,* 85–190.

Hurria, A. (2007). Incorporation of geriatric principles in oncology clinical trails. *Journal of Clinical Oncology, 25,* 5350–5351.

Hurria, A., Li, D., Hansen, K., Sujata, P., Gupta, R., Neslon, C., et al. (2009). Distress in older patients with cancer. *Journal of Clinical Oncology, 27,* 4346–4350.

Hwang, S. Y., Park, E. H., Shin, E. S., & Jeong, M. H. (2009). Comparison of factors associated with atypical symptoms in younger and older patients with acute coronary syndromes. *J Korean Medical Science, 24*(5), 789–794.

Iwamoto, R. (2001). Radiation therapy. In S. Otto (Ed.), *Oncology nursing* (pp. 606–636). Philadelphia: Mosby.

Jemal, A., Murray, T., Samuels, A., et al. (2003). Cancer statistics, 2003. *CA, A Cancer Journal for Clinicians, 53,* 5–26.

Jemal, A., Siegel, R., Ward, E., et al. (2009). Cancer statistics, 2009. *CA, A Cancer Journal for Clinicians.* Retrieved December 12, 2010, from http://caonline.amcancersoc.org/cgi/content/full/caac.20006v1?ikey=0cabd33f34e5c256

Jett, K. (2008). Chronic diseases late in life. In P. Ebersole, P. Hess, T. Touhy, K. Jett, &. A. Luggen. *Toward healthy aging* (7th ed., pp. 222–268). St. Louis, Missouri: Mosby Elsevier.

Johnson, T., & Dang, D. (2006). Taking medications. In C. Mensing (Ed.), *The art and science of diabetes self-management education* (pp. 689–703). Chicago: American Association of Diabetes Educators.

Joslin Diabetes Center. (2007). *Guideline for the care of the older adult with diabetes.* Boston: Joslin Diabetes Center.

Kagan, S. H. (2008). Ageism in cancer care. *Seminars in Oncology Nursing, 24*(4), 246–253.

Kemeny, M. M. (2004). Surgery in the older patient. *Seminars in Oncology, 31,* 175–184.

Kulkarni, K. (2006). Monitoring. In C. Mensing (Ed.), *The art and science of diabetes self-management education* (pp. 297–319). Chicago: American Association of Diabetes Educators.

Kumar, A., Soares, L. P., Balducci, L., & Djulbegovic, B. (2007). Treatment tolerance and efficacy in geriatric oncology: A systemic review of phase III randomized trials conducted by five National Cancer Institute–sponsored cooperative groups. *Journal of Clinical Oncology, 25,* 1272–1276.

Leeman, J. (2007). Interventions to improve self management: Utility and relevance for practice. *Diabetes Education, 32*(4), 571–583.

Lloyd-Jones, D., Adams, R., Carnethon, M., De Simone, G., Ferguson, B., Flegal, K., . . . Hong, Y. (2009). Heart disease and stroke statistics—2009 update. *Circulation, 119*(3), e21–e181.

Lorber, D. (2006). Macrovascular disease in diabetes. In C. Mensing (Ed.), *The art and science of diabetes self-management education* (pp. 475–510). Chicago: American Association of Diabetes Educators.

Mahon, S. (2005). Screening and detection for asymptomatic individuals. In C. Henke-Yarbro, M. Hansen-Fogge, & M. Goodman (Eds.), *Cancer nursing: Principles and practice* (6th ed., pp. 108–125). Sudbury, MA: Jones & Bartlett Learning.

Merck Manuals Online Medical Library. Available at http://www.merckmanuals.com/professional/index.html

Monson, K., Litvak, D. A., & Bold, R. J. (2003). Surgery in the aged population: Surgical oncology. *Archives of Surgery, 138,* 1061–1067.

Mullooly, C. (2006) Physical activity. In C. Mensing (Ed.), *The art and science of diabetes self-management education* (pp. 297–319). Chicago: American Association of Diabetes Educators.

Muss, H. B., Biganzoli, L., Sargent, D. J., & Aapro, M. (2007). Adjuvant therapy in the elderly: Making the right decision. *Journal of Clinical Oncology, 25,* 1870–1875.

National Comprehensive Cancer Network. (2010) *About the NCCN guidelines for patients.* Fort Washington, PA: Author. Retrieved December 12, 2010, from http://www.nccn.com/patient-guidelines.html

National Heart, Lung, and Blood Institute. (2008). *Fact book fiscal year 2008.* Washington, DC: U.S. Department of Health and Human Services. Retrieved December 12, 2010, from http://www.nhlbi.nih.gov/about/factbook-08/FactBookFinal.pdf

National Institute of Diabetes and Digestive and Kidney Diseases. (NIDDK, 2010). *Diabetes overview.* Bethesda, MD: Author. Retrieved December 12, 2010, from http://diabetes.niddk.nih.gov/dm/pubs/overview/

Neufeld, R. R., Libow, L. S., Foley, W. J., Dunbar, J. M., Cohen, C., & Breuer, B. (1999). Restraint reduction reduces serious injuries among nursing home residents. *Journal of the American Geriatrics Society, 47*(10), 1202–1207.

Odencrants, S., Ehnfors, M., & Ehrenberg, A. (2008). Nutritional status and patient characteristics for hospitalised older patients with chronic obstructive pulmonary disease. *Journal of Clinical Nursing, 17*(13), 1771–1778.

Repetto, L. (2003). Greater risks of chemotherapy toxicity in elderly patients with cancer. *Journal of Supportive Oncology, 1,* 18–24.

Resnick, B., & McLeskey, S. W. (2008). Cancer screening across the aging continuum. *American Journal of Managed Care, 14,* 267–276.

Riefkohl, E., Bieber, H., Burlingame, M., Lowenthal, D., Rodin, M., & Mohide, S. (2007). A practical approach to geriatric assessment in oncology. *Journal of Clinical Oncology, 25,* 1936–1944.

Rubenstein L. Z., & Josephson, K. R. (2002). The epidemiology of falls and syncope. In R. A. Kenny & D. O'Shea (Eds.), *Falls and syncope in elderly patients: Clinics in geriatric medicine.* Philadelphia: Saunders 141–158.

Ruggiero, L., Wagner, J., & de Groot, M. (2006). Understanding the individual: Emotional and psychological changes. In C. Mensing (Ed.), *The art and science of diabetes self-management education* (pp. 59–86). Chicago: American Association of Diabetes Educators.

Saltzein, S. L, Behling, C. A., & Baergen, R. N. (1998). Features of cancer in nonagenarians and centenarians. *Journal of the American Geriatrics Society, 46,* 994–998.

Schols, A. M., & Gosker, H. R. (2009). The pathophysiology of cachexia in chronic obstructive pulmonary disease. *Current Opinion in Supportive and Palliative Care, 3*(4), 282-287.

Schwartz, R. N. (2006). *Pharmacologic issues* [Online exclusive]. In D. G. Cope & A. M. Reb (Eds.), *An evidence-based approach to the treatment and care of the older adult with cancer* (pp. 91–101). Pittsburgh, PA: Oncology Nursing Society.

Selvin, E., Coresh J., & Brancati, F. (2006). The burden and treatment of diabetes in elderly individuals in the U.S. *Diabetes Care, 29*(11), 2415–2420.

Sheinfield-Gorin, S., Gauthier, J., Hay, J., Miles, A., & Wardle, J. (2008). Cancer screening and aging: Research barriers and opportunities. *Cancer, 113*(Suppl. 12), 3493–3504.

Spector, T. D., & MacGregor, A. J. (2004). Risk factors for osteoarthritis: Genetics. *Osteoarthritis Cartilage, 12*(Suppl. A), S39–S44.

Spollett, G. (2006). Type 2 diabetes across the lifespan. In C. Mensing (Ed.), *The art and science of diabetes self-management education* (pp. 297–319). Chicago: American Association of Diabetes Educators.

Steil, C. F. (2006). Pharmacologic therapies for glucose management. In C. Mensing (Ed.), *The art and science of diabetes self-management education: A desk reference for healthcare professionals* (pp. 321–355). Chicago: American Association of Diabetes Educators.

Terret, C., Castel-Kremer, E., Albrand, G., & Droz, J. P. (2009). Effects of comorbidity on screening and early diagnosis of cancer in elderly people. *Lancet Oncology, 10,* 80–87.

Terret, C., Zuliam, G., Naiem, A., & Albrand, G. (2007). Multidisciplinary approach to geriatric oncology patient. *Journal of Clinical Oncology, 25,* 1876–1881.

Tinetti, M. E., Liu, W. L., & Ginter, S. F. (1992). Mechanical restraint use and fall-related injuries among residents of skilled nursing facilities. *Annals of Internal Medicine, 116*(5), 369–374.

Tinetti, M. E., Speechley, M., & Ginter, S.F. (1988). Risk factors for falls among elderly persons living in the community. *New England Journal of Medicine, 319*(26), 1701–1707.

Townsley, C. A., Pond, G. R., Oza, A. M., et al. (2006). Evaluation of adverse events experienced by older patients participating in studies of molecularly targeted agents alone or in combination. *Clin Cancer Res, 12,* 2141–2149.

Townsley, C. A., Selby, R., & Siu, L. L. (2005). Systematic review of barriers to the recruitment of older patients with cancer onto clinical trials. *Journal of Clinical Oncology, 23,* 3112–3124.

Trask, P. C., Blank, T. O., & Jacobsen, P. B. (2008). Future perspectives on the treatment issues associated with cancer and aging. *Cancer, 113*(Suppl. 12), 3512–3518.

U.S. Department of Health and Human Services. (2004). *The health consequences of smoking: A report of the surgeon general.* Washington, DC: Author. Retrieved December 9, 2010, from http://www.surgeongeneral.gov/library/smokingconsequences/

Vrezas, I., Elsner, G., Bolm-Audorff, U., Abolmaali, N., & Seidler, A. (2010). Case-control study of knee osteoarthritis and lifestyle factors considering their interaction with physical workload. *International Archives of Occupational and Environmental Health, 83*(3), 291–300.

Walter, L. C., Bertenthal, D., Lindquist, K., & Konety, B. R. (2006). PSA screening among elderly men with limited life expectancies. *Journal of the American Medical Association, 296,* 2336–2342.

Walter, L. C., Eng, C., & Covinsky, K. E. (2001). Screening mammography for frail older women. *Journal of General Internal Medicine, 16,* 779–784.

Walter, L. C., Lindquist, K., & Covinsky, K. E. (2004). Relationship between health status and use of screening mammography and Papanicolaou smears among women older than 70 years of age. *Annals of Internal Medicine, 140,* 681–688.

Wasil, T., & Lichtman, S. M. (2005). Clinical pharmacology issues relevant to the dosing and toxicity of chemotherapy drugs in the elderly. *Oncologist, 10,* 602–612.

Wedding, U., Röhrig, B., Klippstein, A., Pientka, L., & Hoffken (2007). Age, severe comorbidity and functional impairment independently contribute to poor survival in cancer patients. *Journal of Cancer Research and Clinical Oncology, 133*(12), 945–950.

Westin, E. H., & Longo, D. L. (2004). Lymphoma and myeloma in older patients. *Seminars in Oncology, 31,* 198–205.

Wise, R. A., & Tashkin, D. P. (2007). Preventing chronic obstructive pulmonary disease: What is known and what needs to be done to make a difference to the patient? *American Journal of Medicine, 120*(8 Suppl. 1), S14–S22.

World Health Organization. (2009). *World health statistics.* Retrieved December 12, 2010, from http://www.who.int/whosis/whostat/EN_WHS09_Full.pdf

Yancik, R., & Ries, L. A. (2000). Aging and cancer in America: Demographic and epidemiologic perspectives. *Hematology/Oncology Clinics of North America, 14,* 17–23.

Zachariah, B., & Balducci, L. (2000). Radiation therapy of the older patient. *Hematology/Oncology Clinics of North America, 14,* 131–167.

Chapter 9

Assessing the Older Adult: What's Different?

Kathryn Blair, PhD, FNP-BC, FAANP

LEARNING OBJECTIVES

- Identify the physiological changes associated with normal aging.
- Recognize the physical presentations associated with normal aging.
- Explain the clinical implications of the physiological aspects of normal aging.
- Describe common laboratory variation associated with aging.
- Explain nursing implications associated with normal aging.
- Understand the role of geriatric assessment teams in the care of the older adult.

In 2000, 12.4% of the United States population consisted of those age 65 and older, and current predictions suggest that this number could double by 2030 (Administration on Aging, 2010; Ferrucci, Giallauria, & Guralnik, 2008). With an aging population, nurses must know the physiological aspects of *normal* aging to correctly interpret the clinical findings and provide a holistic approach to health promotion and health care. This chapter highlights the typical alterations of aging and provides tools to assess, interpret, and mediate these alterations.

Many theoretical models have been used to explain normal aging. A recent model highlights aging as a progressive decline in homeostasis, a reaction between injury and repair, with aging representing accumulated molecular damage (Kirkwood, 2005). No one can stop aging, but nurses can help to reduce the injury component of aging by providing education (e.g., smoking cessation, routine exercise, weight control) and facilitating the maintenance of homeostasis.

Although aging adults experience many normative changes that may affect the ability to care for self and maintain independence, aging does not have to mean growing frail or ill. Nurses are in a pivotal position to help older adults adapt to the aging process and maintain functional capacity and independence. To accomplish these goals, nurses must recognize that although physical examination of an older adult is similar to that of a young adult, interpretation of the findings may be different. Also, nurses must be able to differentiate normative variations of aging from pathological changes. Armed with this information, nurses can equip older adults with the skills they need to experience healthy aging.

Nurses must be able to differentiate normative variations of aging from pathological changes.

Growing Older Means Change

Aging means adjustment and adaptation. The older adults who are most likely to remain healthy and active are those who learn that, with the proper tools, physiological and physical changes are not insurmountable.

Sensory Changes

Physiological and assessment changes of the senses are often subtle. Indeed, many older adults do not recognize the change until there is an unexpected consequence (Table 9-1).

TABLE 9-1 Summary of Normative Sensory Changes and Effects

SENSE	CHANGES	EFFECTS
Taste	■ Decreased salivation ■ Decreased olfactory sense ■ Reduction of papillae ■ Atrophy and thinning of epithelium	■ Decreased gustatory sensitivity ■ Increased threshold for sodium
Smell	■ Decreased receptors and olfactory bulb fibers ■ General deterioration in CNS processing functions ■ Changes in olfactory epithelium	■ Decreased olfactory sensitivity ■ Decreased ability to discriminate between smells
Hearing	■ Acoustic nerve and inner ear structures malfunction of the organ of Corti ■ Loss of hair cells in ampulla ■ Stiffness in tympanic membrane ■ Increased cerumen	■ Presbycusis (high-frequency hearing loss) ■ Poor word comprehension and discrimination ■ Alteration in balance ■ Conductive hearing loss
Vision	■ Changes in retina ■ Cornea more spherical and lens more rigid	■ Altered visual acuity and peripheral vision ■ Reduction in dark adaptation ■ Decreased depth perception ■ Reduction in contrast sensitivity ■ Reduced accommodation

Taste

Alterations in taste or gustatory function occur normally with aging (Bhutto & Morley, 2008) and are not noticed until the older adult has a change in appetite or notices a condition known as anorexia of aging (see Chapter 7). Changes in the function of taste buds are only one aspect of the decline in taste. Some researchers argue that reduced taste sensitivity may stem mainly from a defect in olfactory sense (Boyce & Shone, 2006).

Physical changes in the aging mouth include a reduction of papillae on the tongue, decreased salivation, missing or worn teeth, and dentures. All of these variations in the mouth contribute to a reduction in taste sensitivity.

Smell

Olfactory sense or sense of smell begins to deteriorate around the seventh decade of life as a result of alterations in the nose and the olfactory nerve. Researchers have identified a reduction of olfactory receptors and olfactory bulb fibers in older adults (Boyce & Shone, 2006; Lafreniere & Mann, 2008).

Expected physical changes in the assessment of the nose would include thinning of the nasal mucosa, increased nasal hair, and decreased function of the olfactory nerve. It is important to note that a more rapid and earlier decline in the sense of smell can occur as a result of smoking, certain medications, and comorbid conditions such as Alzheimer's and Parkinson's disease.

Hearing

Diminished auditory function or hearing is common among older adults and begins as early as the sixth decade of life. The most common form of hearing change is presbycusis, which is a sensorineural hearing loss. Sensorineural hearing loss results from a malfunction of the acoustic nerve (cranial nerve VIII). Typically, sensorineural hearing loss involves high-frequency hearing loss and difficulty with speech comprehension.

When hearing loss results from an inner ear malfunction, the affected person may have trouble with word discrimination. In this scenario, hearing aid devices may be useful; however, if the hearing loss is from nerve damage (cranial nerve VIII) or brain injury, then hearing devices will be of little value (Stenklev, Vik, & Laukli, 2004).

Sensorineural hearing loss may be compounded by a conductive hearing loss that may have occurred during the middle adult years (ages 40 to 50). Often a conductive hearing loss is a result of chronic exposure to loud noises such as iPods, chronic ear infections, and environmental noises from work in construction or airports (Kozak & Grundfast, 2009).

In addition to hearing, the inner ear plays a significant role in maintaining a sense of balance (Matsumura & Ambrose, 2006). With aging, the older adult may experience a change in vestibular function culminating in alterations in balance.

The ear examination would reveal physical changes such as increased hair and cerumen (wax) in the canal. Dullness and stiffness in the tympanic membrane can be observed, which may contribute to a conductive hearing loss. Assessment of hearing via the Weber and Rinne tests (tuning fork tests) would reflect changes consistent with a sensorineural hearing loss and/or conductive hearing loss.

PERSONAL PERSPECTIVE
The Secret to Aging Well

Ruth is 87 and, as she says, "I'm not getting old, I *am* old." For certain, she is a very old soul, full of wisdom. She speaks openly and pragmatically about aging and what it takes to age well. "Everything is diminishing," she says. "Everything—my hearing, my sight, my smell, my taste. Everything. But not to the point that I can't still enjoy those things. I'm one of the lucky ones. There are some people, unfortunately, that lose a lot of their abilities—sight or speech or hearing—and it's not easy for them. And I sympathize with them, but even a lot of those people are not negative. To continue to enjoy the things that we are offered is to keep participating. It's too easy to say, 'Oh, I'm tired.' Leave tired for later if there's something good going on now. We have wonderful concerts here. They're just an hour, so if you're tired you can listen to a beautiful concert, and then rest!"

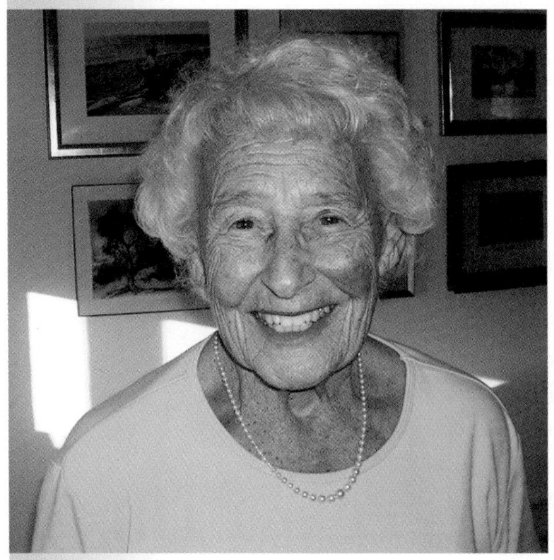

"I think being involved and stimulated," Ruth continues, "is one of the most necessary things that an person can do as they get older. I take all the classes. I go to everything offered here at Tower One. I enjoy it so much. I think attitude has a great deal to do with it, too. There are people who are very unhappy. But I kind of feel, though I may be wrong, that those that are negative and unhappy, were that way all their lives. Losing your husband didn't make you negative. It might have made you unhappy for a long time. It didn't make you negative in all your approaches to all you see—from the food we eat to the sunshine we look at during the day. They don't see the sunshine and they don't see the beautiful sunsets that we've been having all week. They never take the time to look at them or appreciate them, and I think as you get older you should really make a point of enjoying everything you can for as long as you can."

About Ruth Ruth Blum is a twice-widowed mother of four wonderful children. Inspired by a personal interest, Ruth worked for many years as the Connecticut State Representative to the March of Dimes National Foundation. She traveled extensively, speaking about the important work of the March of Dimes and organizing groups to help raise funds for children affected by polio. Ruth has been living at an assisted-living facility for over 3 years. She says that at the time she made the switch from living in her own home she realized she "wasn't getting any younger" and "needed a support system." Ruth calls the move the wisest choice of her life and takes advantage of the many activities offered there.

Lorri B. Danzig, MS, CSL

Vision

A variety of functional and structural changes occur in the eye during the aging process. Changes in ocular perfusion and in retinal pigment epithelial cells can increase the risk of age-related macular degeneration and a loss of central vision (Ehrlich et al., 2008). The corneal curvature decreases, and the inability of the lens to compensate for this change can alter visual acuity. This alteration in visual acuity can be further compounded by neuronal changes in the brain (Artal et al., 2003; Matsumura & Ambrose, 2006).

Along with functional changes in the eye, physical changes may alter the assessment. Common changes include yellowing of the sclera, clouding of the lens, decreased tearing, reduced pupil size, slower pupil response, presbyopia (decreased accommodation), and a reduction in visual fields by confrontation (peripheral vision).

Systems Changes

When systems are affected by aging, the changes are more recognizable by the older adult and provider. Many times the changes affecting systems will result in some alteration in the elder's ability to function or maintain homeostasis.

Integumentary System

The skin is the body's largest organ and has multiple functions that are altered by aging. The primary functions of skin include protection from the environment, maintenance of fluid and electrolytes, temperature regulation, and sensory perception. One important function of the skin that has garnered recent attention is vitamin D production. Current evidence suggests that the skin's ability to synthesize the provitamin calcidiol (25-hydroxycholecalciferol) decreases with age (Venning, 2005).

The aging process of the skin is a combination of environmental and genetic causes. Certain behaviors such as smoking and repeated sun exposure will cause premature aging of the skin.

Common changes in the skin include the loss of collagen and elasticity, resulting in sagging and a wrinkled appearance. Additional alterations include thinning of the dermal layer, resulting in increased risk of injury and slower healing.

The nails and hair are considered part of the integumentary system and undergo similar changes. The hair loses color and thins. Nails typically become thin and grow more slowly (Table 9-2).

Evaluation of the skin and nails involves inspection and palpation. Multiple changes may be visible, such as wrinkling, loss of elasticity, thinning of the epidermis, and age spots (senile lentigines).The hair typically becomes gray secondary to a decline melanocyte function. Many older adult men develop male pattern baldness, and postmenopausal women commonly have an increase in facial hair.

Pulmonary System

With aging, the pulmonary system's ability to ward off infection tends to decline. Pulmonary infections result from mechanical alterations (such as reduced cough reflex and a decline in ciliary function) and a decrease in the lung's innate immune response (Katial & Zheng, 2007).

Externally, the chest wall becomes more barrel-like and, in many cases, changes in the aging spine (kyphosis) contribute to pulmonary alterations as well (Table 9-3). These external variations result in decreased lung compliance and recoil, increasing the work of breathing (Duthie, Katz, & Malone, 2007).

Internal structural changes include a reduction in the number of alveoli as well as a decrease in alveolar surface area and capillary beds. Aging results in a 50% decline in the functional capacity of alveoli

TABLE 9-2 Summary of Normative Integumentary Changes and Effects

CHANGES	EFFECTS
■ Reduction of collagen	■ Wrinkling and reduced elasticity
■ Thinning of dermal layer	■ Increased risk for injury and slower healing
■ Redistribution of fat	
■ Decreased melanocytes	■ Irregular pigmentation ■ Increased risk of UV exposure ■ Graying of hair
■ Decreased function of sweat glands	■ Reduction in thermal regulation
■ Redistribution of hair	■ Thinning of scalp hair ■ Decreased body hair ■ Increased facial hair (women) ■ Decreased facial hair (men)

TABLE 9-3 Summary of Normative Pulmonary Changes and Effects

CHANGES	EFFECTS
■ Kyphosis and barrel chest	■ Increased work of breathing
■ Reduced recoil of lungs	■ Fatigue with normal activities
■ Decreased alveolar surface area ■ Decreased capillary beds	■ Decrease in perfusion-ventilation resulting a reduced compensatory response to hypercapnia and hypoxia
■ Decreased cough reflex	■ Pooling of secretions and unprotected airway
■ Decreased ciliary function	■ Increased risk for infection

to exchange oxygen and carbon monoxide, resulting in a ventilation-perfusion defect (Minaker, 2007). The combined effect of these changes is an impaired response to hypercapnia (increased CO_2 level) and hypoxia (Mason, Murray, Broaddus, & Nadel, 2005).

Assessment of the pulmonary system will reveal changes in the external appearance of the chest wall, possible spinal curvature (kyphosis), and decreased respiratory expansion. Lung sounds and diaphragmatic excursion should remain unchanged; however, diagnostic tests that evaluate internal function (such as spirometry) may change, reflecting a decreased lung capacity.

Cardiovascular System

Normative changes in the cardiovascular system are difficult to separate from pathological changes. For example, the left atrium dilates as a normative process and may result in atrial fibrillation, a pathological condition, which in turn causes hemodynamic changes via pulmonary vein dilation (Pan et al., 2008). Vascular stiffness predisposes to left ventricular stiffness and impaired diastolic filling; together these changes predispose the older adult to developing heart failure (Minaker, 2007; Thomas & Rich, 2007).

The structure of the heart can change during aging in the absence of disease. The valves of the heart become stiffer and often result in functional murmurs. The muscle volume in both ventricles increases, and there is a decrease in the pacemaker cells (Aronow, 2006). Hypertrophy of the heart muscle and loss of pacemaker cells cause a decrease in maximal heart rate and maximal cardiac output (Table 9-4). The combination of these changes results in increased left ventricular end diastolic pressure, left atrial enlargement, and increased atrial pressure contributing to heart failure and atrial arrhythmias (Cademartiri, LaGrutta, de Feyter, & Krestin, 2008 Thomas & Rich, 2007).

Aging can transform the arterial and venous systems. Arterial changes include increased arterial

TABLE 9-4 Summary of Normative Cardiovascular Changes and Effects

CHANGES	EFFECTS
■ Thickening and stiffening of the left ventricular wall	■ Delayed left ventricular filling ■ Increased systolic pressure
■ Loss of pacemaker cells	■ Slowing heart rate ■ Postural hypotension ■ Arrhythmias
■ Decreased β-adrenergic reactivity	■ Decrease in vasodilation
■ Thickening and stiffening of heart valves	■ Murmurs
■ Dilation of aorta and thickening of aortic walls, medial walls calcify	■ Increased systolic pressure
■ Arterial medial wall thickening	■ Increased systolic pressure
■ Decreased arterial elasticity	■ Increased pulse pressure
■ Endothelial dysfunction	■ Predisposition for arterial disease

wall thickness, reduced arterial elasticity, and decreased β-adrenergic reactivity (Cademartiri et al., 2008; Lakatta, Wang, & Najjar, 2009). The consequences of these changes include increased systolic blood pressure and decreased capacity for arterial dilation. The most common venous system changes include reduced valve function and reduced tone, resulting in varicosities.

Cardiovascular assessment will reveal several variations as a result of the older adult's physiological changes. Apical pulse may be displaced laterally, heart rate will be slower, peripheral pulses may be decreased, and systolic blood pressure may be elevated. Murmurs from valvular stiffness and extracardiac sounds (S_4) from reduced ventricular compliance are common findings.

EVIDENCE FOR PRACTICE
Aging and Atrial Fibrillation

Purpose: To identify structural changes, specifically in the pulmonary veins (a common site for ectopy), which may contribute to the genesis of atrial fibrillation, a common cardiac arrhythmia in older adults.

Sample: The study included 180 subjects from younger than age 40 to older than age 80 with a mean age of 56 ± 12 years (standard deviation). All were evaluated for coronary artery disease and arrhythmias. All were found to be in sinus rhythm and without evidence of coronary artery disease as defined by less than 50% stenosis.

Methods: Measurement of left atrium, left ventricle, and pulmonary veins diameters.

Results: Pulmonary veins and left atrium were increased in diameter after age 50, but the differences between ages 70 and 80+ years were not significant.

Implications: Structural changes may influence the development of atrial arrhythmias, and, therefore, left atrium and pulmonary vein changes may be predictors for future development of atrial arrhythmias after age 50.

Resource: Pan, N., Tsao, H., Chang, N., Chen, Y., & Chen, S. (2008). Aging dilates atrium and pulmonary veins for the genesis of atrial fibrillation. *Chest, 133,* 190–196.

Gastrointestinal System

Most healthy older adults will experience some problems with the gastrointestinal (GI) tract. Common changes—such as slowed gastric emptying, reduced gastric acid production, increased colon transit time, and fluctuations in GI hormones—may contribute to a variety of conditions that plague the older adult, such as dysphagia (difficulty swallowing), anorexia, and constipation (Bhutto & Morley, 2008; Morley, 2007). Reduced hydrochloric acid in the stomach can result in a reduction in iron, vitamin B_{12}, calcium, and vitamin D absorption. These nutritional deficiencies can alter bone and muscle strength and red blood cell production (Table 9-5).

Liver function also changes with aging. Blood flow to the liver and liver volume decreases about 30% with a decline in the P450 enzyme system, which results in altered drug metabolism (Junaidi & Di Bisceglie, 2007; Morley, 2007). The aging liver has slower regeneration capabilities; therefore, older adults face a slower recovery after a toxic or viral insult (Junaidi & Di Bisceglie, 2007).

The change in physical assessment of the GI tract or abdomen is subtle. There may be increased fat deposition on the abdomen, as well as reduced muscle tone. The skin may lack normal turgor. Bowel sounds may be slower and anal tone diminished.

Genitourinary System

Like many organs, the kidneys undergo multiple structural and functional changes during the aging process. The kidneys atrophy, blood flow declines, and the glomerular filtration rate is reduced (Telda & Friedman, 2008). These changes have a significant impact on the older adult's ability to clear drugs and maintain fluid and electrolyte balance. Older adults tend to have less ability to conserve sodium with salt restriction and have less ability to concentrate urine when water is restricted.

The bladder may decrease in size and strength of contraction, resulting in frequent voiding and incomplete emptying. With a delay in sodium excretion, nocturia can be a problem (Minaker, 2007).

Atrophic changes of the external genitalia in women can result in frequent urinary tract infections and, with pelvic relaxation, urinary incontinence can be a concern as well. For men, the enlarging prostate

TABLE 9-5 Summary of Normative Gastrointestinal Changes and Effects

CHANGES	EFFECTS
■ Substance P depletion	■ Reduced cough response ■ Decreased swallowing reflex
■ Prolongation of oropharyngeal phase	■ Dysphagia and silent aspiration
■ Small increase in distal esophageal pressure	■ Longer duration of acid reflux
■ Delayed gastric emptying	■ Increased colon diameter
■ Increased colon transit times	■ Constipation
■ Decreased gastric acid production	■ Atrophic gastritis ■ Decreased absorption of vitamin B_{12}, vitamin D, iron, and calcium
■ Decreased bacterial flora	■ Increased risk of *Clostridium difficile* diarrhea
■ Increased GI hormones: gastrin, cholecystokinin, pancreatic polypeptide, somatostatin	■ Increased gastric acid secretion ■ Increased satiation ■ Increased gallbladder and pancreatic enzyme secretion ■ Inhibited pancreatic secretion ■ Inhibits gut secretion, intestine motility and peptide hormone secretion
■ Weakening colonic muscular wall	■ Constipation ■ Fecal incontinence ■ Development of diverticuli
■ Reduction in liver volume ■ Decline in P450 enzyme	■ Altered drug metabolism
■ Increase in lithogenicity of bile salts	■ Increased propensity for gallstones

can cause a decreased urine stream and incomplete emptying of the bladder.

Although there are no overt physical assessment signs of renal changes, the impact of these changes is important for nurses to recognize. The kidneys play an important role in maintaining fluid and electrolyte homeostasis and the removal of toxins and drugs.

Neurological System

A decline in cognitive function is universal as individuals age (Drachman, 2006); however, the degree and rate of decline are variable among older adults. This alteration in function is associated with a selective loss of neurons (Carlson et al., 2008). Although there is a gradual loss of neurons, older adults retain long-term memory, comprehension, and general knowledge. However, short-term memory and the ability for new learning and coordination decline.

Evidence shows that neuronal connections play a significant role in altering the effect of neuronal loss. High-functioning older adults reorganize brain functions and recruit different areas in the brain when performing similar tasks as compared with younger adults (Cabeza, Anderson, Locantore, & McIntosh, 2002; Reuter-Lorenz, 2002).

The effects of neuronal loss are not limited to a decline in cognitive function; they also affect the autonomic nervous system and neurotransmitters. Changes in the autonomic nervous system can result in decreased cortisol and increased catecholamine levels, which alters the normal compensatory mechanisms in the older adult. Alterations in neurotransmitters culminate in short-term memory deficits, changes in sleep patterns, and reduced motor function (Stanley, Blair, & Beare, 2005).

Physical examination of the neurological system will reveal considerable variations among older adults. In general, the response times when performing rapid alternating movements will be slower secondary to changes in neurotransmitters

(Minaker, 2007) and deep tendon reflexes may be diminished because of changes in tendons and slower neuronal conduction. Cognitive function is altered, and the older adult may need more time to respond to questions or commands and to learn new information. Older adults may experience a decrease in vibratory sense in the absence of peripheral neuropathy. Changes in some cranial nerve functions, such as decreased hearing, alterations in taste, and reduction in visual acuity, are common (see the section on sensory changes earlier in the chapter).

Musculoskeletal System

The musculoskeletal system is affected by aging in two major ways: bone health and movement problems. Bone strength is decreased through alterations of bone density and bone quality, commonly known as osteoporosis, resulting in an increased risk for fractures in the older adult (Pietschmann, Rauner, Sipos, & Kerschan-Schindl, 2009). Loss of the inner portion of the bone, or trabecular bone loss, begins in vertebrae and the ends of long bones when bone reabsorption exceeds bone formation—as early as age 30. Loss of the outer shell, or cortical bone loss, begins at about age 45 to 50. In both cases, women experience more bone loss than men, especially after menopause. Like skin changes, bone changes may be hastened by several variables, including inadequate calcium and vitamin D intake, smoking, lack of weight-bearing exercise, and taking certain medications (e.g., steroids).

Additional normative changes include the long-term effects of aging on joints. Those most often affected are the weight-bearing joints, such as the spine, hips, and knees, although other joints can also be affected, such as those of the hands and shoulders. The aging process often results in changes in the joint surfaces, such as a loss of cartilage and connective tissue, which culminate in an alteration of normal joint function and joint deformity. The most common endpoint of these joint changes is osteoarthritis, which is predicted to be the fourth leading cause of disability in older adults by 2020 (Pinn, 2006; Woolf & Pfleger, 2003).

Movement is controlled by an interrelationship between the muscular, skeletal, and neurological systems. Muscles, tendons, and ligaments are responsible for movement and strength but are dependent on an intact neurological system. As muscles age, changes include a loss of fibers, a decrease in muscle regeneration, and stiffening of the tendons and ligaments. In addition, contraction force and maximal muscle strength is reduced as a result of decreased muscular and neural function (Aagaard, Magnusson, Larsson, Kjaer, & Krustrup, 2007). As with the other systems, the aging process of the musculoskeletal system can be accelerated by poor nutrition, sedentary behaviors, and the absence of weight-bearing exercise to prevent muscle loss.

Physical assessment of the musculoskeletal system demonstrates significant normative variations. The gait and posture of the older adult are the most obvious (i.e., slower gait and possibly a stooped posture), with changes in muscle mass and strength being more subtle. Joint deformity, stiffness, and essential tremors are additional features common in the older adult.

Laboratory Changes in Aging

For the most part, there are no significant changes in laboratory data in the older adult; however, some changes are directly affected by the physiology of aging. For example, altered kidney function results in a reduced renal threshold for glucose, and reduced muscle mass results in decreased creatinine clearance (Beers, Jones, Berlwits, Kaplan, & Porter, 2006). Differences in complete blood count in the older adult include decrease hemoglobin, platelet count, and lymphocyte count (Cheng, Chan, Cembrowski, & vanAssendelft, 2004). The decrease in hemoglobin is caused by a 50% reduction in erythropoietin production and a reduction in the dietary intake and absorption of iron. Other changes in lab values may result from such comorbid conditions as diabetes, hypertension, obesity, and physical inactivity (Table 9-6).

Vitamin D deficiency is a common problem in older adults and has been ignored until recently. The problems associated with this deficiency include muscle weakness, poor muscle strength, osteomalacia (softening of the bones), and increased risks for falls. A recent review indicated that one third of older adults over age 65 experienced a fall related to muscle weakness (Venning, 2005).

Less common changes associated with aging that may or may not affect lab values are increased parathyroid hormone, which factors in the maintenance of normal levels of phosphorus and calcium (Minaker, 2007); reduced levels of renin and

TABLE 9-6 Summary of Laboratory Changes

LAB TEST	CHANGE
Alkaline phosphatase	Increased
Calcium	Decreased
Cholesterol	Increased
Clotting factors VII and VIII	Increased
Complete blood count	Decreased hemoglobin level
	Decreased platelet count
	Decreased lymphocyte count
	Increased granulocyte count
Creatinine clearance	Decreased
Vitamin D (25-hydroxycholecalciferol)	Decreased
Phosphorus	Decreased
Triiodothyronine (T_3)	Decreased

aldosterone, which affect fluid balance; and an 85% to 90% reduction in dehydroepiandrosterone, which may play a role in impaired immune function (Minaker, 2007).

Nursing Implications and Interventions

As discussed, multiple sensory and system changes occur during the normal aging process. Nurses must understand the implications of these changes before they can facilitate adaptation to these transformations.

For example, implications of reduced taste sense include reduced nutritional intake and an increased amount of salt on food, which can lead to fluid overload and possibly aggravate heart failure. Consequences of a decline in sense of smell could include the inability to smell smoke, natural gas leaks, or spoiled food. The interrelationship between olfactory and gustatory sense is evident in that dentures and altered chewing impacts olfaction and similarly reduction in olfaction results in reduced taste discrimination (Mattes, 2002). Ultimately, changes in smell and taste impact dietary selection and nutritional status and may contribute to a functional decline in older adults (Murphy, 2008).

Nurses can encourage the older adult to use spices instead of salt to increase the flavor of food. The color and presentation of food can improve the older adult's appreciation for meals. Also, social interaction during meals can improve overall nutrition. Education regarding high-nutrient foods is important.

For changes in olfaction, nurses can suggest that the older adult install gas and smoke detectors and date food to avoid ingesting spoiled food.

The consequences of hearing and vestibular loss for the older adult include social isolation, reduction in cognitive processes, inability to hear alarms or the telephone, and an increased risk of falls because of a loss of balance (Matsumura & Ambrose, 2006; Stenklev, Vik, & Laukli, 2004). Nursing strategies to manage an auditory deficit would include teaching the patient to face the speaker (over time most older adults become successful in lip reading) and to avoid trying to converse with extraneous noise. To increase home safety, nurses can advise using phone adapters (amplification and light signals), installing handrails to adapt to disequilibrium, and observing the home for hazards that increase the risk of falling (e.g., throw rugs and inadequate lighting). Teaching older adults to rise slowly from a recumbent or sitting position also may reduce the risk of disequilibrium and falling.

Functional changes that may result from visual sensory changes include a decline in contrast sensitivity, reduced pupil size (miosis), reduced dark adaptation, and impaired motion detection in the peripheral fields (Matsumura & Ambrose, 2006). These changes can increase the risk of falls and increase the risk of accidents when driving at night.

Nurses can encourage annual eye examinations to detect cataracts, glaucoma, and macular degeneration. Nurses also can examine the home environment for hazards associated with visual changes. For example, suggest installation of adequate nightlights and reflective strips on the stairs. Explain that the older adult will experience changes in adaptation from light to dark areas and depth perception, so caution should be used when entering a dark room or when going down steps. Nurses also can prepare older adults to decrease nighttime driving by offering alternative modes of transportation.

Skin changes that occur with aging cause more than simply cosmetic effects. For example, with age, injury may result from minimal trauma. Nurses can help older adults adapt to this change by advising increased skin protection—such as by limiting sun exposure and direct injury to the integrity of the skin. The collagen cannot be replaced, but educating the older adult to routinely moisturize the skin and to avoid hot showers and harsh soaps will help maintain skin integrity. Recommending an annual examination to identify skin cancers is extremely important. Because the skin is important for thermal regulation, nurses should help older adults understand that their decreased ability to sweat may increase the need to protect against heat exposure. Suggesting fans and adequate hydration should help reduce this risk.

Nurses can assist older adults in adapting to pulmonary changes by encouraging exercises that will increase endurance and reduce fatigue. Through education, nurses can teach older adults to recognize signs and symptoms of respiratory infections and seek early intervention. Nurses should also encourage age-appropriate immunizations, such as the pneumococcal vaccine and annual influenza vaccine, to boost the immune system.

The overall effect of cardiovascular changes reduces older adults' homeostatic capacity (Minaker, 2007). This translates into postural hypotension, cardiac instability, and reduced compensatory mechanisms. A few strategies to enhance cardiovascular function include exercising, monitoring cholesterol level, maintaining normal weight, and maintaining adequate hydration.

Nurse cannot halt the inevitable loss of neurons in the neurological system, but they can help older adults learn to compensate for these changes. For example, encouraging older adults to remain engaged in social activities and to make lists to overcome short-term memory loss are two strategies. Also, encouraging new learning (such as learning a new language or taking a course at a local college) will enhance neuronal connections that will reduce a decline in cognitive function.

Nurses cannot stop the normal aging process but can help older adults prepare for and adapt to the transformations of aging while minimizing influences that speed aging.

Awareness of changes in the musculoskeletal system should prompt nurses to become proactive in helping older adults age successfully. Through weight-bearing exercises, weight control, and weight training, the older adult can maintain bone and muscle strength. Maintaining adequate calcium and vitamin D levels can play an important role in reducing falls and maintaining muscle strength. Nurse can help older adults prevent falls by ensuring adequate lighting in the home and installing hand rails, especially in the bathroom and on stairs.

Nurses cannot stop the normal effects of aging but can help older adults prepare for and adapt to the transformations associated with aging while minimizing the influences that speed the aging process, such as smoking, alcohol consumption, a sedentary lifestyle, poor nutrition, and social isolation. Nurse should be proactive agents to promote healthy aging by helping older adults maintain functional capacity and independence through continued exercise, healthy diet, social interaction, and avoidance of injury.

Geriatric Assessment Teams

Nurses need to be able to appreciate not only the physical variations associated with aging but also the social, economic, psychological, and spiritual changes. Although nurses have traditionally been educated to care for the whole patient, the complexity of caring for older adults requires an interdisciplinary approach.

Geriatric assessment teams are interdisciplinary teams composed of health care providers, family members, and the older adult. The specific composition of the team depends on the needs or goals of the individual person (Dyer et al., 2003). The professional nurse and advanced practice nurse, whether in the hospital or community setting, play a critical role in identifying the goals and the members of the team needed to meet these objectives.

Health care providers on the team typically include professionals from nursing, medicine, physical therapy, social work, and pharmacy, to name a few. All of these professionals have expertise in a specific area; for example, a pharmacist may be concerned only with medications, and a dietitian is concerned with nutrition. The nurse coordinates the activities of these other professionals and keeps the patient as the center of the team.

Nurses armed with knowledge of the normative changes associated with healthy aging can be proactive and intervene before a crisis. They can also help assess and manage changes that are not normative with aging. No one can halt the aging process, but nurses can assist older adults in adapting to these changes and remaining as healthy and independent as possible.

KEY POINTS

- Normative physical and physiological changes of aging can impact an older adult's ability to age successfully.
- Nurses can facilitate successful aging by helping the older adult adapt to these changes.
- Nurse should understand the clinical implications of physiological changes to avoid misinterpreting the clinical findings.
- Interpretation of physical findings should be tempered with the knowledge of the normative changes associated with aging.
- Sensory changes in normal aging interfere with the ability to care for self.
- Changes in gustatory and olfactory sense can lead to poor or undernutrition.
- Visual changes can increase the risks for falls and accidents.
- Auditory changes can lead to social isolation.
- Exercise and adequate nutrition can help the older adult adapt to changes in pulmonary, cardiovascular, musculoskeletal, and neurological changes.
- Nurses are key members of the geriatric assessment team.

CRITICAL THINKING ACTIVITIES

1. Place cotton in your ears, go to a crowded place, and try to have a conversation with a friend. Imagine that an older adult may experience the same effect. How would you help an older adult adapt to this change in hearing?
2. Interview an independent-living 65-year-old and an 85-year-old. Compare and contrast the differences in adaptation each person has had to make to remain independent.
3. Talk to your friends and identify their greatest concerns about growing old. Identify your own concerns about growing old.
4. Talk to a health care provider about his or her concerns in caring for older adults. What does this provider consider when designing a plan of care?
5. Interview staff at a senior center and identify activities that keep elders active.

CASE STUDY | *MRS. FRANK*

Mrs. Betty Frank is an 84-year-old woman who lives alone in her own home. Her husband died about 5 years ago. Mrs. Frank has two sons. One son lives in the same town, and the other lives in a different town about 50 miles away. Mrs. Frank continues to drive her car; however, she does not like to drive at night. Although she wears glasses, she feels the lights of the oncoming traffic are too bright.

Mrs. Frank talks to her friends daily on the phone and attends church weekly. She likes to be engaged in the church, but many church activities take place in the evening. Mrs. Frank also thinks she would like to do some volunteer work at the local hospital, but she says she "just can't remember like I used to." She also has chronic back pain from an accident and arthritis.

Mrs. Frank asks you what she might do to improve her memory and maintain her stamina.

1. Identify some of the normative changes of aging that have affected Mrs. Frank. How has this older adult adapted to them?
2. What would you recommend to encourage continued adaptation?
3. What strategies could help Mrs. Frank improve her memory?
4. What would you suggest to help improve her stamina?

REFERENCES

Aagaard, P., Magnusson, P. Larsson, B., Kjaer, M., & Krustrup, P. (2007). Mechanical muscle function, morphology, and fiber type in lifelong trained elderly. *Medicine and Science in Sports and Exercise, 39*(11), 1989–1996.

Administration on Aging. (2010). *Projected future growth of the older population.* Retrieved November 15, 2010, from http://www.aoa.gov/AoARoot/Aging_Statistics/future_growth/future_growth.aspx#state

Aronow, W. S. (2006). Heart disease and aging. *Medical Clinics of North America, 90,* 849–862.

Artal, P., Guirao, A., Berrio, E., Piers, P.,& Sverker, N. (2003). Optical aberrations and the aging eye. *International Ophthalmology Clinics, 43,* 63–77.

Beers, M., Jones, T., Berlwits, M., Kaplan, J. & Porter, R. (Eds.). (2006). *The Merck manual of geriatrics* (3rd ed.). Retrieved November 15, 2010, from http://www.merck.com/mkgr/mmg/home.jsp

Bhutto, A., & Morley, J. W. (2008). The clinical significance of gastrointestinal changes with aging. *Current Opinion in Clinical Nutrition and Metabolic Care, 11,* 651–660.

Boyce, J. M., & Shone, G. R. (2006). Effects of ageing on smell and taste. [Electronic version]. *Journal of Postgraduate Medicine, 82,* 239–241.

Cabeza, R., Anderson, N., Locantore, J., & McIntosh, A. (2002). Aging gracefully: Compensatory brain activity in high-performing older adults. *Neuroimage, 17,* 1394–1402.

Cademartiri, F., la Grutta, L., de Feyter, P. J., & Krestin, G. P. (2008). Pathophysiology of the aging heart. *Radiology Clinics of North America, 46,* 653–662.

Carlson, N., Moore, M., Dame, A., Howieson, D., Silbert, L. Quinn, J., . . . (2008). Trajectories of brain loss in aging and the development of cognitive impairment. *Neurology, 70,* 828–833.

Cheng, C., Chan, J., Cembrowski, G., & vanAssendelft, O. (2004). Complete blood count reference interval diagrams derived from NHANES III: Stratification by age, sex, and race. *Laboratory Hematology, 10,* 42–53.

Drachman, D. A. (2006). Aging of the brain, entropy, and Alzheimer disease. *Neurology, 67,* 1340–1352.

Duthie, E., Katz, P., & Malone, M. (2007). *Practice of geriatrics.* Philadelphia: Saunders-Elsevier.

Dyer, C., Hyer, K., Feldt, K., Lindemann, D., Whitehead, J., Greenberg, S., . . . (2003). Frail older patient care by interdisciplinary teams: A primer for generalists. *Gerontology and Geriatrics Education, 24,* 51–61.

Ehrlich, R., Harris, A., Kheradiya, N., Winston, D. M., Ciulla, T. A., & Wirostko, B. (2008). Age-related macular degeneration of the aging eye. *Clinical Interventions in Aging, 3,* 473–482.

Ferrucci, L., Giallauria, F., & Guralnik, J. M. (2008) Epidemiology of aging. *Radiologic Clinics of North America, 46,* 643–652.

Junaidi, O., & Di Bisceglie, A. (2007). Aging liver and hepatitis. *Clinics in Geriatric Medicine, 23,* 889–903.

Katial, R., & Zheng, W. (2007). Allergy and immunology of the aging lung. *Clinics in Chest Medicine, 28,* 663–672.

Kirkwood , T. B. (2005). Understanding the odd science of aging. *Cell, 120,* 437–447.

Kozak, A., & Grundfast, K. (2009). Hearing loss. *Otolaryngologic Clinics of North America, 42,* 79–85.

Lafreniere, D., & Mann, N. (2008). Anosmia: Loss of smell in the elderly. *Otolaryngologic Clinics of North America, 42,* 123–131.

Lakatta, E. G., Wang, M., & Najjar, S. (2009). Arterial aging and subclinical disease are fundamentally intertwined at the macroscopic and molecular levels. *Medical Clinics of North America, 93,* 583–604.

Mason, R., Broaddus, C., Murray, J., & Nadel, J. (Eds.). (2005) *Murray and Nadel's textbook of respiratory medicine* (4th ed.). Philadelphia: Saunders-Elsevier.

Matsumura, B. A., & Ambrose, A. F. (2006). Balance in the elderly. *Clinics in Geriatric Medicine, 22,* 395–412.

Mattes, R. (2002). The chemical senses and nutrition in aging: Challenging old assumptions. *Journal of the American Dietetic Association, 102,* 192–196.

Minaker, K. (2007). Effects of aging on specific organs and systems. In L. Goldman & D. Ausiello (Eds.), *Cecil medicine* (23rd ed.). Philadelphia: Saunders-Elsevier.

Morley, J. E. (2007). The aging gut: Physiology. *Clinics in Geriatric Medicine, 23,* 757–767.

Murphy, C. (2008). The chemical sense and nutrition in older adults. *Journal of Nutrition for the Elderly, 27,* 247–263.

Pan, N., Tsao, H., Chang, N., Chen, Y., & Chen, S. (2008). Aging dilates atrium and pulmonary veins for the genesis of atrial fibrillation. *Chest, 133,* 190–196.

Pietschmann, P. Rauner, M., Sipos, W., & Kerschan-Schindl, K. (2009). Osteoporosis: An age-related and gender-specific disease—A mini-review. *Gerontology, 55*(1), 3–12.

Pinn, V. (2006). Past and future: Sex and gender in health research, aging experience, and implications for musculoskeletal health. *Orthopedic Clinics of North America, 37,* 513–521.

Reuter-Lorenz, P. (2002). New visions of the aging mind and brain. *Trends in Cognitive Sciences, 6,* 394–400.

Stanley, M., Blair, K., & Beare, P. (2005). *Gerontological nursing: Promoting successful aging with older adults* (3rd ed.). Philadelphia: Davis.

Stenklev, N. C., Vik, O., & Laukli, E. (2004). The aging ear: An otomicroscopic and tympanometric study. *Acta Otolargology, 124,* 69–76.

Telda, F., & Friedman, E. (2008). The trend toward geriatric nephrology. *Primary Care Clinics in Office Practice, 35,* 515–530.

Thomas, S., & Rich, M. W. (2007). Epidemiology and prognosis of heart failure in the elderly. *Clinics in Geriatric Medicine, 23,* 1–10.

Venning, G. (2005). Recent developments in vitamin D deficiency and muscle weakness among elderly people. *British Medical Journal, 330,* 524.

Woolf, A., & Pfleger, B. (2003). Burden of major musculoskeletal conditions. *Bulletin of the World Health Organization, 81,* 646–654.

Chapter 10

Staying Physically Fit as We Age

Paula E. Papanek, Ph.D., MPT, FACSM, and Jean W. Lange, PhD, RN, FAAN

LEARNING ACTIVITIES

- List the physical, psychological, and health-promoting benefits of exercise training.
- Describe national goals and guidelines for activity among older adults.
- Discuss considerations in designing an exercise program for older adults.
- Explain ways to monitor exercise intensity and indications of overexertion.
- Discuss strategies to promote exercise as a life-long behavior.

Fitness can be described as a condition that helps us look, feel, and do our best. More specifically, it is: "The ability to perform daily tasks vigorously and alertly, with energy left over for enjoying leisure-time activities and meeting emergency demands. It is the ability to endure, to bear up, to withstand stress, to carry on in circumstances where an unfit person could not continue, and is a major basis for good health and well-being" (President's Council on Physical Fitness and Sports, 2010). Several *Healthy People 2020* national goals address the need to increase the proportion of people at all ages who exercise regularly. This can be as simple as walking for a few minutes each day.

Many older adults have active lifestyles that help them optimize functioning. It is not uncommon today to see people passing their 100th birthday while still driving a car and living independently. Successful aging is greatly enhanced by regular exercise.

Unfortunately, not everyone leads an active lifestyle. In fact, in America, only about one fourth of people exercise regularly, and 250,000 deaths are associated with inactive lifestyles (President's Council on Physical Fitness and Sports, 2010). Sixty percent of all Americans are at risk for premature disability or death related to inactivity, and an estimated 2.5 million will die prematurely in the next 10 years. This number exceeds the combined number of deaths from substance abuse, firearm injuries, motor vehicle accidents, and sexually transmitted disease.

Adults over age 55 spend only 3% to 4% of their time engaged in sports, recreation, or physical activity, compared with 56% to 58% of time spent watching television (Fig. 10-1). Only one in four adults over age 55 engages in regular exercise and, by age 85, this percentage declines to less than 10%. Fifty-eight percent of adults over age 65 report that they find it very difficult or they are unable to do one of the following: walk one-quarter mile; climb 10 steps without resting; stand or sit for 2 hours; stoop, bend, or kneel; reach overhead; grasp or handle small objects; lift or carry 10 pounds; or push or pull large objects (Fig. 10-2).

Estimates suggest that for individuals to live independently, they must at least be able to walk 1,000 feet and carry packages weighing 6.7 pounds. Given the percentage of aging adults with limited functional capacity, many may be on the verge of losing their independence. Inactivity leading to decreased strength, endurance, and balance is a principle cause of functional loss. In addition, 42% of adults age 75 and older have a chronic condition that limits their ability to perform their usual daily activities.

Given these statistics, it is not surprising that many consider inactivity to be the second largest threat to public health. National efforts to increase the health of its citizens have targeted exercise as a major factor in reducing chronic disease and disability. In this chapter, we discuss the many benefits of exercise, along with some guidelines and resources for helping older adults stay active safely.

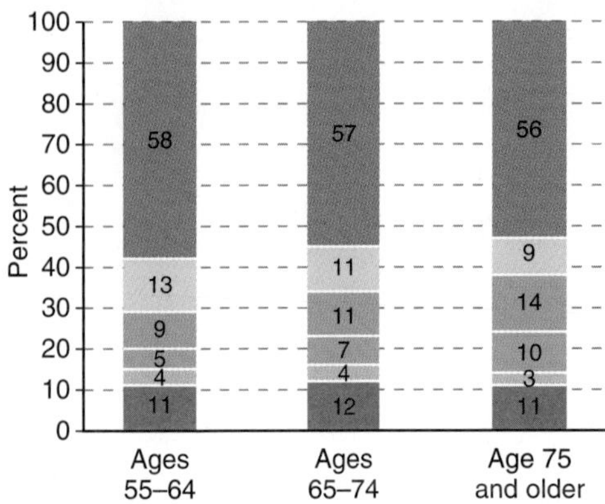

Figure 10-1 *(From Bureau of Labor Statistics. (2008). American time use study. Retrieved November 15, 2010, from http://www.bls.gov/tus/)*

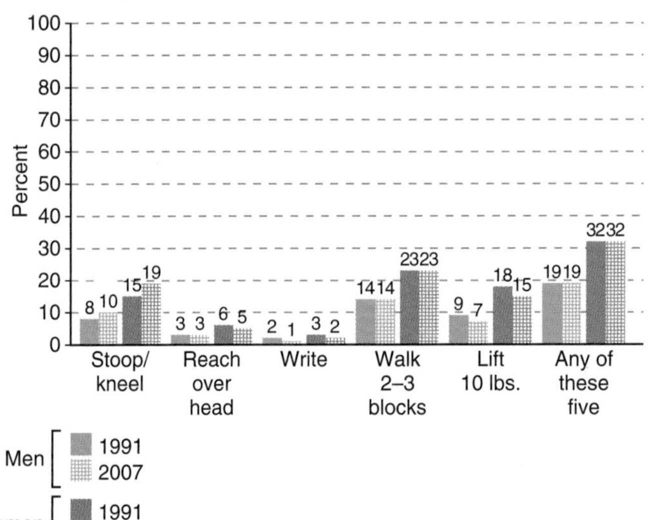

Figure 10-2 *(From Centers for Medicare and Medicaid Services, Medicare Current Beneficiary Survey; https://www.cms.gov/LimitedDataSets/11_MCBS.asp)*

The Role of Exercise in Aging Successfully

Physical changes that are often associated with aging are not necessarily inevitable. For example, aging can be associated with gradual and progressive declines in physiological function that reduce functional and aerobic capacities. Capacity is further reduced by exercising for less time and at a lower intensity. Inactivity leads to loss of skeletal muscle mass (sarcopenia) and a simultaneous increase in the percentage of body fat (Doherty, 2003). It is important to recognize that such age-related declines are not true for all older adults. Decline in physical function varies such that some adults in their late 50s seem much older than those in their late 70s. That is, some adults experience decline while others appear to age more successfully. Physical activity can help to reverse the trend toward decline and lower the risk of chronic disease (Booth, Gordon, Carlson, & Hamilton, 2000; DiPietro, 2001).

Successful aging is commonly defined as having the physical, cognitive, and financial resources to do the things one desires without pain or disease.

Healthy or successful aging is commonly defined as having the physical, cognitive, and financial resources to do the things one desires without pain or disease for as long as one lives (Rowe & Kahn, 1997). This implies a relative freedom from cardiovascular ailments—such as hypertension, stroke, and vascular diseases—pulmonary and metabolic diseases, osteoporosis, and dementia. Healthy aging also implies having the strength, flexibility, and endurance to perform tasks associated with independent living, such as carrying groceries, doing household tasks, climbing stairs, and getting into and out of a chair or bed. Appropriate, adequate exercise can help older adults optimize their physical functioning and independence, key elements of aging successfully.

Benefits of Exercise

Exercise helps us gain better endurance, strength, balance, and flexibility (National Institutes of Health, 2010). Endurance, or aerobic, activities increase the efficiency of cardiac and respiratory function so that simple daily tasks such as gardening, playing with grandchildren, and carrying laundry or groceries become easier. Exercises that use large muscle groups in a continuous movement such as water aerobics, bicycling, brisk walking, or dancing improve endurance.

Strength training exercises increase skeletal and muscle strength, as well as balance. Strengthening exercises help older adults improve their ability to lift objects, climb stairs, or walk longer distances without fatigue. Strength training includes exercises such as Pilates, weight lifting, and resistance training.

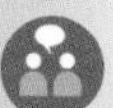

PERSONAL PERSPECTIVE
Keeping Fit

Ellsworth is age 74 and lives in an assisted-living apartment building in urban New Haven, Connecticut. "The first three weeks, maybe a month, that I was living here," he says, "it was a little depressing, because I hadn't encountered people with disabilities so much on a daily basis. I mean the canes, walkers, wheel chairs, sometimes complaining so much. You know it's a little difficult to get used to, but having dealt with a lot of older people on not such a daily basis, it wasn't such a shock. It just took some adjusting to. It could have been depressing, and was at some times, but I looked at the brighter side of things." Ellsworth didn't only look at the brighter side, he took action, organizing a weekly exercise class, he says, "to get some people to do some things they didn't think they could do, and to complain less."

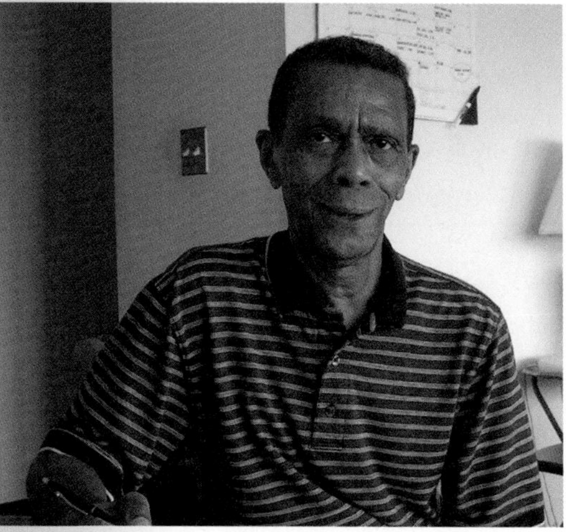

For Ellsworth, exercise is not solely a key to physical fitness. "Exercise," he says, "makes me feel good emotionally because my whole body is relaxed. Very rarely am I hurting while

I'm exercising because I'm not straining or breathing heavily or even sweating a great deal. I'm just keeping my body active, and when I go to bed at night, I'm more relaxed. I'm looser. I have very few aches and pains. I go to bed at a regular time and get up at a regular time and I sleep well, and I attribute it to eating well and exercising." Ellsworth's trim appearance, his strength, and his flexibility testify to the fact that he is one who walks his own talk. Asked the key to staying physically fit, he responds: "Simply, stay active. I walk a lot. I exercise daily. I lead an exercise class once a week, sometimes twice a week. I walk stairs occasionally. I read enough to keep my mind active. I participate in things like trivia, things to make me think, to question my memory and whatnot." Today, exercising his body and his brain are a way of life for Ellsworth, and the benefits of this lifestyle are readily apparent in this high-energy, engaging man.

About Ellsworth Ellsworth Lindsey is the divorced father of five children, and he now has seven grandchildren. Before retiring he had a varied career that included work as a head waiter at the Woodbridge Country Club, furniture salesperson, manager of a senior center lunch program, and line dancing teacher. After retirement, Ellsworth actively gave back to his community, taking on the role of manager of the soup kitchen at his church. At the assisted-living complex where he now resides, Ellsworth leads an exercise class and is affectionately referred to as "The Mayor" because of his readiness to help, be involved, and get things done.

Lorri B. Danzig, MS, CSL

Exercises that help with balance also help to improve posture and decrease the risk of falling. Tai Chi is a good example (Komagata & Newton, 2003). Finally, stretching before and after exercising improves flexibility and reduces the risk of injury. Flexibility improves range of motion, making it easier to turn one's head while driving, reach overhead, or bend down to put on shoes or socks. Yoga is a good example of an exercise that improves flexibility, as well as balance and muscle strength. Other exercises designed to stretch various muscle groups are available online and through exercise specialists.

Older adults benefit from all forms of exercise (Box 10-1). In fact, the importance of regular physical activity in aging successfully is indisputable (Booth, Gordon, Carlson, & Hamilton, 2000; Rowe & Kahn 1997; Warburton, Nicol, & Bredin, 2006). Quality of life improves with exercise not only because exercise helps reduce the risk of chronic disease but also because exercise increases cardiovascular reserve and endurance, strengthens skeletal muscles, reduces fatigue, and decreases body fat (American College of Sports Medicine Position Stand, 1998). Improved balance can also be achieved through exercise. These improved capacities help to reduce fall risk and maintain independence in performing activities of daily living, such as bathing, dressing, and doing household chores. Regular physical activity also helps preserve bone mineral density, which decreases the risk of osteoporosis and fractures.

Exercise has psychological benefits as well. Physical activity is associated with a sense of well-being and decreases the risk of cognitive decline, dementia, and clinical depression (Chodzko-Zajko & Moore, 1994; Strawbridge, Deleger, Roberts, & Kaplan, 2002). Those who lead an active lifestyle also tend to

BOX 10-1 Benefits of Exercise

- Increased endurance and stamina
- Increased muscle mass and strength
- Enhanced flexibility and range of motion
- Higher basal metabolic rate and energy levels
- Improved balance and kinesthetic awareness
- Decreased blood pressure
- Improved sleep
- Improved glucose regulation
- Improved thermoregulation
- Decreased body fat percentage, increased lean tissue, and better weight management
- Improved lipid control (total cholesterol, high- and low-density lipoproteins, triglycerides)
- Increased bone mineral density (decreased risk of osteoporosis)
- Decreased risk of falls
- Reduced onset and severity of coronary artery disease, stroke, diabetes, and hypertension
- Fewer aches and pains
- Improved relaxation
- Reduced stress, depression, and anxiety
- Improved quality of life, life satisfaction, and self-esteem

Adapted from U.S. Surgeon General's Report. (1996). Guidelines for promoting physical activity among older persons. http://www.cdc.gov/nccdphp/sgr/index.htm

sleep better, experience less stress, and report a better quality of life than those who are inactive. Nurses can safely promote regular physical activity in older adults to help them achieve successful aging.

The overall goal of exercise training is to provide the maximum benefit at the lowest possible risk of injury and to do so in a progressive manner that allows the body to adapt to each new exercise demand.

Goals of Exercise

The overall goal of any exercise training program is to provide the maximum benefit at the lowest possible risk of injury and to do so in a progressive manner that allows the body to adapt to each new exercise demand. Recommendations for physical activity vary with the patient's particular goals and medical history. For example, a person whose goal is to prevent osteoporosis or improve leg strength will need an exercise program heavy on resistance training, whereas a person whose goal is to control hypertension or body weight will need an exercise program heavy on aerobic exercise. When weight reduction is desired, exceeding minimal recommended amounts of activity will usually be required.

Exercise programs for the older adult population ideally should target cardiovascular endurance, muscular strength and endurance, flexibility, and balance. Older adults who previously have been sedentary or who have physical or medical limitations should always consult their health care provider before beginning an exercise program. An exercise physiologist or physical therapist can assist in designing prescriptions tailored to meet individual goals.

Guidelines for Adults

In 2008, the Department of Health and Human Services published evidence-based *Physical Activity Guidelines for Americans* that incorporated recommendations from the American College of Sports Medicine (ACSM) and the American Heart Association (U.S. Department of Health & Human Services, 2008).

General guidelines for adults also apply to those age 65 and older except when they have limiting chronic or physical conditions. In these cases, older adults should be as physically active as their abilities allow and avoid inactivity. The following recommendations are designed for the average healthy adult to maintain health and reduce the risk of chronic disease.

- Exercise for at least 2½ hours per week at moderate intensity or 75 minutes per week at a vigorous intensity using aerobic activities that use large muscle groups in continuous motion (such as swimming, running, or biking).
- Perform aerobic activity in at least 10-minute durations that are spread throughout the week.
- For additional health benefits, increase to 5 hours (300 minutes) a week of moderate-intensity aerobic physical activity, 2½ hours a week of vigorous physical activity, or an equivalent combination of both.
- Incorporate muscle-strengthening activities of all major muscle groups performed two or more days per week (U.S. Department of Health & Human Services, 2008).

Guidelines for Older Adults

In addition to the exercise guidelines published by the Department of Health & Human Services, which are intended for healthy adults of all ages, the National Institutes of Health (2010) and American Heart Association (2010a) suggest guidelines for exercise in older adults. Most of these are also good recommendations for people of any age. Again, before starting an exercise program, older adults should have a physical examination and exercise test to determine baseline health status and individual tolerance to activity.

Older adults lose some muscle elasticity as they age and can be more prone to injury. Older adults should warm up by slowly stretching major muscle groups, beginning activity slowly, and increasing the intensity gradually. Stretching is performed after a period of warm-up activity by lengthening to the point of tension and holding a muscle. To prevent injury, it is important not to stretch to the point of pain. A trained exercise specialist can teach patients how to safely warm up and stretch before exercising.

Exercising safely includes attending to apparel and the environment where the exercise will occur. Clothing should be breathable and allow freedom of movement. Shoes that are comfortable and provide good support will reduce the likelihood of injury. Temperature extremes can also pose risks. Older adults may easily become dehydrated because the thirst signal diminishes with aging. It is a good idea to carry water and drink every 15 minutes, especially when exercising in hot, humid conditions. In addition, the body's ability to thermoregulate through sweating or vasoconstriction becomes less effective; therefore, it is important to dress appropriately; avoid exercising during extreme temperatures; and drink fluids before, during, and after exercise.

Environmental safety is another important consideration. When walking or jogging, older adults should choose a route that is relatively smooth to reduce the risk of falling. Exercising with another person can help people stay motivated, provide an opportunity for socialization, and decrease the vulnerability of being alone. If exercising alone, advise older adults to consider walking during the day, when lighting is better, and at times or locations where there is less traffic. Walking in a public place such as a shopping mall may be a safer choice for some while also having the advantage of climate control. Carrying a cell phone is a good way to call for help if the need arises.

The Nurse's Role in Promoting Exercise

Most adults today are aware of the need to incorporate more physical activity into their lives, but few if any understand how to do so safely. As we age, the benefits of being physically active become more important while risk of injury associated with exercise increases. That is, cardiovascular, pulmonary, metabolic, and orthopedic disorders are more prevalent in the aging populations than in younger populations. Fear of injury is often a concern of patients when exercise and active lifestyles are discussed. Although exercise or activity may cause musculoskeletal injuries, it is the risk of sudden and acute cardiovascular events that is more frightening to many older adults.

These risks are real; the likelihood of myocardial infarction is significantly greater during physical than sedentary activity. It is similarly accurate that risk of injury or heart attack increases with aging. It is also well established, however, that being sedentary is detrimental to healthy aging. Efforts to educate middle-aged and older adults on the negative effects of a sedentary lifestyle are more important than ever. According to Exercise is Medicine (2010a), all health care providers are urged to incorporate discussions about exercise into *every* patient interaction. The goal of all health professionals is to promote moderate, safe levels of activity such that people of all ages will reap the documented benefits of exercise. To achieve this goal requires effective screening, appropriate risk stratification, and adherence to basic guidelines for safety.

All health care providers are urged to incorporate discussions about exercise into every patient interaction.

Nurses have an important role in helping patients understand the benefits that even a modest program of regular exercise can have. Decreasing the time spent being sedentary is as important as increasing the amount of time spent being physically active. The overall goal is to get people moving. This basic concept is an important message that is often underemphasized by health care providers despite strong evidence to suggest that when medical professionals counsel patients about physical activity, activity increases (Elley, Kerse, Arroll, & Robinson, 2003). Assessing activity habits, teaching about exercise benefits, and promoting and following up on a specific exercise plan positively impact patient behavior.

The importance of nursing's role in promoting the national activity agenda and exercise is underscored by the recently announced web-based initiative called *Nurses' Action Guide* for exercise in adults. This initiative is a result of a partnership between the American College of Sports Medicine and the Preventative Cardiovascular Nurses Association. The *Nurses' Action Guide* is a free resource available as part of the Exercise is Medicine initiative (http://www.exerciseismedicine.org/nurses.htm). The guide provides specific information to assist in determining whether a patient is capable of exercising independently. It also suggests templates for exercise prescription and referrals (Exercise is Medicine, 2010b).

Nurses can partner with older adults and their support network to assess resources, limitations, and opportunities for safe exercise. Examples of questions the nurse might ask include:

- Are there any physical, sensory, cognitive, or resource barriers to starting a physical activity program?
- Does the patient have a history of falling, or is he or she on medications such as antihypertensives that may induce orthostatic changes or affect balance?
- What medical diagnoses should be considered?
- Does the patient have risk factors for heart disease or symptoms of underlying but undiagnosed cardiac, respiratory, or metabolic disease (Boxes 10-2 and 10-3)?

BOX 10-2 Risk Factors for Cardiovascular Disease

- Age (over age 45 for men, 55 for women)
- Postmenopause or posthysterectomy in women
- Smoking
- Hypertension (blood pressure exceeding 140/90 mm Hg) or therapy with antihypertensive medication
- Elevated cholesterol (above 200 mg/dL), low-density lipoprotein (above 160 mg/dL), or triglyceride level (above 150 mg/dL)
- More than 20 pounds overweight or a body mass index above 30
- Family history of a first-degree male relative under age 55 or female relative under age 65 with a myocardial infarction or cardiac surgery
- Abnormal fasting glucose level or impaired glucose tolerance test confirmed on at least two separate occasions
- Sedentary lifestyle (exercising <30 minutes 3 days per week for the past 3 months)

BOX 10-3 Signs and Symptoms of Cardiovascular, Pulmonary, and Metabolic Disease

- Pain or discomfort in the chest, neck, jaw, arms, or other areas associated with ischemia
- Shortness of breath at rest or with mild exertion
- Syncope
- Orthopnea
- Paroxysmal nocturnal dyspnea
- Dependent edema
- Heart palpitations or tachycardia
- Heart murmur
- Intermittent claudication
- Unusual fatigue
- Shortness of breath during usual activities
- Excessive thirst, hunger, or frequent urination

From American Heart Association. (2010b). Understand your risk of heart attack. Retrieved November 15, 2010, from http://www.heart.org/HEARTORG/Conditions/HeartAttack/UnderstandYourRiskofHeartAttack/Understand-Your-Risk-of-Heart-Attack_UCM_002040_Article.jsp

- Is the older adult steady on his or her feet, or would chair exercises be a safer alternative to a walking program?
- Should exercise be supervised to avoid the risk of injury?
- Is the environment safe for an older adult to walk alone?
- Are their family members, friends, or neighbors living nearby who might help? What transportation is accessible?
- What options are available in the community that might also provide an opportunity for an older adult who is living alone to socialize with others?
- Are there exercise programs tailored to older adults available at a local YMCA or senior center?
- Are costs of organized programs covered by insurance or do finances present a barrier?
- Does joint pain that limits movement need to be better managed to facilitate mobility?
- What does the older adult enjoy doing so that he or she will be more likely to feel motivated to continue an activity?
- When should patients be referred to their health care provider for exercise recommendations or referral to an exercise expert such as a physical therapist or physiologist?

Many older adults enjoy a more positive physical, social, and mental sense of well-being when they are active. For patients with limited endurance, daily activity can be divided into shorter periods, such as taking short walks each morning and evening.

With a little creativity and planning, increased activity can often be integrated easily into daily life. Finding the right fit that matches safety and capacity with the type of activity is key to sustaining exercise as a lifelong activity. Suggestions for helping patients start and sustain an exercise program are listed in Box 10-4. Understanding some of the basic concepts about exercise can also help nurses be better prepared to promote exercise among their patients.

BOX 10-4 Suggestions for Helping Patients Get Active and Keep Moving

- Choose activities that are fun, suit your needs, and can be done year-round.
- Find a friend or companion to exercise with you if it will help you stay on a regular schedule and add to your enjoyment.
- Integrate exercise into your daily routine.
- Exercise at the same time each day so that it becomes a regular part of your lifestyle.
- Monitor your progress in a diary or journal. Include the days you exercise, distance traveled or length of time exercised, and how you felt after each session.
- If you miss a day, plan a make-up day.

Strength Training

Strength training helps increase muscle strength and power and bone mineral density. These benefits also help to improve physical functioning and reduce the risk of falling (Hughes et al., 1995; Morey, Pieper, & Cornoni-Huntley, 1998; Province et al., 1995).

Examples of muscle strengthening exercises include resistance training, weight-bearing calisthenics, and stair climbing. A basic strength-training program includes 1 to 3 sets of 8 to 15 repetitions at a weight corresponding to 65% to 85% of maximal ability. Resistance training targets eight major muscle groups: shoulders, chest, back, abdomen, arms (biceps and triceps), forearms, and upper and lower legs (gluteals, hamstrings, quadriceps, calves). Effective strength training requires exercising for at least two nonconsecutive days each week (Nelson et al., 2007).

Building a well-designed, individualized resistance training program requires knowledge and adequate training in skeletal muscle anatomy and physiology, testing, and program design. A certified fitness trainer or exercise physiologist should be consulted to teach patients proper exercise techniques and to determine the correct amount of weight. Performing strength training exercises correctly is more important than performing exercises at a higher intensity or weight with incorrect form that can lead to serious injury. Regular follow-up is also needed to adjust the program in keeping with changes in fitness level or health status (Brachle & Earle, 2008).

Aerobic Exercise

Aerobic exercise improves cardiovascular and respiratory efficiency and is linked to a reduction in the risk for chronic disease. Patients should be taught how to judge their exercise intensity, evaluate their tolerance to physical activity, and recognize the warning signals of overexertion. Moderate intensity exercise is defined as at least 10 minutes of activity that increases heart and respiratory rates and produces sweating. Typically, this is equivalent to a brisk walk for a middle-aged, healthy adult. A person's rating of perceived exertion (RPE) is often evaluated using a 10-point scale, where 0 represents no exertion (e.g., sitting or resting) and 10 represents maximal effort. Moderate activity would equate to a 3 to 4 exertion rating. Another easy way that patients can gauge whether they are exercising at a moderate level of intensity is with the *talk test.* Patients exercising at a moderate level should be able to speak in a fluid, uninterrupted stream of conversation without difficulty. Vigorous activity such as jogging results in rapid breathing and substantially larger increases in heart rate when compared with activity of moderate intensity. Using the 10-point RPE scale, vigorous activity would be assessed greater than 5 to 7 rating as described with such words as *somewhat hard* or *hard.* Talking tends to be in short phrases of three to four words interrupted with breathing. Sweating is more noticeable and may be heavy. In general, performing exercise in the recommended range of 3-5 on the 10-point RPE scale will result in an effective yet safe workout for the majority of adults.

Balance Training

Proprioception, or our ability to sense how our body moves in relation to itself, can become less accurate as we age. Reaction time also tends to slow somewhat with aging. Collectively, these changes can affect balance and increase the risk of falling. Two easy tests of balance include the Berg balance test, and the Get Up and Go test. The Berg test has been validated for use in predicting fall risk among older adults. The scale measures patients' ability to perform 14 different tasks safely, efficiently, and without assistance (Berg, Wood-Dauphinee, Williams, & Maki, 1992). The Get Up and Go test is also useful to screen for fall risk. Patients are observed for their ability to sit and stand without using their arms for support, to stand with eyes closed, and to walk steadily (Mathias, Nayak, & Isaacs, 1986; available at http://www.aan.com/practice/guideline/uploads/273.pdf.

Like fitness testing, balance testing provides quantification of deficits and improvement in response to training. Any activity that challenges balance can be used to improve balance. The key is to select exercises that are similar to activities the patient regularly performs and to challenge balance limits safely, that is, tip but not fall over. For example, many older adults are unsteady standing on one leg. A functional balance exercise might ask a patient to stand with feet comfortably apart and facing the instructor. Ask the patient to stand in place with arms out and palms facing up and hold this position for several minutes. Assess for sway and stability. If stable, this exercise can be repeated with eyes closed. Gradually, patients progress to longer periods, narrower stance and even a single-leg stand without loss of balance. This exercise must be done with someone who can catch the person if he or she should begin to fall. Group activities such as Tai Chi and yoga effectively combine strength and balance training. Balance training is an important component of a comprehensive exercise plan for the aging adult and requires little or no equipment.

Before a patient starts a new exercise program or physical activity, the first consideration should be whether the person has an acute or chronic condition that limits physical activity or increases the risk for injury.

Components of an Exercise Prescription

General exercise guidelines are for healthy adults and those with chronic conditions not associated with physical activity. These guidelines exclude a significant portion of the geriatric or adult population with movement-related disorders and physical limitations.

Primary care nurses serve as a pivot entry point into the medical system and as such are well positioned to identify when referrals to exercise specialists are needed (Box 10-5). Before a patient starts a new exercise program or physical activity, the first consideration should be whether the person has an acute or chronic condition that limits physical activity or increases the risk for injury. Patients with an orthopedic condition, neurological condition, acute injury, change in mobility status, or history of falling will benefit from a thorough evaluation.

For individuals with no limitations or serious medical problems, general recommendations include gradually and progressively increasing activity levels within the comforts and limits of the individual. Determining baseline activity patterns and fitness level provides a starting place for the exercise plan. What are the patient's goals and needs? Does the person need aerobic activity more than balance training? Is the person already active with a walking program but now desires a prescription that emphasizes muscular strength? What type of activities does the person enjoy or dislike? Does the person want competitive exercise, group activity, or individual activity? For example, someone who enjoys the outdoors may prefer nature hikes versus another person who is very social but lives alone (Fig 10-3). The latter may prefer group activities offered by the local YMCA or senior center.

For patients with physical or medical limitations, a more formal exercise prescription can be tailored to a patient's needs. Usually, exercise prescriptions are determined by a trained professional, such as a physical therapist, exercise physiologist, or medical specialist. Exercise prescriptions include four components: frequency, mode, intensity, and duration.

Frequency refers to the number of repetitions in a set of strength training exercises, or the number of times per week to perform an exercise. *Mode* is the type of exercise—for example, walking, swimming, calisthenics, or dancing. The mode is chosen according to

BOX 10-5 The Role of Physical Therapists

Although it is clear that all adults, regardless of age or primary or secondary medical conditions, will benefit from a more active lifestyle, it is equally clear that some patients require skilled rehabilitation services. Physical therapists are uniquely trained in the care and rehabilitation of acute and chronic orthopedic conditions and injuries as well as in the unique needs of the geriatric population. Physical therapists help restore function, improve mobility, relieve pain, and prevent or limit permanent physical disabilities in patients with injuries or disease. Physical therapist services are a cost-effective way to restore, maintain, and promote overall fitness and health, and are covered by most third party payors.

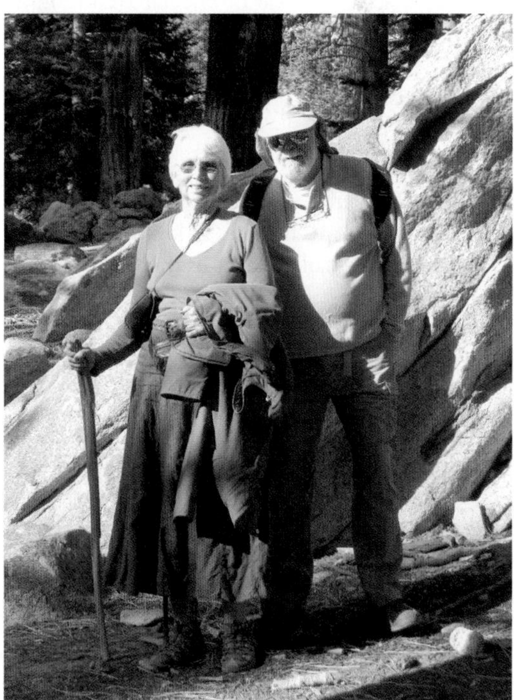

Figure 10-3 For those who enjoy the outdoors, an exercise prescription might include hikes chosen to match individual fitness levels.

patient preference and the desired goal (e.g., to increase strength, balance, endurance, or flexibility; to decrease weight). Asking someone to perform water aerobics is not a good choice if he or she does not have access to a pool or is afraid of the water. Selection of the appropriate mode should consider the patient's likes and dislikes, availability or access, and type of stimulus. *Intensity* is the level of difficulty at which exercise is performed. Moderate intensity exercise is considered to be 30 minutes per day, 5 days per week. Vigorous intensity exercise is associated with additional health benefits but may carry greater risk for injury. Intensity can be quantified using the RPE scale. *Duration* defines the length of time the activity is to be performed.

Regular exercise increases tolerance for higher levels of intensity, so exercise prescriptions need to be periodically evaluated and updated by a trained professional. Progression may be accomplished by increasing the number of repetitions or sets, increasing the weight load, or changing to a more challenging exercise. Progression in aerobic or cardiorespiratory conditioning may include increasing the total time exercised, decreasing rest between exercises, or increasing the pace. An exercise prescription for a previously sedentary person designed to improve aerobic or cardiovascular conditioning might take the following approach:

- Week 1—Walk for 10 minutes at low intensity (RPE of 3 or less) twice daily, 2 days of the week.
- Week 2—Progress to 3 days per week.
- Week 3—Progress to 4 days per week.
- Week 4—Walk 10 minutes at low to moderate intensity twice daily, 5 days of the week.

After 4 weeks without pain or discomfort, the patient might be instructed to walk for 20 minutes at low to moderate intensity daily, for 3 to 5 days of the week.

Exercise that is both safe and appropriate for one person may not be safe and appropriate for another person. The complexity of tailoring prescriptions to individual needs requires a trained professional who can safely assess capacity, establish the prescription, regularly reassess, and progress appropriately, ensuring safety and technique.

Additional Safety Considerations

Safety is an important consideration in the aging population. Exercise programs must consider individual limitations or restrictions, as well as the safety of equipment and environment. All equipment must be stable to prevent falls and injuries. Stand-by assist, grab bars on walls, and floor mats to cushion falls can help to prevent injury. It is also important to ensure that exercise space is clear of obstacles and that there is adequate seating and water available.

Adults should be taught to monitor their RPE to make sure the appropriate intensity is achieved during training and activity. Use of the RPE helps to decrease risks from overexertion and provides an easy method to compensate appropriately when the environmental conditions have changed or when recovering from an illness. Patients also can be taught to monitor intensity of effort by counting their heart rate from either the radial or carotid pulse. For a quick estimate of beats per minute, the patient can count with a second hand for 6 seconds and add a zero to the value. For patients who have decreased vision or sensation, who have an irregular heart rate, or who take certain medications (such as beta blockers), the talk test or RPE may be better methods to monitor exertion levels.

Signals of overexertion include pain or pressure in the chest, neck, shoulder, or arm; dizziness; nausea; profuse sweating; muscle cramps; significant pain in the joints, feet, ankles, or legs; or being out of breath and unable to talk. Patients should be taught to recognize these signals, stop exercising immediately, and seek assistance. If symptoms persist or get worse despite stopping exercise, patients should be instructed to access the emergency response system (e.g., by calling 911). If symptoms resolve when exercise stops, activity should not be resumed until after consulting with the primary provider.

Sustained exercise at the appropriate intensity will lead to higher fitness levels. After a few weeks, patients who exercise regularly will notice that they can exercise longer and faster than before at the same RPE. Teaching patients to understand their body's response to exercise empowers them to safely monitor and adjust their exercise workload.

In the event of injury or a medical event, it is important to have a safety plan in place. This is particularly important when older adults exercise alone or outside the home, in parks, or in malls. Identification that includes medical conditions and emergency contact information should always be accessible. One of the best ways to enhance safety, as well as help sustain interest, in continued exercise is by having an exercise partner (buddy) or group. An exercise buddy can help determine exercise intensity with the talk test and provide feedback regarding workload. They can also observe changes on a daily basis that often go unnoticed. And buddies can provide competition and commitment, two things that increase long-term adherence to an exercise program.

The American College of Sports Medicine and the American Medical Association have designed Exercise is Medicine (2010a, 2010b) to provide health professionals with resources to help people of all ages increase their activity levels. Resources include access to contemporary guidelines, provider links, and educational materials designed for patients and professionals. The goal of Exercise is Medicine is to give health care providers the resources they need to educate all patients at every visit about exercise.

Conclusion

When exercise is a routine part of life, older adults reap powerful benefits from an active lifestyle. Health care providers play a pivotal role in educating, evaluating, and referring older adults to resources that support a safe and routine program of exercise. The evidence is clear that "motion is lotion" for our physical and mental well-being. No other population demonstrates this as clearly as those facing the challenges of an aging body. Physical activity helps preserve our independence in later years and allows us continue to enjoy the things that make life worth living. Some might say that regular exercise is the fountain of youth.

KEY POINTS

- Nursing professionals can serve as role models and educators for the national guidelines for physical activity and a healthy lifestyle.
- Nursing professionals can capture teachable moments to review healthy lifestyle objectives, review coronary artery disease risk factors, and discuss the role of physical activity in successful aging.
- Regular physical activity provides broad health benefits and increases functional capacity.
- Increasing physical activity decreases all-cause morbidity and mortality and increases quality of life in aging and older adults.
- National guidelines recommend 30 minutes of moderate intensity exercise performed 5 days per week for a total of 150 minutes per week as tolerated for adults up to age 65 without physical limitations.
- A large percentage of the geriatric population has physical limitations and will benefit from increased physical activity and decreased sedentary time, but they are simultaneously at an increased risk for sudden myocardial infarct and sudden death.
- Nurses can partner with older adults and their support network to assess resources, limitations, and opportunities for safe exercise.
- For older adults with physical or medical limitations, an exercise prescription should define the frequency, mode, intensity, and duration of recommended exercise in gently increasing levels as tolerance increases.
- The complexity of tailoring prescriptions to individual needs requires a trained professional who can safely assess capacity, establish the prescription, regularly reassess, and progress appropriately, ensuring safety and technique.
- Use of the RPE helps to decrease risks from overexertion and provides an easy method to compensate appropriately when the environmental conditions have changed or when recovering from an illness.

CRITICAL THINKING ACTIVITIES

1. You are teaching a group of older adults at the local senior center about goals of exercise. How would you explain the difference between aerobic, strength training, and balance or flexibility exercises?
2. Your home care patient wants to start exercising more frequently so that she is no longer short of breath with light housework. What types of activities would you suggest? What safety considerations would you convey?
3. Arrange to observe a supervised cardiac rehabilitation session and meet with the exercise therapist to discuss how goals are set for each patient.
4. You are about to discharge your 55-year-old patient following a myocardial infarction. As a busy executive, Mr. Wu has no time for exercise. How would you describe to him the benefits of exercise?
5. The nurse administrator tells you that residents at an assisted-living facility want to start a walking club. What environmental considerations would you suggest the nurse administrator consider?

CASE STUDY | *MARY*

Mary is 78 years old, and she walks the mall for exactly 30 minutes 3 days each week with her sister, Angie, age 72, who picks her up. After walking, they get coffee and often run errands on their way home. Mary is very proud that they have done this now for a whole year, missing only the holiday season when the mall is way too busy and she is afraid she will get knocked down. This year, they are going to walk earlier in the morning because the mall has started a program for early walkers; they plan to keep walking even on holidays. Mary reports that at first she was very tired and used a cane, but now, the 30 minutes fly by as they talk the entire time they are walking, and she no longer uses the cane for her walks.

1. You are delighted that Mary and Angie are active. How can you progress them?
2. In what ways could you quantify the intensity of Mary's exercise?
3. What could you add to Mary's routine that would be beneficial on the days she does not walk?

REFERENCES

American College of Sports Medicine Position Stand. (1998). Exercise and physical activity for older adults. *Medicine & Science in Sports & Exercise, 30,* 992–1008.

American Heart Association. (2010a). *Exercise tips for older Americans.* Retrieved November 15, 2010, from http://www.heart.org/HEARTORG/GettingHealthy/PhysicalActivity/GettingActive/Exercise-Tips-for-Older-Americans_UCM_308039_Article.jsp

American Heart Association. (2010b). *Understand your risk of heart attack.* Retrieved November 15, 2010, from http://www.heart.org/HEARTORG/Conditions/HeartAttack/UnderstandYourRiskofHeartAttack/Understand-Your-Risk-of-Heart-Attack_UCM_002040_Article.jsp

Berg, K. O., Wood-Dauphinee, S. L., Williams, J. T., & Maki, B. (1992). Measuring balance in the elderly: Validation of an instrument. *Canadian Journal of Public Health, 83,* S7–S11.

Booth, F. W., Gordon, S. E., Carlson, C. J., & Hamilton, M. T. (2000). Waging war on modern chronic diseases: Primary prevention through exercise biology. *Journal of Applied Physiology, 88*(2), 774–787.

Brachle, T. R., & Earle, R. W. (Eds.). (2008). *Essentials of strength training and conditioning* (3rd ed.). Champaign, IL: Human Kinetics.

Bureau of Labor Statistics. (2008). *American time use study.* Retrieved November 15, 2010, from http://www.bls.gov/tus/

Chodzko-Zajko, W. J., & Moore, K. A. (1994). Physical fitness and cognitive function in aging. *Exercise and Sport Sciences Reviews, 22,* 195–220.

DiPietro, L. (2001). Physical activity in aging: Changes in patterns and their relationship to health and function. *Journal of Gerontology Series A: Biological Sciences and Medical Sciences, 56*(Suppl.), 13–22.

Doherty, T. J. (2003). Physiology of aging. Invited review: Aging and sarcopenia. *Journal of Applied Physiology, 95,* 1717–1727.

Elley, C. R., Kerse, N., Arroll, B., & Robinson, E. (2003). Effectiveness of counseling patients on physical activity in general practice: Cluster randomized controlled trial. *British Medical Journal, 326,* 793–799.

Exercise is Medicine. (2010a). *Physicians and health care providers.* Retrieved November 15, 2010, from http://www.exerciseismedicine.org/physicians.htm

Exercise is Medicine. (2010b). *Nurses' action guide.* Retrieved November 15, 2010, from http://www.exerciseismedicine.org/nurses.htm

Hughes, V. A., Frontera, W. R., Dallal, G. E., Lutz, K. J., Fisher, E. C., & Evans, W. J. (1995). Muscle strength and body composition: Associations with bone density in older subjects. *Medicine & Science in Sports & Exercise, 27,* 967–974.

Komagata, S., & Newton, R. (2003). The effectiveness of Tai Chi on improving balance in older adults: An evidence-based review. *Journal of Geriatric Physical Therapy, 26*(2), 9–16.

Mathias, S., Nayak, U. S. L., & Isaacs, B. (1986). Balance in elderly patients: The "Get Up and Go" Test. *Archives of Physical Medicine and Rehabilitation, 67,* 387–389.

Morey, M. C., Pieper, C. F., & Cornoni-Huntley, J. (1998). Physical fitness and functional limitations in community-dwelling older adults. *Medicine & Science in Sports & Exercise, 30,* 715–723.

National Institutes of Health. (2010). *Exercise and physical activity for older adults.* Retrieved November 15, 2010, from http://nihseniorhealth.gov/exerciseforolderadults/printerFriendly.html?selectedTopics=selectTopic&howtogetstarted=How+to+Get+Started&print=Confirm+print+selection

Nelson, M. E., Rejeski, W. J., Blair, S. N., Duncan, P.W., Judge, J.O., King, A.C., . . . (2007). Physical activity and public health in older adults: Recommendation from the American College of Sports Medicine and the American Heart Association. *Medicine & Science in Sports & Exercise, 39*(8), 1435–1445. Available online at http://www.acsm.org/AM/Template.cfm?Section=Home_Page&Template=/CM/ContentDisplay.cfm&ContentID=7789

President's Council on Physical Fitness and Sports. (2010). *Fitness fundamentals: Guidelines for personal exercise programs.* Washington, DC: US Department of Health and Human

Services. Retrieved November 15, 2010, from http://www.fitness.gov/fitness.htm

Province, M. A., Hadley, E. C., Hornbrook, M. C., Lipsitz, L. A., Miller, J. P., Mulrow, C. D., . . . Wolf, S. L. (1995). The effects of exercise on falls in elderly patients: A pre planned meta-analysis of the FICSIT Trials. Frailty and Injuries: Cooperative Studies of Intervention Techniques. *Journal of the American Medical Association, 273*(17), 1341–1347.

Rowe, J. W., & Kahn, R. L. (1997) Successful aging. *Gerontologist, 37*(4), 433–440.

Strawbridge, W. J., Deleger, S., Roberts, R. E., & Kaplan, G. A. (2002). Physical activity reduces the risk of subsequent depression for older adults. *American Journal of Epidemiology, 156,* 328–334.

U.S. Department of Health and Human Services. (2008). *Physical activity guidelines for Americans.* Retrieved November 15, 2010, from http://www.health.gov/paguidelines/guidelines/default.aspx#toc

Warburton, D. E., Nicol, C. W., & Bredin, S. S. (2006). Health benefits of physical activity: The evidence. *Canadian Medical Association Journal, 174*(6), 801–809.

Chapter 11

Assistive Technology to Optimize Physical Functioning

Kinsuk Maitra, PhD, OTR/L

LEARNING OBJECTIVES

- Identify the role of occupational therapy in the care of older adults.
- Describe assistive devices that can be used to optimize independence.
- Discuss the value of driver rehabilitation programs for older adults.
- Consider how nurses can collaborate with occupational therapists to enhance the care of older adults.

Activities of daily living (ADLs) and instrumental activities of daily living (IADLs) are everyday activities that fill our time from when we awaken until we go to sleep at night. In older adults, these activities can range from grooming and eating to taking medications and managing finances. The ability to take care of oneself is important in promoting health, wellness, and quality of life and has implications for self-identity, social relationships, and well-being.

Chronic diseases or trauma may occur as we age and may cause impairments or limitations that interfere with the ability to perform ADLs and IADLs (Bonder & Dal Bello-Haas, 2009). Not surprisingly, research indicates that older adults with disabilities need more time to accomplish self-care tasks. A decline in functioning also may lead to increased dependence on others and on the health-care system (Bonder & Dal Bello-Haas, 2009).

As health-care providers, how can we help the aging population retain as much independence as possible? How can we make life easier for our patients despite the challenges that illness and aging can pose? Assistive technology involves devices or services that can help make tasks less challenging for patients. The Assistive Technology Act of 1998 (amended 2004) defines technology as "any item, piece of equipment or product system whether acquired commercially, off the shelf, modified, or customized that is used to increase, maintain, or improve functional capabilities of individuals with disabilities." These devices may include, but are not limited to, hearing aids, communication devices, stair lifts, wheelchairs, adapted computers, and van conversions. Also included in assistive technology are home modifications and adaptations such as ramps or grab bars placed in hallways or bathrooms (State of Oklahoma, 2009).

Assistive technology is a device or service that can help make tasks less challenging.

Occupational therapists (OTs) can be a valuable resource in helping patients preserve their independence. OTs are educated to evaluate a patient's environment, whether at work or at home, and to determine which modifications or devices may help the person adjust to their physical limitations. OTs teach patients how to use appropriate assistive devices in ways that optimize their physical functioning (American Occupational Therapy Association [AOTA], 2008). Nurses can collaborate with OTs to ensure that assistive technology is used correctly and that the goals of therapy are met. Nurses play an important role in assessing when patient safety may be enhanced by the use of assistive devices and in monitoring patients' adaptation to this new technology. The goal of this chapter is to discuss the sensory and physical impairments most commonly experienced by older adults and to illustrate how assistive technology can help older adults maximize independence in their daily functioning.

Sensory Impairment

More than 12 million people in the United States currently live with low vision (National Eye Institute, 2008). Low vision is defined as visual impairment that cannot be corrected with surgery, glasses, or contact lenses and is severe enough to interfere with the performance of everyday activities. In contrast to those who are blind, people with low vision still have some useful sight (Lighthouse International, 2009). Low vision includes loss of visual acuity or sharpness, reduced field of vision, marked light sensitivity, visual distortion, or a loss of the ability to see contrast. Low vision may result from birth defects, injuries, the natural aging process, or a complication of disease.

"Low vision care is a coordinated and collaborative system of discrete services designed to maximize independence and quality of life for individuals with low vision" (Lueck, 2004, p. 3). Low vision care includes restoring function by enhancing impaired vision, teaching strategies to compensate for the impaired vision, and providing the patient with a full range of educational and rehabilitation support systems and services. Low vision care is provided by a full team of varying practitioners, including optometrists, ophthalmologists, and OTs (Lueck, 2004). Nursing plays an important role in the care of patients with low vision by recognizing the need for referral. Any change in or loss of vision, as well as symptoms such as flashing lights, clouded vision, or floating objects, should be evaluated by a physician trained in diseases of the eye (ophthalmologist).

Reading becomes more challenging for most older adults, and good lighting is crucial for those with low vision. Reading material should be positioned to minimize glare or shadows that can exacerbate poor vision. To reduce shadows, place lighting overhead and opposite to the side on which the person is working. Glare can be minimized by placing shades on windows, wearing tinted glasses or a brimmed hat and covering shiny surfaces (Kalish, 2009).

Environmental modifications may also be needed to ensure the safety of those with impaired vision. Strategies include teaching patients to minimize clutter to reduce fall risk, prepare for a task by gathering all essential items at once, and store belongings in single versus multi-item rows rather than in vertical stacks so that all objects remain visible and are less likely to fall (Kalish, 2009).

Many visual aids can help patients with low vision to adapt and are widely available through catalogs and online resources. For instance, brightly colored tape can be used to highlight thresholds or steps, and stickers with bumps can be used to mark settings on appliances. Increased contrast by using distinct shades of light and dark can also help the visually challenged discriminate during tasks. For example when setting the table, use a white plate on top of a dark placemat; when pouring beverages, place light-colored beverages such as milk into dark-colored cups. Electronic magnification using closed circuit television (CCTV), although expensive, offers magnification and improved visual fields and can also be used to enhance reading, writing, and small tasks. Unfortunately these devices are not portable and may be too costly for many patients.

Using patterns to organize objects can also be an effective strategy to compensate for low vision. For example, the clock method involves placing food groups at specific locations on the plate. When vegetables are always placed at 12 o'clock and meat at 6 o'clock, people can readily identify what food they are eating. Using a system such as the clock method helps people identify boundaries and serves as a system of organization (Kalish, 2009).

People with visual limitations often learn to use other senses to compensate (Table 11-1). Assistive devices that depend on other nonimpaired senses can be very helpful, such as a clock that "says" what time it is, or a calculator with an auditory component. Liquid-level indicators can make a sound to indicate that the liquid being poured has reached a certain level, thus signaling the patient to stop pouring (Kalish, 2009).

Environmental safety is a key concern for older adults with low vision. When assessing the home of a person with impaired vision, attention should be paid to lighting and the font size of wording on appliances or everyday items. Appliances with small text, such as an oven temperature knob, may need that to be adapted so the numbers are more clearly identifiable. It is also important not to rearrange furniture or items without the patient's knowledge or consent.

TABLE 11-1 Assistive Technology for Persons with Visual Impairments

ADAPTIVE DEVICE	NAME/TYPE	APPROXIMATE COST	USE
Hand-held magnifiers	3x Aspheric	$40.00	These lightweight and easy-to-carry magnifiers aid in daily reading.
	4x Aspheric	$32.00	
	5x Aspheric	$32.00	
	6x Aspheric	$32.00	
	7x Aspheric	$32.00	
LED hand-held magnifiers	3.5x Aspheric	$68.00	These LED-equipped magnifiers provide additional light for enhanced reading.
	3x Aspheric	$68.00	
	4x Aspheric	$60.00	
	5x Aspheric	$60.00	
	6x Aspheric	$60.00	
	7x Aspheric	$58.00	
	8x Aspheric	$58.00	
	10x Aspheric	$54.00	
	12x Aspheric	$54.00	
	14x Aspheric	$54.00	
LED stand magnifiers	3x 100x50	$92.00	The stand on this product allows the magnifier to rest on top of the reading material.
	3x 100x75	$96.00	
	4x 100x75	$64.00	
	5x 100x75	$64.00	
	6x 100x75	$64.00	
	7x 100x75	$60.00	
	8x 100x75	$60.00	
	10x 100x75	$56.00	
	12x 100x75	$56.00	
	14x 100x75	$56.00	
Computer screen magnifier	Computer screen enlarger for 17–19 inch screens	$49.95	These can magnify up to 1.5 times the original source. The magnifier hangs from or attaches to the computer monitor or laptop screen.
	Flatscreen LCD monitor magnifier, 17–19 inch screens	$44.95	
	Widescreen laptop magnifier, 15.4-inch screen	$39.95	
	Widescreen laptop magnifier, 14.1-inch screen	$39.95	
	LCD monitor magnifier, widescreen	$44.95	

TABLE 11-1 Assistive Technology for Persons with Visual Impairments—cont'd

ADAPTIVE DEVICE	NAME/TYPE	APPROXIMATE COST	USE
Screen magnification software	ZoomText Magnifier	$395	This program enlarges everything on the computer screen.
Screen reader	ZoomText Magnifier/ Reader	$595	In addition to enlarging everything on the computer screen, this program also reads the text on the screen.
	JAWS	$895	JAWS reads on-screen information through a synthesized voice.
	Braille Sense	$5,495	Braille Sense provides simultaneous voice output with refreshable Braille.
Portable electronic magnifiers—closed circuit televisions (CCTVs)	SensView	$825	The SensView, has a 4.3-inch widescreen LCD display. The user can zoom from 4x up to 22.5x.
	Looky	$695	The Looky electronic magnifier has a 3.5-inch LCD display and can zoom from 3x to 8x.
	Amigo	$1,695	The Amigo has a 6.5-inch viewing screen and can zoom from 3.5x to 14x.
Electronic magnifiers—CCTV	Merlin 17 inch Merlin 19 inch Merlin 22 inch	$2,595 $2,795 $2,995	These CCTVs have a screen that pivots horizontally and vertically and can be used with a computer. Magnification is from 2.4x to 77x.
Talking word processor	Read: OutLoud	$299	This provides the individual with access to any text the user needs to read.
Portable notetaker	Type 'n Speak 2000	$1,495	This portable notetaker is available in many languages.
Writing and marking aids	Check Writing Guide	$4.00	This guide can be used with a standardized check.
	Signature Guide	$4.00	The signature guide is small enough to fit into a pocket or wallet.
	Envelope Writing Guide	$4.00	Aids in writing on a 4 1/8 x 9 1/2 inch envelope.
	Letter Writing Guide	$4.00	Provides a layout for 8 1/2 x 11 inch unlined paper.

Continued

TABLE 11-1 Assistive Technology for Persons with Visual Impairments—cont'd

ADAPTIVE DEVICE	NAME/TYPE	APPROXIMATE COST	USE
Large print organizers	The Big Print Check Register	$6.75	Additional space allows for easier writing while larger print eases reading.
	Large Print Check Deposit Register	$6.50	
	Jumbo Print Calendar	$6.95	
	EZ Giant Print Address Book	$12.95	
Telephone	Big Button and Braille Telephone	$40.00	This telephone has large buttons, a loud ringer, and a ringing indicator and is hearing aid compatible.
Caller ID	Talking Caller ID	$56.00	This caller ID can announce up to 50 callers according to the recorded name or telephone number.
Talking watch	Tel-Time IV Talking Watch Unisex	$13.00	This black, talking watch comes with a plastic adjustable band and uses a female voice.
Digital recorder	Olympus Digital Recorder with Voice Guid-ance: 2GB Memory	$299.99	Record up to 530 hours of audio.
Braille printer	Romeo Attaché	$1,995	This printer allows the user to print in Braille.

Several options are available to aid those with impaired hearing. One way to help is to provide visual prompts as a notification system. For example, provide a telephone that flashes a light for incoming calls. For additional assistive devices for persons with hearing impairments, see Table 11-2.

Physical Impairment

Older adults with physical changes that impact the performance in daily activities can often benefit from assistive devices and environmental modification (Bonder & Goodman, 1995). Decreased dexterity and coordination can make fine motor tasks such as placing a plug in a wall socket or cutting with a knife more challenging (Bonder & Goodman, 1995). Vestibular changes can affect balance and increase the risk of falls. Decreased muscle fibers and muscle mass can make it more difficult to get out of a chair and slow a person's walking speed. Impaired mobility and agility can also present a safety hazard. Assistive devices and environmental adaptations can improve safety and help older adults regain independence in self-care, work, and leisure activities. Functional improvement in these areas can translate into economic, social and personal gains.

Assistive devices and environmental adaptations can improve safety and help older adults regain independence in self-care, work, and leisure activities.

TABLE 11-2 Assistive Technology for People with Impaired Hearing

ADAPTIVE DEVICE	NAME/TYPE	APPROXIMATE COST	USE
Headset amplifier	Reizen Super Ear 120 dB Gain Hearing Enhancer for Hard of Hearing	$39.95	Amplifies sound at a distance of up to 100 feet.
	Pocketalker Ultra with Lightweight Headphones	$142.95	Amplifies sound closest to the listener and reduces background noise.
Portable phone amplifier	Clearsounds IL95 Portable Phone Amplifier	$38.44	Drastically increases listening volume, making speaker easier to hear.
Telecommunication device	Porta View 20 Junior	$239.99	Provide text output from the telephone.
	Porta Printer 2000 Standard	$359.10	
Alerting system	Deaf/Blind Vibrating Call Kit	$507.70	24-hour alerting system can transmit signals from a doorbell, telephone, smoke detector, and personal receiver, all at the same time.
Door beacon	The Door Beacon – Door Knock Sensor	$29.70	Device flashes when it senses a knock on the door.
Vibrating pager	Tactile Telephone Ring Pager	$159.95	Pager shakes when receiving an incoming call.

Dressing

Dressing is one example of a self-care activity that may become more difficult or frustrating for aging adults with limited range of motion or joint mobility because it involves reaching, bending, and fine motor grasping. Button hooks, zipper pulls, and elastic shoelaces can assist those with limited grasp or poor fine motor coordination. Adapted button hooks allow for single-handed buttoning and assist those who have deficits in fine motor coordination or who may use only one hand effectively. These hooks come in a variety of lengths and with variable grip sizes. The wire hook is threaded through the button hole; the button is then grasped by the wire and pulled back through the hole. Zipper pulls are an additional aid to those with impaired fine motor control (Fig 11-1A). Pulls come in a variety of styles, such as a plastic grip with a hook on the end that attaches to the zipper tab or a 1-inch ring with a snap hook attached to the zipper tab. Elastic shoelaces can make it easier to secure shoes when older adults cannot bend sufficiently and are also beneficial for single-handed people or for those with arthritis.

Other assistive devices for dressing include sock aids (Fig. 11-1B), long-handled shoe horns, dressing sticks, and reachers. A sock aid is made of plastic attached to two long rope handles. The person places a sock over the flexible part of the aid to open the top of the sock. The person then drops the aid to the floor while still holding the two rope handles. The foot is slipped into the sock opening, and the person pulls upward with the two handles to allow the foot to slip into the sock and out of the sock aid. A sock aid is very valuable because it can accommodate most foot sizes and sock styles. Long-handled shoe horns reduce bending and stress to the spine or joints. These come in a variety of lengths to accommodate various heights and arm lengths. A dressing stick helps those with limited range of motion don and doff clothing (Fig. 11-1C). It can also be used to push or pull objects. Its design is a wooden handle with a small C-hook on one end and a large

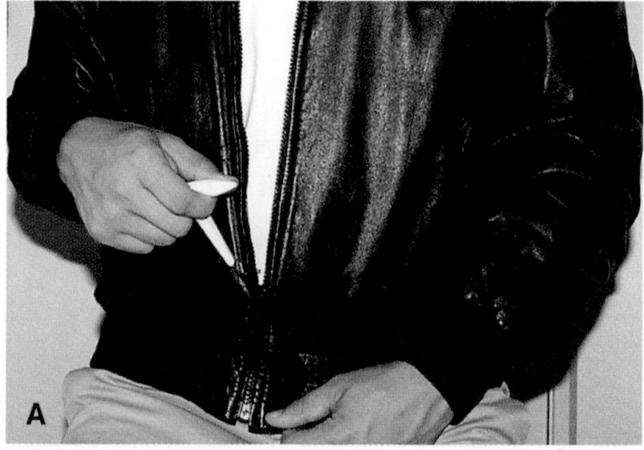

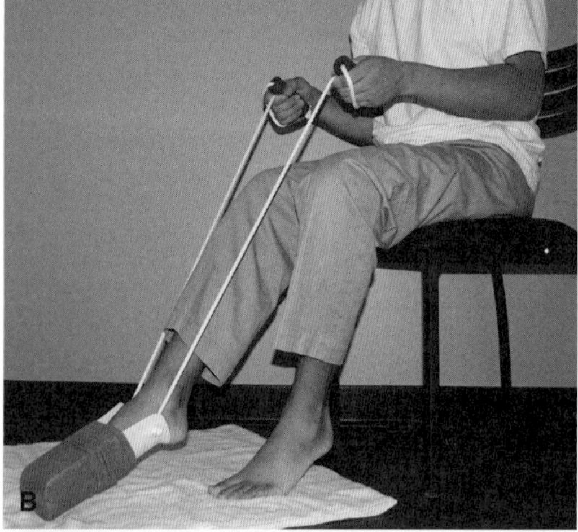

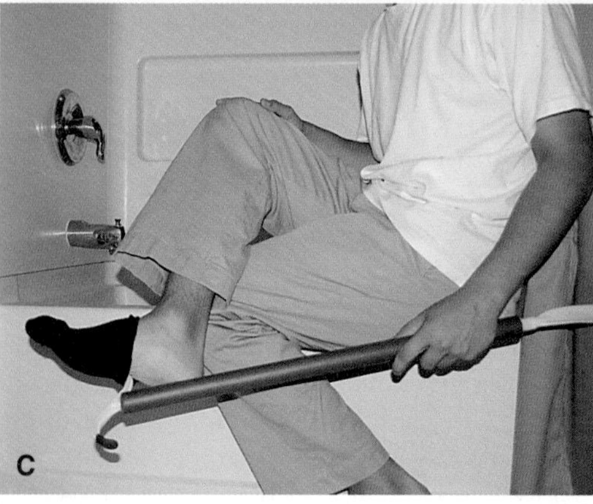

Figure 11-1 Dressing aids include zipper pulls (A), sock aids (B), and dressing sticks (C).

push/pull hook on the other end. Reachers also assist in dressing or picking up various household items. On one end of the reacher is the jaw hook that is operated by a power grip located at the other end. Adaptive equipment for dressing is especially beneficial for older adults who experience poor fine motor control and/or limited reach (Cook & Polgar, 2008).

Eating

Adaptive technology can also help a person compensate when his or her ability to eat safely and efficiently is compromised. Side effects of disease, such as the tremors of Parkinson's disease, hand or arm weakness following a stroke or traumatic injury, or decreased fine motor control, can make eating very difficult. A patient with tremors can benefit from such devices as weighted utensils and cups that provide an opposing force to the affected hand. Rubber placemats and rubber-bottomed bowls and plates help to stabilize food containers and reduce spills. Adaptive devices that increase grip function include utensils with enlarged handles, utensil holders, and universal cuffs. The universal cuff is an adjustable band secured around the palm of the hand that helps provide a secure grasp on various handle shapes and sizes. Slots in the band help hold silverware or other utensils such as a toothbrush, pen, pencil, brush, and comb. When upper body range of motion is limited in the neck, elbow, or shoulder, long plastic straws and feeding tools that swivel are often beneficial.

OTs can be very helpful in evaluating feeding ability and recommending suitable adaptive devices or compensatory techniques. Compensatory techniques might include getting assistance from another person in the household or modifying the environment (Pendleton & Schultz-Krohn, 2006). Difficulty eating can be worsened by poor body positioning or posture. More upright positioning can decrease pressure on the upper gastric area, while lowering the chin while swallowing can decrease choking. A patient's ability and desire to use an assistive device and the cost of the equipment are critical to this assessment.

Toileting

Toileting is a very private activity; therefore, it is important to preserve as much independence as possible. The need for assistance depends on a variety of factors, such as lower extremity strength, range of motion, balance, and fine motor coordination. OTs can help nurses tailor a toileting program for patients and/or caregivers in the natural or home environment. Adaptive equipment to aid in the toileting process may include raised toilet seats, grab bars, personal wiping mechanisms, and toilet seat lifting and lowering devices. Raised toilet seats come in a variety of heights and allow a person to sit comfortably without having to expend unnecessary energy to reach or rise from a toilet seat that is too low. Grab bars provide stability during seating and standing. Bars should be installed at the appropriate height for the patient and near the toilet to ensure safety and ease of transfer.

Personal wiping mechanisms are adaptive devices that allow those with physical disabilities and mobility challenges to toilet more independently. Those who have trouble bending or have limited use of their hands and arms can use a personal wiping device to thoroughly clean the perineal area.

Another adaptive device for those with difficulty toileting is a toilet seat lifting and lowering device. For those with decreased strength, limiting their ability to lower down to or rise up from a toilet seat, a toilet seat lift is optimal. It installs easily on most toilets and requires no permanent modifications.

Grooming

Grooming is an important part of self-care; it not only promotes proper hygiene but also helps one feel and look their best. Grooming includes such activities as bathing, brushing and flossing teeth, drying and combing hair, shaving, and nail care. Arthritis, decreased strength, range of motion or endurance, a stroke, poor balance, or low vision can make these tasks increasingly difficult. Adaptive devices can simplify and reduce the energy and dexterity required for many grooming tasks so that individuals can remain independent for as long as possible. Some of these adaptive devices are designed to alter the environment so that the aging adult can perform the task safely and more easily, while other devices adapt an existing grooming tool.

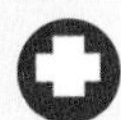

FOCUS ON SAFETY

Shaving Shaving is one task of grooming that can be very dangerous if incorrect equipment is used. Rather than a straight-edged razor, an electric razor is a safe and simple way to avoid injury. Electric razors are available in waterproof versions that can safely be used in the shower. A straight-edged razor may also be modified with a longer handle to help patients shave lower extremities, and handles can be enlarged to make them easier to grasp.

Washing one's hair and body typically requires the ability to stand for long periods and have dexterity in bending and reaching that can be both time consuming and tiring. Fatigue, decreased balance and flexibility, limited endurance, low vision, and poor fine motor control create challenges for bathing. Adaptive equipment in the bath or shower can provide a safer and less taxing way to bathe. Nonslip mats and grab bars reduce slippage and provide stability in tubs and showers, which decreases fall risk. Grab bars can also ease transfers into and out of the shower or tub. A shower chair enhances stability as well as decreases the energy expended in bathing. Long-handled sponges make reaching difficult areas such as the back and lower extremities possible for patients with decreased flexibility or poor fine motor control. A leg lifter can be used in combination with a shower chair to help older adults reach their lower extremities without needing to bend or balance on one leg while cleaning their feet.

Adaptive equipment is also available for grooming tasks such as brushing teeth or hair, nail care, and shaving. Electric toothbrushes are simple and readily available devices that eliminate the need to perform the small motor movements required to properly brush one's teeth. In addition, electric toothbrushes have larger handles that are easier to grasp. If a patient prefers to use a traditional toothbrush, building up the handle size can make the toothbrush easier to hold. Flossing with a floss pick with a plastic wand can also help those who lack the coordination to complete this task.

Hair care is an activity that requires significant range of motion. Using lightweight, plastic brushes and combs requires less energy than heavier wooden tools. A long-handled brush or comb can help those with limited range of motion to reach behind the head. The handles of these tools can also be built up to make it easier to grasp these items. A mounted hairdryer or hairdryer stand can ease the task of hair drying and leave hands free for styling.

Nail care is an important part of grooming but a task that is often overlooked. Nail clippers can be modified with longer handles, larger grips, or wider clipping surfaces to meet patients' needs. Scrub brushes to clean under the nails can be modified so that the handle loops around the hand and eliminate the need to grip the brush. A scrub brush can also be mounted to the sink or shower wall to allow operation with one hand.

Many assistive devices for grooming are available in local stores (Table 11-3). This allows patients to simplify their grooming tasks affordably and discretely. Simple changes in the environment and tools used can allow older adults to remain independent longer while looking and feeling their best. Nurses can help patients identify resources to obtain these devices, as well as monitor their use at home.

TABLE 11-3 Assistive Technology for Persons with Physical Impairments

ADAPTIVE DEVICE	NAME/TYPE	APPROXIMATE COST	USE
Button hook	Button Aid	$4.25	Allows one to get a secure, cushioned grip on hard-to-hold buttons. The built-up handle features flexible ribbing that adapts to any grip.
Zipper pull	Eagle Creek I.D. Zipper Pull Set	$4.95	This makes it easier to grasp to zipper a jacket or coat more easily.
Elastic shoe laces	Perma-Ty Elastic Shoelaces	$5.95	These allow shoes to slip on and off like loafers.
Sock aid	Sock Aid with Foam Grip	$10.95	Allows the sock to be pulled onto the foot easily and independently.
Long-handled shoe horn	Telescopic Shoehorn	$13.75	Provides excellent reach for those who find bending difficult.
Dressing stick	Dressing Stick	$3.59	Ideal for persons with limited arm movement or decreased hip flexion.
Reacher	E-Z Assist Reacher-20 inch	$11.95	Helps pick items up from the floor or can be used to remove socks.
	E-Z Assist Reacher-26 inch	$13.95	
	E-Z Assist Reacher-32 inch	$14.50	
Weighted utensils	Heavy Weighted Utensils	$7.90	Provides opposing force to help stabilize the hand when eating.
	K Eatlery Weighted Utensils	$9.35	
Raised toilet seat	Hi-Loo Raised Toilet Seat	$49.95	Allows for great accessibility and stability. Assists in lowering to or rising up from toilet.
	Raised Toilet Seat with Lock	$44.25	
Grab bars	Chrome Grab Bars	$11.79	Provides a nonslip place to grab on to stabilize in the shower.
	Economy Suction Grab Bar	$9.95	
	Suction Cup Grab Bars	$63.95	
Shower bench	Portable Shower Bench	$39.95	Allows person to sit while showering to increase safety and decrease fatigue in the shower.
	Bariatric Bath Bench	$48.50	
	Corner Shower Seat	$119.00	

TABLE 11-3 Assistive Technology for Persons with Physical Impairments—cont'd

ADAPTIVE DEVICE	NAME/TYPE	APPROXIMATE COST	USE
Nonslip mats	Slip-X Massage Bath Mat	$8.95	Improves traction and safety on slippery surface of shower or tub floor.
	Slip-X Extra Long Deluxe Bath Mat	$9.95	
	Non-Slip Safety Treads	$2.95	
Long-handled sponge	Buff Sponge-22 inch	$3.10	For those with limited range of motion, the long handle allows one to easily reach back, feet, etc.
	Long Handle Bath Brush	$5.95	
Electric toothbrush	Oral-B Vitality Precision Clean Electric Toothbrush	$21.19	Eliminates the need for small, delicate movements to brush one's teeth. The handles are also built up so that they are easier to grip.
	Oral-B Sonic Complete Electric Toothbrush with Charger-S200	$69.99	
	Sonicare Xtreme E3000 Power Toothbrush	$28.99	
	Sonicare Essence Base Model-5300	$68.99	
	Phillips Sonicare Flexcare Toothbrush	$136.99	
	Water Pik Sensonic Profes-sional Toothbrush	$79.99	
Long-handled brush/comb	ETAC Long Reach Comb	$12.95	Makes it possible to comb and brush hair even if one can only lift the hand to shoulder height.
	ETAC Long Reach Hair Brush	$12.95	
Hair dryer stand	Hair Dryer Stand	$16.95	Holds hair dryer upright so that both hands are free for styling. Also elim-inates the need to lift hair dryer for duration of drying.
Long-handled nail clippers	Long Reach Toenail Cutters	$10.95	Designed to assist those who have swollen finger joints or difficulty bending.
Easy grip clippers	Nail Clippers with Suction Cup Base	$17.95	Easy to use for people with limited finger strength, limited dexterity, or tremors.
	Table-Top Nail Clippers	$16.95	

Continued

TABLE 11-3 Assistive Technology for Persons with Physical Impairments—cont'd

ADAPTIVE DEVICE	NAME/TYPE	APPROXIMATE COST	USE
Electric razor	Panasonic Pro-Curve Triple Blade Shaving System	$53.99	Helps people avoid cuts and nicks. The handles are also larger, so they are easier to grip.
	Panasonic Vortex Pro-Curve Triple Blade HydraClean System	$80.99	
	Orbix REV 360 Razor	$29.65	
	Norelco 7810	$77.99	
	Panasonic Close Curves Pivot Action Ladies Shaving System	$39.99	
	Close Curves Wet/ Dry Ladies Shaver	$19.99	

Cognitive Impairment

During the normal aging process, the rate of processing information slows, but significant decline in cognitive functioning is not expected (Bonder & Dal Bello-Haas, 2009). Significant regression in cognition due to dementia, however, does affect one's ability to live and perform ADLs and IADLs safely. Dementia is a deterioration of cognitive functioning that impacts one's ability to meet the intellectual demands of their daily life.

Although there are many types of dementia, there is no specific test designed to diagnose these disorders. The diagnosis is based on behavioral changes that can have a big impact on a person's ability to accomplish daily activities, make decisions using good judgment, solve problems, or recall recent events. Patients with dementia can forget where they are or how to get where they want to go, especially in unfamiliar surroundings. Dementia can present as a slow, progressive decline or as an acute onset of impairments in memory, orientation, task initiation or sequencing, and judgment. These impairments can put patients at risk who fail to recognize or address safety hazards in the home, for example, forgetting to turn off the stove before leaving the house. When cognitive impairment is a concern, home safety should always be evaluated. Safety modifications also need to match the cognitive capacity of the patient. For example, although fire alarms or extinguishers and emergency phone numbers may be readily accessible, they are not useful if the homeowner is unable to use them appropriately.

A thorough assessment is an important first step in identifying areas of concern for the patient, as well as caregivers and other residents. Assessing cognitive status to determine a baseline as well as to identify other health problems that may limit performance of ADLs and IADLs is an important role of health care providers. Such comprehensive assessments often require an interprofessional team of geriatricians, social workers, occupational or physical therapists, nutritionists, and nurses. Regular reevaluation will be needed to assess the appropriateness of modifications when disease or decline is expected to be progressive.

Assistive technology can be helpful to patients with memory problems. Older adults with multiple medical diagnoses are often taking several medications at different times of day. To help these patients remember to take each medication on time, a personal digital assistant or memory aid can be useful. A personal digital assistant allows the patient, nurse, or caregiver to set a number of alarms to serve as patient reminders. Patients who have trouble remembering how to complete the steps of an activity (e.g., warming a meal in the microwave oven) may benefit from visual aids or lists that cue the proper sequencing. When there is concern about turning off appliances such as an iron or stove, automatic shut-off devices can be used to reduce the risk of injury. Some appliances include an automatic shut-off feature (e.g., coffee makers, irons, toaster ovens), or a shut-off device can be installed.

Disorientation is a common problem among patients with dementia. This is especially a concern at night, when patients awaken in a dark room without visual cues to help them remember where they are. Movement-sensitive lighting can help prevent falls and injuries by orienting patients to their surroundings. These lighting devices can turn on room, hallway, or bathroom lights to illuminate a safe path at night. Patients with dementia may become disoriented to the point of leaving their residence and becoming lost outdoors. An alarm system can warn other household members when a confused person wanders out of the home.

The complexity of any adaptive technology must be consistent with a patient's capacity to manipulate the equipment and to learn about its appropriate use. Making several changes at once may further confuse or disorient a patient with dementia, so careful planning and assessment are essential. Whether a patient can continue to live safely in his or her environment is an important consideration in which nurses play a key role. During home visits or history taking, nurses have the opportunity to identify concerns regarding patient safety or functioning and to address their needs by coordinating patient care with other team members.

Adaptive Technology in the Environment

Home Modifications

About 37 million Americans are age 65 or older, a number that the U.S. Census Bureau (2004) estimates will rise to 54 million by the year 2020. Currently, only about 5% of these older adults live in nursing homes (Federal Interagency Forum on Aging Related Statistics, 2008; Bonder & Dal Bello-Haas, 2009). Although older adults now live at home longer, these homes are often ill equipped to support declining health (Sabata, Shamberg, & Williams, 2008). Climbing stairs, stepping in and out of tubs, reading fine print, or buttoning clothes can become increasingly challenging as sensory, cognitive, and physical impediments develop.

Home modifications can create safer and more satisfying environments for older adults choosing to age in place. Many home safety checklists are available to help nurses and caregivers assess the safety of an older adult's living environment. Safety should always be the first consideration in any home assessment. According to the Joint Commission, which accredits health care organizations, a complete home assessment should address four key areas: environmental/mobility safety, bathroom safety, fire safety, and electrical safety (Anemaet & Moffa-Trotter, 1999).

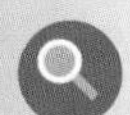

EVIDENCE FOR PRACTICE
Home Modifications

Purpose: To look at the impact home modifications have on self-rated ability in everyday life from multiple aspects for people aging with disabilities.

Sample: There were 73 subjects with approved referrals, scheduled to receive home modifications. Also included were 41 subjects waiting for their approval applications.

Methods: The subjects related their ability in everyday life using the Patient-Clinician Assessment Protocol. This assessment provides information on the patients' self-rated independence, difficulty, and safety in everyday life. Subjects filled out the assessment at baseline and the follow-up. Home modifications were installed (after an OT or physician addresses the problems the individual encounters in everyday life and certifies the need for modification, and then is approved by professionals at Agency for Home Modifications).

Results: Subjects who received home modifications reported a statistically significant increase in their self-rated ability in everyday life, specifically in tasks related to self-care. Home modifications have a direct impact on self-rated ability in everyday life, particularly impacting level of difficulty and safety.

Implications: There is a need to expand the assessments of everyday life abilities for people living in their own home environments to address problems specific to ADLs/IADLs.

Reference: Petersson, I., Lilja, M., Hammel, J., & Kottorp, A. (2008). Impact of home modification services on ability in everyday life for people ageing with disabilities. *Journal of Rehabilitation, 40,* 253–260.

A complete home assessment should address four key areas: environmental/mobility safety, bathroom safety, fire safety, and electrical safety.

The ability to move safely in one's environment means sufficient space to navigate, furniture that is easy to get into and out of, and belongings that are easily reached. Stairs, thresholds, and loose carpeting can be hazardous to people who have trouble climbing or use mobility aids such as walkers and wheel chairs. Evaluating the environment therefore includes ensuring that hallways are sufficiently wide to allow for wheelchairs, lighting is adequate, possessions on counter tops are reachable, furniture is accessible, and cords or rugs do not pose a fall risk. A goal of home assessment is to determine improvements that can be made to optimize safe and independent functioning. Falls often occur in bathrooms; therefore, it is important to observe how easily and steadily the older adult accesses the tub, toilet, and shower. Loose, long, or frayed electrical cords or several appliances plugged into one electrical outlet create fall and fire hazards. Installing smoke, carbon monoxide, and fire alarms may provide sufficient warning for an older adult to exit the home in an emergency. Ready access to emergency telephone numbers, as well as up-to-date fire extinguishers, are also important considerations but are only useful if the homeowner knows how and when to use them.

When assessing a home, it is important to observe the patient performing ADLs and IADLs in the environment and to elicit the patient's help in identifying any difficulties he or she may have. Modifications can then be jointly planned to incorporate patient preferences and financial resources (McCullagh, 2006). If new symptoms arise or functioning declines abruptly, the older adult should be seen by a physician for further evaluation.

An OT is a useful referral when a home-dwelling older adult faces physical, cognitive, or sensory challenges. OTs can recommend assistive technology that enhances the older adult's performance of daily activities and helps prolong independence. When determining what modifications are needed, expectations about recovery or progressive decline are important considerations. Mobility impairments such as those experienced after hip replacement surgery may be temporary, while impairment due to a stroke or arthritis may require more permanent modifications. Cognitive or perceptual limitations will influence the design of any home modification.

Modifications should be adaptable to all members of a household, who often have varying abilities. Such "universal designs" must be easy to use, require little energy, pose little hazard, and be efficient, comfortable, aesthetically pleasing, and size-appropriate for everyone (Connell et al., 2008). An example of the universal design concept is replacing doorknobs that are difficult to turn with levered handles that are useful for people with decreased hand strength, as well as anyone carrying bags of groceries into the house. They are attractive and do not stand out as a modification. Other common examples using the principles of universal design include no-step entryways, single-story living, widened doorways or hallways that can accommodate a wheelchair, open floor space, nonslip surfaces on floors and bathtubs, thresholds that are flush with the floor, and rocker light switches (American Association of Retired Persons, 2010). Designs with universal characteristics are more likely to be used because they are stigma free while being useful to patients and families alike.

Environmental changes do not always require new devices. Simple alterations such as raising the height of or rearranging existing furniture, delivering groceries or meals to the home, performing activities while seated instead of standing, or using proper body mechanics that minimize fatigue can enable older adults to remain living well and independently for longer periods of time (Box 11-1). Arranging items on shelves or other storage areas that the patient can reach increases accessibility at no cost. Installing ramps, grab bars, raised toilet seats, bedside commodes, and shower chairs or benches are lower-cost modifications that enhance stability.

BOX 11-1 Recommendations for Proper Body Mechanics

- Tighten your stomach muscles to support your spine. Do not hold your breath.
- Lift with your legs instead of the small muscles of your back.
- Bring the load as close as possible to your body to prevent lower back strain.
- Maintain the curves of your spine. Keep your body in an upright position while squatting to pick up loads.
- Turn with your feet, not your back. In other words, pivot your body rather than twisting it.
- Push loads instead of pulling them.
- Ask for help if a load is too heavy.

The use of assistive domotics conserves energy by allowing the person to control multiple electronic devices remotely from one keypad, Internet site, or mobile device.

Some home functions can also be automated using home automation or assistive domotics. The use of assistive domotics conserves energy by allowing the person to control multiple electronic devices remotely from one keypad, Internet site, or mobile device. For example, to help wheelchair-bound patients or those with limited reach, a single remote control can assist with operating lights, television, radio, ceiling fans, HVAC (Heating, Ventilating, and Air conditioning) systems, alarm systems, sprinkler systems, motorized curtains, and music systems. Remote keyless entry systems can also be programmed to let residents see who is at the door before opening it remotely. Assistive domotic systems can also monitor and communicate physiological measurements such as vital signs and data from implanted cardiac devices. Voice reminder systems can cue patients about upcoming doctor appointments or medication times, as well as everyday activities such as turning off the stove, closing blinds, locking doors, or eating meals (Cook & Polgar, 2008). Assistive domotics help older adults with disability remain at home more safely and comfortably.

Although advances in technology can help older adults function more independently, more sophisticated devices can be cost prohibitive. A primary consideration therefore is to design modifications that are least costly and affordable to the individual. In the United States, residents pay for approximately 80% of all home modifications, repairs, and renovations (Fagan, 2007). Various programs and services pay for the remaining 20%. This financial responsibility presents a barrier to modifications for many who would otherwise benefit. OTs can often recommend programs and services in the community that supply assistive equipment at little or no cost. Senior centers or the local American Cancer Society often will loan portable equipment such as canes, walkers, electric beds, commodes, and wheelchairs. When extensive home modification is needed to create a safe home environment, moving to a residential setting such as assisted living that is designed with the safety needs of older adults in mind may be a more feasible alternative.

Work Modifications

Our aging demographics have led to changes in retirement benefits such that older adults are working longer than ever before. More than half of older adults between ages 65 and 69 work outside the home. At age 70, nearly 40% continue to work, and one in five older adults is working at age 80 (U.S. Census Bureau, 2010). Regardless of age, occupation, or disability, almost all employees can benefit from assistive technology and devices in the workplace. Assistive technology can help prevent work-related disabilities as well as enable persons with disability to continue meeting job performance requirements.

Ergonomics is the science of coordinating the design of devices, systems, and physical working conditions with the capacities and requirements of the worker. Put simply, "ergonomics reduces the risk of injury by adapting the work to fit the person instead of forcing the person to adapt to the work" (University of Texas at San Antonio, n.d.). Older adults with chronic disease are more vulnerable to workplace injury. Work-related musculoskeletal disorders are the single largest class of worker's compensation claims, followed by carpal tunnel syndrome affecting the hands (U.S. Department of Labor, 2009). Twenty-two percent of workplace injuries, most commonly to the back or shoulders, are due to overexertion, especially while lifting. Two key factors that contribute to disability in the workplace include failure to use good body mechanics and poor posture (see Box 11-1). Other factors that contribute to musculoskeletal, nerve, or other injury include prolonged standing or sitting, bending at the waist, wrist flexion or extension, elbow extension without support, and turning or holding the head to one side. Motions that compress a body part against a surface, are repetitive without rest or variation, or require frequent reaching, working overhead, or lifting heavy objects all put workers at risk for injury (Centers for Disease Control and Prevention, n.d.). Office space may need to be modified to accommodate the disabilities (Table 11-4). Filing systems and office supplies should be within reach. The fit of chairs and desks can be individualized to promote good posture. Many employers consult specialists in occupational therapy, seating technology, and engineering regarding workplace redesign to minimize worker's compensation issues and loss of work days (Troy, Cooper, Robertson, & Grey, 1997). In addition, the Americans with Disabilities Act (ADA) of 1990 guarantees the right

TABLE 11-4 Workspace Problems and Possible Solutions

WORKSPACE AREA	POSSIBLE PROBLEM	POSSIBLE SOLUTIONS
Computer monitor	Eye strain Neck and shoulder pain	■ Clean computer screen. ■ Adjust screen brightness. ■ Place monitor directly in front of user at eye level. ■ Avoid twisting neck to see screen. ■ Place monitor within arms' length of user. ■ Tilt monitor back 10 to 20 degrees. ■ Place monitor in area with minimal glare.
Chair adjustment	Back pain Increased pressure on intervertebral discs Pooling of blood in feet and legs	■ Avoid staying in same position for extended length of time. ■ Shift weight periodically. ■ Alternate between standing and sitting. ■ Adjust chair height so feet rest on the floor or a footrest. ■ Adjust chair so knees are level with or slightly lower than hips. ■ Adjust armrests so elbows are bent at 90-degree angle and resting at user's sides. ■ Adjust chair height so wrists are in neutral position and resting on a rounded tabletop edge. ■ Adjust armrest heights so elbows rest lightly on armrests to avoid nerve injuries. ■ Use a chair of appropriate dimensions, usually 18 inches wide by 15 by 17 inches deep. ■ Make sure chair has a soft edge behind the knees. ■ Keep 2 to 3 inches between the seat edge and backs of knees. ■ Make sure chair provides low- and middle-back support. ■ If needed, use towel or lumbar pad to support lumbar curvature.
Desktop surface	Nerve injuries (such as carpal tunnel syndrome) Wrist, forearm, and hand injuries	■ Adjust desk to elbow height so elbows can rest lightly on desktop. ■ Clear area beneath desk to allow leg stretching and movement. ■ Place frequently used objects within arms' reach to prevent reaching, bending, or twisting. ■ Adjust desk height so keyboard is 1 to 2 inches above thighs.

TABLE 11-4 Workspace Problems and Possible Solutions—cont'd

WORKSPACE AREA	POSSIBLE PROBLEM	POSSIBLE SOLUTIONS
		■ Adjust keyboard distance so within arms' reach of user. ■ Adjust height of keyboard so shoulders are relaxed. ■ Adjust height of keyboard so arms are parallel to floor. ■ Avoid placing hands on mouse when not in use. ■ Avoid excessive flexion or extension of wrists, and try to maintain a neutral position. ■ Place mouse next to and at same height as keyboard.
Lighting	Eye strain Double vision Dry eyes Eye fatigue	■ Position computer away from lighting to avoid glare. ■ Close window treatments to avoid glare. ■ Use a no-glare screen. ■ Paint walls medium or dark color to avoid glare. ■ Do not paint walls with a reflective finish. ■ Reduce overhead lighting. ■ Use indirect lighting.

of persons with disabilities to equal opportunity of employment in any business with 15 or more employees and also requires that employers make reasonable accommodations such as acquiring or modifying equipment or devices (U.S. Department of Justice, 2005; U.S. Equal Employment Opportunity Commission, 2009).

Driver Rehabilitation

The ability to drive is embedded in American culture. It connotes freedom to go where we want when we want. Thus, losing driving privileges is considered by many older adults to be a major loss that transforms their lives and marks the beginning of dependency and isolation. As of 2008, nearly one third of licensed drivers were over age 65 (U.S. Department of Transportation, 2010). This proportion is expected to increase as the Baby Boomer population ages because, in 2008, 40% of licensed drivers were ages 45 to 54.

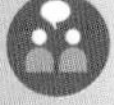

PERSONAL PERSPECTIVE
Independence Lost

"I can't do what I'd like to do. I can't walk. Well, it's difficult to walk. It's difficult to get around," says Ed, age 95. He continues, "I have that chair. It's an automatic chair, and that takes me a lot of places, and I've got a walker besides that. But it's tough . . ." Ed is dealing with what he says has been the most significant loss associated with his aging—the inability to walk on his own. "I'm not independent," he says. "I depend on my chair or my walker to get around. I can't get up and dance. We have music here. Some people are dancing. I'd love to do that, but I hesitate because I'm afraid I'll fall flat on my face. I guess that's what I miss more than anything. But I manage, somehow."

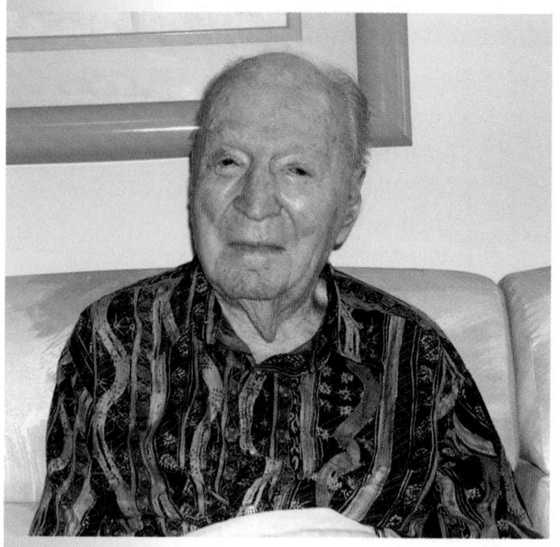

Ed is fortunate. He doesn't have to manage alone. He lives in a lovely assisted-living apartment with his wife of 68 years. Gertrude is 93. "My wife takes pretty good care of me," Ed says, "and if I've got any problems, I've got this thing around my neck that I can use in case of emergency. It gives Gertrude a little more independence, too. She hesitates to go away and leave me alone. I like to see her go [play cards] because she's tied up here with me all the other time and this gives her a little recreation, too."

Independence is precious to Ed, as illustrated by his story about the loss of his driver's license. "Just recently," he says, "my license expired . . . I sent in my application with a check for fifteen dollars and for a long time I never heard from them. Finally, after maybe three or four or five months, I don't know, quite a long time, they sent me back my check along with the examination I had for my eyes. They said it wasn't sufficient. So I went to my ophthalmologist and he filled out another form, and we sent it in with another check for fifteen dollars, and I still haven't heard from them. And I always say I'm going to call them up and ask them why they haven't at least let me know why they haven't returned my check, or at least told me why they don't give me a license. Though I wouldn't drive anyway, probably, at this point. Because my reflexes aren't like they used to be, and I wouldn't want to hurt anybody."

Despite his recognition that he can no longer drive safely, Ed very much wants that license in his wallet. Why? "Just to give me some independence," he says. "I'd like to be able to drive if I wanted to. I probably would get a car but Gert says, 'Why buy a car? You don't want to drive it anyway.' So I haven't bought a car. But it's tough without one, because we've always had one. Just to go to a store and back. Little things."

About Ed Edward Lerman's 40-year career as a dentist included service during World War II. A Major in the U.S. Army, Ed traveled to bases across the United States tending to the dental needs of our service men and women. After the war, Ed's private practice grew, though it was not his sole interest in life. Encouraged by his wife Gertrude, he took blocks of time off every year so that they could travel the world. His dentistry skills carried him to Israel where, for 2 months each year for 6 years, he served as a volunteer dentist on a kibbutz. Ed is a family man with an abundance of love for his two children. Today, only his daughter survives, and although she lives at a distance, they remain close. Ed also receives great joy from his grandchildren and great grandchildren. Some years ago, Ed was an avid golfer. Today, he enjoys watching a good television show.

Lorri Danzig, MS, CSL

> *Losing driving privileges is considered by many older adults to be a major loss that transforms their lives and marks the beginning of dependency and isolation.*

Facilitating conversations about driver safety among older adults, families, and caregivers is an important role of the nurse. Nurses can help patients identify community resources and refer to other health professionals who are skilled in evaluating their needs (Ekelman et al., 2009). When questions about whether changes in hearing, vision, mental processing, or physical capacity are affecting an older adult's driving performance, referral to a driver rehabilitation program can help determine a person's ability to drive safely. Driver specialists perform a battery of assessments including a comprehensive clinical assessment of sensory and functional impairment, a driving history, and an "on-road" evaluation of the individual's judgment and reaction time (Justice Institute of British Columbia, 2007; Kartje, 2006). The driving history should be obtained from someone who has driven with the older adult or observed his or her driving. Information gathered regarding the older adult's driving history should include frequency, length, and duration of trips; location of trips; types of roadways used; whether the individual drives at night, during rush hour, or in adverse conditions; whether he or she uses a navigator or has caregivers who can drive; familiarity with roadways; caregiver's perception of the older adult's driving skill; whether the individual transports passengers; any near misses, crashes, or tickets; and whether the individual has gotten lost while driving (Carr, 2000). Conditions such as cognitive or sensory loss, dementia, alcoholism, cardiopulmonary disease, arthritis, sleep apnea, and other diseases can all affect a person's driving ability. Further information may be obtained from the Hartford Insurance Web site (http://hartfordauto.thehartford.com/Safe-Driving/Car-Safety/Older-Driver-Safety/warning-signs.shtml), as well as the AAA seniors Web site (http://www.aaaseniors.com/howtohelp/threekeys/understand).

Training with adaptive devices can improve driver safety for some people. Safety includes the driver and passengers, as well as others on the road. OTs trained in driver rehabilitation can play an important role in evaluating limitations and training older adults to use adaptive devices to improve their driving performance (AOTA, 2004). Adaptations can be made to the car itself so that older adults with low vision can more easily read information on a dashboard modified with larger characters or a brighter display (Imbeau, Wierwille, Wolf, & Chun, 1989). To reduce glare, a small windshield rake angle and low dashboard reflectance can provide a clearer image of the road (Schumann, Flannagan, Sivak, & Traube, 1997).

Modifications for older adults with arthritis may include a built-up steering wheel, as well as larger knobs for dials and buttons. Cars designed with controls on the steering wheel eliminate the need to reach and help keep eyes focused on the road. For an older adult with poor depth perception, adapted cruise control can be installed. This cruise control adjusts to the speed and distance of the car ahead. Another option is to install a collision avoidance system. These systems use sensors to monitor the car's surroundings and sound an alarm to prevent a collision.

Navigation systems and their placement can minimize getting lost. Placement of these devices should not block the driver's view or require him or her to look away from the road. A study in which older adults used "heads-up displays" while driving resulted in more correct turns and shorter response times (Mollenhauer, Dingus, & Hulse, 1995; Steinfeld & Green, 1995). Dingus and colleagues (1997) reported that navigation systems giving turn-by-turn instructions as route guidance are better than those giving full route information at once. According to this same study, redundancy of auditory and visual information also resulted in better performance in older adult driving (Dingus et al., 1997). Highly technological modifications such as these can be expensive, however, so cost must be considered when determining appropriate solutions.

In addition to teaching drivers how to use adaptive devices, driver training teaches participants how to avoid high-risk situations. These situations include driving on high-speed roadways and driving at night or in poorly lit areas. Well-lit intersections have been found to significantly reduce vehicle crashes (Staplin, Lococo, Byington, & Harkey, 2001). Some driver rehabilitation programs such as the driver safety program offered by the American Association of Retired Persons (AARP) are tailored to common driving challenges experienced by older adults. One example of a strategy taught to address reduced response time is to keep sufficient distance when stopping behind another vehicle so that the driver can see the rear wheels of the car in front of him or her. Other general recommendations can be found in Box 11-2.

Environmental modifications could also improve driver safety. Older adults are at greater risk for driving fatalities than any other age group. Deaths from motor vehicle accidents increase markedly between ages 70 and 74 and continue to rise as we age (Insurance Institute for Highway Safety, 2008). Nurses play an important role in advocating for change to improve road safety, as well as to promote more accessible public transportation options. In a study conducted by Chrysler, Carlson, and Hawkins (2002), older adults were tested to see how well and at what distance they could read different colored

BOX 11-2 Driving Tips for Older Adults

- Exercise regularly to increase strength and flexibility.
- Ask your doctor or pharmacist to review medicines—both prescription and over-the counter—to reduce side effects and interactions.
- Have eyes checked by an eye doctor at least once a year. Wear glasses and corrective lenses as required.
- Drive during daylight and in good weather. Find the safest route with well-lit streets, intersections with left turn arrows, and easy parking. Plan your route before you drive.
- Leave a large following distance behind the car in front of you.
- Avoid distractions in your car, such as listening to a loud radio, talking on your cell phone, texting, and eating in the car.
- Think about potential alternatives to driving, such as riding with a friend or using public transit, that you can use to get around.

From Centers for Disease Control and Prevention (n.d.). Older adult drivers: Fact sheet. Retrieved from http://www.cdc.gov/MotorVehicleSafety/Older_Adult_Drivers/adult-drivers_factsheet.html

signs while driving at night. Participants had difficulty reading orange-colored signs such as those used in construction zones. Larger signs placed overhead and those treated with retroreflective sheeting have also been shown to increase visibility among older adult drivers (Staplin, Lococo, Byington, & Harkey, 2001). Redundant signs, signs placed well in advance, and large lettering with high contrast are signage modifications that could improve visibility for all drivers. Traffic signals with a large, black background behind the signal provide contrast, which helps drivers see the signal color and also reduces daytime glare. A longer yellow light increases stopping time for drivers with slower response times (Staplin, Lococo, Byington, & Harkey, 2001).

Roadway design can also impact driving safety. Lane markings that are in poor condition are especially difficult for low-vision drivers to see and increase the risk that they will encroach into other lanes and fail to follow turn pathways (Florida Department of Transportation, 2002). Sharp angles greater than 90 degrees are difficult for drivers with reduced peripheral vision or neck immobility to navigate safely. Retroreflective markings on medians can increase visibility of intersections or where a lane is divided (Staplin, Lococo, Byington, & Harkey, 2001). Rumble strips installed before stops help warn the driver to begin braking. Much could be done to address these safety concerns.

Rosenbloom (2003) proposed that to fully address driving safety among older adults, improving roadway conditions is insufficient. He argues that age-appropriate driver rehabilitation courses must be developed and implemented. Self-tests that allow older drivers to examine their own competence in a noncoercive manner may encourage older adults to voluntarily seek out training programs. Driver rehabilitation programs should also work with communities to identify ways to expand the community's transportation services. Lack of adequate public transportation contributes to keeping older adults driving even when they themselves believe they are no longer safe (Rosenbloom, 2003). Comprehensive community planning is needed to design better alternatives to independent transportation that are accessible to all. OTs can provide valuable insight when planning for the needs of an aging community (AOTA, 2006).

The older adult population is on the rise with an increasing demand for services that can sustain optimal independence and quality of life. Driving is merely one area that needs to be addressed with this population; however, it is an important need. Because the American culture places such an emphasis on driving as an indicator of independence, older adults will not hand over their licenses easily. Nurses must work with other health providers to ensure that older drivers are capable of and safe in operating motor vehicles. Facilitating conversations about driver safety among older adults, families, and caregivers is an important role of the nurse. Nurses can help patients identify community resources and refer to other health professionals who are skilled in evaluating their needs.

Conclusion

Assistive technology can have a positive impact on many aspects of a person's life: in the home, workplace, and community. Adaptive equipment can optimize functioning and make it possible for older adults to retain independence and improve their quality of living. OTs are an important part of the health care team in identifying appropriate technology and environmental modifications that are consistent with an older adult's limitations. A collaborative approach among health care providers will yield the best possible solution to each patient's needs.

KEY POINTS

- The ability to perform ADLs and IADLs is important in promoting health, wellness, and quality of life, as well as in serving as an important tool in promoting self-identity in older adults.
- Aging can interfere with performance of ADLs due to various health issues.
- OTs can use assistive technology to make tasks easier for older adults and promote independence.
- Multiple changes in vision occur due to the natural aging process and can be made easier through the use of assistive technology and environmental modifications.
- Physical impairments such as vestibular changes, decreased muscle mass, and loss of dexterity and coordination can limit older adults in many aspects of their daily functioning; however, there are many devices that can be used to help persons with physical impairments.
- Assistive technology can benefit persons with cognitive impairments by aiding with issues such as memory, orientation, initiation, sequencing, and judgment.
- OTs are skilled in assessing home and work environments and promoting effective performance of ADLS and IADLs with the use of assistive technology to prevent injury.
- Driver rehabilitation is an important aspect in promoting the independence of older adults.
- Many adaptations can be made to the vehicle as well as to the community to ensure safety on the road for the older adult.
- Nurses play an important role in collaborating with other health team members to advocate for personal and environmental modifications that optimize the safety and well-being of older adults in the home, workplace, and community.

CRITICAL THINKING ACTIVITIES

1. If cost is an issue making accessibility of dressing aids to your patient difficult, can some of these aids be homemade? How?
2. Go to a local drug or multipurpose store in your area. What assistive devices can you find that could be used to simplify activities of daily living?
3. Use one of the home safety checklists available from the North Carolina Area Agency on Aging Web site (http://www.fullcirclecare.org/caregiverissues/general/safety.html#check) to evaluate potential safety hazards in your own home or that of an aging parent or relative.

CASE STUDY | *CASEY*

Casey is a 61-year-old man with rheumatoid arthritis (RA). RA is a chronic, inflammatory, systemic disease that manifests in the joints. Symptoms of RA that can affect driving are limited range of motion, decreased muscle strength, and stiffness. His wife passed away 5 years ago and he does not have any children who live in the area. Casey is currently living alone with his beloved 8-year-old dog but is having increasing difficulty dressing, getting in and out of a chair or bed, and preparing meals. Casey is still able to drive and wants to live in his home long as possible. Casey's children are concerned about whether he is safe to remain living alone. His general physician expresses concern about Casey's symptoms and their affect on his ability to operate a vehicle.

1. What factors would you assess in determining whether Casey can continue to live safely at home?
2. What modifications could be made to the home environment to help Casey remain in his home?
3. How might the use of adaptive equipment be beneficial for Casey?
4. You decide to request a referral to Occupational Safety to assess Casey's driving ability. What adaptations might an OT make to the vehicle to ensure Casey's independence with driving?

REFERENCES

American Association of Retired Persons. (2010). *Why do you need universal design*? Retrieved from http://www.aarp.org/home-garden/housing/info-04-2010/why-do-you-need-universal-design.html, **April, 6, 2011**.

American Occupational Therapy Association. (2004). *Tips for living: Keeping older drivers safe.* Retrieved from http://www.aota.org/Consumers/consumers/Adults/OlderDrivers/35123.aspx?FT=.pdf, **April 6, 2011**.

American Occupational Therapy Association. (2006). *Modify your home for independence.* Retrieved from http://www.aota.org/Consumers/consumers/Adults/HomeMods.aspx, April 6, 2011

American Occupational Therapy Association. (2008). *Maintaining quality of life with low vision.* Retrieved from http://www.promoteot.org/AI_LowVision.html

Anemaet, W. K., & Moffa-Trotter, M. E. (1999). Promoting safety and function through home assessments. *Topics in Geriatric Rehabilitation, 15,* 26–55.

Assistive Technology Act of 1998, as amended (2004). PL 108-364, § 3, 118 stat 1707.

Bonder, B. R., & Dal Bello-Haas, V. (2009). *Functional performance in older adults* (3rd ed.). Philadelphia, PA: Davis.

Bonder, B. R., & Goodman, G. (1995). Preventing occupational dysfunction secondary to aging. In C. A. Trombly (Ed.), *Occupational therapy for physical dysfunction* (pp. 391–404). Baltimore, MD: Williams & Wilkins.

Carr, D. B. (2000). The older adult driver. *The Washington manual: Geriatrics subspecialty consult* (pp. 59–65). St. Louis, MO: Lippincott, Williams & Wilkins.

Centers for Disease Control and Prevention. (1997). *Elements of Ergonomics –A primer based on workplace evaluations of musculoskeletal disorders.* Retrieved from http://www.cdc.gov/niosh/docs/97-117/ , April 6, 2011.

Chrysler, S. T., Carlson, P. J., & Hawkins, H. G. (2002). *Nighttime legibility of ground-mounted traffic signs as a function of font, color, and retroreflective sheeting type* (FHWA Report #FHWA/TX-03/1796-2). College Station: Texas Transportation Institute.

Center for universal design: Environments and products for all people . (2008). Retrieved from http://www.design.ncsu.edu/cud/about_ud/udprincipleshtmlformat.html#top, April 6, 2011.

Cook, A. M., & Polgar, J. M. (2008). *Cook & Hussey's assistive technologies: Principles and practice* (3rd ed.). St. Louis, MO: Mosby.

Dingus, T. A., McGhee, D. V., Manakkal, N., Carney, C., & Hankey, J. M. (1997). Human factors field evaluations of automotive headway maintenance/collision warning devices. *Human Factors, 39,* 216–229.

Ekelman, B. A., Stav, W. B., Baker, P., O'Dell-Rossi, P., & Mitchell, S. (2009). Community Mobility. In B. R. Bonder & V. Dal Bello-Haas (Eds.), *Functional performance in older adults* (3rd ed., pp. 332-385). Philadelphia, PA: Davis.

Fagan, L. A. (2007). Funding sources for home modifications. *Home and Community Health Special Interest Section Quarterly, 14*(3), 1–3.

Federal Interagency Forum on Aging Related Statistics. (2008). *Older Americans 2008: Key indicators of well-being.* Retrieved from http://www.aoa.gov/agingstatsdotnet/Main_Site/Data/Data_2008.aspx , April 6, 2011

Florida Department of Transportation. (2002). *Elder roadway user program test sections and effectiveness study* (Project 669535, contract # BB-901). Miami, FL: Guerrier & Fu.

Imbeau, D., Wierwille, W. W., Wolf, L. D., & Chun, G. A. (1989). Effects of instrument panel luminance and chromaticity on reading performance and preference in simulated driving. *Human Factors, 31,* 147–160.

Insurance Institute for Highway Safety (IIHS). (2008). *Fatality facts, Older people.* Arlington (VA): IIHS. Retrieved from http://www.iihs.org/research/fatality_facts_2008/olderpeople.html, April 6, 2011

Justice Institute of British Columbia. (2007). *On road driving assessment of older adults: A review of the literature.* British Columbia, Canada: Kowalski & Tuokko.

Kalish, T. (2009, June 28). *Occupational therapy in low vision rehabilitation presented in Interventions II.* Rush University, Chicago, IL.

Kartje, P. (2006). Approaching, evaluating, and counseling the older driver for successful community mobility. *OT Practice,* 11 (19) 13–17.< Lighthouse International. (2009). *All about low vision.* Retrieved from http://www.lighthouse.org/medical/low-vision-defined/, April 6, 2011

Lueck, A. H. (2004). *Functional vision: A practitioner's guide to evaluation and intervention.* San Francisco, CA: AFB Press.

McCullagh, M. C. (2006). Home modifications. *American Journal of Nursing, 106,* 54–63.

Mollenhauer, M. A., Dingus, T. A., & Hulse, M. C. (1995). *The potential for advanced vehicle systems to increase the mobility of elderly drivers.* Iowa City: University of Iowa.

National Eye Institute. (2008). *Prevalence of blindness data tables [NEI Statistics and Data].* Retrieved from http://www.nei.nih.gov/eyedata/pbd_tables.asp

Pendleton, H. M., & Schultz-Krohn, W. (2006). *Pedretti's occupational therapy practice skills for physical dysfunction* (6th ed.). St. Louis, MO: Mosby.

Petersson, I., Lilja, M., Hammel, J., & Kottorp, A. (2008). Impact of home modification services on ability in everyday life for people ageing with disabilities. *Journal of Rehabilitation, 40,* 253–260.

Rosenbloom, S. (2003). Older drivers: Should we test them off the road? *Access, 23,* 8–13.

Sabata, D. B., Shamberg, S., & Williams, M. (2008). Optimizing access to home, community, and work environments. In M. Radomski & C. Latham Trombly (Eds.), *Occupational therapy for physical dysfunction* (6th ed., pp. 951–973). Baltimore, MD: Lippincott Williams & Wilkins.

Schumann, J., Flannagan, M. J., Sivak, M., & Traube, E.C. (1997). Daytime veiling glare and driver visual performance: Influence of windshield rake angle and dashboard reflectance. *Journal of Safety Research, 28,* 133–146.

Staplin, L., Lococo, K., Byington, S., & Harkey, D. (2001). *Highway design handbook for older drivers and pedestrians* (Publication No. FHWA-RD-01-103). Washington, DC: U.S. Department of Transportation, Federal Highway Administration.

State of Oklahoma. (2009). *Assistive technology for older adults.* Retrieved from http://www.ok.gov/abletech/Publications/Assistive_Technology_for_Older_Adults.html

Steinfeld, A., & Green, P. (1995). *Driver response times to full-windshield heads-up displays for navigation and vision enhancement* (Technical Report UMTRI-95-29). Ann Arbor: University of Michigan Transportation Research Institute.

Troy, B., Cooper, R., Robertson, R., & Grey, T. (1997). An analysis of work postures of manual wheelchair users in the office environment. *Journal of Rehabilitation Research & Development, 34,* 151–161.

University of Texas at San Antonio. (n.d.). *Environmental health, safety & risk management: Successful solutions start with safety.* Retrieved from http://www.utsa.edu/Safety/?section=workplace&page=ergonomics

U.S. Census Bureau. (2004). *U.S. interim projections by age, sex, race, and Hispanic origin.* Retrieved from http://www.census.gov/ipc/www/usinterimproj/

U.S. Census Bureau. (2010). *Current population survey, annual social and economic supplement.* Retrieved from http://www.census.gov/cps/, April 6, 2011. U.S. Department of Justice, Civil Rights Division, Disability Rights Section. (2005). *A guide to disability rights laws.* Retrieved from http://www.ada.gov/cguide.htm, April 6, 2011

U.S. Department of Labor, Bureau of Labor Statistics. (2009). *Nonfatal occupational injuries and illnesses requiring days away from work.* Retrieved from http://www.bls.gov/news.release/osh2.nr0.htm , April 6, 2011

U.S. Department of Transportation, Federal Highway Administration, Office of Highway Policy Information, Highway Statistics. (2010). *Our nation's highways: 2010.* Retrieved from http://www.fhwa.dot.gov/policyinformation/pubs/pl10023/fig4_3.cfm, **April 6, 2011**

U.S. Equal Employment Opportunity Commission. (2009) *Disability discrimination.* Retrieved from http://www.eeoc.gov/laws/types/disability.cfm April 6, 2011

The author gratefully acknowledges the Rush Occupational Therapy graduate class of 2010 for their assistance in writing this chapter and Alexandria L. Janezic for editorial support.

Chapter 12

Optimizing Rest and Sleep Patterns

Jean Lange, PhD, RN, FAAN

LEARNING OBJECTIVES

- Discuss the incidence of sleep disorders among older adults.
- Describe factors that place older adults at risk for sleep disorders.
- List criteria for assessing the presence of a sleep disorder.
- State the potential adverse consequences of sleep disorders.
- Plan care that minimizes the risk for sleep disruption in older adults.

Incidence

Most adults (67%) believe that sleep is as important to their health and well-being as diet and exercise (National Sleep Foundation, 2009). On average, we need about 8 hours of sleep (American Academy of Family Physicians, 2005). However, a survey of older adults living at home found that less than half actually get this much rest (National Sleep Foundation, 2003). What's more, one third of older adults living at home have chronic sleep disorders (Ross, 2009). Older people living in residential settings have even more difficulty sleeping. By some estimates, more than half of older adults in assisted living or long-term care facilities report being sleep deprived (Chaperon, Farr, & LoChiano, 2007; St. George, Delbaere, Williams, & Lord, 2009). The National Sleep Foundation (2003) reports that nearly two thirds of older adults report having some of the symptoms associated with sleep disorders, with a higher incidence among older women (Ancoli-Israel & Ayalon, 2006).

Nearly two thirds of older adults report some of the symptoms of sleep disorders.

Sleep and Aging

Given the prevalence of symptoms reported by older adults, you may wonder whether sleep problems are just a normal part of aging. Sleep patterns do change as we age; for example, older people tend to go to sleep earlier in the evening and wake up earlier in the morning. This is due to alterations in our circadian rhythms (Paredes et al., 2009). The anterior hypothalamus controls circadian rhythms, which regulate hormone secretion, core body temperature, and sleep patterns. Aging alters the circadian rhythms of melatonin, serotonin, thermoregulatory responses, and sleep-wake cycles (Parades et al., 2009). The sleep-wake cycle responds to changes in core body temperature and the release of melatonin and serotonin, as well as external light through our retinal sensors. As we age, levels of melatonin and serotonin are lower and we become more sensitive to light so that we awaken more easily. Core body temperature also tends to drop earlier in the evening, causing older adults to fall asleep earlier and awaken sooner.

Sleep occurs in several stages of lighter (known as rapid eye movement) and deeper, more restful sleep. Time spent in the deepest and lightest stages of sleep changes somewhat starting in middle adulthood but stabilizes in most people by age 60. Hours of productive sleep (actual time spent asleep versus being in bed but awake) do decrease for many adults as they age (Ancoli-Israel & Ayalon, 2006). Despite this change, however, 75% of older adults say that their sleep quality remains good to excellent (National Sleep Foundation, 2003).

For many older adults, sleep actually becomes more consistent after they are no longer working. Whereas working adults tend to "catch up" on weekends after getting less sleep on working days, hours of sleep for older adults over age 55 tend to be more stable (Fig. 12-1). Research suggests that genetics may play a role in our sleep patterns. In

Percentage of Day That People Age 55 and Older Spent Doing Selected Activities on an Average Day, by Age Group, 2006

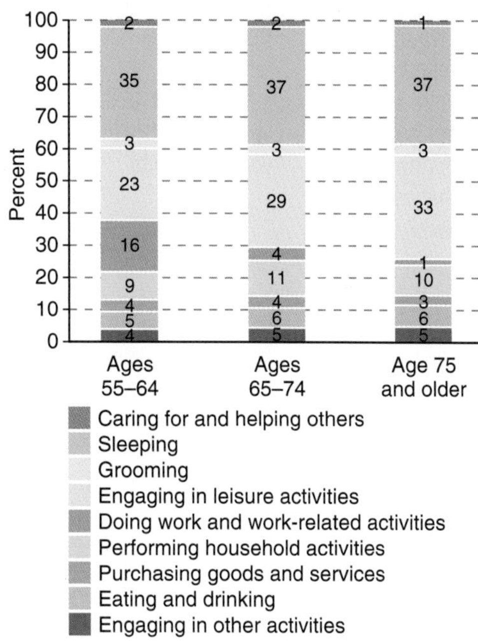

Note: "Other activities" includes activities such as educational activities; organizational, civic, and religious activities; and telephone calls. Chart includes people who did not work at all.
Reference population: These data refer to the civilian noninstitutionalized population.
Source: Bureau of Labor Statistics, American Time Use Survey.

Figure 12-1 *(From Federal Interagency Forum on Aging-Related Statistics. (2010). Older Americans 2010: Key indicators of well-being. Washington, DC: U.S. Government Printing Office.)*

summary, sleep patterns do change in most people as they age; however, insomnia (difficulty falling or staying asleep) is not a normal consequence of aging (Cole & Richards, 2007).

Older adults who report sleep problems typically do so because of a change in their ability to sleep rather than the actual number of hours slept. Common complaints include trouble falling asleep, frequent nocturnal awakening or waking too early and being unable to fall asleep again, snoring or breathing pauses (also symptoms of apnea), a tingling feeling or repeated jerking movements in the legs (also a symptom of restless leg syndrome), and feeling unrested upon awakening (National Sleep Foundation, 2003). A summary of common sleep disorders appears in Table 12-1. Imagine how you would feel about your ability to perform on an exam after waking up several times the night before, or being unable to fall asleep until 3 a.m. because you were worrying about feeling underprepared.

When nighttime sleep is inadequate, people sometimes compensate by napping during the day. Boredom can also contribute to daytime napping. However, significant sleeping during the day can contribute to poor sleep quality at night (St. George et al., 2009). You may have noticed that some older adults seem to take several naps during the day, even falling asleep in a chair, and wonder if this is true of most older people. Research shows that although the percentage of older adults who nap does increase slightly with age, it is by no means the norm. In fact, only about one-quarter of those ages 74 to 85 nap during the day. Napping incidence does tend to be higher among older adults living in residential care settings. Those with vision and hearing losses are also more likely to nap. In fact, older adults who are hearing impaired nap twice as much (Asplund, 2005). Nearly half of men and 35% of women experience some hearing loss by age 65 (Fig. 12-2). Helping older adults stay engaged can help reduce the boredom of inactivity and provide sources of stimulation that may improve their mental well-being, as well as their sleep quality (National Sleep Foundation, 2003; St. George et al., 2009).

TABLE 12-1 Sleep Impairment Syndromes

SYNDROME	SYMPTOMS	AT-RISK INDIVIDUALS	CONSIDERATIONS	TREATMENT
Periodic limb movements in sleep (PLMS)	Five or more repeated leg jerks or kicks per hour during sleep that cause awakening	PLMS in older adults is estimated at 45%, versus 5%–6% in younger adults	Patients may not be aware of their leg jerks. Bed partners are often able to better describe symptoms that some patients experience in the daytime	Dopamine agonists (e.g., ropinirole, pergolide, pramipexole)
Restless legs syndrome (RLS)	Uncomfortable sensations including tingling, prickling, or crawling feelings in the legs that diminish with movement	RLS increases significantly with age, with women affected twice as often as men	Assess for anemia, uremia, and peripheral neuropathy	Dopamine agonists (e.g., ropinirole, pergolide, pramipexole)
Rapid eye movement behavior disorder	Vigorous or violent motor movement during light sleep (rapid eye movement stage) of which patients are often unaware	More common among older men	May be associated with Parkinson's disease, dementia, tricyclic antidepressants, fluoxetine, monoamine oxidase inhibitors, or withdrawal from alcohol or sedatives	Clonazepam
Sleep-disordered breathing (SDB)	Loud snoring or incomplete or absent respirations during sleep causing awakening, hypoxia, and daytime sleepiness	Incidence averages 10% in middle-aged adults versus 20% in adults over age 60	Snoring may interfere with being able to sleep with a partner. SDB increases risk of hypertension and cardiac and pulmonary diseases	Positive airway pressure devices or surgery in extreme cases

Adapted from Ancoli-Israel, S., & Ayalon, L. (2006). Diagnosis and treatment of sleep disorders in older adults. *The American Journal of Geriatric Psychiatry, 14*(2), 95–103.

Consequences of Sleep Disturbance

Sleep deprivation can have a major impact on how people feel about their ability to function and their attitude about life. Poor sleep can have both physical and cognitive effects, including fatigue, difficulty focusing, slower response times, memory problems, decreased balance, decreased ability to perform tasks, and increased daytime sleepiness (Ancoli-Israel, 2005; Blackwell et al., 2006; Smyth, 2008; Yaggi, Araujo, & McKinlay, 2006). Excessive daytime sleepiness may even cause a person to fall asleep

Percentage of People Age 65 and Older Who Reported Having Any Trouble Hearing, Any Trouble Seeing, or No Natural Teeth, by Sex, 2006

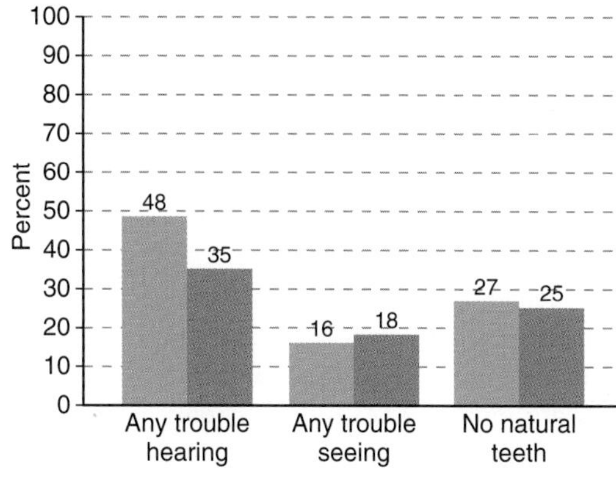

Men
Women

Note: Respondents were asked, "Which statement best describes your hearing without a hearing aid: good, a little trouble, a lot of trouble, deaf?" For the purposes of this indicator, the category "Any trouble hearing" includes "a little trouble, a lot of trouble, and deaf." Regarding their vision, respondents were asked, "Do you have any trouble seeing, even when wearing glasses or contact lenses?" The category "Any trouble seeing" also includes those who in a subsequent question report themselves as blind. Lastly, respondents were asked, in one question, "Have you lost all of your upper and lower natural (permanent) teeth?"
Reference population: These data refer to the civilian noninstitutionalized population.
Source: Centers for Disease Control and Prevention, National Center for Health Statistics, National Health Interview Survey.

Figure 12-2 *(From Federal Interagency Forum on Aging-Related Statistics. (2010). Older Americans 2010: Key indicators of well-being. Washington, DC: U.S. Government Printing Office.)*

while reading, watching television, conversing, or driving. Daytime sleepiness has cognitive, social, and occupational consequences that threaten personal safety, as well as the ability to keep a job or maintain relationships.

Chronic sleep loss also compromises endocrine and immune function, making individuals more prone to infections and poor healing. Studies show that older adults who sleep less than 5 to 6 hours per night are at greater risk for obesity, hypertension, diabetes, depression, and heart disease (Patel et al., 2008; Smyth, 2008). In addition, older adults who are not well rested tend to have more medical problems and report more falls, which put them at risk of injury (Endeshaw, 2009; Hill, Cumming, Lewis, Carrington, & Le Couteu, 2007; National Sleep Foundation, 2003; St. George et al., 2009; Teo, Briffa, Devine, Dhaliwal, & Prince, 2006).

Imagine that you are a home care nurse discussing a medication regimen with a new patient. You learn that the patient takes a diuretic at 9 a.m. and 9 p.m. to control her hypertension. The patient also tells you that she has trouble falling asleep after getting up to go to the bathroom as many as three times each night. How might you help this patient improve her sleep? What safety concerns might you have?

Precipitating Factors

How can nurses identify which patients are at greatest risk for sleep deprivation? Some of the most common factors related to difficulty sleeping include having to get up to go to the bathroom and having unrelieved pain (Endeshaw, 2009; National Sleep Foundation, 2003). Diuretics used to treat hypertension or cardiac disease, urinary tract infections, prostate problems, and high intake of caffeine can cause nocturia. Many chronic medical conditions produce uncomfortable symptoms such as pain, esophageal reflux, or difficulties breathing that are hard to control and can interfere with sleep. As many as 30% to 50%

of patients with chronic arthritis, pulmonary or cardiac disease, prostate disorders, or diabetes experience sleep disorders. Patients recovering from a stroke, cancer, or joint replacement are also at risk for insomnia (Ancoli-Israel & Ayalon, 2006). Psychological factors such as worrying, feeling anxious or depressed, or taking medications to treat other health problems may also precipitate sleep disorders (Boxes 12-1, 12-2, and 12-3) (Ouellet & Morris, 2006; Ross, 2009).

Patients with dementia, especially those living in nursing homes, exhibit a much higher rate of sleep disturbance than older adults in general, and their symptoms are more severe. Although only about 5% of adults over age 65 live in nursing homes, about 17% of adults over age 85 reside in such settings. (See Fig. 5-2 in Chapter 5.) These adults are commonly awake more often and for longer periods, while sleep quality and quantity are decreased. Daytime napping is very common because patients with severe dementia rarely experience a single hour of uninterrupted sleep in a 24-hour period. Family members caring for a patient with dementia at home require support services such as respite care or day care to manage the physical and psychological challenges of caregiving. Behaviors associated with sleep deprivation are often the reason why family members ultimately choose to place their loved one in a residential care setting. The long-term care environment, however, commonly worsens symptoms when lighting, noise, and timing of care at night is not managed effectively. In addition, many institutionalized patients spend most of their waking hours in bed. To better address their needs, many long-term care agencies have created specialty

BOX 12-1 Factors Associated with Sleep Disturbance

- Anxiety
- Caffeine intake
- Coughing
- Daytime napping
- Depression
- Diuretics
- Dyspepsia
- Dyspnea or orthopnea
- Headache
- Hot flashes
- Incontinence
- Neuropathy
- Nocturia
- Pain
- Psychotropic medications
- Stress
- Tinnitus
- Vision or hearing loss

BOX 12-2 Medical Conditions Associated with Insomnia

- Angina
- Apnea
- Arthritis
- Cancer
- Cerebral vascular accident
- Congestive heart failure
- Dementia
- Diabetes
- Fibromyalgia
- Gastroesophageal reflux
- Hypertension
- Hyperthyroidism
- Hypothyroidism
- Inactivity
- Joint disease
- Menopause
- Neuromuscular conditions
- Obesity
- Obstructive pulmonary disease
- Parkinson's disease
- Peripheral vascular disease
- Prostate disease
- Renal disease
- Restless leg syndrome
- Ulcers
- Urinary tract infection

BOX 12-3 Medications That May Interfere with Sleep

- Alpha blockers
- Antidepressants`
- Antidepressants with stimulating effects
- Antihistamines with stimulating effects
- Antiparkinsonian drugs
- Beta blockers
- Bronchodilators
- Calcium channel blockers
- Central nervous system stimulants
- Decongestants
- Diuretics
- Dopamine agonists
- Hormone therapy (e.g., corticosteroids, thyroid hormone replacement)
- Monoamine oxidase inhibitors
- Psychotropics
- Reuptake inhibitors

units for patients with dementia (Ancoli-Israel & Ayalon, 2006).

Changes in older adults' lives can also contribute to problems with sleeping. Perhaps your patient has recently lost the ability to drive and is now homebound, has recently lost a spouse, or is experiencing financial stress from unpaid medical bills. Important life changes and stressors such as these are cues to the nurse to ask questions about how rested the patient feels. In each of these situations, think about which health profession might best help the patient. Identifying patients who may be at risk for sleep disorders can help nurses to make appropriate referrals to health professionals who can help patients and families better manage these situations.

Risk Assessment

Sleep problems are often overlooked by health-care providers. Early recognition of sleep disorders provides an opportunity for intervention that can minimize the impact on patient functioning. Tools are available to help nurses assess whether a sleep disorder may be present.

- The Pittsburgh Sleep Quality Index (PSQI) asks 18 questions about the quality, duration, use of sleep aids, sleep disruptions, and daytime functioning over the last month (Buysse, Reynolds, Monk, Berman, & Kupfer, 1989). The PSQI has been tested with older adults and can be completed in about 10 minutes (Smyth, 2008).
- The Epworth Sleepiness Scale (Johns, 1991) is a screening tool that asks older adults to consider tiredness in eight situations to determine when daytime sleepiness is significant enough to warrant referral.
- The Functional Outcomes of Sleep Questionnaire (Weaver et al., 1997) poses 30 questions that assess the impact of disorders of excessive sleepiness on five domains of everyday living (Smyth, 2008).

These tools are useful to identify adults who should be referred for evaluation and to monitor the effectiveness of treatment. Both the PSQI and Epworth Sleepiness Scale are available through the "Try This" series published by the Hartford Institute for Geriatric Nursing (http://consultgerirn.org/resources). The Functional Outcomes of Sleep Questionnaire is available through the American Thoracic Society at http://qol.thoracic.org/sections/instruments/fj/pages/fosq.html.

Treatment

The most important treatment of sleep disorders is to identify and eliminate underlying causes (Ross, 2009). Because bright light is the most influential external regulator of our circadian rhythm, increasing light exposure during the early hours of darkness may help older adults achieve a more normal sleep cycle. Lowering lights during sleeping hours can help to reduce nighttime waking. Low-intensity night lights can also help to prevent falls in older adults who rise at night to urinate or to orient older adults who may otherwise be confused upon awakening. Modifying environmental factors in assisted-living or long-term care settings (such as decreasing hallway noise, lowering bright lights, or not awakening residents at night for routine care) may help to improve sleep quality of older adult residents. (See the accompanying "Evidence for Practice" box.) Encouraging moderate exercise programs such as yoga has also been shown to improve sleep quality in older adults (Chen et al., 2009; King et al., 2008). Unfortunately only 1 in 5 adults over age 65 exercises regularly, while only 1 in 10 does so by age 85 (Fig. 12-3).

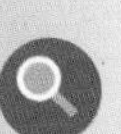

EVIDENCE FOR PRACTICE
Investigating Sleep Disturbance

Purpose: This pilot study compared circadian rhythms (core temperature, rest/activity pattern, melatonin level, sleep percentage, and daytime sleepiness) between adult groups living independently and in long-term care facilities.

Sample: Ten cognitively intact, English-literate older adults living in an apartments or a long-term care facility were recruited from each setting ($n = 20$). Patients taking hypnotic or antipsychotic medications or diagnosed with a sleep disorder or psychosis were excluded. The setting for the study was a midwestern, continuing care retirement community.

Methods: A quasi-experimental, repeated measures design was used to examine differences in rhythmic and sleep variables. Light and rest/activity were measured continuously for 48 hours using an Actilume/Actigraph wristwatch. Temperatures were measured using a secured axillary temperature probe. Melatonin was measured from saliva samples taken every 4 hours while awake, day and night. The Stanford Sleepiness Scale was used to measure sleepiness at each wake interval. Sleep percentage was estimated by actigraphy. Participants recorded when they took medications and ate meals and the types of activities they participated in during the 48-hour period.

Results: Temperature, rest/activity, and melatonin levels were unrelated to age. Long-term care facility residents tended to be older and sleep more, have more daytime sleepiness, and have lower variation between day and night core temperatures than apartment dwellers. Apartment dwellers were more active and had more defined circadian rhythms. Highest melatonin and sleepiness levels of the long-term care facility residents occurred during breakfast. Nighttime light exposure was significantly greater among long-term care facility residents.

Implications: Compared with apartment-dwelling residents, long-term care facility residents lack the necessary changes in core temperature, melatonin levels, and activity to establish consistent sleep-wake cycles. Long-term care facility residents were less active, slept longer, and experienced more nighttime light exposure that could interfere with productive rest. Further investigations are needed to explore whether the higher incidence of daytime sleepiness is related to the decreased activity levels observed among the long-term care facility residents in this sample. The role of environmental variables in long-term care facilities on the sleep patterns of residents needs to be investigated. The results suggest that use of night lighting and lower activity levels may adversely affect the quality of sleep among long-term care facility residents.

Reference: Chaperon, C. M., Farr, L. A., & LoChiano, E. (2007). Sleep disturbance of residents in a continuing care retirement community. *Journal of Gerontological Nursing, 33*(10), 21–28.

People who have a strong social network, feel financially secure, and have an active lifestyle are less likely to report sleep disturbances (National Sleep Foundation, 2003). Nurses must do a comprehensive assessment of patients' economic, social, medical, and psychological state to identify and remediate factors that may contribute to sleep loss. When a medication used to treat illness is suspected to cause insomnia, the nurse should notify the health-care provider. Adjusting the dosage of medications that contribute to sleep problems or trying alternative treatments may be effective.

Sleep disturbances that persist despite attempts to eliminate the underlying cause typically are treated with a combination of medication and behavior therapy. The goal of behavior therapy is to adjust sleep routines to a more normal pattern through education, lifestyle change, and modifications to the patient's environment. Poor sleep habits include spending too much time in bed; having an irregular sleep schedule; getting inadequate bright-light exposure during the day; sleeping in an environment that is too bright, too noisy, or too hot or cold; and drinking alcohol or caffeinated beverages too close to bedtime (Ancoli-Israel & Ayalon, 2006, pp. 98–99). Effective strategies to improve sleep include establishing a regular bedtime schedule, keeping an active daytime lifestyle, and performing relaxation exercises to encourage falling asleep.

Prescribed medications such as benzodiazepine receptor agonists and melatonin receptor agonists are safe for most older adults and can be a useful adjunct to behavior modification therapy. Over-the-counter (OTC) sleep aids include antihistamines and herbal supplements such as valerian root and melatonin (Ross, 2009). It is important in planning effective care to consider what prescribed medications, OTC remedies, and other strategies the patient is currently trying and their effectiveness. Patients taking OTC products or prescribed medications may experience side effects or interactions with other medications they take. This can lead to additional problems such as confusion, changes in bowel and bladder function, arrhythmias, or an increased risk of falling. A more detailed discussion about prescription and OTC medications or herbal supplements used to treat sleep disorders is provided in Chapter 15.

Treatment of sleep disorders in patients with dementia is highly challenging. Establishing a schedule of uninterrupted nighttime sleep is especially important for institutionalized patients. Medications commonly prescribed for these patients, such as sedative-hypnotics and antipsychotics, can worsen the symptoms of dementia and sleep deprivation. Effective strategies to manage these symptoms include limiting bright night lights, minimizing hallway noise during the night, and avoiding waking patients for nighttime treatments. Limiting their

Percentage of People Age 45 and Older Who Reported Engaging in Regular Leisure Time Physical Activity, by Age Group, 1997–2006

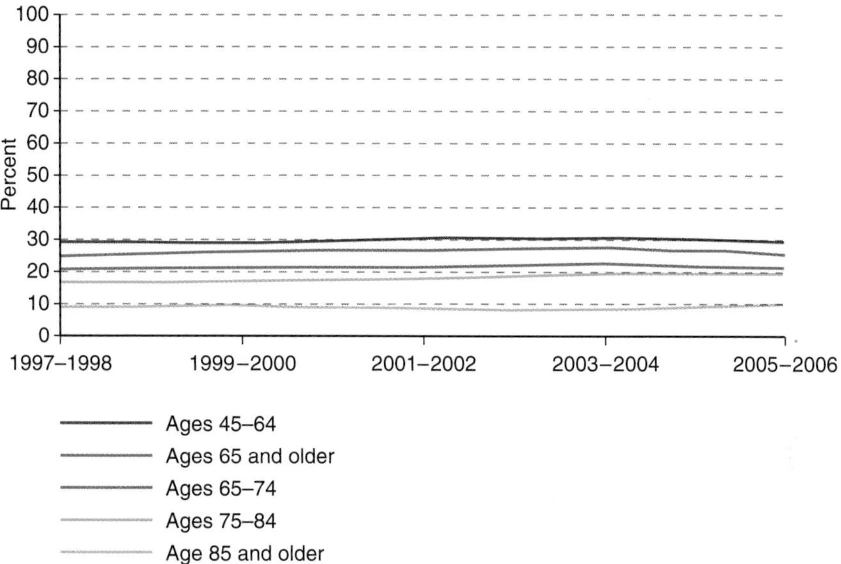

Note: Data are based on 2-year averages. "Regular leisure time physical activity" is defined as "engaging in light-moderate leisure time physical activity for greater than or equal to 30 minutes at a frequency greater than or equal to 5 times per week, or engaging in vigorous leisure time physical activity for greater than or equal to 20 minutes at a frequency greater than or equal to 3 times per week."
Reference population: These data refer to the civilian noninstitutionalized population.
Source: Centers for Disease Control and Prevention, National Center for Health Statistics, National Health Interview Survey.

Figure 12-3 *(From Federal Interagency Forum on Aging-Related Statistics. (2010). Older Americans 2010: Key indicators of well-being. Washington, DC: U.S. Government Printing Office.)*

time spent in bed during the day and encouraging physical activity in the daily routine are also beneficial in controlling symptoms of insomnia in these patients (Ancoli-Israel & Ayalon, 2006).

Sleep disturbance is not a natural consequence of aging, but rather a treatable condition (Ancoli-Israel, 2005).

Summary

Although sleep patterns change as we age, sleep problems are not a normal consequence but are more likely due to environmental, physical, or medical conditions. Sleep disturbances negatively impact quality of life and put patients at risk for additional health problems. Nurses need to identify patients who may be at risk and identify possible underlying causes through a comprehensive assessment. Screening tools can be useful in identifying patients in need of referral. Behavior therapy and medication can be effective in treating sleep disorders.

KEY POINTS

- Nearly two thirds of older adults report having some of the symptoms associated with sleep disorders.
- Although sleep patterns change as we age, insomnia is not a normal consequence of aging.
- Sleep complaints are typically due to changes in the ability to sleep rather than the actual number of hours slept.
- Daytime napping is higher among older adults living in residential care settings and those with vision and hearing loss.

- Poor sleep adversely affects social, physical, mental, and cognitive functioning.
- Uncontrolled symptoms (such as pain or nocturia), medical or psychosocial problems, and medications can contribute to sleep disturbance.
- Patients with dementia, especially those living in long-term care facilities, have a much higher rate of sleep disturbance than older adults in general, and their symptoms are more severe.
- Nursing home environments worsen symptoms when lighting, noise, and timing of care at night are not managed effectively.
- A comprehensive assessment using sleep assessment tools facilitates identification of high-risk people in need of evaluation and treatment, and contributing factors that require modification.
- Modifying environmental factors that contribute to sleep disruption in assisted-living or long-term care settings may help to improve the sleep quality of older adult residents.
- Older adults who live independently, engage in moderate exercise, and are socially active and financially secure are less likely to report sleep disturbances.
- Sleep disturbances that persist despite attempts to eliminate the underlying cause are typically treated with a combination of medication and behavior therapy.

CRITICAL THINKING ACTIVITIES

1. Imagine you are assigned to care for a patient in a long-term care setting. You enter the patient's room at 7:30 a.m. with a plan to help the person bathe and dress before breakfast starts at 8 a.m. You cannot understand why the patient angrily refuses your help. Later, you learn from the nurse that this patient was complaining of unrelieved pain most of the night. How might this information affect your plan of care for the day?
2. Use one of the sleep assessment tools to interview an older relative or patient to whom you are assigned. Discuss the outcome of your assessment with this person, and explore possible contributing factors. Suggest that the person convey significant results to health care provider.

CASE STUDY | *MRS. McDONALD*

Mrs. McDonald (whom everyone called Mrs. McD) never enjoyed watching television very much, although it was her husband's typical evening activity. Mrs. McD would lie on the couch to read and soon fall asleep. Her husband went to bed around 10 p.m. and often was unsuccessful in waking his wife to join him. Mrs. McD would awaken after several hours of sleep around 3 a.m. She usually would go to the bathroom and then stay up to read because she could not fall back to sleep. By 6 a.m., when her husband woke for work, Mrs. McD was tired again and would go into the bedroom to sleep for a while longer. Upon arising at about 9 a.m., she would fix a pot of coffee and sip this throughout the day as she completed her household chores.

As Mrs. McD passed through menopause, she was diagnosed with hypertension. She began taking a diuretic and now found herself needing to get up two or three times each night to urinate. Mrs. McD complained of feeling tired most mornings and was not very enthusiastic about going places with her retired husband, who had developed an interest in hiking. Mr. McD began to do more things alone, and Mrs. McD became lonely and depressed. She feared that her husband was no longer interested in their relationship.

1. What symptoms of sleep disturbance is Mrs. McD exhibiting?
2. What lifestyle patterns may be contributing to Mrs. McD's sleep problems?
3. What further information should you seek to thoroughly assess her sleep problem?
4. What elements of a plan of care would help Mrs. McD deal with her sleep disturbance?
5. How might you include Mr. McD in the plan of care? Consider other disciplines with whom it may be beneficial to collaborate.

REFERENCES

American Academy of Family Physicians. (2005). Information from your family doctor: Sleep changes in older adults. *American Family Physician, 72*(7), 1315–1316.

Ancoli-Israel, S. (2005). Sleep and aging: Prevalence of disturbed sleep and treatment considerations in older adults. *Journal of Clinical Psychiatry, 66*(Suppl. 9), 24–30.

Ancoli-Israel, S., & Ayalon, L. (2006). Diagnosis and treatment of sleep disorders in older adults. *American Journal of Geriatric Psychiatry, 14*(2), 95–103.

Asplund, R. (2005). Sleep and sensory organ functions in the elderly. *Sleep and Hypnosis, 7*(2), 68–76.

Blackwell, T., Yaffe, K., Ancoli-Israel, S., Schneider, J. L., Cauley, J. A., Hillier, T. A. . . . (2006). Poor sleep is associated with impaired cognitive function in older women: The study of osteoporotic fractures. *The Journals of Gerontology Series A: Biological Sciences and Medical Sciences, 61A*(4), 405–410.

Buysse, D. J., Reynolds III, C. F., Monk, T. H., Berman, S. R., & Kupfer, D. J. (1989). The Pittsburgh sleep quality index: A new instrument for psychiatric practice and research. *Journal of Psychiatric Research, 28*(2), 193–213.

Chaperon, C. M., Farr, L. A., & LoChiano, E. (2007). Sleep disturbance of residents in a continuing care retirement community. *Journal of Gerontological Nursing, 33*(10), 21–28.

Chen, K.M., Chen, M.H., Chao, H.C., Hung, H.M., Lin, H.S., & Li, C.H. . . . (2009). Sleep quality, depression state, and health status of older adults after silver yoga exercises: Cluster randomized trial. *International Journal of Nursing Studies, 46*(2), 154.

Cole, C., & Richards, K. (2007). Sleep disruption in older adults. *American Journal of Nursing, 107*(5), 40–49.

Endeshaw, Y. (2009). Correlates of self-reported nocturia among community-dwelling older adults. *The Journals of Gerontology Series A: Biological Sciences and Medical Sciences, 64A*(1), 142-148.

Hill, E. L., Cumming, R. G., Lewis, R., Carrington, S., & Le Couteur, D. G. (2007). Sleep disturbances and falls in older people. *The Journals of Gerontology Series A: Biological Sciences and Medical Sciences, 62A*(1), 62–66.

Johns, M. W. (1991). A new method for measuring daytime sleepiness: The Epworth sleepiness scale. *Sleep, 14,* 540–545.

King, A., Pruitt, L., Woo, S., Castro, CM., Ahn, D.K., Vitiello, M.V. . . . (2008). Effects of moderate-intensity exercise on polysomnographic and subjective sleep quality in older adults with mild to moderate sleep complaints. *J Gerontol A Biol Sci Med Sci, 63A*(9), 997–1004.

National Sleep Foundation. (2003). *2003 sleep in America poll.* Retrieved December 3, 2010, from http://www.sleepfoundation.org/sites/default/files/2003SleepPollExecSumm.pdf

National Sleep Foundation. (2009). *2009 sleep in America poll.* Retrieved December 3, 2010, from http://www.sleepfoundation.org/sites/default/files/2009%20Sleep%20in%20America%20SOF%20EMBARGOED.pdf

Ouellet, N., & Morris, D. L. (2006). Sleep satisfaction of older adults living in the community: Identifying associated behavioral and health factors. *Journal of Gerontological Nursing, 32*(10), 5–11.

Paredes, S., Marchena, A., Bejarano, I., Espino, J., Barriga, C., Rial, R.V. . . . (2009). Melatonin and tryptophan affect the activity-rest rhythm, core and peripheral temperatures, and interleukin levels in the ringdove: Changes with age. *The Journals of Gerontology Series A: Biological Sciences and Medical Sciences, 64A*(3), 340–350.

Patel, S. R., Blackwell, T., Redline, S., Ancoli-Israel, S., Cauley, J.A., Hillier, T.A. . . . Stone, K.L. (2008). The association between sleep duration and obesity in older adults. *Int J Obes. 32,* 1825–1834.

Ross, S. (2009). Sleep disorders: A single dose administration of valerian/hops fluid extract (dormeasan) is found to be effective in improving sleep. *Holistic Nursing Practice, 23*(4), 253.

Smyth, C. (2008). Evaluating sleep quality in older adults. *American Journal of Nursing, 108*(5), 42.

St. George, R., Delbaere, K., Williams, P., & Lord, S. (2009). Sleep quality and falls in older people living in self- and assisted-care villages. *Gerontology, 55*(2), 162–168.

Teo, J., Briffa, K., Devine, A., Dhaliwal, S., & Prince, R. (2006). Do sleep problems or urinary incontinence predict falls in elderly women? *Australian Journal* of *Physiotherapy, 52*(1), 19–24.

Weaver, T. E., Latzner, A. M., Evans, L. K., Maislin, G., Chugh, D.K., Lyon, K. . . . Dinges, D.F.. (1997). An instrument to measure functional status outcomes for disorders of excessive sleepiness. *Sleep, 20,* 835–843.

Yaggi, H. K., Araujo, A. B., & McKinlay, J. B. (2006). Sleep duration as a risk factor for the development of type 2 diabetes. *Diabetes Care, 29,* 657–661.

Chapter 13

Intimacy, Sexuality, and Aging

Pamela S. Brown, M.A., A.B.D.

LEARNING OBJECTIVES

- Define intimacy.
- Define sexuality.
- List and evaluate two myths/stereotypes about sexuality in older adults.
- Recognize normal changes in sexual function.
- Describe gender-related differences in age-related sexual functioning.
- Recognize diseases and/or medications that may interfere with sexual functioning.
- Identify two sexually transmitted infections, the method of prevention, and treatment.
- Describe the PLISSIT model and demonstrate its use in discussing sexuality with older adults as a health professional.
- Explain the Patient's Bill of Rights regarding privacy within the Federal Nursing Home Reform Act of 1987 (NHRA 1987).

What is intimacy? Is intimacy the same as sexuality, or are they different? Many times when discussing intimacy, people mean only physical intimacy or sexual acts. But intimacy is so much more. To be intimate involves physical communion with another person, but it also involves intellectual or emotional closeness or unity. Thus, intimacy has three components. Each component may be experienced separately with another person, or two or all three of the components may be shared with another person.

Neither is sexuality just a physical sexual sharing; it is about our feelings and beliefs about ourselves; what it is to be male, female, or transgendered; and how we relate to and express sexual feelings to those of the same and opposite genders. Our sexuality is shaped by the cultural, religious, and family environments that we experienced throughout our lives.

When thinking about sexual acts, society often views physical sexual sharing as only for persons who are young, passionate, lustful, and physically attractive—in other words, not for those who are old. But sexuality is not only for the young. Research reveals that most older adults maintain interest in sex and desire for sexual activity and intimacy, albeit at decreased levels (Lindau, Leitsch, Lundberg, & Jerome, 2007). In the future, older adults as a group probably will have an even higher sustained interest in sex and a higher frequency of participating in sexual acts as social acceptance and the perception takes hold that sexuality is normal among older adults (Hillman, 2008).

As we age, we may continue to have a desire for intercourse, oral sex, masturbation, passionate kissing, public displays of affection, and intimate touching. As a health care professional, it is important for you, more than most, to be familiar with your older adult patients' emotional and physical health. Unfortunately, there are only a handful of programs in the United States that educate older adults on healthy sexuality and sexual behaviors (see resource section for more information). You may be the only person in your older patient's life who can provide accurate and reliable sexual health information. This chapter will help you, as a health care professional, understand the myths and realities about sexuality in older adults, normal changes in sexual functioning, sexual dysfunction and its treatment, the loss of a partner and its effect on sexuality, privacy in residential settings, and sexually transmitted disease.

You may be the only person in your older patient's life who can provide accurate and reliable sexual health information.

Myths and Stereotypes

Older adults are often stigmatized by myths and stereotypes simply by being old. One of the most prevalent areas where society perpetuates ageist attitudes is the realm of sexuality. The term *dirty old man* is an intersection of two –isms: ageism and sexism. Older men are often referred to as dirty old men if they are perceived as being sexually active or interested in sexual activity (Saporta, 1991, p. 333). Older women are often called *old hags* or *old crows.* Richlin (2005) says that these terms were used to describe old women in Roman satirical prose, often exaggerating their repulsiveness by their age and decrepitude. Old women commonly were portrayed as drinking too much and regularly offering younger men money for sexual favors. Richlin states that these "repulsive stereotypes give women a set of boundaries, warning them that certain types of women can expect only mockery and revulsion for manifestations of sexuality, even for existence."

Ideas and beliefs about older adult sexuality have been passed down from generation to generation via cultural and social norms, religious ideologies, and even from comedic representations of older adults in the media. These types of ageist sexual attitudes pervade our society so intensely that many older adults see themselves as sexless, asexual, or too old for sexual activity, which can lead to a self-fulfilling prophecy. Gerontologist/sexologist Alex Comfort (1977) describes this as "bewitchment by expectation," noting that the notion of asexuality "which they had when they were younger became a blueprint for their own aging" (p. 191).

Another stereotype of the older adult is the "myth of the sexy oldie" (Gott, 2005, p. 8). This stereotype is the polar opposite of the asexual older adult. Gott says "the key messages underpinning this stereotype are that 'being sexual' is fundamental to mental and physical well-being at any age, but particularly as a means to stave off old age" (Gott, 2005, p. 24). In other words, there is an obligation for the older adult to maintain sexuality and sexual attractiveness and to continue to maintain the ability to participate in sexual intercourse. However, existing in a social atmosphere that extols youthfulness as sexually attractive and ignoring other types of physical sexual behavior that brings pleasure and intimacy again limits and stereotypes those who cannot or do not wish to participate in becoming a sexy oldie. Thus, those who cannot meet the criteria for sexual attractiveness, those who do not participate in heterosexual intercourse, or those who do not have rampant sexual desire may be labeled as abnormal or unhealthy.

The sexy oldie stereotype then further marginalizes those who have a disability, who do not have a sexual partner, or who participate in non-heterosexual sexual activity. Hinchliff and Gott (2008, p. 67) note how these ideologies, whereby all people want sex (sexual intercourse) and sexual intercourse is important to all older adults, "neglect the actuality that sexual intercourse can be detrimental to well-being, for example when it is non-consensual or transmits sexual infections." Obviously this statement debunks the proposal that sex is always good for you. The sexy oldie myth also reinforces the power of other stakeholders in the world of sexuality medicalization: the pharmaceutical industry.

Age-Related Changes in Sexual Functioning

There is great heterogeneity among age-related changes in the sexual reproductive system. It is not an absolute that a particular change will or will not occur. Poor nutrition, certain medications, or disease in other parts of the body may contribute to some changes. As health care professionals, we must also understand that each instance of sexual activity is dependent upon such factors as the environment, the partner, and the time since the last sexual experience, as well as independent of other incidences. Each patient should be evaluated on an individual level, and no assumptions should be made concerning age-related sexual changes without medical and medication history and discussion with the patient about his or her current emotional and psychological health. Each person ages because of, or in spite of, his or her genetic makeup, environmental exposures throughout life, race, socioeconomic status, and health care availability. Therefore, there is no one-size-fits-all aspect to aging and thus no normal or abnormal aging process as it pertains to intimacy and sexuality.

It is important as a health care professional to be familiar with the components and functions of the reproductive system before considering age-related changes in sexual function. The following sections briefly review the male and female reproductive systems along with common age-related changes.

There is no one-size-fits-all aspect to aging and thus no normal or abnormal aging process as it pertains to intimacy and sexuality.

Men

Male Reproductive System Review

The testes are oval shaped and produce spermatozoa (sperm cells). They also secrete the male sex hormones, chiefly testosterone. These hormones control the appearance of secondary sex characteristics, such as body hair on the pubic area, the face, and the armpits. Testosterone is also responsible for the growth and development of the body and behavior.

The scrotum, which is often referred to as the scrotal sac, suspends from the pubis in the front of the pelvis. The scrotum is a soft, thin-walled pouch that encloses and supports the testes and is composed of skin and fibrous material. A midline septum divides the scrotum into a left and right half, so each testis has its own pouch. It is the scrotum's job to control the "climate" for the testes because the production of sperm is highly dependent upon an appropriate temperature. In warm temperatures the scrotum is more loose or flaccid and allows the testes to hang lower, away from the body's heat. In colder temperatures the scrotum pulls the testes up close to the body and thus closer to the heat source. Temperature regulation is important for normal sperm production. The testes should be at a slightly cooler temperature than the body for normal production.

The penis contains three columns of erectile tissue, the urethra, and several veins and arteries. Two of the columns of erectile tissue are the corpus cavernosa, and one column is the corpus spongiosum.

The prostate gland is located just below the bladder and surrounds the upper end of the urethra. This gland produces and secretes an alkaline fluid containing the enzymes fibrinolysin and acid phosphatase, which is significant in activating the sperm. Secretions from the prostate gland make up about 15% of the semen.

The Cowper's glands or bulbourethral glands are about the size of a pea and are located on either side of the urethra, just below the prostate gland. These glands also produce an alkaline fluid that assists in neutralizing acid in the urethra before contractions in the ejaculatory ducts push the sperm cells through. This fluid protects sperm cells from acidic urine that could be in the urethra. It also aids in the lubrication of the penis through release of precoital fluid.

Two seminal vesicles located behind the urinary bladder and just above the prostate gland produce about two thirds of the semen. The thick secretion from the seminal vesicles' inner layer contains such substances as fructose, water, and alkaline materials. The water in this substance helps to dilute the sperm cells so that they have more motility. The fructose provides energy to the sperm, producing more active swimming toward the ovum. Again, the alkaline materials protect the sperm, neutralizing acid in the urethra and in the woman's reproductive system.

A duct system moves the sperm from the testes to the outside of the body. The system includes the epididymis, ductus deferens (vas deferens), and ejaculatory duct. The ejaculatory duct ejects semen, which contains spermatozoa and various fluids, into the urethra before the sperm cells and fluid exit the body through ejaculation.

Age-Related Changes

As a man ages, his testes may decrease in size and weight. This may be caused by a decrease in the testosterone levels or other factors such as poor nutrition or disease. Fewer viable sperm may also be produced and the motility, or movement, of the sperm may decrease. In spite of this change, most men do continue to produce enough viable sperm to fertilize ova and produce offspring well into older age.

Age-related changes appear to account for the gradual decline in the quickness of penile erection. These changes may appear as early as age 30 to 40. However, organic factors are often responsible for these changes. Atherosclerosis is the most common cause (Schiavi, 1999, p. 124).

Age-related changes in the prostate are often apparent by age 40, when the lining and muscle layer of the prostate gland become thinner. Benign prostatic hyperplasia (BPH) is an enlargement of the prostate gland that occurs on a microscopical level in almost half of American men by age 60. However, BPH usually does not affect sexual functioning. More information on BPH can be found in the urological literature.

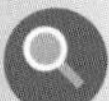

EVIDENCE FOR PRACTICE
Physical Health and Sexuality

Purpose: This study examined the association between sexuality (sexual activity and quality of sexual life) and self-rated physical health among middle-aged and older adults and estimated the average remaining years of sexually active life gained as a result of good health status.

Sample: Two samples were used in this study. The first included 3,032 adults (51.5% women, 48.5% men) ranging in age from 25 to 74 years. The second sample was composed of 3,005 older adults (51.6% women, 48.4% men) age 57 to 85. A majority of respondents in both samples were identified as heterosexual; among the middle-aged sample, 97.8% of women and 97.1% of men reported "being sexually attracted only to the opposite sex," and among the older sample, 95% of women and 96.4% of men reported only heterosexual contacts during their lifetime.

Methods: A secondary data analysis was conducted using data from two large, nationally representative and cross-sectional health surveys (the National Survey of Midlife Development in the United States [MIDUS] and the National Social Life, Health, and Aging Project [NSHAP]). Analyses measured prevalence of sexual activity, quality of sexual life, interest in sex, and the average number of remaining years of sexually active life (referred to as sexually active life expectancy) and determined the relationship between these outcomes and self-rated physical health.

Results: At all ages, men were more likely than women to be sexually active, report a good-quality sexual life, and be interested in sex. These differences were greatest among the 75- to 85-year-old age group (38.9% of men were sexually active, compared with 16.8% of women); of those sexually active, 70.8% of men versus 50.9% of women had a good sexual life, and 41.2% of men compared with 11.4% of women were interested in sex. Both men and women reporting very good or excellent self-rated health were significantly more likely to be sexually active than those reporting fair or poor health. Among sexually active respondents, good health was also significantly associated with interest in sex, frequent participation in sexual activity in men, and a good-quality sexual life among men and women in the midlife cohort. Sexually active life expectancy was greater for men than women in all age groups. At age 30, men had an average of 34.7 remaining years of sexually active life, while women had 30.7 remaining years. At age 55, men had 14.9 to 15.3 years and women had 6 years; for this age group, however, men in very good or excellent health gained 5 to 7 years of sexually active life compared with counterparts in fair or poor health, while healthy women gained 3 to 6 years compared with women in poor or fair health.

Implications: Sexual activity, quality sexual life, and interest in sex were higher for men than for women across all ages. This gender disparity and its implication for health merits further investigation. Sexual activity, quality of sexual life, and interest in sex were also significantly and positively associated with health in middle and older age. Sexually active life expectancy was longer for men, but men lost more years of sexually active life than women as a result of poorer health. More research is needed to understand the relationship between self-rated health; sexual activity, interest, and quality; and sexually active life expectancy.

Reference: Lindau, S. T., & Gavrilova, N. (2010). Sex, health, and years of sexually active life gained due to good health: Evidence from two U.S. population-based cross sectional surveys of ageing. *British Medical Journal, 340,* c810.

Male Climacteric

The male climacteric, or male menopause, is a controversial topic in biological, psychological, and sociological spheres. The medical profession, particularly endocrinologists, acknowledges that testosterone levels decline during the aging process; however, it does not decrease as severely as estrogen levels decrease in women during menopause. Some research professionals, such as sociologists, note that andropause, or male menopause, may be the medicalization of an issue that used to be considered a part of normal life events, such as childbirth. With recent television advertisements such as "Do you have Low Testosterone" (http://www.isitlowt.com), the topic of the male climacteric is moving further into the mainstream medical community than it once was. Testosterone replacement therapy (TRT) may be an option for some men, but it is as controversial a topic as male menopause.

Age-Related Disorders

Prostate cancer is the leading cause of new male cancers in the United States and the second most common cause of cancer deaths in men, with more than 215,000 estimated new cases in 2010 and about 32,000 deaths (American Cancer Society, 2010a). In men over age 60, prostate cancer is the most common cause of cancer death (Carroll, 2009, p. 161). Prostate cancer occurs most often in men in their 60s to 80s. In fact, according to the National Cancer Institute (2005) the main risk factor is being over age 65. It is rare for a man under age 45 to have the disease. One of the most common symptoms of prostate cancer is difficulty having an erection. This is yet another reason underscoring the importance of discussing a patient's sexual health and activity.

Women

Female Reproductive System Review

The vulva, or pudendum, is composed of the mons veneris (also known as the mons pubis), labia majora, labia minor, vestibule, clitoris, and perineum. The mons veneris/mons pubis is the fatty tissue located over a women's pubic bone. Extending downward from the mons and backward to the perineum is the labia majora or the outer lips. The labia majora is pigmented and covered with hair. The labia minora, or the inner lips, are smaller and are located between the labia majora and the vestibule. The two folds of the labia minora join at the clitoris to form the prepuce. The labia minora does not have hair follicles like the labia majora and also serves to protect the vagina and urethra.

The vagina leads inward to the cervix, which is the lower portion of the uterus that contains the opening into the uterus. The vagina is thin-walled, about 4 inches long, and in most women tilts toward the back, forming a 90-degree angle with the uterus, which is usually tilted forward. The uterus is a pear-shaped organ located between the bladder to the front and the rectum to the back. It is suspended by four sets of ligaments that hold it in place. Menstruation is the releasing of the uterine lining if no pregnancy has begun during the previous menstrual cycle.

Each of the two ovaries are roughly the size and shape of an almond, about 1.5 inches long. They are located on either side of the uterus near the fallopian tubes and are held in place by ligaments. Ovaries are the repositories of oocytes (ova/eggs) and thus are the primary reproductive organ in women. They also produce the female sex hormones estrogen and progesterone.

Age-Related Changes

The term climacteric is often used synonymously with menopause, which is an incorrect use of the term. The climacteric period in a woman's life commonly begins in the 40s and includes both physiological and psychological changes. It is during the climacteric period that menstrual periods fluctuate and begin to change. Often the first sign is a cycle/period that does not include ovulation. These changes result from a decreased production of estrogen and progesterone by the ovaries.

Menopause has occurred when a 1-year period passes without menstruation. According to the National Institute on Aging (2010), the current average age for menopause in the United States is 51, although it may occur at any time between 45 and 55.

Women may also experience surgical or medical menopause. Surgical menopause occurs as a result of a bilateral oophorectomy (ovariectomy), or surgical removal of both ovaries, often in response to ovarian, uterine, or endometrial cancer. However, it also may be performed because of uterine fibroids, endometriosis, infection, or together with a hysterectomy. A hysterectomy is the surgical removal of the uterus and does not induce surgical menopause. Other illnesses/diseases such as colon cancer or rectal cancer also may involve a removal of the ovaries. Medical menopause may occur as a result of chemotherapy or radiation therapy.

Other age-related changes include graying and thinning of pubic hair, a decrease in the size and weight of ovaries and uterus, a slight decrease in the size of external genitalia from loss of subcutaneous fat and elastic tissue, and an up to 50% decrease in the size of the uterus within 15 years of menopause. The uterus may eventually shrink to as small as 2 cm.

Age-Related Disorders

Some of the best known age-related reproductive disorders in women include uterine prolapse or hernia, atrophic vaginitis, vaginal infection and irritation, urinary incontinence, and cancer of the cervix, uterus, ovaries, or breast.

Prolapse and Hernia When the supporting ligaments of the ovaries and uterus lose some of their elasticity, the uterus may tip backward and move into the lower abdominal cavity. If the uterus lowers too much, it may slide down into or through the vagina. This is known as uterine prolapse. The same loosening of ligaments and fibrous tissue also may occur with other pelvic organs, such as the bladder or intestine, allowing hernias to form. A cystocele is a herniation of the bladder into the vagina, and a rectocele is a herniation of a portion of the large intestine into the vagina. These three conditions are influenced by reduced estrogen levels and repetitive childbirth. Surgery is often recommended and can be successful in mitigating the problems.

Atrophic Vaginitis Women who have lower estrogen levels may develop atrophic vaginitis, or inflammation of the vaginal walls. As women age, the vaginal walls shrink slightly in size and become thinner, drier, and less elastic. The fragile vaginal walls may be more easily irritated by sexual intercourse or other irritants. Estrogen suppositories, creams, or oral medications may be prescribed to relieve the symptoms. However, if unexplained vaginal bleeding occurs, cancer should be ruled out.

Vaginal Infection and Irritation Vaginal infections also may become more common in older women because cells lining the vagina contain and release less glycogen, causing less acidic material to be produced by the healthy bacteria. The thinning of the vaginal walls also increases the frequency of bladder or urethral irritation. Inflammation or cystitis may result from agitation of the vagina during sexual intercourse. Women who develop postmenopausal cystourethritis from sexual intercourse may want to consider using a vaginal lubricant during sex and voiding afterward (Cardozo, 1996, p. 129). Conditions such as diabetes and fibroids should also be ruled out.

Water-soluble, glycerin- and alcohol-free over-the-counter lubricants may be helpful, such as Astroglide Natural, Astroglide Glycerin & Paraben Free, and Yes. Some women are sensitive to chemical additives or fragrances in lubricants and have opted to use the pure natural oils such as vitamin E, coconut oil, almond oil, or apricot oil. It is highly recommended by many sexual health educators that older women do not use any products containing cinnamon, mint, menthol, or warming lubricants, such as Durex's Tingle or Sylk's Sensation. It is also recommended that a woman should try a small amount of lubricant a few hours before sexual intercourse to determine if it is the right blend for her. Some women may also feel comfortable using an estrogen vaginal cream such as Premarin if both they and their physician are in agreement. As a health-care professional, you should familiarize yourself with the latest lubricants, as well as the latest research and products containing estrogen.

Cervical Cancer The peak age of cervical cancer incidence is 55 to 60, with most new cases developing between ages 40 and 60 (Dallred & Burke, 2006, p. 32). Several risk factors may place older women at more risk for cervical cancer in the years to come. It is currently thought that infection with the human papillomavirus (HPV) is necessary for most types of cervical cancer to develop (Dallred & Burke, 2006, p. 32). But for older women, the most important risk factor may be having sexual intercourse at an early age. Other risk factors include having sexual intercourse with uncircumcised men, having multiple sex partners, having sex with men who have had multiple sexual partners, smoking or exposure to second-hand smoke, using oral contraceptives for more than 5 years, having multiple full-term pregnancies, having lower socioeconomic status, and being exposed to diethylstilbestrol (DES) in the womb. Women who have a first-degree relative (mother, sister, or daughter) who has been diagnosed with adenocarcinoma or squamous cell carcinoma of the cervix have double the risk of developing cervical cancer, compared with women without a family history (Cancer Research UK, n.d.).

Uterine Cancer Also known as endometrial cancer, uterine cancer occurs most often in women between ages 50 and 64, usually after menopause. The main initial symptom is usually vaginal bleeding, either between menstrual periods or after menopause. Pain during intercourse also may be an early warning signal. Uterine cancer is the most common of all female reproductive cancers.

Ovarian Cancer Accounting for about 3% of cancers in women, ovarian cancer is the ninth most common cancer among women and ranks fifth in cancer deaths (American Cancer Society, 2010c). Early detection is difficult because symptoms may be vague and not disease-specific. Age is one of the greatest risk factors for ovarian cancer, with half of ovarian cancers found in women over age 63 (American Cancer Society, 2010d). Ovarian cancer is rare in women under age 40. There is also a familial risk factor; heredity accounts for up to 10%

of ovarian cancer cases (American Cancer Society, 2010d). Studies are continuing on a possible link between ovarian cancer and postmenopausal hormone therapy.

Breast Cancer Breast cancer is another form of cancer in which age is a risk factor. About two of three invasive breast cancers occur in women age 55 or older (American Cancer Society, 2010b). Breast cancer is second only to lung cancer as the highest incident rate of cancer in women. Ongoing investigations are exploring the possible links among postmenopausal hormone therapy, hormone replacement therapy, and breast cancer.

Urinary Incontinence Urinary incontinence is a reduced ability to control the bladder, resulting in accidental loss of urine (National Institute of Diabetes and Digestive and Kidney Disorders, 2004b). Estimates suggest that 13 to 17 million Americans experience urinary incontinence (National Institute of Diabetes and Digestive and Kidney Disorders, 2004a; Resnick, 1998), and women with type 1 diabetes have an increased risk of this disorder (Sarma et al., 2009). About twice as many women over age 65 have urinary incontinence as men over age 65. The incidence for women over age 65 is an estimated 1 in 5, while the incidence among older men is 1 in 10 (Lifford, Curhan, Hu, Barbieri, & Grodstein, 2005).

Although urinary incontinence is a disorder of the excretory system, the symptoms may have profound effects on a woman's ability to feel sexual, because urine loss may occur during sexual activity (National Institute of Diabetes and Digestive and Kidney Disorders, 2007).

Discussing Sex Using the PLISSIT Model

It is important as a health-care professional to know and identify your level of comfort in providing information and intervention in the realm of sexual issues. The PLISSIT model (Annon, 1974) is an excellent tool to use when discussing sexual topics with older adults. The model not only identifies the level of intervention the patient needs but also can help the health-care professional identify his or her own comfort level. Many health-care professionals are comfortable in the first three levels.

Permission

The first level of the PLISSIT model, permission begins with the health-care professional asking the patient for permission to discuss sexuality and sexual issues. Often health-care professionals make the first move to initiate discussion as clients/patients may not be comfortable in addressing their concerns. Approaching the patient also implies that sexual information is a normal and natural conversation with patients and also implies that other clients/patients may have had these concerns as well. This allows the patient an open-door opportunity to discuss any of his or her sexual concerns.

Limited Information

The next step, limited information, gives the health-care professional the opportunity to share factual sexual information with the patient. The information should be specifically directed toward the patient's concerns and relate to the patient's particular illness and how the illness may affect sexual function. Information can be given to dispel myths and erroneous advice or facts, as well as pharmacological effects on sexual functioning. The information also may include basic anatomy and physiology of the reproductive organs affected. Information for illness support groups may also be given. It is important for the patient to know that there are others in similar situations. Some support groups will provide informational handouts or brochures to physician offices if requested.

Along with providing limited information, the health-care professional should also know his or her limits of knowledge when presenting information. We encourage you to maintain your competence in these topics. Continuing education credits are often offered at nursing conferences or online and can be helpful in keeping you up to date with the latest informational resources.

Specific Suggestions

The third step in the model, specific suggestions, goes further than the limited information step. Beyond basic, broad information, the third step provides an opportunity for the health-care professional to assist the patient in setting specific individualized objectives or goals. This step may or may not include the patient's partner. Education provided at this level should be more than pamphlets and resource sheets. This step could include education on adaptive equipment, positioning during sexual intercourse, and alternative methods of sexual satisfaction.

It is desirable for the health-care professional who moves into this step to have graduate course work in sexuality and sexual health or ongoing work toward a specialized certificate. The health-care professional working at step 3 should also be able to refer the patient to other providers who may be more prepared to move on to step 4 or convey more specific individualized information or therapy to the patient, the patient's partner, or both. Information on programs, such as the American Association of Sex Educators, Counselors, and Therapists, is located in the resource section on the CD-ROM for this chapter.

Intensive Therapy

The fourth and final step of the PLISSIT model is intensive therapy. Often, general health-care professionals refer patients to a more specialized physician, such as a psychologist, psychiatrist, nurse practitioner, sex coach, or other specialized physician, for material included in step 4. The health care professional should consider the referred specialist to be part of the patient's medical management team and should coordinate medical management and therapy with that professional. Intensive therapy may be needed for the psychological demands of illness, the particular relationship, or long-term sexual problems. It is also a good idea to know ahead of time whether there are sexuality counselors or therapists certified by the American Association of Sex Educators, Counselors, and Therapists in your area.

Sexual Dysfunction and Treatment

There is no absolute consensus among medical practitioners and researchers for defining sexual dysfunction. Moreover, the past 20+ years have narrowed the term to more of a medical model of physical malfunctioning rather than also including the psychological aspects of sexual dysfunction. In this chapter, we refer to sexual dysfunction as sexual problems involving all aspects of the inability to achieve sexual function, whether physiological, psychological, or pharmaceutical. The causal knowledge of sexual problems, regardless of origination, is of utmost importance for health care professionals. It is essential to realize that the three factors may act alone or in tandem, creating a complex situation for the health care professional. It is often a difficult task to untangle one problem from another.

Chronic illness is one of the leading causes of sexual problems in older adults. Illnesses such as arthritis, depression, diabetes, heart disease, high blood pressure, incontinence, Parkinson's disease, and mental illness may contribute to physical decline, causing a decline in sexual functioning and sexual interest. Medications used to treat these chronic conditions may also contribute to declining sexual desire and function. Chronic illness is also the easiest area of intervention for a health care professional.

Currently, more than 200 medications are known to cause sexual side effects, with new information being obtained with each pharmacological research study. Such side effects are the number one reason for noncompliance with drug regimens. For example, it is estimated that more than 25% of erectile dysfunction may actually be medication related. Some medications may cause decreased sexual desire or arousal, absent arousal, delayed or nonexistent orgasm, and ejaculatory problems (i.e., painful, retrograde, or absent). Studies have implied that many patients do not receive information about the effects of medications on sexual function (Walker, Osgood, Richardson, & Ephross, 1998). By providing information about a patient's illness and how it or a medication may affect sexual functioning, you can help to allay fears and debunk myths about sexual behavior and illness. Consult a sexual pharmacology text or search the Internet for the most up-to-date information on a drug's sexual side effects.

One example of an illness that can affect sexual functioning is diabetes. Diabetes is a major problem in the aging community and affects sexual function in many ways. More than 12 million adults age 60 and older have diabetes, accounting for more than 23% of this age group, and the numbers are growing (Centers for Disease Control and Prevention, 2008b). One of the main risk factors for type 2 diabetes is age. For older adults with diabetes, comorbid conditions may include heart disease, high blood pressure, kidney disease, diabetic neuropathy, autonomic polyneuropathy, and a high cholesterol level.

Diabetes is linked to sexual problems in both men and women and has been recognized as the leading organic cause of erectile dysfunction, also known as impotence (Deacon, Minichiello, & Plummer, 1995). Poor glycemic control can cause temporary erectile dysfunction, but often, once blood glucose levels are controlled, erectile ability resumes. Diabetes can cause hardening and narrowing of blood vessels in both men and women. This reduces blood flow to the penis, preventing an erection or preventing an erection firm enough for penetration. In women, a parallel process occurs in which blood flow to the vaginal walls is inadequate, causing dryness and difficulty with intercourse. Limited blood flow to the clitoris may also cause difficulty in achieving orgasm. Much more research is needed in the area of female sexual problems caused by diabetes.

Treatment options for men with diabetes and erectile dysfunction vary. For some men, oral medication such as sildenafil (Viagra), tadalafil (Cialis), or vardenafil (Levitra) may be an option. Other options may include intracavernosal injection therapy, in which medication, usually alprostadil, is injected directly into the penis to stimulate an erection. Alprostadil suppositories may also be available. Check with the patient's physician or a pharmaceutical representative to learn more about these medications, because several are currently off the market. Another option is a vacuum erection device, which may be battery powered or manual and which allows blood to be pulled into the corporal columns. Because penile hematoma may occur with improper use, only medically approved vacuum devices should be used, and patients should be educated on proper use and safety. For some patients, another alternative might be a penile implant or prosthesis.

In women, the problem of dryness may be addressed through prescribed therapy, over-the-counter aids, or homeopathic remedies. Other problems, such as chronic yeast infections, bladder infections, and microcirculation issues, can affect a woman sexually as well and should be investigated.

It is best to use a team approach when working with patients who have chronic illnesses. You, the physician, the patient, perhaps the partner, and often a counselor may need to look at all aspects of the person's physical, psychological, and pharmaceutical needs. It may be up to you as the health care professional to determine if the patient's sexual problems are related to an illness or to a medicine used to treat the illness. Approach the diagnosis with caution and be sure to first rule out other causes. Review medication benefits with the patient. Other treatment options may include lowering the dosage, changing to a different medication, allowing the patient to take a drug holiday (not recommended with blood pressure medications) or adding an antidote medication, such as Viagra.

Loss of a Partner

For both women and men across the lifespan, interest in sex and sexual behaviors decreases when no desirable partner is available (Wasow & Loeb, 1979). However, very little information exists in research literature on sexuality in older adults after the loss of a partner, whether the loss is from divorce or death. Even in sexuality textbooks, widowhood or divorce among adults commonly merits little more than a single paragraph of coverage. When widowhood is mentioned, it is most often within the context of widow(er)'s syndrome, a term attributed to Masters and Johnson. Widow's syndrome is commonly used to describe a woman who has had no sex for a long time and who has atrophy of the vaginal walls and reduced amounts of lubrication. Widower's syndrome is used commonly to describe a man who has been able to function sexually with his previous partner, but then may be unable to have intercourse with a new partner because of anxiety, guilt, or other psychological issues. The relationship between the loss of partner and decreased sexual activity is further underscored by a belief of many current cohorts of elders that sexual behaviors and intimacy are appropriate only in marriage (DeLemater & Moorman, 2007). Engaging in sexual relationships with others after losing a partner may therefore feel wrong, or older men and women may worry about being judged by family, friends, and even health care professionals.

In one recent study (Ginsberg, Pomerantz, & Kramer-Feeley, 2004), 60% of older adult participants identified the lack of a partner as the most important obstruction to sexual experiences. Many women stop sexual activity because of the death of their partner. Gott and Hinchliff (2003, p. 1621) note that "current partner status ... coupled with the fact that most thought they would not be sexually active again in their lifetime ... emerged as the most significant determinants of their views toward sex." Gott and Hinchliff also found that some women who had been satisfied with marital sexual relations expressed fear that they would compare a new partner to their previous spouse.

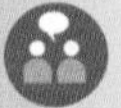

PERSONAL PERSPECTIVE
Octogenarians on Intimacy

"I think at this point I've had it with physical intimacy with a lover," says Ruth Landau Levy Cohen, age 88. "I did have it, but that was more than two years ago, and enough is enough. My husband is gone—my real husband, who I was married to for fifty years. We were young, I was in love with him tremendously. We had a real intimacy. The second time I married, I really didn't want to get married, but we were very good friends, we became intimate and we started to travel all over the world, and I was very, very lonely, extremely lonely. He really wanted me to marry him and it's a wonderful thing that I did."

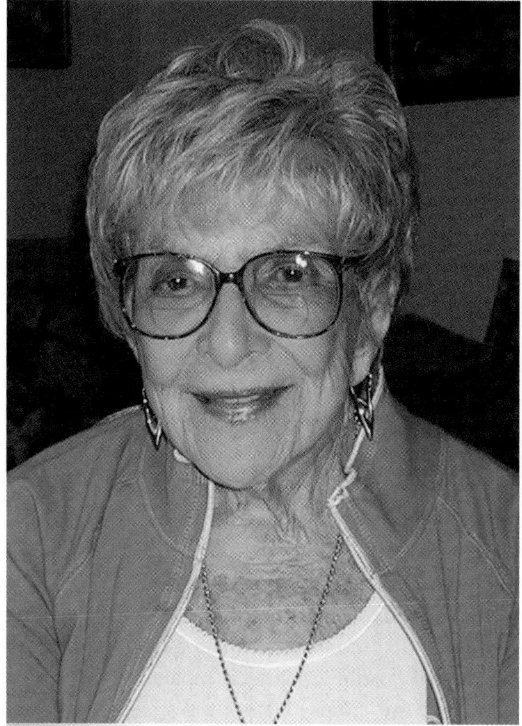

"Now I have intimacies with so many wonderful women," Ruth continues. "I talk with them every week, every other week. Here in the building, there is a certain intimacy I've developed with certain people here. And you feel it. You feel when you like someone and someone likes you, but you can't feel that way with everyone."

Ruth Blum, also an octogenarian and pictured in Chapter 9, adds her insights on intimacy to the conversation. "I think the need for a person to be loved or supported in some way, or have attention paid to them, never ever goes away," she offers in her quiet philosophical tone. "It might diminish as you get older," she continues, "but there is a need to have affection. It doesn't have to be a sexual affection. It could be that someone looks at you in a very special way, or asks you to dance at one of the programs, and that's all I really need. But, I list it as one of the needs. That may be over emphasizing, but I feel it really is."

"Intimacy to me," she goes on after a thoughtful pause, "is a very intimate relationship that you might have with someone, or a very verbal exchange with personal things that you don't usually talk to everyone about. You might have one person, and it might be someone of the opposite sex, where you can talk about what a wonderful relationship you had with your husband and he could talk about his relationships too. And you appreciate each other. If it entails a good night kiss, wonderful, and I appreciate it. But I don't want anyone to think that as people get older they don't have these needs. They do. I laugh at the people who say, 'oh who needs it, who cares, so what?' They're not honest, I don't think. Either that, or they can't express themselves. It makes them feel awkward."

About Ruth Landau Levy Cohen Ruth Landau Levy Cohen is mother to three children and loving grandma to three grandchildren. Her first marriage of 50 years ended with the death of her much beloved husband. She was fortunate to once again find companionship in a second marriage, which lasted until the passing of her spouse 10 years later.

Ruth has always loved music and for many years gave piano lessons from her home. Later, certified as a substitute teacher, she taught all subjects to children in kindergarten through high school. As a younger woman, Ruth was very active in the parent-teacher association, synagogue, and a number of philanthropic organizations. Ruth has a passion for American politics and avidly follows the news. Asked what she loves, she replies "Bible stories!! I love to read them and analyze them. They are so fascinating."

About Ruth Blum Ruth Blum is a twice-widowed mother of four wonderful children. Inspired by a personal interest, Ruth worked for many years as the Connecticut State Representative to the March of Dimes National Foundation. She traveled extensively, speaking about the important work of the March of Dimes and organizing groups to help raise funds for children affected by polio. Ruth has been living at an assisted-living facility for over 3 years. She says that at the time she made the switch from living in her own home she realized she "wasn't getting any younger" and "needed a support system." Ruth calls the move the wisest choice of her life and takes advantage of the many activities offered there.

Lorri B. Danzig, MS, CSL

However, this was not the case with all of the participants. Gott and Hinchliff also stated that one woman in particular indicated her sex life had become better since the death of her husband as she was able to explore sexual experiences that were taboo with her spouse. Brown and Ewen (2011) concur with Gott and Hinchliff, finding in a qualitative research project that some women do have gratifying sexual experiences with men after divorce or the death of their partner and find a freedom that they did not have in the past. Further, men and women who lose a partner may continue to satisfy sexual desires through masturbation; however, access to information from health care professionals or access to products may be hindered by the social stigma of masturbation.

It is apparent that more research needs to be conducted on the topic of sexuality, older adults, and partner loss whether through divorce or death. Gott and Hinchliff say there are barriers in studying sexuality and aging, whether methodologically or because of the sensitive nature of the topic. Brown and Ewen (n.d.) also agree, stating that barriers exist in qualitative sexuality and aging research, particularly within close communities, where a perception exists that speaking with researchers may indicate participation or a willingness to participate in sexual activity.

Privacy in Residential Settings

Privacy issues vary with the older adult's particular living situation, whether it be home-based, community-based, assisted living, or long-term care facility. The important point to remember is that no matter where an older adult lives, privacy is paramount in facilitating sexual expression. In fact, it is such an important issue that the Federal Nursing Home Reform Act of 1987, part of the Omnibus Budget Reconciliation Act (1987), includes a Resident's Bill of Rights [42 U.S.C. § 1396r(c)(1)(a)(iii)] whereby each resident has a right to privacy, and even more important, a right to having his or her private space respected (e.g., knocking on doors and asking permission to enter) (Braun, 2004, p. 12-4.2). The Nursing Home Reform Act also states that a resident has the right to receive visitors at reasonable hours and the right for visitors to have reasonable access to the resident (Helewitz, 2001, p. 65).

The Resident's Bill of Rights also allows residents to choose their roommates, live with a spouse, and have a right to privacy with whomever they wish to be private and, during that privacy, to expect both visual and auditory privacy (Feldkamp, 2003). Facilities that violate these rights are subject to citations, investigations of complaints, fines, or sanctions. Remedies may include monetary penalties, in-service training, a ban on admissions, or termination of Medicaid and Medicare participation (Braun, 2004). Sadly, many nursing facilities and even less restrictive settings, such as assisted-living residences, do not adhere to these privacy rights by not allowing patients to lock their rooms, or staff may not allow residents enough time, after knocking, to invite them into the room (Knaplund, 2009; Morgan, 2009). According to Knaplund, federal statutes are often ignored, and some nursing facilities notify the families if two competent residents begin a sexual relationship. The nursing facility staff may frown upon and discourage sexual expression among residents (Box 13-1).

In addition, Béphage (2008) includes lack of information on sexuality issues, religious or sociocultural backgrounds of the staff or residents, and ageist attitudes. Many nursing homes are designed with an institutional model of long-term care, usually similar to a hospital, where the rooms are situated along a hallway with a centrally located nursing station. This model may also have semiprivate rooms with only a curtain separating residents. However, the *culture change* movement has been gaining momentum and is working toward a deinstitutionalization of long-term care facilities. With a more person-centered care focus, the resident's environment is changing and enabling more choice and freedom. This change is seen in such aspects as dining options, where there are more dining choices such as buffet, restaurant, or family-style meals, and often at different times throughout the day. Residents also may determine their daily schedule, such

BOX 13-1 Barriers to Sexual Expression in Residential Living Facilities

- Lack of privacy
- Lack of a willing and able partner
- Mental illness
- Physical limitations
- Attitudes of staff
- Attitudes of family members
- Adverse effects of medications
- Feelings of being unattractive
- Erectile dysfunction in men
- Dyspareunia in women

Hajjar, R., & Kamel, H. (2004). Sexuality in the nursing home, part 1: Attitudes and barriers to sexual expression. J Am Med Direct Assoc, 5(2 Suppl), S42–S47.

as when they wish to rise, sleep, and bathe. More facilities are transforming their semiprivate rooms into private ones. This one simple change may allow for more privacy for sexual expression.

A variety of sexually expressive behaviors may be observed in long-term care or nursing facility residents. Studies in long-term care settings such as assisted-living facilities and nursing homes found several examples of sexual expressions, such as holding hands, kissing, and touching. This also includes mutual or solitary erotic or sexual activity, such as masturbation (Béphage, 2008; Frankowski & Clark, 2009). Sexual intercourse also may take place between residents.

"Viagratization" also has had a significant impact on the sexuality of the aging population (Kingsberg, 2000). The Baby Boomer generation does not follow one-time societal norms in the same way that previous generations have, and the probability that aging Baby Boomers will engage in sexual activity is high. Social changes such as divorce have also left more singles in the aging population, and new relationships form with sexual intercourse not being as taboo as in previous generations (Kingsberg, 2000).

It is important that nurses and other health care professionals in long-term care residences treat sexual expression and intimate relationships between residents with respect and take steps to preserve their dignity. The unfortunately common use of elderspeak, in which staff members at long-term facilities talk to the residents as though they were children rather than with respect and deference to age, is stigmatizing and inappropriate (Dobbs et al., 2008; Pasupathi & Lochenhoff, 2002). One study revealed that sexuality is yet another way in which elders are stigmatized in long-term care; findings showed that residents' actions and intimate relationships become the fodder of passing conversation, often with patronizing tones (Frankowski & Clark, 2009). Earlier in the chapter we addressed using the PLISSIT model. It would be a useful tool in long-term care settings in approaching a patient to discuss sexual expressions.

The staff should take care to help residents overcome barriers to sexual expression in long-term care settings (Hajjar & Kamel, 2004) These steps include adding a sexual history and assessment to the resident's care plan, providing sexual information and counseling to interested residents, and educating both the staff and families on the sexual needs of the residents. Geriatric sexual education for staff and families could improve understanding of residents' sexual needs, as well as skin hunger, which is the physiological and psycho-emotional need to be touched, to have contact with another person. In addition, resources are available to help long-term care facilities address intimacy, sexual expression, and sexual behaviors. Finally, it is important that the staff of long-term care settings not automatically assume that all residents are heterosexual, and when matters pertaining to sexuality and intimacy arise, care should be taken to address both homosexual and heterosexual issues.

Sexually Transmitted Infections

Older adults who are sexually active have a significant risk of contracting sexually transmitted infections (STIs). However, this group is less likely than younger adults to know or believe that they are at risk. They also are less likely to use condoms or to get tested for STIs. In addition, elders are less likely than younger patients to be diagnosed with STIs by physicians (Lindau, Leitsch, Lundberg, & Jerome, 2006). Underdiagnosis of STIs in older adults is attributed to stereotypes by health practitioners that older adults do not have sex and therefore are not at risk; mistaking symptoms for normal age-related changes; and hesitation by physicians, other health-care providers, and older adults themselves to inquire about sexual behavior and changes (Feldman, 1994). Research has also found that older adults are categorically excluded from clinical trials investigating prevention and treatment of STIs, in effect placing this group at additional risk (Levy, Ding, Lakra, Kosteas, & Niccolai, 2007).

The risk of contracting STIs is of even greater concern for lesbian, gay, bisexual, and transgender (LGBT) older adults compared with heterosexual elders. This is in part because of additional barriers that LGBT older adults encounter, including the tendency to conceal their sexual orientation or gender identify for fear of being stigmatized, having limited choices of amenable health-care providers and physicians, and seeing providers who ignore their sexuality or fail to provide appropriate prevention information (Cahill, South, & Spade, 2000).

HIV/AIDS

Older adults are one of the fastest growing segments of the population with HIV/AIDS. About 28% of those living with AIDS are over age 50, and the numbers are rising, with estimates that more than 50% of the HIV/AIDS population will be over age 50 by 2015 (Myers, 2009). About 15% of new

AIDS cases occur in people over age 50 (Centers for Disease Control and Prevention, 2008a). But in many cases, older adults with AIDS are newly identified rather than newly infected. In adults over age 50 with AIDS, infection occurred at a younger age, but people are living longer or "aging in" through the use of highly active antiretroviral therapy (HAART) and other medical treatment.

Actual rates of HIV/AIDS are higher than reported for the over-50 age group through misdiagnosis, under-reporting, or lack of knowledge among health-care professionals that this group is at risk. The misconception that adults over age 50 are not sexually active takes a particularly dangerous turn when it comes to HIV/AIDS and contributes both to inaccuracy in the numbers and to the universally unacknowledged and untreated phenomenon of geriatric HIV/AIDS (Calasanti & Slevin, 2001).

The most common way that women acquire HIV is through heterosexual sex with an HIV-infected man.

The most common way that HIV-positive women acquire HIV is through heterosexual sex with an HIV-infected man (Centers for Disease Control and Prevention, 2010). Women over age 50 who may have been in a long-term relationship may have a difficult time negotiating their partners' use of a condom (Lorber, 2000). Asking for condom use during sexual intercourse may infer mistrust in the monogamy of the partner or an admission of their own breach of monogamy and may lead to anger or even violence by the partner (Neundorfer, Harris, Britton, & Lynch, 2005). Older women are less likely than younger women to insist upon condom use (Neundorfer, Harris, Britton, & Lynch, 2005). Indeed, it may not even occur to women currently over 50 to ask about a partner's sexual history or about condom use because pregnancy prevention was the main reason that most in this age cohort used condoms, and most are now through menopause (Villarosa, 2003). In a study of 377 women, only 26% of those who had a main partner used condoms more than half of the time during vaginal or anal intercourse (Lorber, 2000).

The tried and true belief over the past three decades has been that biologically, older women are at more of a risk for STIs because of reduced vaginal lubrication and thinning of the vaginal wall. But new advances in technology are telling researchers more about HIV transmission in women. Researchers at Northwestern and Tulane Universities have recently discovered that HIV may enter a woman's body without vaginal thinning, atrophy, or other openings such as from herpes virus lesions. Research has shown "for the first time that the HIV virus does indeed penetrate a woman's normal, healthy genital tissue to a depth where it can gain access to its immune cell targets" (Northwestern University, 2008).

Herpes Simplex

The herpes simplex virus (HSV) is a virus in the family known as herpesviruses. This includes the Epstein-Barr virus, which causes mononucleosis, and the varicella zoster virus, which causes chickenpox and shingles (American Social Health Association, 2010). About 67 million Americans are infected by the herpes simplex virus, about 45 million having herpes simplex virus-2 (HSV-2) (National Institute of Allergy and Infectious Diseases/NIAID, 2009).

HSV-2 is the most common STI in older women (Wilson, 2006). It is often believed that herpes simplex virus-1 (HSV-1) affects only the face and not the genitals, but this belief is false. Both HSV-1 and HSV-2 may be genital or oral and be spread through sexual contact. More than 85% of those with HSV-2 are unaware that they are infected (Gilbert & Wyand, 2009). Contrary also to myths is that HSV is caused by having sex with multiple partners. Anyone who has ever had any sexual relationship, oral/genital, genital/genital, oral/anal, or genital/anal, is at risk for HSV.

Kissing and skin-to-skin contact can also transmit HSV-1 and HSV-2. Fever blisters and cold sores are terms that people commonly associate with an oral herpes outbreak. It is thought that most people acquire HSV-1 when they are infants or children from relatives' kisses (American Social Health Association, 2010). About 90% of the U.S. population over the age of 50 has HSV-1.

Blood tests are available to determine if a person has HSV, and some tests can be used to determine if the virus is HSV-1 or HSV-2. A convenient herpes blood test reference guide is available from the American Social Health Association at http://www.ashastd.org/pdfs/HerpesBloodTestGuide.pdf.

Currently, there is no cure for herpes. It is not necessary to treat herpes outbreaks or the virus with medication, but there are medications available to keep the lesions from recurring. The Food and Drug Administration has approved three prescription antiviral drugs and one OTC drug to lessen the outbreaks and control symptoms (Table 13-1). These three antiviral medications are usually used to treat outbreaks in the genital area, but they often may be prescribed for oral outbreaks as well. They may be taken episodically or daily for suppressive therapy. For episodic use, the drug is taken at the first sign or prodrome of the outbreak. The prodrome is an itching, tingling, or painful sensation in the area where the recurrent lesion will develop. Each person has their own prodromal signals, and it may take time for the person to learn either the signals or the triggers of the outbreak. Triggers are also highly individualized and may include overexposure to ultraviolet light, friction in the genital area, physical or emotional stress, illness, and poor diet. Suppression therapy typically is used by those who have multiple outbreaks each year and has been shown to lessen recurrence by at least 75% (American Social Health Association, 2010).

KEY POINTS

- Despite stereotypes to the contrary, older adults can maintain interest in sex and an active sexual life.
- Myths and stereotypes about aging and sexuality can lead to a hesitation of older patients to discuss questions, symptoms, or other concerns with health care professionals.
- Age-related changes to the reproductive system can create difficulties for older adults to engage in sexual activity.
- Sexual dysfunction is often related to the presence of chronic disease, such as diabetes. Acute conditions such as yeast or bladder infections can also result in sexual dysfunction.
- Older adults can benefit from products such as lubrication to improve their sexual experiences.
- It is vital for nurses and other health care practitioners to communicate with older patients about sexuality and intimacy.
- The PLISSIT model exists to help health-care professionals communicate with older adults about intimacy and sexuality.
- Losing one's sexual partner can result in decreased interest in sex or feelings of guilt or shame when entering into a new sexual or intimate relationship.
- The ability to engage in intimate or sexual relationships can be greatly hindered after a move into a long-term care setting such as assisted living or a nursing home.
- Staff of long-term care settings are required by the Federal Nursing Home Reform Act of 1987 to respect resident privacy, but often this privacy is compromised.
- Most long-term care settings do not consider intimate or sexual relationships in the development of care plans.

TABLE 13-1 Drugs for Treating Herpes Simplex Virus

acyclovir (Zovirax)	Inhibits both HSV-1 and HSV-2 Available in pill, ointment, and cream form Available as generic form
valacyclovir (Valtrex)	Uses acyclovir as its active ingredient Reduces HSV transmission by 50% May provide greater protection when used with a condom
penciclovir (Denavir)	Most effective when used as early as possible after outbreak May reduce duration of viral shedding Available in cream form
famciclovir (Famvir)	Uses penciclovir as its active ingredient Stops HSV from replicating Taken less often than either acyclovir or valacyclovir
docosanol (Abreva)	The only approved OTC treatment for HSV Blocks cell entry by virus May speed lesion healing time Not approved for genital lesions

HSV, herpes simplex virus; OTC, over-the-counter.

- Older adults are at risk for sexually transmitted infections.
- Underdiagnosis or misdiagnosis of sexually transmitted infections is prevalent in our health care system.
- Homosexual relationships exist among older adults. Health care professionals should not assume all older patients are heterosexual.
- Older adults are at risk for contracting sexually transmitted infections because of generational attitudes and lack of education about protected sex and underdiagnosis of sexually transmitted infections by health care professionals.
- GLBT elders may be at increased risk for contracting sexually transmitted infections because they are hesitant to discuss sexual activity for fear of being stigmatized.
- Older adults are one of the fastest growing segments of the HIV/AIDS population.
- Twenty-eight percent of persons living with HIV/AIDS are over age 50.

CRITICAL THINKING ACTIVITIES

1. Discuss your idea of intimacy and sexuality. How does your concept differ from your classmates? Are the differences based on familial ideals, sociocultural, religious?
2. Find a greeting card, an advertisement in a magazine, or a YouTube video that depicts sexuality and aging in a positive/negative light. Bring it to class. Discuss the implications of the stereotypes of aging and sexuality.
3. Watch a movie such as *Something's Gotta Give* (2003), *About Schmidt* (2002), *The Notebook* (2004), *The Birdcage* (1996), *Ruth and Connie: Every Room in the House* (2002), or *Letters to Juliet* (2010). Discuss the aspects of the older adult characters' sexuality.
4. Visit the condom/lubricant section of a drug store or an adult store. If possible, bring different condoms/lubricants to class. Open the products and pass them around to see the difference in condom sizes (length/width) and the different types of lubricant. Which ones are water-based, and what are the implications of that difference?
5. Participate in a role-play exercise with another student. One of you plays the role of a nurse at a community health center. The other plays the role of an older patient who has just entered into a new relationship and wants to begin a sexual relationship with the partner. As the patient, how do you begin this conversation? As the nurse, what questions do you ask this patient? What information and resources can you offer?

CASE STUDY | *MR. BUCKLEY*

Mr. Buckley recently moved into the assisted-living residence in which you work as an RN. He is always friendly and wanting to strike up a conversation when you visit him in his room, and over the past few weeks you've developed a good relationship with him. One day, you knock and enter through Mr. Buckley's door and find him sitting in his recliner with no pants on, apparently masturbating. Embarrassed, you hurry out of the room and tell him you'll come back later.

A few hours later, you return to Mr. Buckley's room and knock on his door. You are sure to wait for his invitation before you enter the room. When he sees you, he apologizes and appears quite upset about the situation. He is afraid that you will tell other staff or his family. As a health care professional, you feel it is your responsibility to put him at ease and reassure him that you will keep the matter between you and him. You have a conversation with him to convey this, and during your talk, Mr. Buckley begins to get teary and tell you that he has been very lonely since moving into the assisted-living facility and misses having a companion.

1. What steps can you take to prevent this embarrassing situation from occurring with other staff and residents in the assisted-living facility?
2. In your conversation with Mr. Buckley, what can you say to reassure him about this embarrassing situation?
3. What questions might you ask Mr. Buckley about his loneliness? What suggestions could you make as a health-care professional?

REFERENCES

American Cancer Society. (2010a). *What are the key statistics about prostate cancer?* Retrieved November 18, 2010, from http://www.cancer.org/Cancer/ProstateCancer/DetailedGuide/prostate-cancer-key-statistics

American Cancer Society. (2010b). *What are the risk factors for breast cancer?* Retrieved November 15, 2010, from http://www.cancer.org/Cancer/BreastCancer/DetailedGuide/breast-cancer-risk-factors

American Cancer Society. (2010c). *What are the key statistics about ovarian cancer?* Retrieved November 15, 2010, from http://www.cancer.org/Cancer/OvarianCancer/DetailedGuide/ovarian-cancer-key-statistics

American Cancer Society. (2010d). *What are the risk factors for ovarian cancer?* Retrieved November 15, 2010, from http://www.cancer.org/Cancer/OvarianCancer/DetailedGuide/ovarian-cancer-risk-factors

American Social Health Association/ASHA (2010a.) *Herpes.* Retrieved November 13, 2010, from http://www.ashastd.org

Annon, J. S. (1974). *The behavioral treatment of sexual problems* (Vol. 1). New York: Harper & Row.

Béphage, G. (2008). Meeting the sexuality needs of older adults in care settings. *Nursing & Residential Care, 10*(9), 448–452.

Braun, J. A. (2004). Portfolio 12: Rights of long-term care facility residents. In H. S. Margolis (Ed.), *The elder law portfolio series* (Vol. 2, Release #21 pp. 12-1 – 12-49). New York, NY: Aspen.

Brown, P., & Ewen, H. (2011; manuscript in preparation). Power and safe sex: Measuring the ability of older women to negotiate condom usage.

Cahill, S., South, K., & Spade, J. (2000). *Outing age: Public policy issues affecting gay, lesbian, bisexual and transgender elders.* New York, NY: The Policy Institute of the National Gay and Lesbian Task Force Foundation.

Calasanti, T. M., & Slevin, K. F. (2001). *Gender, social inequalities and aging.* New York: AltaMira Press.

Cancer Research UK. (n.d.) *Cervical cancer risks and causes.* Retrieved November 18, 2010, from http://www.cancerhelp.org.uk/type/cervical-cancer/about/cervical-cancer-risks-and-causes

Cardozo, L. (1996). Postmenopausal cystitis. *British Medical Journal, 313*(7050), 129.

Carroll, J. L. (2009). *Sexuality now: Embracing diversity* (3rd ed.). Belmont, CA: Wadsworth.

Centers for Disease Control and Prevention. (2008a). *HIV/AIDS among persons ages 50 and older.* Atlanta, GA: Author. Retrieved December 3, 2010, from http://www.cdc.gov/hiv/topics/over50/resources/factsheets/over50.htm

Centers for Disease Control and Prevention. (2008b). *National diabetes fact sheet, 2007.* Atlanta, GA: Author. Retrieved December 4, 2010, from http://www.cdc.gov/diabetes/pubs/pdf/ndfs_2007.pdf

Centers for Disease Control and Prevention. (2010). *HIV/AIDS and women.* Atlanta, GA: Author. Retrieved December 4, 2010, from http://www.cdc.gov/hiv/topics/women/index.htm

Comfort, A. (1977). *A good age.* London: Mitchell Beazley.

Dallred, C., & Burke, C. (2006). Cervical cancer screening in older women. *Clinical Journal of Oncology Nursing, 10*(1), 31–33. doi:10.1188/06.CJON.31-33

Deacon, S., Minichiello, V., & Plummer, D. (1995). Sexuality and older people: Revisiting the assumptions. *Educational Gerontology, 21*(5), 497–513.

DeLemater, J., & Moorman, S. M. (2007). Sexual behavior in later life. *Journal of Aging and Health, 19,* 921–945.

Dobbs, D., Eckert, J. K., Rubinstein, B., Keimig, L., Clark, L. J., Frankowski, A. C., . . . (2008). An ethnographic study of stigma and ageism in residential care or assisted living. *Gerontologist, 48,* 517–526.

Feldkamp, J. (2003). Navigating the uncertain legal waters of resident sexuality. *Nursing Homes Long Term Care Management, 52*(2), 62.

Feldman, M. (1994). Sex, AIDS, and the elderly. *Archives of Internal Medicine, 154*(1), 19–20.

Frankowski, A. C., & Clark, L. J. (2009). Sexuality and intimacy in assisted living: Residents' perspective and experiences. *Sexuality Research and Social Policy, 6,* 25–37.

Gilbert, L., & Wyand, F. (2009). Genital herpes education and counseling: Testing a one-page 'FAQ' intervention. *Herpes Journal of the IHMF, 15*(3), 51–56.

Ginsberg, T. B., Pomerantz, S. C., & Kramer-Feeley, V. (2005). Sexuality in older adults: Behaviours and preferences. *Age & Ageing, 34*(5), 475–480.

Gott, M. (2005). *Sexuality, sexual health and ageing.* New York, NY: Open University Press.

Gott, M., & Hinchliff, S. (2003). How important is sex in later life? The views of older people. *Social Science & Medicine, 56*(8), 1617. doi:10.1016/S0277-9536(02)00180-6

Hajjar, R., & Kamel, H. (2004). Sexuality in the nursing home, part 1: Attitudes and barriers to sexual expression. *Journal of the American Medical Directors Association, 5*(2 Suppl.), S42–S47.

Helewitz, J. (2001). *Elder law.* Albany, NY: West Legal Studies/Thomson Learning.

Hillman, J. (2008). Sexual issues and aging within the context of work with older adult patients. *Professional Psychology Research & Practice, 39*(3), 290–297.

Hinchliff, S., & Gott, M. (2008). Challenging social myths and stereotypes of women and aging: Heterosexual women talk about sex. *Journal of Women & Aging, 20*(1/2), 65–81.

Kingsberg, S. A. (2000). The psychological impact of aging on sexuality and relationships. *Journal of Womens Health and Gender-Based Medicine, 9*(1), 33–39.

Knaplund, K. S. (2009).The right of privacy and America's aging population. *Denver University Law Review, 86*(2), 439–456.

Levy, B. R., Ding, L., Lakra, D., Kosteas, J., & Niccolai, L. (2007). Older persons' exclusion from sexually transmitted disease risk-reduction clinical trials. *Sexually Transmitted Diseases, 34,* 541–544.

Lifford, K. L., Curhan, G. C., Hu, F. B., Barbieri, R. L., & Grodstein, F. (2005). Type 2 diabetes mellitus and risk of developing urinary incontinence. *Journal of the American Geriatrics Society, 53,* 1851–1857. doi: 10.1111/j.1532-5415.2005.53565

Lindau, S., Leitsch, S., Lundberg, K. L., & Jerome, J. (2006) Older women's attitudes, behavior, and communication about sex and HIV: A community-based study. *Journal of Womens Health, 15,* 747–753.

Lindau, S. T., Schumm, L. P., Laumann, E. O., Levinson, W., O'Muircheartaigh, C. A., & Waite, L. J. (2007). A study of sexuality and health among older adults in the United States. *New England Journal of Medicine, 357,* 762–774.

Lorber, J. (2000). *Gender and the social construction of illness.* New York, NY: AltaMira Press.

Myers, J. (2009). Growing old with HIV: The AIDS epidemic and an aging population. *Journal of the American Academy of Physician Assistants, 22*(1), 20–24.

Morgan, L. (2009). Balancing safety and privacy: The case of room locks in assisted living. *Journal of Housing for the Elderly, 23,* 185–203.

National Cancer Institute. (2005). *What you need to know about prostate cancer.* NIH Publication No. 05-1576. Bethesda, MD: National Institutes of Health, U.S. Dept. of Health & Human Services. Retrieved November 15, 2010, from http://www.cancer.gov/cancertopics/wyntk/prostate.pdf.

National Institute of Allergy and Infectious Diseases /National Institute of Health. (2009). *Genital herpes.* Retrieved December 7, 2010, from http://www.niaid.nih.gov/topics/genitalHerpes/Pages/default.aspx

National Institute of Diabetes and Digestive and Kidney Diseases. (2004a). *Urinary incontinence in women.* Retrieved November 15, 2010, from http://kidney.niddk.nih.gov/kudiseases/pubs/uiwomen/index.htm

National Institute of Diabetes and Digestive and Kidney Diseases. (2004b). *Urologic diseases dictionary.* Retrieved November 15, 2010, from http://kidney.niddk.nih.gov/kudiseases/pubs/udictionary/

National Institute of Diabetes and Digestive and Kidney Diseases. (2007). *Urinary incontinence in women* (NIH Publication No. 08-4132). Washington, DC: U.S. Government Printing Office.

National Institute on Aging. (2010). *Menopause.* Retrieved November 15, 2010, from http://www.nia.nih.gov/healthinformation/publications/menopause.htm

Neundorfer, M. M., Harris, P. B., Britton, P. J., & Lynch, D. A. (2005). HIV risk factors for midlife and older women. *Gerontologist, 45*(5), 617–625.

Northwestern University. (2008, December 17). New way men can transmit HIV to women. *ScienceDaily.* Retrieved November 15, 2010, http://www.sciencedaily.com/releases/2008/12/081216133436.htm

Pasupathi, M., & Lochenhoff, C. F. (2002). Ageist behavior. In T. D. Nelson (Ed.), *Ageism: Stereotypes and prejudice against older persons* (pp. 201–246). Cambridge, MA: MIT Press.

Resnick, N. (1998, December 16). Improving treatment of urinary incontinence. *Journal of the American Medical Association, 280*(23), 2034–2035.

Richlin, A. (2005). Invective against women in Roman satire. In P. A. Miller (Ed.), *Latin verse satire: An anthology and critical reader* (pp. 375–386). New York, NY: Routledge.

Saporta, S. (1991). Old maid and dirty old man. The language of ageism. *American Speech, 66.3,* S, 333–334.

Sarma, A., Kanaya, A., Nyberg, L., Kusek, J., Vittinghoff, E., Rutledge, B., Cleary, P., Gatcomb, P., Brown, J., and Diabetes Control and Complications Trial/Epidemiology of Diabetes Interventions and Complications Research Group (DCCT/EDIC). (2009). Risk factors for urinary incontinence among women with type 1 diabetes: Findings from the epidemiology of diabetes interventions and complications study. *Urology, 73*(6), 1203–1209.

Schiavi, R. C. (1999). *Aging and male sexuality.* Cambridge, UK: Cambridge University Press.

Villarosa, L. (2003). Raising awareness about AIDS and the aging. *New York Times,* July 8. Retrieved November 15, 2010, from http://query.nytimes.com/gst/fullpage.html?res=9901E0D6173DF93BA35754C0A9659C8B63&sec=health&pagewanted=print

Walker, B., Osgood, N., Richardson, J., & Ephross, P. (1998). Staff and elderly knowledge and attitudes toward elderly. *Educational Gerontology, 24*(5), 471.

Wasow, M., & Loeb, M. (1979). Sexuality in nursing homes. *Journal of the American Geriatrics Society, 27,* 73–79.

Wilson, M. G. (2006). Sexually transmitted diseases in older adults. *Current Infectious Disease Reports, 8*(2), 139–147.

Chapter 14

Healthy Eating

Ruth E. Johnston, MS, RD, LD, and Ronni Chernoff, PhD, RD, FADA

LEARNING OBJECTIVES

- Describe major changes that occur in the body due to normal aging.
- Outline major nutrient needs of older adults.
- Identify micronutrient needs of older adults.
- Discuss factors involving older adults' hydration and fiber needs.
- Recommend healthy eating tips.

Being healthy, happy, and productive. Those are major life goals for virtually everyone, no matter what their age. Indeed, this wish continues to be true even as we age into that category of life known as old age. Data are clear that our lifestyle choices will make a substantial difference in our ability to achieve the goals of being happy, healthy, and productive as we age.

The fact is, continued health and productivity will depend in part on whether we avoid smoking, eat a variety of foods in moderation, exercise regularly, and socialize in a meaningful way with family and friends. This approach to life is recommended in the *Steps to a Healthier US* and given context in *Older Americans 2010: Key Indicators of Well-Being* (Federal Interagency Forum on Aging-Related Statistics, 2010; Welman, 2007). In 2007, the U.S. Surgeon General wrote that "healthful eating habits prolong the independence of older adults by helping them to maintain their hearing and vision, cognitive abilities, physical strength and endurance. In addition, good nutrition and routine physical activity promote health by lowering the risk for heart disease, stroke, cancer, diabetes, and osteoporosis" (Moritsugu, 2007). Many of the chronic diseases and infirmities faced by older adults can be prevented by good nutrition. In this chapter, we focus on diet and nutrition for older adults.

Normal Changes

The further we move through the aging process, the more dissimilar we may become. Although one person may be 80 years old but appear to be 15 years younger, another person might be 70 years old and appear to be 10 years older. This difference manifests in part by how our choices and habits influence the normal changes of aging. As we grow older, our bodies and organs naturally start to lose function. However, the rate of that loss is not fixed or predetermined. Our genetic history, our habits and choices, and our life experiences determine, in part, the rate at which we age.

Certain changes are inevitable as we get older. Lean body mass decreases, total body water decreases, bone density declines, and the percentage of adipose tissue increases (Fig. 14.1). Also, skin turgor declines and subcutaneous fat decreases. The functionality of organs begins to decline. Blood vessel elasticity decreases, along with heart muscle strength and the kidneys' ability to filter waste products and excrete salt. In the endocrine system, hormone production decreases, which contributes to decreased glucose tolerance. Starting in our 20s, we lose about 1 cm of height per decade from decreased bone density and the vertebral compression that occurs with aging.

Some of the normal changes of aging have a direct effect on nutrition, such as when sensory changes affect a person's oral intake. For example, the blending of smell, taste, and somatosensation (the feel of texture and temperature) contribute to the enjoyment of eating. As we age, the loss of any of these senses alone or in combination can decrease dining pleasure. Although a total loss of taste (ageusia) is rarely a result of aging, there is evidence that taste sensation changes. The largest to smallest changes are in the threshold for salt, bitterness (i.e., citric acid), and sweet (sugar). Also with aging, the sense of smell may be reduced (hyposmia) or lost completely (anosmia). Aging adults are more susceptible to a loss of smell than to a loss of taste. Thirst sensitivity is also compromised in the aging person (Duffy & Chapo, 2006).

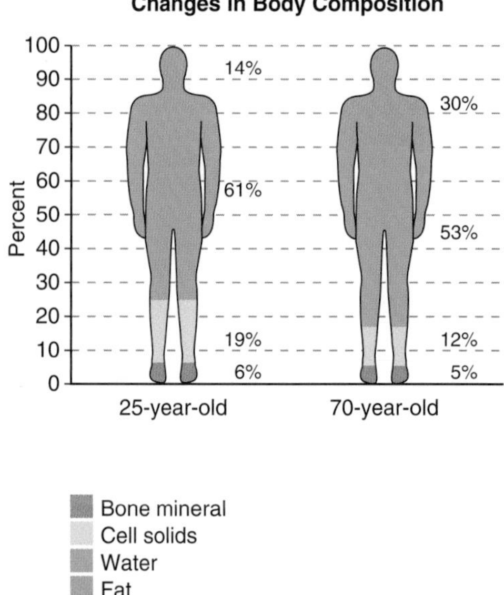

Figure 14-1 Differences in body composition with aging.

There doesn't appear to be a change in somatosensation with age with regard to eating.

Having good dentition is important no matter how old we are. However, with aging, oral health may have major consequences. Not being able to chew (masticate) food well enough will limit the types of foods a person can consume and thus limit the variety of nutrients that can be ingested. Also, adequate saliva production is needed during mastication. If an older adult has dentures, it is important that they be checked routinely for proper fit. Removing dentures for an hour or two during each 24-hour period will help avoid the loss of bone on which the dentures rest. This is one reason that some people remove their dentures while they sleep (Johnston & Chernoff, 2003).

Macronutrient Needs

The calorie needs of the aging adult decline from mid-life onward. A decline in muscle mass, which is the most metabolically active part of the body, along with a less active lifestyle is believed to be the major reason that calorie needs decrease. With the Baby Boomer generation reaching the beginning of their retirement years, however, less activity will not necessarily remain the norm. Maintaining an active lifestyle is an important part of healthy living practices.

A good rule of thumb for maintaining weight is to provide 30 to 35 calories per kilogram of body weight. If weight gain is desired, then adding 500 to 1000 calories per day will produce 1 to 2 pounds of weight gain per week. If weight loss is the goal, then subtracting 500 to 1000 calories per day will produce 1 to 2 pounds of weight loss per week. The body mass index, or ideal weight to height ratio, is between 18 and 24 for healthy aging adults (Box 14-1) (Duffy & Chapo, 2006).

With decreased caloric needs, one might expect lower protein needs as we age. However, the amount of nitrogen retained by the body decreases as calorie intake declines; therefore, one must ensure an adequate intake of protein to provide a positive nitrogen balance. The recommended daily amount of protein is 0.8 grams per kilogram of body weight for adults. This covers the minimum amount needed to prevent a loss of body protein. Loss of muscle mass is called *sarcopenia.* Aging adults can reduce the risk of sarcopenia by participating in resistance training along with consuming an adequate amount of protein (Campbell & Leidy, 2007).

Some older adults have a decrease in appetite as they age, a change that may be worsened by chronic disease conditions that also affect appetite. Most recent studies indicate that 1.0 to 1.5 grams of protein per kilogram of actual body weight is more appropriate for healthy aging adults. As long as there

BOX 14-1 Calculating Body Mass Index

Body mass index (BMI) gives a quick indicator of whether a patient is underweight, normal weight, overweight, or obese. The higher one's BMI, the greater the risk of disease and disability. The National Heart Lung and Blood Institute has an online BMI calculator at http://www.nhlbisupport.com/bmi/ along with a downloadable app. If you'd rather calculate BMI manually, use one of these formulas:

$$\text{BMI} = \frac{(\text{Weight in pounds}) \times 703}{\text{Height in inches}}$$

$$\text{BMI} = \frac{(\text{Weight in kilograms})}{\text{Height in meters}}$$

A patient whose BMI is below 18.5 is probably underweight. If BMI is 18.5 to 24.9, the patient is normal weight. A patient whose BMI is 25.0 to 29.9 is overweight. And one whose BMI is 30.0 or above is obese. Keep in mind that BMI may overestimate body fat in people with a very muscular build. It may underestimate body fat in those who have lost muscle.

A complete assessment of weight and health risks should include BMI, waist circumference (greater than 35 inches for women or 40 inches for men indicates increased health risk), and a consideration of diseases and conditions associated with obesity.

is good kidney function and good fluid intake, elderly people can increase their protein intake above 1.0 grams per kilogram of body weight (Wolfe, Miller, & Miller, 2008).

The need for carbohydrates remains the same as we grow older. The aging adult should obtain 55% to 60% of daily calories from carbohydrates. Keep in mind, however, that glucose tolerance may decline with age. A stable serum glucose level can be maintained through exercise and eating complex rather than simple carbohydrates. In other words, including more whole grains and limiting simple sugars is recommended (Chernoff, 2006).

Recommendations for fat requirements remain the same as well for aging adults. About 30% of daily calories may come from fat, particularly monosaturated and polyunsaturated fats rather than saturated and partially hydrogenated fats. Eliminating fat is not recommended because doing so would also eliminate essential fatty acids, which the body cannot produce on its own. Fat also helps attain satiety, or the feeling of fullness after eating (Chernoff, 2006).

Micronutrient Needs

Vitamin A

The physiological functions of vitamin A include the formation and maintenance of healthy teeth, bones, mucous membranes, skin, visual pigments, cell differentiation, and gene regulation. There doesn't seem to be an issue with older adults consuming adequate amounts of vitamin A. (Good food sources include liver, sweet potatoes, carrots, and leafy green vegetables.) Some foods are supplemented with vitamin A, and many dietary supplements also include vitamin A. The Dietary Reference Intake (DRI) for those age 65 and above is 900 mcg/day for men and 700 mcg/day for women. Vitamin A is a fat-soluble vitamin and, thus, can be retained in the body. The tolerable upper intake level is 3000 mcg/day (U.S. Department of Agriculture, 2010a).

Vitamin D

Vitamin D is a fat-soluble vitamin important for bone development and the maintenance of serum calcium levels. It aids in the absorption of calcium and phosphorus, as well as in the maintenance of calcium homeostasis, immune function, and colon health (Duyff, 2006). Vitamin D–fortified milk is the major source of the vitamin in the American diet. Some deep-sea fish, such as salmon and mackerel, are also good sources of vitamin D.

Our bodies synthesize vitamin D after exposure to the sun, but many older adults avoid the sun for fear of skin cancer. Many others live in areas where sunlight is limited. Others develop an intolerance of lactose, or lactase deficiency, and may omit dairy products from their diet. Therefore, some elderly people are at risk of vitamin D deficiency (Johnston & Chernoff, 2003; U.S. Department of Agriculture, 2010a).

The DRI for adults ages 51 to 70 is 10 mcg/day and, for those age 70 and over, 15 mcg/day. For older adults who spend inadequate time in the sun or consume too few foods high in vitamin D, a supplement in the range of 400 to 600 International Units per day is recommended. This can be taken alone or with a calcium supplement. Supplementation is especially beneficial during the winter months (Suter, 2006).

Vitamin E

Another fat-soluble vitamin is vitamin E (tocopherol), which is an antioxidant that helps the body use vitamin K. It also has a function in the formation of red blood cells. Sources of vitamin E include spinach, other green leafy vegetables, asparagus, vegetable oil, and olives. The DRI for vitamin E is 15 mg/day for older adults. Few have trouble meeting this nutritional need.

Vitamin K

Vitamin K is important in blood coagulation. For adults age 70 and older, the DRI is 90 mcg/day for men and 120 mcg/day for women. Spinach, cabbage, cauliflower, and soybeans are good food sources of Vitamin K.

B Vitamins

Thiamine

Thiamine or vitamin B_1 in its role as a coenzyme assists in the conversion of carbohydrate into energy. It is necessary for heart function and nerve cells. The DRI is 1.1 mg/day for older women and 1.2 mg/day for older men. Sources of thiamine include fortified bread, cereal, and pasta; whole grains; lean meats; dairy products; fruits and vegetables; and dried beans.

Riboflavin

Riboflavin or vitamin B_2 is important for the production of red blood cells and for body growth. It functions as a part of coenzymes involved in oxidation and reduction reactions. It works in combination with other B vitamins. The DRI for riboflavin in adults over age 70 is 1.1 mg/day in women and 1.3 mg/day in men. Cereal and dairy products are good sources of riboflavin.

Niacin

Niacin, also known as vitamin B_6, is the coenzyme in nicotinamide adenine dinucleotide (NAD) and nicotinamide adenine dinucleotide phosphate (NADP), which are the metabolically active forms of niacin. The DRI for niacin in adults age 70 and over is 14 mg/day for women and 16 mg/day for men. Recommended food sources of niacin include meat, fish, legumes, and some cereal products.

Pyridoxine

Vitamin B_6 includes pyridoxine found in plant foods and pyridoxal and pyridoxamine found in animal foods. It functions as a cofactor in metabolism and is important in the synthesis of neurotransmitters. The DRI for vitamin B_6 in adults age 70 and over is 1.7 mg/day for men and 1.5 mg/day for women. Whole grains, legumes, nuts, meats, and poultry provide good sources of vitamin B_6.

Cobalamin

Vitamin B_{12}, also known as cobalamin, is another cofactor in metabolism. It is importance in the formation of red blood cells and in the maintenance of central nervous system function. For adults over age 70, the DRI is 2.4 mcg/day. Vitamin B_{12} can be found in fortified cereals, milk, eggs, cheese, red meats, organ meats, oysters, and salmon.

The risk of vitamin B_{12} deficiency is increased in older adults for several possible reasons. For one, some sources of vitamin B_{12}—such as red meat and organ meats—have been cut out of many elders' diets as a way to reduce saturated fats. Also, the cost of red meat, as well as the need for good dentition to chew it, can be prohibitive to some older Americans. Further, with age comes a higher incidence of achlorhydria, which is an absence of or reduced production of gastric acid needed for the proper pH level in the stomach, and reduced production of intrinsic factor, which is needed to disconnect B_{12} from its protein carrier so that the body can absorb it. The combination of achlorhydria and less intrinsic factor increases the risk of vitamin B_{12} deficiency (Suter, 2006).

Folate

Folate is another B-complex vitamin that functions as a cofactor in metabolism and acts with vitamin B_{12} to form red blood cells. As with vitamin B_{12}, reduced or absent gastric acid production can decrease the absorption of folate. The DRI for those age 70 and older is 400 mcg/day. Green leafy vegetables and fortified foods are good food sources of folate.

Vitamin C

Vitamin C or ascorbic acid is needed for skin integrity, including healthy teeth and gums, with its role in the formation of collagen. Vitamin C also aids in the absorption of iron. The DRI for adults age 70 and older is 75 mg/day for women and 90 mg/day for men. Food sources of vitamin C include citrus fruits and juices, broccoli, white and sweet potatoes, strawberries, and cantaloupe.

Minerals

Except for iron, there are no major changes in the need for minerals with the aging process. As we age, we store more iron, particularly in women after menopause.

The presence of osteoporosis in aging adults does indicate a need to monitor calcium intake and blood levels. As previously mentioned, if one develops an intolerance to any or all dairy products, calcium intake may become inadequate. In these cases, supplementation is indicated. The DRI for calcium in those age 70 and older is 1200 mg/day. In addition to dairy products, salmon, sardines, turnip greens, and kale are good sources of calcium.

Water and Fiber

The hydration status of the aging adult can be labile; therefore, it is very important to maintain good hydration. Water plays multiple roles. It is needed for good renal function to rid the body of the waste products in the urine. During a fever, increasing water intake will aid in bringing down body temperature because the fluid acts as a thermal buffer. Water also functions in the maintenance of cellular integrity and in the dilution of medications.

A rule of thumb is to consume 1 ounce (30 mL) of water per kilogram of body weight per day (alternatively, 1 mL of fluid per kilocalorie consumed per day). Fluid requirements also can be met by juices and fruits with high water content.

The two stimuli that trigger the body to recognize thirst are cellular dehydration and hypovolemia. However, as we age, our thirst sensitivity decreases. Knowing the signs and symptoms of dehydration is essential. Among these are increased body temperature, confusion, sunken eyes, swollen tongue, low blood pressure, decreased urine output, and dark yellow urine (Chernoff, 2006).

Fiber needs remain the same as we age, but the sources of fiber may need to change in keeping with mastication abilities. The role of fiber is to provide bulk that promotes peristalsis, which are rhythmic contractions that move food through the gastrointestinal tract. It is imperative that older adults consume adequate fluids along with the fiber to avoid impaction. Whole grain cereals and breads, nuts, and fresh fruits and vegetables are good sources of fiber. The DRI for fiber in those age 70 and older is 20 to 30 grams daily.

Diet Tips

Although the traditional thought that three meals a day is ideal, smaller and more frequent meals may be appropriate for aging adults. A recent study by Zizza, Tayie, and Lino (2010) indicated that intake of vitamin A, vitamin C, beta carotene, and vitamin E increased. Careful selection should be made to choose low-calorie, nutrient-dense foods to avoid gaining weight if that is an issue of concern. Some aging adults find themselves consuming less volume as they decrease their activity levels. This increases the risk of consuming inadequate amounts of their nutritional needs (Chernoff, 2006).

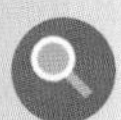

EVIDENCE FOR PRACTICE
Benefits of Snacking

Purpose: The purpose of this study was to examine the association between snacking frequency and older adults' daily intakes of vitamins, carotenoids, and minerals.

Sample: The study included respondents older than age 65 at the time of their interview and were part of the 2,065 participants in the 2003–2006 National Health and Nutrition Examination Survey.

Methods: The study used cross-sectional data from the NHNE Survey, which was a multistage, stratified representative probability sample. Using linear regression to adjust for multiple covariates, adjusted mean intakes and standard errors for each vitamin, carotenoid, and minerals were estimated. The data included age, sex, race/ethnicity, education, income, body mass index, and total energy intake.

Results: As snacking frequency increased, daily intakes of vitamins A, C, E, and beta carotene increased. Older adults' daily intakes of magnesium, copper, and potassium also increased as snacking frequency increased. However, the older adults' daily intake of selenium decreased. Snacking frequency was not associated with daily intakes of B-complex vitamins, vitamin K, lycopene, phosphorus, iron, or zinc.

Implications: Residential facilities, rehabilitation facilities, feeding centers, and long-term care facilities could use wise snacking choices as a practical way to help meet the nutritional needs of their residents.

Reference: Zizza, C. A., Ariswalla, D. D., & Ellison K. J. (2010). Contribution of snacking to older adults' vitamin, carotenoid, and mineral intakes. *Journal of the American Dietetic Association, 110*(5), 768–772.

Grains

Whole grains, breads, and cereals include whole wheat, brown rice, oats, corn, barley, or other cereal grains. Some products may have bran added to them for increased fiber. Refined bread and cereal products may have B vitamins added back to the product in a process called enrichment. Serving sizes vary according to the food chosen. One-half cup of oatmeal, 3 cups of popcorn, 1 cup of whole wheat cereal flakes, one-half cup of brown rice, or one slice of bread all equal an individual serving. Including up to six servings a day is recommended. Whole grain intake has been inversely related to the development of the metabolic syndrome in adults (U.S. Department of Agriculture, 2010b).

Vegetables

This group includes any vegetables or 100% vegetable juices. Including a variety of vegetables with an assortment of colors, such as dark green, yellow, orange, and red, is an easy way to include the best mix of vitamins and nutrients. As with fruit, the vegetables can be fresh, frozen, canned, or dried. Five to seven servings a day of fruits and vegetables are recommended. Dried beans and peas overlap into this food group, as well as the meat and beans food group (U.S. Department of Agriculture, 2010b).

Fruits

The fruit group includes 100% fruit juices or any fruit that is fresh, canned, frozen, or dried. Fresh fruits that are deep in color, such as berries and melon, are the healthiest choice. As with the grain group, a serving size depends upon the chosen item. As mentioned previously, citrus fruits and juices are an excellent source of vitamin C. Five to seven servings a day of fruits and vegetables are recommended (U.S. Department of Agriculture, 2010b).

Milk Products

Two servings a day of dairy products, including milk, yogurt, and cheese, provide calcium and protein in the diet. Eight ounces or 1 cup of milk is considered a serving. Choosing low-fat or no-fat products will aid with heart health (U.S. Department of Agriculture, 2010b).

Beans and Meat

The beans and meat group includes dried beans, nuts and seeds, fish, poultry, meat, and eggs. Again, choosing lower-fat products equates to heart-healthy choices. Meats provide protein, B vitamins, and iron, which are important in a healthy diet. Fish, nuts, and seeds can provide omega 3 fatty acids and polyunsaturated and monounsaturated fats. Some nuts provide essential fatty acids, which the body does not make on its own. Two servings a day are recommended from the meat and beans group. Two ounces of meat or one-half cup of beans are considered a serving size (U.S. Department of Agriculture, 2010b).

Oils and Fats

For heart health, advise patients to choose less-saturated liquid vegetable oils over more-saturated solid fats (Fig. 14-2). Healthy oils include canola, safflower, sunflower, corn, olive, soybean, peanut, and cottonseed. Avocado, palm, coconut, and fish oils are higher in saturated fat. Choosing oils or tub margarines with no trans fats and with healthy vegetable oils as the first ingredient is preferred. Choosing more saturated fats such as butter, lard, shortening, or stick margarine with hydrogenated vegetable oil as the first listed ingredient and products containing trans fats are not recommended. Also suggest that patients look for salad dressings that contain the healthier oils. Urge older adults to use fats sparingly for sautéing or stir frying as part of a heart-healthy regimen (U.S. Department of Agriculture, 2010b).

Alcohol

The effects of alcohol on older adults vary largely with amount consumed. Heavy daily or episodic consumption is, of course, harmful in a variety of ways. And thanks to the general aging of the U.S. population, alcohol abuse may be a growing problem

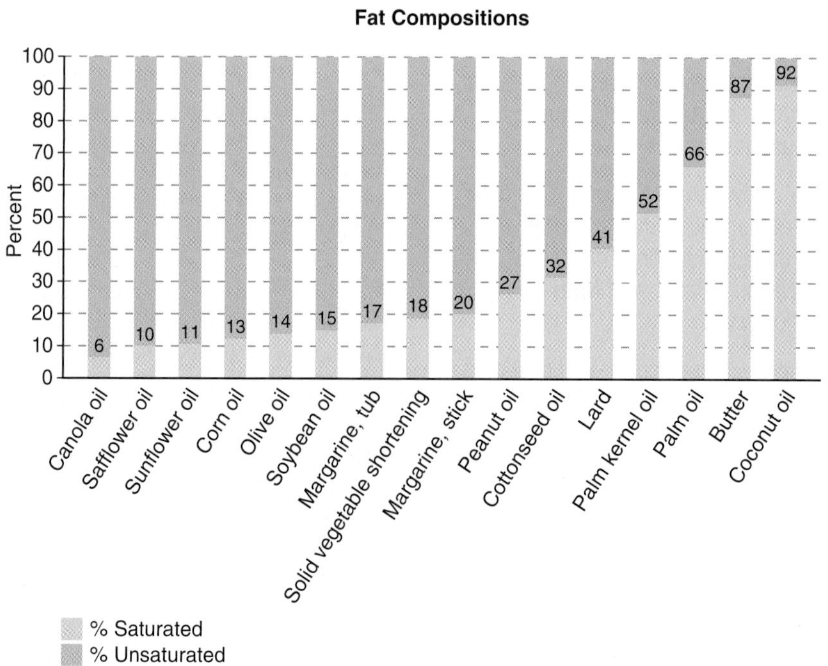

Figure 14-2 *(From the National Heart Lung and Blood Institute, Washington, DC.)*

(Ferreira & Weems, 2008). On the other hand, routine consumption of moderate amounts of alcohol may produce positive effects. Snow indicates that these benefits may not appear until middle age for women and possibly later for men (Snow et al., 2009). And someday, an anti-inflammatory compound in red wine, known as resveratrol, may help reduce the risk of heart disease.

Supplements

Randomized controlled studies have found that nutritional supplements may be helpful when dietary intake of certain nutrients is not adequate. They may even help in reducing the risk of stroke, depression, and macular degeneration. However, studies report less evidence that supplements can delay cardiovascular disease, cancer, and age-related cognitive changes. Making small changes in the intake of fatty fish and fish oil could reduce the risk of sudden cardiac death. And fish oil supplements at high doses can help lower serum triglyceride levels (Buhr & Bales, 2009, 2010).

Above all, keep in mind that dietary supplements are not regulated in the ways that drugs are regulated. The maker of a dietary supplement is not required to prove the product is safe or effective before marketing it (National Center for Complementary and Alternative Medicine, 2010). However, supplements—especially herbal supplements—may have powerful effects. They may mimic drug effects, and they may interact with prescribed drugs. Always urge patients to tell health-care providers about any dietary supplements they take.

Summary

Because our energy needs decrease as we age, it can be a challenge to meet macronutrient and micronutrient needs in fewer calories. Age-related changes indicate a need to increase calcium, vitamin D, folate, vitamin B_6, vitamin B_{12}, and riboflavin. More research is indicated to evaluate whether there are age-related changes affecting the nutritional needs of vitamin K and niacin.

Appropriate carbohydrate, protein, fat, vitamin, and mineral needs plus adequate hydration and a good fiber intake will provide for nutritionally healthy aging. Participating in an active lifestyle, including exercise and socializing, completes the prescription for healthy aging. Except for the previously mentioned nutritional supplements, other supplements are not routinely recommended. A general multivitamin would be reasonable for the aging adult.

Choosing a diet low in calories and high in nutrient-dense foods, along with a routine exercise regimen, choosing not to smoke, and having a happy lifestyle is what Everitt and colleagues (2006) recommend as the path to delay aging. Kennedy (2006) agrees that starting a healthy diet early in life and maintaining regular exercise with a focus on prevention is the way to promote wellness. Samples of questions to ask and tools for evaluating the aging adult's diet can be found in *Duyff's Complete Food and Nutrition Guide* (Duyff, 2006).

KEY POINTS

- As we age, we have less lean body mass and total body water and decreased bone density while we have a higher percentage of fat.
- The largest sensory change we experience is a decrease in smell.
- With aging, calorie needs decrease and protein needs increase.
- Carbohydrate, fat, water, and fiber needs remain the same.
- Age-related changes affect the needs for calcium, vitamin D, folate, vitamin B_6, vitamin B_{12}, and riboflavin.
- Snacking can be beneficial to the aging adult.
- Good dental health is an important part of good nutrition.
- Variety in food choices includes a rainbow of colors in fruits and vegetables.

CRITICAL THINKING ACTIVITIES

1. Picture yourself at age 80. What shape will you be in physically? Where will you live? A city? A town? A rural area?
2. Will you be able to prepare your own meals? Do you have arthritis? If you cannot prepare meals, how will you ensure that you are eating well?
3. Will you be able to purchase your own groceries? If yes, do you have the income to purchase the foods you need and want? If not, how will you obtain your groceries?
4. Are you still driving? If not how do you get to the grocery store?
5. Will you still have all of your own teeth, or will you have dentures? If you have dentures, when

will be the last time you got a new pair or had your current dentures fitted? Do you need changes in the texture or consistency of food to eat it?

6. Do you have any chronic diseases that require a special diet? Do you need to limit sodium, salt, concentrated sweets, sugar, or certain types of fat in your diet?
7. Do you live alone? Do you invite family, friends, or neighbors to eat with you? Do you accept invitations to eat with family, friends, or neighbors?

CASE STUDY | *JOHN D*

John D is a 75-year-old man who was diagnosed with hypertension and diabetes 15 years ago. Since that time, John's wife has been responsible for all grocery shopping and food preparation. Four months ago, John's wife died, and John is now living alone in the one-level home they shared for 40 years. His two children and their families live within 15 miles. Since his wife's death, John has been eating his midday meal, Monday through Friday, at a local diner. Usually, he has the blue plate special. This commonly is chicken and dumplings, beef stew, a Rueben sandwich, or a hamburger and French fries. He usually has a piece of cake or pie for dessert. For breakfast, John has toast and coffee at home. For supper, he has cold cereal and milk. In the refrigerator, he has eggs, hot dogs, lunch meat, canned biscuits, whole milk, buttermilk, ice cream, cookies, and some frozen dinners he heats in the microwave. He also keeps bananas and orange juice on hand.

Although John has lost 10 pounds since his wife's death, he still weighs 190 pounds. At 5 feet 8 inches, his current weight gives him a body mass index of 28.9—about 25 pounds over his ideal weight. He walks from his home to the mailbox at the end of the sidewalk daily. He gets little exercise other than this. Although his children live nearby, they are busy with their families. They talk to him about three times a week, and they visit about once a month. John can drive, has his own car, and can do his own grocery shopping.

1. What do you see as risks in John's routine diet?
2. What social issues do you think would affect his food intake?
3. What does John need to omit from his diet?
4. What does he need to add to his routine food intake?

REFERENCES

Administration on Aging. (2010). *Profile of older Americans.* Washington, DC: U.S. Department of Health & Human Services. Retrieved December 13, 2010, from http://www.aoa.gov/AoARoot/Aging_Statistics/Profile/index.aspx

Buhr, G., & Bales C. W. (2009) Nutritional supplements for older adults: Review and recommendations—Part 1. *Journal of Nutrition for the Elderly, 28*(1), 5–29.

Buhr, G., & Bales, C.W. (2010) Nutritional supplements for older adults: Review and Recommendations – Part 2. *Journal of Nutrition for the Elderly, 29*(1) pp 42-71.

Campbell, W. W., & Leidy, H. J. (2007). Dietary protein and resistance training: Effects on muscle and body composition in older persons. *Journal of the American College of Nutrition, 256*(6), 696S–703S.

Chernoff, R. (Ed.). (2006). *Geriatric nutrition: The health professional's handbook* (3rd ed.). Sudbury, MA: Jones & Bartlett Learning.

Chernoff, R. (2006). Carbohydrate, fat, and fluid requirements in older adults. In R. Chernoff (Ed.). *Geriatric nutrition: The health professional's handbook* (3rd ed., pp. 23–30). Sudbury, MA: Jones & Bartlett Learning.

Duffy, V. B., & Chapo, A. K. (2006). Smell, taste, and somatosensation in the elderly. In R. Chernoff (Ed.), *Geriatric nutrition: The health professional's handbook* (3rd ed., pp. 115–162). Sudbury, MA: Jones & Bartlett Learning.

Duyff, R. L. (2006). For mature adults healthful eating! In R. Duyff (Ed.), *American Dietetic Association complete food and nutrition guide* (pp. 458–478). Hoboken, NJ: Wiley.

Everitt, A. V., Hilmer, S. N., Brand-Miller, J. C., Jamieson, H. A., Truswell, A. S., Sharma, A. P., . . . Le Couteur, D.G. (2006). Dietary approaches that delay age-related diseases. *Journal of Clinical Interventions in Aging, 1*(1), 11–31.

Federal Interagency Forum on Aging-Related Statistics. (2010). *Older Americans 2010: Key indicators of well-being.* Washington, DC: Author. Retrieved December 10, 2010, from http://www.agingstats.gov/agingstatsdotnet/Main_Site/Data/2010_Documents/Docs/OA_2010.pdf

Ferreira, M. P., & Weems, M. K. (2008). Alcohol consumption by aging adults in the United States: Health benefits and detriments. *Journal of the American Dietetic Association, 108*(10), 1668–1676.

Johnston, R. E., & Chernoff, R. (2003). Geriatrics. In L. Matarese & M Gottschlich (Eds.), *Contemporary nutrition support practice: A clinical guide* (pp. 376–383). St. Louis, MO: Saunders.

Kennedy, E. T. (2006). Evidence of nutritional benefits in prolonging wellness. *American Journal of Clinical Nutrition, 83*(4), 410S–414S.

Moritsugu, K. P. (2007). Healthy aging starts with healthful eating. *Journal of the American Dietetic Association, 107*(5), 723.

National Center for Complementary and Alternative Medicine. (2010). *Using dietary supplements wisely.* Washington, DC: National Institutes of Health. Retrieved December 13, 2010, from http://nccam.nih.gov/health/supplements/wiseuse.htm

Snow, W. M., Murray, R., Ekuma, O., Tyas, S., & Barnes, G. E.. (2009). Alcohol use and cardiovascular health outcomes: A comparison across age and gender in the Winnipeg health and drinking survey cohort. *Age and Ageing, 38,* 206–212.

Suter, P. (2006). Vitamin, metabolism and requirements in the elderly: Selected aspects. In R. Chernoff (Ed.), *Geriatric nutrition: The health professional's handbook* (3rd ed., pp. 31–76). Sudbury, MA: Jones & Bartlett Learning.

Welman, N. S. (2007). Prevention, prevention, prevention: Nutrition for successful aging. *Journal of the American Dietetic Association, 107*(5), 741–743.

Wolfe, R. R., Miller, S. L., & Miller K. B. (2008). Optimal protein intake in the elderly. *Clinical Nutrition, 27,* 675–684.

U.S. Department of Agriculture. (2010a). *Interactive DRI for healthcare professionals.* Retrieved November 9, 2010, from http://fnic.nal.usda.gov/nal_display/index.php?info_center=4&tax_level=2&tax_subject=256&topic_id=1342

U.S. Department of Agriculture. (2010b). *MyPyramid.gov: Steps to a healthier you.* Retrieved December 13, 2010, from http://www.mypyramid.gov/

Zizza, C. A., Ariswalla, D. D., & Ellison, K. J. (2010). Contribution of snacking to older adults' vitamin, carotenoid, and mineral intakes. *Journal of the American Dietetic Association, 110*(5), 768–772.

Zizza, C. A., Tayie, F. A., & Lino, M. (2007). Benefits of snacking in older Americans. *Journal of the American Dietetic Association, 107*(5), 800–806.

Chapter 15

Using Medications Safely and Effectively

Chris Shea, PharmD, CGP, and Heather Townsend

LEARNING OBJECTIVES

- Appreciate the significant risks that prescription and over-the-counter (OTC) medications pose for older adults.
- Distinguish the differences between adverse drug events and common side effects.
- Discuss the age-related physiological changes that place older adults at risk for medication-related problems.
- List specific medications that are potentially harmful to older adults.
- Describe ways to help older adults improve the daily management of their medications.

Adverse Drug Events

The increasing longevity among older adults in recent years has resulted in part from advancements in pharmacology. However, in addition to extending life and improving its quality, drugs also may result in adverse events and side effects. What's more, adverse drug effects disproportionately affect older adults. Although older adults make up less than 15% of the American population, they use more than 30% of the drugs prescribed and sustain 33.6% of severe adverse drug events (Malone & Bhandary, 2001).

A serious adverse drug event, as defined by the Food and Drug Administration (FDA), is one that results in death, disability, or hospitalization; is life-threatening; or requires intervention to prevent harm. If adverse drug events were classified as a distinct disease, it would be ranked as the fifth leading cause of death in the United States. The FDA reported in 2007 that adverse drug events more than doubled between 1998 and 2005, as did the deaths associated with those adverse events (Moore, Cohen, & Furberg, 2007). More than 465,000 serious adverse drug events were reported during that time, and the number of fatal adverse drug events increased from 5,519 to 15,107. Although almost 1,500 drugs were linked to adverse drug events, 43.6% of those adverse events resulted from only 51 drugs.

If adverse drug events were classified as a distinct disease, it would be ranked as the fifth leading cause of death in the United States.

Of the top 15 drugs linked most often to *fatalities,* four are opioid pain relievers and three are antipsychotics (commonly used in older adults to treat behaviors related to dementia). Tylenol (acetaminophen) was number 5 on the list. The top 15 drugs linked most often to *disability* or *serious outcomes* included estrogens, insulin, antidepressants, cholesterol-lowering drugs, and anticoagulants. Many of the drugs identified in fatal or serious events also top the list of most prescribed drugs. As you can see, older adults carry a disproportionate burden of the adverse drug events (Moore, Cohen, & Furberg, 2007) (Box 15-1).

So, what is a side effect, and how might it differ from an adverse drug event? Side effects may also be serious, but most often they are well-documented, unintended events that can occur even when a drug is maintained at what would be considered an acceptable or normal dose. Many times a side effect resolves at a lower dose; in some cases, however, the drug may need to be stopped completely.

BOX 15-1 Identifying Inappropriate Drugs

Two resources are available to help nurses and other health care providers identify drugs that may be inappropriate for adults over age 65. The Beers criteria were created by a panel of pharmacists and geriatric experts. They list medications that may be ineffective, may pose an unnecessary risk, or should be avoided because a safer alternative exists. Dose, duration, and possible interaction with other diseases or conditions are also considered. The Beers list includes more than 40 drugs or classifications of drugs, the concerns about each drug, and a rating for the degree of risk (Fisk et al., 2003). See the "Try This" series for a copy of this list (http://consultgerirn.org/uploads/File/trythis/try_this_16_1.pdf).

More recently, the *Screening Tool of Older Persons' Potentially Inappropriate Prescriptions* (STOPP) was developed for adults over age 65 (Hamilton, Gallagher, & O'Mahony, 2009). STOPP includes drugs with adverse effects that were clearly related to the hospital admission of 715 older adults (Gallagher & O'Mahony, 2009).

In a comparison of the Beers and STOPP lists, Gallagher and O'Mahony reported that the "STOPP criteria identified a significantly higher proportion of Irish patients requiring hospitalization as a result of PIM [potentially inappropriate medications]-related adverse events than Beers's criteria" (p. 673).

To compare an adverse drug event to a side effect, let's take a look at the common anti-inflammatory and pain-relieving medication ibuprofen. Some adverse drug events associated with ibuprofen could be gastrointestinal (GI) bleeding, myocardial infarction, stroke, congestive heart failure, and kidney damage. Some common side effects of ibuprofen are nausea, abdominal pain, headache, dizziness, fluid retention, and bruising. Despite the evidence supporting the link between medications and longevity, there is the obvious concern that many of these medications can be as harmful as they are helpful.

Age-Related Physiological Changes

The aging body can be both very dynamic and frail. Older adults often have little or no physiological reserve, which is the body's ability to respond under stress. Reduced physiological reserve may affect the body as a whole or an individual organ's ability to continue functioning under stress. As a natural part of aging, physiological reserves begin declining in the 40s, a decline that may produce profound changes by the time people reach their 60s and 70s (Resnick & Marcantonio, 1997). Many factors can diminish physiological reserve in addition to the normal aging process. For example, smoking diminishes respiratory and cardiovascular reserve. A stroke may diminish neurological reserve. Medications also may be a significant source of added stress that can tip an older adult from a healthy state to an unhealthy one (Walston, Hadley, & Ferrucci, 2006).

Keep in mind that physiological and chronological age may be inconsistent. How many times have you been surprised to find out how old or young a person really was? If you could look inside the body, you would likely find the same scenario. You might be surprised to find that age-related changes may vary between organ systems in the same person. For example, one person may have decreased kidney function and a fully functional liver. We especially need to be mindful of these age-related changes when drugs are introduced into the system. A particular organ system may be operating well enough to maintain adequate function until an added drug stresses the system. To help explain this process, the following sections look at what the body does to drugs (the pharmacokinetics) and what changes take place in the body to alter its ability to process those drugs (the pharmacodynamics).

Altered Pharmacokinetics

Pharmacokinetics is what the body does to a medication and is composed of four basic actions:

- *Absorption:* How the drug gets into the body
- *Distribution:* Where the drug goes once it gets into the body
- *Metabolism:* How the drug is processed by the body
- *Excretion:* How the drug is eliminated from the body

Absorption

A drug can enter the body via several avenues: orally, buccally (via the oral mucosa), topically, rectally, and parenterally (subcutaneously, intramuscularly, and intravenously). Age-related changes in absorption rarely present a clinical challenge, and adverse drug events rarely result from altered drug absorption.

Distribution

Once a drug gets into the body, it either travels to fatty tissue or remains in the body's fluid compartments (circulatory system and fluid around the cells). If a drug favors fatty tissue (such as the antianxiety drug diazepam), it will travel out of the circulatory system and concentrate in the fatty tissues. On the other hand, if a drug favors the fluid compartment (such as the antihypertensive atenolol), it will preferentially remain in the bloodstream and in the fluid that surrounds the cells.

As we age, we have a 25% to 30% increase in body fat and a corresponding decrease in body water and lean muscle mass, which may affect drug actions. Consequently, drugs that concentrate in fatty tissues may take significantly longer to exit the body, and the duration of action for those drugs may be significantly extended. In drugs that prefer the fluid compartment, serum concentrations can be greatly increased. In either scenario, age-related alterations in distribution can lead to significant adverse drug events and increase the risk that an older adult could develop adverse effects at doses that are therapeutic in other age groups.

Metabolism

The liver is the main site of drug metabolism (Table 15-1). Although other tissues contain many of the same enzymes involved in metabolism, these enzymes are much more concentrated in the liver. The rate at which a drug is metabolized varies greatly among people and may be influenced by several factors, including genetics and the physiological changes of aging. Blood flow to the liver can decrease by up to 50% in older adults, which can dramatically decrease the initial processing of some drugs (known as first-pass metabolism) and thus extend their duration of action. Also, the enzyme system responsible for metabolizing medications is more easily saturated (Merck Manuals, 2010).

Typically, metabolism inactivates a drug. However, there are instances in which metabolism alters the drug, rendering it an active substance rather than an inactive one. Also, when a drug undergoes processing by the liver, by products or metabolites are often formed that may be active or inactive.

TABLE 15-1 Commonly Prescribed Medications Extensively Metabolized by the Liver

CLASS	MEDICATIONS	CONCERN
Acid reducers	Proton pump inhibitors: Prilosec, Nexium, Acidphex	Headache, dizziness, abdominal pain, nausea, back pain
Analgesics	Acetaminophen	Worsen liver function
	Tramadol	Dizziness, somnolence, seizure, nausea, vomiting, irritability
Anticoagulants	Coumadin	Accumulation: increase bleeding risk
Anticonvulsants	Depakote	Worsen liver function, tremors, dizziness, somnolence, nervousness, abdominal pain
Antidepressants	Amitriptyline	Anticholinergic SE, cardiovascular toxicities, falls
	Celexa, Lexapro, Prozac, Paxil, Zoloft	Accumulation: fatigue, confusion, anorexia, tremors, nausea, agitation, irritability, insomnia
	Effexor, Cymbalta	Accumulation: hypertension, fatigue, confusion, anorexia, tremors, nausea, agitation, irritability, insomnia
Antidiabetics	Metformin	Accumulation: headache, nausea, diarrhea, lactic acidosis
	glyburide, glipizide	Accumulation: prolonged hypoglycemia, diarrhea, nausea, headache

TABLE 15-1 Commonly Prescribed Medications Extensively Metabolized by the Liver—cont'd

CLASS	MEDICATIONS	CONCERN
Antihyperlipidemics	Statins: Lescol, Lipitor, Pravachol, and Zocor	Worsen liver function, muscle pain and weakness
Antihypertensives	Verapamil	Accumulation: bradycardia, hypotension, dizziness, edema, severe constipation
	Amlodipine	Accumulation: hypotension, dizziness, edema, nausea, fatigue
Antiinflammatory analgesics	Naproxen, Celebrex	Accumulation: increased potential for renal failure, GI upset, ulcers, GI bleeding, edema
Antipsychotics	Risperdal, Seroquel, Zyprexa	Accumulation: sedation, dizziness, tremor, tachycardia
Anxiolytics	Benzodiazepines: diazepam, lorazepam, clonazepam	Accumulation: increased sedation, weakness, falls and fractures

GI, gastrointestinal; SE, side effects.

From Potentially harmful drugs in the elderly: Beers list and more. (2007, September). *Pharmacist's Letter/Prescriber's Letter, 23*(9):230907. Retrieved from http://www.pharmacistsletter.com/(S(d5v5aw55o12014i4jhsksm3f))/pl/ArticleDD.aspx?rn=1&cs=&s=PL&pt=6&fpt=56&dd=230907&pb=PL#dd

Active metabolites can exert either desired or undesired actions in the body.

Drugs can be processed by several different mechanisms in the liver, all of which ultimately prepare the drug for excretion. Many drug-drug interactions take place here and result from each drug competing for the liver's attention. For example, suppose that drug A and drug B are both introduced into the body. Both require metabolism by the liver before they can be inactivated and packaged for excretion. However, drug A has preference in the liver for metabolism over drug B. Therefore, while drug A is being processed by the liver, drug B continues to circulate in the system, exerting its effects at a higher concentration than desired and for a longer duration than desired. This higher concentration and longer duration of action can stress the body beyond its physiological reserve and lead to a side effect or adverse drug effect. Having an appreciation for possible drug-drug interactions can help anticipate and avoid drug-related issues in older adults.

Excretion

Once a drug is absorbed and distributes to either the fatty tissues or fluid compartments and is metabolized by the liver, the last step is where and how the drug is eliminated from the body. Most drugs and their active or inactive metabolites are excreted by the kidneys. This elimination can become problematic with age because the most dramatic consequences of age-related physiological changes are often experienced in the kidneys (Table 15-2). Blood flow to the kidneys decreases by about 10% per decade, and overall kidney function declines by nearly 50% by age 75 to 80. This decrease in kidney function corresponds with a decreased ability to excrete medications and metabolites, which in turn can lead to the accumulation of these substances and an increased risk of elevated serum drug levels, side effects, and adverse effects.

Altered Pharmacodynamics

Pharmacodynamics is the physiological response to a drug or, more simply, what the drug does to the body. Because of age-related changes, some drug effects are increased and some are decreased. Older adults typically become much more sensitive to drugs because of these pharmacodynamic changes. The central nervous system often becomes the most vulnerable as the blood-brain barrier becomes more permeable. Several drug classes impact the central nervous system and may produce a profound response to what would otherwise be considered a normal dose in a younger patient.

For example, opioid analgesics can produce the same level of pain relief in an elderly patient as in

TABLE 15-2 Common Medications That Require Dose Adjustments in Diminished Kidney Function

CLASS	MEDICATION	CONCERN
Acid reducers	Zantac Pepcid	Accumulation: confusion
Analgesics	opioid and opioid like: meperidine, propoxyphene, tramadol, morphine, codeine	Accumulation: sedation, drowsiness, dizziness, lethargy, fatigue, confusion, respiratory depression, seizure
Antiarrhythmics	Digoxin	Accumulation: anorexia, visual changes, bradycardia
Antibiotics	Cipro	Accumulation: tendonitis and tendon rupture increased risk in those > 60, agitation, confusion
	Keflex, Bactrim	Accumulation: nausea, vomiting, liver damage
Antidepressants	Effexor, Cymbalta	Accumulation: hypertension, fatigue, confusion, anorexia, tremors, nausea, agitation, irritability
Antidiabetic	Metformin	Accumulation: headache, nausea, diarrhea, lactic acidosis
	Glyburide, glimepiride	Accumulation: prolonged hypoglycemia, diarrhea, nausea, headache
Antifungal	Fluconazole	Accumulation: dizziness, seizures
Antigout	Allopurinol	Accumulation: nausea, diarrhea, somnolence
Antihistamines	Cetirizine, loratadine, fexofenadine	Nervousness, fatigue, malaise
Antihypertensives	Atenolol	Accumulation: bradycardia, hypotension
Cholesterol-lowering agents	Statins: Crestor, Mevacor, Pravachol	Accumulation: headache, nausea, diarrhea, muscle pain/weakness
Anti-inflammatory analgesics	meloxicam, naproxen, piroxicam	Worsening renal function, edema, dyspepsia, abdominal pain, nausea, vomiting

a younger patient but may require half the dose. This is especially true for drugs designed to act on the central nervous system, such as antidepressants, sedatives, and antipsychotics. When adding a new drug to an older adult's regimen, the adage of *start low and go slow* is one of the best ways to minimize the risk of adverse effects or side effects. If the initial dose is started low and adjusted slowly, it may provide time to respond before an adverse effect or side effect becomes overwhelming to the system.

Drugs Potentially Harmful in Older Adults

As you can see, many drugs may be harmful to or inappropriate in older adults. Many drugs have been identified as potentially harmful based on their pharmacokinetic and pharmacodynamic characteristics, by accumulating in the body, providing an extended duration of action, or crossing the blood-brain barrier more easily (Table 15-3). In addition to these characteristics, drugs with anticholinergic activity often top the list of drugs that pose harm to older adults.

TABLE 15-3 Potentially Harmful Medications for Use in Geriatric Patients

CLASS	MEDICATION	CONCERN
Analgesics	Darvocet (propoxyphene w/ acetaminophen)	Accumulation leading to potential cardiovascular toxicities
Antidepressants	Elavil (amitriptyline) Sinequan (doxepin) Tofranil (imipramine)	Anticholinergic activity, cardiovascular toxicities
	Prozac (fluoxetine)	Extended duration of action, agitation, insomnia, anorexia
Antihistamines	Benadryl (diphenhydramine), Vistaril (hydroxyzine)	Anticholinergic activity
Antihypertensives	Alpha 1 blockers: Cardura(doxazosin), Minipress (prazosin), Hytrin (terazosin)	Hypotension, falls
Antipsychotics	Zyprexa (olanzapine)	Glucose dysregulation
Anxiolytics	Long-acting benzodiazepines: Librium (chlordiazepoxide), Valium (diazepam)	Prolonged sedation, confusion, falls, fractures, respiratory depression
	Short-acting benzodiazepines: Xanax (alprazolam) Ativan (lorazepam) Serax (oxazepam)	Sedation, confusion, falls, fractures
Corticosteroids	Prednisone, prednisolone, etc.	Worsening glucose control in patients with diabetes
Muscle relaxants	Soma (carisoprodol), Flexeril (cyclobenzaprine), Skelaxin (metaxalone), Robaxin (methocarbamol)	Anticholinergic activity
NSAIDs	Aleve, Naprosyn (naproxen), Feldene (piroxicam) Motrin, Advil (ibuprofen)	GI bleeding, ulcers, renal failure, hypertension, heart failure, MI
Stimulant drugs	Amphetamines, methylphenidate	Hypertension, myocardial ischemia, CNS stimulation, appetite suppression, seizures
Urinary drugs	Ditropan (oxybutynin) Detrol (toterodine)	Anticholinergic activity
Supplements	Iron (ferrous sulfate > 325 mg daily) Calcium	Constipation

CNS, central nervous system; GI, gastrointestinal; MI, myocardial infarction; NSAIDs, nonsteroidal antiinflammatory drugs.

Adapted from Fick, D. M, Cooper, J. W., Wade, W. E., Waller JL, Maclean JR, Beers MH. (2003). Updating the Beers criteria for potentially inappropriate medication use in older adults. *Archives of Internal Medicine, 163,* 2716–2724, and Potentially harmful drugs in the elderly: Beers list and more. (2007). *Pharmacist's Letter/Prescriber's Letter, 23*(9), 230907. Retrieved from http://www.pharmacistsletter.com/(S(d5v5aw55o12014i4jhsksm3f))/pl/ArticleDD.aspx?rn=1&cs=&s=PL&pt=6&fpt=56&dd=230907&pb=PL#dd

Acetylcholine is a neurotransmitter found in many body systems, including the cardiovascular system, GI tract, urinary tract, respiratory tract, and central nervous system. Drugs that block the effects of acetylcholine are called anticholinergics. Some drugs are designed specifically as anticholinergics, such as those used to treat urinary incontinence (Ditropan or Detrol). However, many others have anticholinergic activity as a side effect to their intended action. Some of the common antidepressants (Paxil, amitriptyline), skeletal muscle relaxants (cyclobenzaprine), antihypertensives (clonidine), and antihistamines (diphenhydramine) have anticholinergic activity.

In many instances these drugs alone would not produce a significant amount of anticholinergic activity. However, it is not uncommon for older adults to be taking multiple drugs with anticholinergic effects. Unfortunately, most of the serious adverse drug events and side effects from anticholinergic activity can manifest in essentially every body system, with the central nervous system impacted the most (Table 15-4).

Lastly, some drugs commonly prescribed to older adults require very close monitoring to maintain a delicate balance between effectiveness and toxicity or another adverse drug event. In other words, these drugs have a narrow range between their benefits and their risks. These drugs, commonly said to have a narrow therapeutic index, include digoxin, warfarin, theophylline, phenytoin, and levothyroxine, among others (Table 15-5). Although normal serum levels have been established for these drugs, older adults may develop toxic effects even at the normal or therapeutic level. Older patients should be cautioned against altering their use of such drugs without consulting the prescriber. They also should be instructed to contact the prescriber or their healthcare provider if they have unexpected changes in weight, mental status, or appetite, or if a new medication is added to the regimen. Drugs with a narrow therapeutic index should never be shared, borrowed, or stored for future use.

Administering Drugs to Older Adults

One of the primary roles a nurse can play in the care of older adults is administering drugs. Providing medications to an older adult can present several challenges depending on the route of administration. These include the oral, enteral, parenteral, mucosal, and percutaneous routes.

TABLE 15-4 Body Systems Adversely Affected by Anticholinergic Medications

SYSTEM	EFFECT	CONCERN
Cardiovascular	Hypotension Palpitations Tachycardia Arrhythmias	Falls, fractures
Urinary tract	Dysuria Urinary retention	Incontinence, increased risk for UTI
Gastrointestinal tract	Constipation Abdominal discomfort Dry mouth/mucous membranes	Toxic megacolon, Perforation leading to peritonitis
Central nervous system	Confusion Delirium Hallucinations Restlessness Drowsiness Dizziness Blurred vision	Falls, fractures

UTI, urinary tract infection.

Adapted from O'Neill, M. J. (2006). *The Merck index: An encyclopedia of chemicals, drugs, and biologicals* (14th ed.). Whitehouse Station, NJ: Merck & Co., Inc. and Potentially harmful drugs in the elderly: Beers list and more. (2007). *Pharmacist's Letter/Prescriber's Letter, 23*(9), 230907. Retrieved from http://www.pharmacistsletter.com/(S(d5v5aw55o12014i4jhsksm3f))/pl/ArticleDD.aspx?rn=1&cs=&s=PL&pt=6&fpt=56&dd=230907&pb=PL#dd

TABLE 15-5 Drugs with a Narrow Therapeutic Index

DRUG	INDICATION	MONITORING PARAMETER AND GOAL	TOXIC EFFECTS (ELEVATED LEVEL)
Digoxin (Rathore et al., 2003)	Heart failure, arrhythmia	Digoxin level *Goal:* 0.5–1.2 ng/mL	Confusion, nausea/vomiting, appetite/weight loss, blurred or yellowing of vision, and arrhythmias
Warfarin	Leg/lung clots, arrhythmia, heart valve replacements	Protime/INR *Goal:* 2–3 (2.5–3.5)	Bleeding
Theophylline	Bronchitis, asthma	Theophylline level *Goal:* 5–15 mcg/mL	Mood changes, muscle cramping/tremors, repetitive vomiting, arrhythmias, and seizure
Phenytoin	Seizure, head trauma	Phenytoin level *Goal:* 10–20 Needs to be corrected for albumin level < 3.7 Corrected level = serum phenytoin level ÷ [(0.1 x albumin) + 0.1]	Altered mental status, slurred speech, appetite/weight loss, nausea/vomiting, falls and unsteady gait, arrhythmia
Levothyroxine	Hypothyroidism	Free T_4, thyroid-stimulating hormone (TSH) *TSH Goal:* 1–3	High level—fatigue, hair loss, sedation, confusion, weight loss or gain Low level—arrhythmias, weight loss, anxiety/agitation

INR, international normalized ratio.
Some information from Pope, N. D. (2009). Generic substitution of narrow therapeutic index drugs. *US Pharmacist, 34*(6; Generic Drug Review Suppl.), 12–19.

Routes of Administration

Oral

The oral route encompasses all drug formulations (tablet, capsule, or liquid) that are provided by mouth and absorbed by the GI tract. This is the preferred route of administration for most drugs because the rate and extent of absorption typically remain very reliable even as we age. However, other routes of administration are used when a patient is unable to take anything orally, possibly due to the inability to swallow, or a drug is not absorbed from the GI tract because of a disease process or the drug's chemical structure.

Enteral

The enteral route also makes use of the GI tract for drug absorption but bypasses the oral route, commonly because the patient is unable to swallow. Many tablets can be crushed or the contents of capsules can be given directly into the stomach by gastrostomy tube (Box 15-2). Providing medications rectally, such as by suppository, is also considered the enteral route because absorption from the GI tract is maintained.

Parenteral

The parenteral route mainly involves administering a drug into a vein (intravenous), muscle (intramuscular), artery (intraarterial), or the fatty tissue beneath the skin (subcutaneous). The parenteral routes are often used when a drug cannot be given via the GI tract, is not absorbed from the GI tract, or would be absorbed too slowly from the GI tract.

Percutaneous

Several drugs are formulated to be given percutaneously or via the skin. Many of these drugs come in the form of a patch and are absorbed slowly and directly through the skin and into the bloodstream.

BOX 15-2 The Rules of Extended Release

Many drugs are formulated to release a dose over an extended period of time (12–24 hours), or they have a special coating (called an enteric coating) that protects the drug from stomach acid. Slow-release and enteric-coated drug formulations should not be crushed before administering them, and patients should be cautioned not to chew them. Crushing or chewing could cause a slow-release drug to be delivered too quickly, placing the patient at risk for adverse effects or toxicity. Crushing an enteric-coated drug may expose it to stomach acid and render it ineffective.

Comprehensive lists of drugs that should not be crushed or chewed are readily available. One such list has been compiled by the Institute for Safe Medication Practices and can be found at http://www.ismp.org/tools/donotcrush.pdf.

Male and female hormones (estrogens, progesterones, and testosterone) are often formulated as patches to slow the rate of metabolism by the liver. A disadvantage to giving drugs percutaneously in older adults is that age-related alterations in the skin can cause the drug to be absorbed erratically, making its effects difficult to predict.

Mucosal

In this route, the drug is absorbed through the oral mucosa, respiratory mucosa (nasal cavity and bronchioles), or vaginal mucosa. Some drugs are designed to be absorbed from the oral mucosa so the drug bypasses the acidic environment in the stomach. However, most drugs designed for mucosal absorption provide action at the site of absorption. Nasal sprays for allergies, inhaled drugs for respiratory diseases, and vaginal suppositories are examples of the types of drugs designed for mucosal absorption. This route can be a challenge in older adults because the mucous membranes may grow less moist, and because older adults are more likely to take drugs that dry the mucous membranes (such as diuretics and anticholinergics). If the mucous membrane is not moist, a mucosal drug probably will not dissolve well or be absorbed optimally.

Five Rights

Above all, remember that the core of accurate drug administration is the five "rights," which include:

- Right patient
- Right drug
- Right dose
- Right time
- Right route

Each is crucial to ensuring patients receive the appropriate drug therapy. Many of the medication errors that result in harm stem from preventable errors in administration.

Particularly for older adults, keep in mind that many drugs have specific times of administration. For example, some drugs used to treat osteoporosis, such as risedronate (Actonel) and alendronate (Fosamax), have very specific times of administration recommended by the manufacturer to maximize the drug's efficacy. Some common cholesterol-lowering medications, known as statins, may require administration at bedtime to coincide with the body's cholesterol production, which occurs primarily when we sleep.

Also, many drugs can be given by different routes. For instance, the antinausea medication promethazine, and many of the opioid pain medications, such as morphine, can be given orally, enterally (by gastrostomy tube), parenterally (intramuscular or intravenous), or rectally. In some cases, as with promethazine, the dose may stay the same regardless of the route of administration. In other cases, as with morphine, giving an oral dose by the intravenous route could be fatal. Remember that accurate drug administration is crucial to limiting adverse drug effects and is one of the nurse's most critical areas of practice.

Managing Self-Medication

Many people, especially older adults, purchase over-the-counter (OTC) medications at their local pharmacies before going to the effort and expense of a medical appointment for such everyday annoyances as aches and pains, heartburn, constipation, insomnia, or the common cold. More than 100,000 OTC medications are available in the United States today, and older adults are their leading consumers, purchasing 40% of all OTC products (Berardi, 2002). About 90% of all patients over age 65 take at least one prescription drug; 50% to 90% take at least one OTC or dietary supplement; and 50% take more than five prescription drugs, OTC products, or supplements (Qato et al., 2008). One in eight older adults (about 13%) takes five or more OTC products or supplements (Qato et al., 2008). About 40% of older adults believe that OTC products are too weak to cause real harm (Roumie & Griffin, 2004).

About 40% of older adults believe that OTC products are too weak to cause real harm.

The use of multiple drugs by older adults is of great concern because of altered pharmacokinetics and pharmacodynamics from impaired kidney and liver function and multiple comorbidities. Self-medication and polypharmacy (the use of multiple medications) increases the risk of adverse drug effects and interactions and may worsen current disease states, including heart disease, prostate enlargement, and glaucoma. It may even cause life-threatening illnesses such as GI bleeding. One nursing facility found that for every $1 spent on medications, another $1.30 was spent on treating adverse drug effects (Zarowitz, Stebelsky, Muma, Romain, & Peterson, 2005).

Efforts should be taken by health professionals to inquire about a patient's use of OTC and dietary and herbal supplements. One study found that less than 5% of all OTC products being taken by those admitted to the hospital were documented (Oborne & Luzac, 2005). Understanding the most common OTC products and their possible interactions and adverse effects will improve the health and safety of older adults by allowing the health professional to better assess and evaluate the patient. OTC products and supplements commonly used by older adults include sleep aids, analgesics, antacids, gastric acid inhibitors, constipation remedies, cough and cold products, and certain herbal supplements.

Sleep Aids

The prevalence of insomnia in the elderly is reported to be 20% to 40% (Sateia, Doghramji, Huari, & Morin, 2000). The National Sleep Foundation (2008) poll found that 9% of respondents used OTC or herbal sleep aids to self-medicate. Most OTC or supplemental sleep aids contain antihistamines such as diphenhydramine or doxylamine, valerian root, and melatonin.

Antihistamines

Antihistamine sleep aids include Unisom, Tylenol PM, Benadryl, Sominex, and Nytol. These products have been proven to reduce the number of awakenings during the night (Glass, Sproule, Herrmann, & Busto, 2008) and to be effective in treating insomnia in those previously not treated when used for less than 2 weeks (Glass et al., 2003; Yudo & Kurihara, 1990). In many people taking antihistamine sleep aids, tolerance to the sedating effects will develop over a few days (Richardson et al., 2002).

Antihistamines may cause substantial adverse effects. These products have high anticholinergic activity, which may result in confusion, hallucinations, weakness, falls, urine retention, constipation, and arrhythmias. They also may cause significant daytime sedation and altered mental status, although this is more common with doxylamine (Unisom) because of its long half-life (Box 15-3). Antihistamines may worsen many disease states, including arrhythmias (such as atrial fibrillation), benign prostatic hypertrophy, glaucoma, and constipation, and they may cause frequent urinary tract infections in older adults.

EVIDENCE FOR PRACTICE
Anticholinergics and Cognitive Decline

Purpose: To determine if drugs with anticholinergic properties contribute to cognitive decline and dementia in community-dwelling older adults.

Sample: The sample included 4,128 women and 2,784 men age 65 or older.

Methods: Cognitive performance, clinical diagnosis of dementia, and anticholinergic use were evaluated at baseline and at 2 years and 4 years. Several cognitive tests were performed to assess different areas and levels of cognitive function. A diagnosis of dementia was determined based on standards of practice and validated by a panel of neurologists. An inventory of all drugs (prescription and OTC) was taken. Medications taken the preceding month were also included. All standard demographic information was collected. Extensive health histories were taken along with information about the extent of alcohol, tobacco, and caffeine use.

Results: The study revealed that 7.5% of the participants were taking anticholinergics, of which 6.9% were taking two anticholinergics and 1.5% were taking three. Twice as many women took anticholinergics as men. Anticholinergic utilization was higher in participants with depression, those with a higher consumption of alcohol, and those with poor mobility. Women were noted to have increased risks for cognitive decline with anticholinergics with increasing age. There was an increase in cognitive decline and dementia in both men and women who continuously used anti-cholinergic medications compared with those who did not. Those who stopped using the anticholinergic decreased the risk of further cognitive decline.

Implications: The use of drugs with anticholinergic properties is associated with an increased risk for cognitive decline and dementia in the elderly population. Discontinuing or at least minimizing the anticholinergic burden can decrease the risk of cognitive decline. Not surprisingly, the risks of taking anticholinergics increase the older and frailer the elderly patient becomes.

Reference: Carrière, I., Fourrier-Reglat, A., Dartigues, J-F., Rouaud, O., Pasquier, F., Ritchie, K., & Ancelin, M.. (2009). Drugs with anticholinergic properties, cognitive decline, and dementia in elderly general population. *Archives of Internal Medicine,* 169(14), 1317–1324.

BOX 15-3 Understanding Half-Life

In simple terms, the half-life of a drug is the length of time it takes for half the drug to be eliminated from the body. For example, if the initial dose of doxylamine is 25 mg, and its half-life is 15.5 hours, 12.5 mg will be left active after 15.5 hours, 6.25 mg after another 15.5 hours, and so on. Essentially, five half-lives are required to eliminate a given drug. It could take up to 77.5 hours (five 15.5-hour periods) to eliminate one dose of doxylamine. Therefore, with a half-life of 15.5 hours associated with doxylamine, you can see why an older adult could easily experience a "hangover" effect well into the next day.

Herbal Products

Two herbal products are widely used to treat insomnia: valerian root and melatonin.

Valerian Valerian root is often recommended to promote sleep in those with restlessness and nervous disturbances of sleep (Klepser & Klepser, 1999). Its mechanism of action is not fully understood but may be similar to that of benzodiazepines (Valium, Ativan) and barbiturates (phenobarbital). Several studies and meta-analysis have evaluated the efficacy of valerian root with varying results. Most studies are of poor quality, with unreliable results (Oxman et al., 2007). Results indicate that valerian root may improve sleep quality and self-assessed improvement in insomnia in a small population of habitually poor sleepers (Klepser & Klepser, 1999; Oxman et al., 2007). Valerian root is typically well tolerated and has few drug interactions. Common side effects are headaches, hallucinations, decreased alertness, and fatigue. Because valerian root is an herbal product, its manufacturing processes and purity are not regulated by the FDA.

Melatonin Melatonin was developed into an extended-release product, ramelteon (Rozerem), and approved in 2005 for treating insomnia (Takeda Pharmaceutical Company Limited, 2010). However, it is still available as an OTC product. Melatonin is a hormone secreted by the pineal gland once the sun goes down to regulate the sleep-wake cycle. It is effective in decreasing the time needed to fall sleep, but it has not been proven effective in maintaining sleep. It often is promoted for use in improving insomnia caused by jet lag or shift work, although data on these uses are limited and inconclusive (Buscemi et al., 2004). Common side effects from melatonin are daytime sedation, vivid dreams, nightmares, and depression. As with valerian root, OTC melatonin is not regulated by the FDA.

Analgesics

Most older adults will take OTC analgesics at some point for headache, aches and pains, or fever. OTC pain medications were used by 52% of older persons in pain in one study (Sawyer, Bodner, Ritchie, & Allman, 2006), and another study reported 78.9% used acetaminophen in the past 6 months (Stumpf, Skyles, Alaniz, & Erikson, 2007). OTC analgesics are usually acetaminophen, nonsteroidal anti-inflammatory drugs (NSAIDs), or aspirin. The World Health Organization (2010) created a pain relief ladder that promotes acetaminophen, NSAIDs, or aspirin as the first step for treatment of pain.

Acetaminophen

Acetaminophen is included in more than 100 products, including Tylenol, Excedrin, Tylenol PM, Vicodin, Norco, and Percocet. In addition, acetaminophen content can vary within each product from 325 mg to 1000 mg. The American College of Rheumatology recommends acetaminophen as the first-line treatment of osteoarthritis because of its effectiveness and tolerability (Altman, Hochberg, Moskowitz, & Schnitzer, 2000). Acetaminophen is also effective in reducing fever but is not effective in reducing inflammation.

The maximum recommended dose of acetaminophen for adults is 4,000 mg in 24 hours (eight 500-mg tablets or twelve 325-mg tablets). Some advocate a lower maximum of 2,000 to 3,000 mg in older adults and those who consume excess alcohol because of their possibly diminished liver function (Borman, 2009; Watkins et al., 2006).

Ingestion of acetaminophen at doses greater than those recommended may cause significant liver toxicity or death. The FDA has recently decided to modify the labels and warnings on OTC acetaminophen-containing products to decrease the risk factors for intentional and unintentional overdose (Borman, 2009). The new suggestions for acetaminophen dosing are that no more than 650 mg be taken at any one time and that no more than 2000 mg be taken in a 24-hour period. Signs of liver toxicity are nausea, vomiting, diarrhea, altered mental status, dark or brown urine, and yellowing of the skin and eyes.

NSAIDs

As with acetaminophen, the use of NSAIDs in those age 65 or older may be as high as 70% (Hawboldt, 2008). NSAIDs include a wide range of drugs, including ibuprofen (Advil, Motrin), naproxen (Aleve), diclofenac, etodolac, indomethacin, and more. Aspirin is similar to NSAIDs and can have the same actions and risks as NSAIDs. Uses for NSAIDs include pain, fever, and inflammation. Low-dose aspirin (81 to 325 mg) is also used for cardiovascular protection.

Although these drugs are effective for many people, they are associated with many adverse effects, especially in older adults. Common and serious adverse effects from NSAIDs include bleeding, heartburn, GI ulceration or bleeding, edema, hypertension, and renal failure. The adverse effects NSAIDs are estimated to cause about 7% to 11% of hospitalizations (Hawboldt, 2008).

NSAIDs also have many disease state and drug interactions. NSAIDs may worsen congestive heart failure, hypertension, chronic kidney disease, gastroesophageal reflux disease, and asthma. One study found that NSAIDs could account for about 20% of hospitalizations for heart failure (Page & Henry, 2000), while another found a 60% increased risk of acute renal failure when taking NSAIDs (Griffin, Yared, & Ray, 2000).

The most common drug interactions are with other antiplatelet/anticoagulant agents, including low-dose aspirin for cardiovascular protection, clopidogrel (Plavix), warfarin (Coumadin), antihypertensive medications (especially diuretics), and ginkgo biloba, which may increase the risk of bleeding.

Because of the risks associated with NSAIDs, older adults should be cautioned to take these drugs only after consulting a physician or pharmacist. They should be avoided in those with congestive heart failure, kidney disease, a history of GI ulcers, or current warfarin therapy.

Antacids and Gastric Acid Inhibitors

OTC products for heartburn and dyspepsia include antacids (Tums, Rolaids, Mylanta); histamine type 2 antagonists (H_2 blockers), including cimetidine (Tagamet), ranitidine (Zantac), and famotidine (Pepcid); and the proton pump inhibitors omeprazole (Prilosec) and lansoprazole (Prevacid).

Antacids

Antacids are fast- and short-acting agents used for acute dyspepsia and heartburn. They contain calcium, aluminum, or magnesium, which act to neutralize gastric acid for 30 minutes to 2 hours (Williams, 2002). Calcium- and aluminum-containing products may cause constipation, whereas magnesium-containing products may cause diarrhea. Magnesium-containing products should be avoided in patients with kidney dysfunction because of the risk of accumulation and toxicity (Williams, 2002). All antacids may decrease the absorption of other drugs, including some antibiotics, thyroid hormones, and osteoporosis drugs. For this reason, antacids should be taken about 2 hours before or after other drugs.

H_2 Blockers

H_2 blockers have a slower onset of action (about 2 hours) and last longer (about 12 hours) than antacids (Williams, 2002). This makes these drugs more appropriate for frequent heartburn or anticipated heartburn due to a meal. These drugs have also been used to prevent and treat GI ulcerations (Malfertheiner, Chan, & McColl, 2009). Cimetidine affects the metabolism of many drugs and therefore has many drug interactions. Important drug interactions to consider with cimetidine are theophylline (Theodur), phenytoin (Dilantin), and warfarin (Williams, 2002).

Proton Pump Inhibitors

Omeprazole (Prilosec OTC) is available for chronic heartburn or dyspepsia. This agent does not work acutely and should not be used as needed for relief as it may take several doses for it to be effective. Once omeprazole has elicited its effect, it will inhibit gastric acid for 3 to 5 days (Berardi, 2002). Omeprazole is also often taken with NSAIDs to prevent GI ulceration and bleeding (Desai et al., 2007).

Like omeprazole, lansoprazole (Prevacid) OTC is also used for frequent heartburn. Prevacid 24HR is a delayed-release OTC formulation that stops the release of most acid into the stomach, with the effects of each once-daily pill lasting 24 hours.

Proton pump inhibitors have been found to heal ulcerations faster than H_2 blockers and are more effective in treating GI bleeding (Gisben et al., 2001). They may result in decreased absorption of iron due to a higher pH in the stomach. Long-term use of omeprazole may also cause some people to have decreased serum vitamin B_{12} levels, leading to anemia. Also, some people develop diarrhea (Berardi, 2002).

OTC antacids, H_2 blockers, and proton pump inhibitors are recommended for occasional or short-term treatment (less than 2 weeks) for heartburn or dyspepsia. Treating heartburn and dyspepsia with OTC products is concerning because it may mask a serious problem, including a stomach bleed, ulcer, or heart attack. OTC products should not be used if the patient has such warning signs as chest pain, vomiting, coughing, or blood in the stool or sputum. A physician should be contacted if these symptoms are present or if these OTC products are needed on a regular basis.

Drugs for Constipation

Many older adults seek OTC constipation products because of the decreased gut motility associated with aging and certain disease states (such as Parkinson's disease). Many constipation products are available OTC, including stool softeners, fiber products, stimulant laxatives, and osmotic laxatives.

Stool Softeners

Stool softeners (docusate) are often used to allow stool to pass more easily. These are especially beneficial in those who should avoid straining, such as those who have had a recent heart attack, in which straining may increase the risk of heart attack in those with weak hearts. Stool softeners are generally benign and do not cause many adverse effects; thus, these agents offer a good first line of therapy for constipation.

Fiber Products

Fiber products (Metamucil) help to regulate the bowel and can be used for both constipation and diarrhea. Fiber in the diet or by OTC products should be used first line for bowel disorders as most older adults will not get enough fiber in their diet. Fiber products often cause gas and bloating.

Laxatives

Stimulant laxatives (sennosides, bisacodyl) and osmotic laxatives (Milk of Magnesia, magnesium citrate, MiraLax) are used to cause a bowel movement within 24 hours. These agents should be used cautiously in older adults because they may cause dehydration and electrolyte (serum sodium, chloride, potassium, and magnesium) disturbances. Many older adults take diuretics or potassium supplements, which may worsen dehydration and electrolyte disturbances caused by laxatives. Magnesium products should be avoided in renal disease due to risk for accumulation and toxicity.

Polyethylene glycol 3350 (MiraLax) is a new OTC osmotic diuretic that can be used safely in older adults. It has no interaction with kidney disease and carries little risk for electrolyte disturbances.

As with OTC heartburn medications, laxatives should not be used frequently or on a regular basis without consulting a physician. Larger problems that frequently cause constipation such as bowel obstructions, cancer, or opioid use should be evaluated before self-medicating.

Cough and Cold Products

Cough and cold products aim at treating the symptoms—cough (guaifenesin, dextromethorphan), runny nose (antihistamines), fever (acetaminophen, NSAIDs), and congestion (phenylephrine, pseudoephedrine). Many cough and cold products contain multiple symptom relievers. Many of these products are not safe in older adults due to comorbid diseases. In addition, many of these products frequently change the active ingredients, and consumers may not be aware of what they are actually taking. It is important for the consumer to always read the active ingredients on the OTC labeling.

Decongestants are commonly taken for cold symptoms. These products are not recommended for use in most older adults due to the risk for worsening hypertension, diabetes, benign prostatic hypertrophy, arrhythmias, heart disease, and glaucoma. They also commonly cause anxiety and insomnia.

Antihistamines (diphenhydramine, chlorpheniramine) are also common in OTC cough and cold products. As discussed previously, these may cause significant adverse effects in older adults, including confusion, falls, sedation, urine retention, and constipation.

Cough and cold products should be used only occasionally. Older adults in particular should be encouraged to discuss the use of OTC cough and cold products with their physician or pharmacist before starting them because of their many risks.

Popular Herbal Products

Herbal products commonly taken by older adults include ginkgo biloba, saw palmetto, and St. John's wort.

Ginkgo Biloba

Ginkgo biloba is reported to be used by 2% to 5% of those over age 65 (Nahin et al., 2009; Qato et al., 2008). It is an herbal product commonly promoted to improve memory and mood, improve peripheral artery circulation, and reduce dementia (Klepser & Klepser, 1999). Clinical trials have shown variable results in improving memory, concentration, and mood. Studies have shown significant improvement in peripheral arterial disease, including increased walking distance, decreased walking time, and decreased reported pain. Current evidence does not support its use in dementia, with no improvement in cognitive symptoms over placebo (Klepser & Klepser, 1999).

Ginkgo biloba's common adverse effects include dizziness, headache, stomachache, and bleeding. There are reports of spontaneous bleeding events, including subdural hematoma (Bent, Goldberg, Padula, & Avins, 2005). Because of the risk of bleeding, ginkgo biloba should not be taken with NSAIDs, aspirin, warfarin, vitamin E, or other products likely to increase bleeding risk (Nahin et al., 2009). Older adults are generally at increased risk for bleeding; thus, the risk of using ginkgo biloba may outweigh any benefits it may have.

Saw Palmetto

Saw palmetto is reported to be used by about 7% of older men with benign prostatic hypertrophy (Qato et al., 2008). This supplement is used to block testosterone production and thus decrease the size of the prostate (Klepser & Klepser, 1999). Saw palmetto may be as effective in improving self-reported symptoms as the prescription drug finasteride (Wilt et al., 1998). Saw palmetto is generally well tolerated and has few reported adverse effects and no known drug interactions. It should not be taken with finasteride (Proscar) or dutasteride (Avodart) because of its similar mechanism of action. Saw palmetto should not be handled by pregnant women.

St. John's Wort

St. John's wort is promoted for the treatment of anxiety and depression. Its mechanism is not fully understood, but it may block serotonin reuptake similar to other antidepressants (Klepser & Klepser, 1999). Clinical evidence for St. John's wort is poor and inconclusive, but the herb may be effective for mild to moderate depression (Klepser & Klepser, 1999). There are many adverse effects associated with St. John's wort, including sedation, confusion, photosensitivity (fair-skinned people are more likely to sunburn), dizziness, and restlessness. This supplement also has some monoamine oxidase inhibitor (MAO-I) activity and therefore has the possibility of causing serious adverse effect if taken with beer, cheese, wine, other antidepressants, dextromethorphan, and many others. St. John's wort also interacts with digoxin and HIV medications. This product is not recommended for self-medication and should only be used under a physician's supervision.

Polypharmacy

Older adults are more likely to have multiple disease states that require close monitoring and thus may see multiple physicians. Each physician may prescribe additional medications, thereby increasing the effects of polypharmacy. It has been reported that about 20% to 50% of older adults have two or more prescribing physicians (Preskorn et al., 2005; Tamblyn, McLeod, Abrahamowicz, & Laprise, 1996). One study reported that about 21% of all respondents had four or more prescribing physicians (Tamblyn, McLeod, Abrahamowicz, & Laprise, 1996).

A study of 5,003 Veterans Administration patients found that, for each additional prescriber, the likelihood of being prescribed eight or more medications doubled (Preskorn et al., 2005). It has been reported that 18% to 26% of all potentially inappropriate drug combinations are a result of prescribing by multiple physicians (Tamblyn, McLeod, Abrahamowicz, & Laprise, 1996). Polypharmacy increases the risk of adverse drug effects in addition to increasing the patient's medical costs. A primary care physician should always coordinate the care for each patient, including all prescribed drugs and OTC products. All older adults also should be encouraged to maintain a complete record of physicians and medications, including prescribed drugs, OTC products, herbal and dietary supplements, and borrowed medications (Box 15-4). These steps will help eliminate unnecessary prescribing and the dangers of polypharmacy.

BOX 15-4 The Dangers of Borrowing and Sharing

The borrowing and sharing of prescription drugs may occur in up to 27% of the overall population, although most studies have been done in people younger than age 44 (Ellis & Mullan, 2009; Goldsworthy, Schwartz, & Mayhorn, 2008). The true incidence of medication borrowing and sharing among older adults may be much higher because older adults take many more drugs and have many more ailments than younger adults. Borrowing and sharing drugs raises many risks of adverse effects and negative health outcomes.

The most common drugs shared or borrowed are allergy medications, analgesics (especially NSAIDs and opioids), antibiotics, and mood-altering medications such as antianxiety drugs and antidepressants (Goldsworthy, Schwartz, & Mayhorn, 2008). Many of these drugs are likely to cause adverse effects in older adults and may cause drug interactions, toxicity, overdose, or antibiotic resistance (Goldsworthy, Schwartz, & Mayhorn, 2008). In addition, borrowing medications may mask health problems and delay the identification and appropriate treatment of the condition.

When educating older adults about their prescribed drugs, always make a point to discourage borrowing or sharing drugs.

Strategies to Support Accurate Use of Medications

About one third to one half of all U.S. patients fail to comply with their prescribed drug regimens. Older adults are challenged with adherence on a daily basis, especially as the number of drugs prescribed increases and memory and cognitive skills decrease. Nonadherence is known to decrease the quality of health care and increase medication costs. It is estimated that failure to comply with medications costs the United States approximately $100 billion annually (Task Force for Compliance, 1993). Medication compliance is a problem in older adults in part because many don't believe the drug is working or needed. Some believe that if one pill is good, two is better, while others believe that all pills cause more harm than good.

Some people may have trouble paying for prescribed drugs or feel that they take too many. The lack of affordability or the perception of overmedication is often the source of medication noncompliance or self-medication in the older adult population. These situations may lead the older adult to several different tactics to lessen the cost or the pill burden. One of the more common strategies of self-medication is to "stretch" the prescription by cutting the pills in half, taking a twice-daily medication once daily, or taking a daily medication every other day.

This method of self-medication could lead to serious health issues. For example, poorly controlled hypertension or elevated blood glucose may not always cause symptoms; therefore, poor glucose control may not be recognized by the patient. Chronic increases in blood pressure and serum glucose level may increase the risk of heart disease, eye complications, and kidney disease.

Be aware that simple comments such as "I just don't think my pills are helping me," "I take too many pills!," or "My pills cost too much" can be clues that self-medication tactics such as "stretching" could be taking place. It is important to identify potential noncompliance or self-medication in older adults.

One study found as many as 42% of older people stockpiled and hoarded medications for later use (Ellis & Mullan, 2009). Storing medications often leads to expired and less potent or inactive medication use. People who take stored medications are less likely to believe in a treatment because they may feel the medication is ineffective (Goldsworthy, Schwartz, & Mayhorn, 2008).

Also keep in mind that many older adults have trouble taking medications because they cannot open the bottles or cannot swallow properly. There are several tools and strategies to improving adherence in these older adults, including dosing strategies, medication packaging and organizers, education techniques, and family and health-care provider involvement.

Prescribing strategies to improve medication adherence include dosing medications infrequently (once daily versus three times daily), using combination products to decrease the number of drugs taken, and dosing medications at key times in the day to cue the patient to take them (such as at bedtime or meals). Appropriate dosing formulations (e.g., solution versus large tablets) should also be prescribed to make sure the patient is physically able to take the drug.

Drugs may be packaged in easy-open bottles or foil packages to ease the strain of obtaining the drug. Daily, weekly, or monthly medication organizers are available at most drug stores to remind patients when to take their medications. Many pharmacists will help organize pill boxes to improve compliance. There are also medication packages that make verbal reminders to alert the patient when the medication is due or in need of a refill.

Education and care coordination among providers, family members or caregivers, and the patient also improves compliance. Education regarding the importance of each drug in maintaining the patient's health and the need for compliance should be stressed. Older adults should also be educated on what to do if they miss a dose or take a drug out of its directed use. For example, if a patient has a drink of alcohol at a social function, he or she may avoid his or her medications altogether because he or she was told not to take them with alcohol. Educating the patient that having one drink is much different than many drinks and that medications should still be taken may improve compliance. Educating the family and caregivers may also improve compliance as they can function as reminders, help organize the patient, and provide support when needed.

One meta-analysis found behavioral approaches, educational approaches, and the combination of both significantly improved adherence with a drug regimen (Peterson, Takiya, & Finley, 2003). However, no method was any better than the others. This evidence suggests that the patient's medication management tools should be specifically tailored to his or her needs to be most effective.

Conclusion

Providing our older adults with a safe and effective medication regimen can prove to be one of the most significant challenges we face in caring for our geriatric patients. Older adults can be inundated with multiple diseases and multiple drug treatments, thereby increasing the risk of adverse drug events, side effect, or interactions. Interestingly, the data available from one of the largest studies on adverse drug events in nursing homes suggest that more than half of adverse events are preventable and that most are associated with monitoring errors. Many adverse events and side effects go unrecognized in older adults because they commonly present as vague or nonspecific complaints or symptoms such as nausea, vomiting, malaise, urine retention, constipation, confusion, delirium, lethargy, and falls (Gallagher & O'Mahony, 2008). Medications should always be considered as a possible cause for any new health-related issue or complaint that arises in an older adult.

KEY POINTS

- Although older adults make up less than 15% of the American population, they use more than 30% of the drugs prescribed and sustain 33.6% of severe adverse drug events.
- The aging process, as well as smoking, chronic diseases, and drugs, affect the body's physiological reserves, which are significantly reduced in even healthy persons by the seventh decade.
- Age-related changes may vary between organ systems within the same person.
- Pharmacokinetics is composed of four basic actions: absorption, distribution, metabolism, and excretion.
- Older adults typically are more sensitive to drugs because of pharmacodynamic changes and may have exaggerated effects. Therefore, new drugs should be started at lower doses and gradually increased to produce the best therapeutic effect with minimal side effects.
- Drugs identified as potentially harmful to older adults are listed in the Beers Criteria Updated (Fick et al., 2003).
- Drugs with a narrow therapeutic index require close monitoring to avoid toxic effects.
- Drugs should never be shared, borrowed, or stored for future use.
- Oral administration is the preferred route for most medications because the rate and extent of absorption typically remains predictable across the lifespan.
- Extended-release drugs should not be crushed because doing so will deliver the full dose all at once and place the patient at risk for adverse drug effects or toxic side effects.
- Crushing an enteric-coated drug may alter its therapeutic effect.
- Parenteral administration may be used when a drug cannot be given via the GI tract, it is not absorbed from the GI tract, or faster absorption is required.
- Age-related alterations in the skin may cause percutaneous medications to be erratically absorbed.
- Administration of sprays or inhalants can dry mucous membranes.
- Older adults are the leading consumers of OTC products used primarily to treat insomnia, pain, heartburn, indigestion, constipation, cough, cold, or fever.
- About 90% of all patients over age 65 take at least one prescription medication; 50% to 90% take at least one OTC product or dietary supplement; and 50% take more than five prescription drugs, OTC products, or supplements in combination.
- Self-medication and polypharmacy increase the risks for adverse drug effects and interactions and

may worsen current disease states (including heart disease, prostate enlargement, and glaucoma) or cause life-threatening illnesses such as GI bleeding.

- Acetaminophen, a common ingredient in OTC products, may cause significant liver toxicity if recommended doses are exceeded or the person has impaired liver function. Recommended dosages for older adults may be lower than those for younger adults.
- Reasons for hospitalizations due to adverse effects of NSAIDs include bleeding, heartburn, GI ulceration or bleeding, edema, hypertension, renal failure, or worsening of underlying chronic diseases.
- Products containing magnesium (including many antacids) should be avoided in patients with kidney dysfunction or taken 2 hours before antibiotics, thyroid medications, or drugs to treat osteoporosis.
- Products to treat constipation—including stool softeners, fiber products, stimulant laxatives, and osmotic laxatives—are used by many older adults because of the decreased gut motility associated with aging.
- Stools softeners or increased fiber through diet or OTC products is the preferred initial treatment for constipation.
- Laxatives may cause dehydration and electrolyte disturbances and should be used cautiously in older adults.
- Decongestants may worsen hypertension, diabetes, benign prostatic hypertrophy, arrhythmias, heart disease, glaucoma, anxiety, and insomnia.
- The anticholinergic activity of antihistamines found in many OTC cold and sleep products may result in daytime sedation, altered mental status, confusion, hallucinations, weakness or falls, urine retention, constipation, and arrhythmias.
- Antihistamines may cause frequent urinary tract infections in older adults and may worsen many disease states including arrhythmias (such as atrial fibrillation), benign prostatic hypertrophy, glaucoma, and constipation.
- Herbal supplements often used by older adults are not regulated by the FDA so that concentrations and absorption rates may vary among manufacturers. Herbal supplements may cause side effects or interact with prescription or OTC medications.
- Prescription borrowing or stockpiling has been reported among 13% to 27% of the adult population and is likely to be much higher in the elderly.
- The most commonly shared or borrowed medications are antiallergy drugs, analgesics (including opioids), antibiotics, and mood-altering medications (antianxiety drugs and antidepressants).
- Medication sharing and borrowing may increase polypharmacy and drug interactions, adverse drug effects, toxicity, overdose, and antibiotic resistance, as well as mask health problems and delay appropriate treatment.
- People who take stored medications are less likely to believe in a treatment because they may feel the medication is ineffective.
- Because many older adults see multiple providers, maintaining a complete record of physicians and drugs may reduce the risk of inappropriate drug combinations and adverse effects.
- One third to one half of all U.S. patients fail to comply with their prescribed drug regimens due to cost, disbelief in drug effectiveness, resistance to drug treatments, experienced side effects, or difficulty managing drug forms and packages.
- Strategies to improve adherence include less frequent doses, timing doses with routines (such as meals or bedtime), using combination products, requesting easy-open containers, using medication organizers, and involving family members in instructions and care coordination.

CRITICAL THINKING ACTIVITIES

1. Imagine that in 2009 you are driving a 1974 four-door sedan. Although you know there are several minor problems with the car, it has no problem getting you where you need to go. Everything seems to be working just fine during the fall, winter, and spring months. Now, summer is here, it is 98ºF outside and you reach over and turn on the air conditioner. You continue on your way for the next 5 miles enjoying the cool stream of air. Low and behold, after about mile 6 you notice the car is losing power and on mile 7, you find yourself sitting on the side of the road with steam coming from under the hood. What just happened and how does this simulate the addition of a prescription or OTC medication to a senior's drug regimen?
2. A 76-year-old man comes into the physician's office for a routine checkup. You take his history and find that he has no specific complaints other than that he simply has not been feeling himself for the past 2 to 3 months. His activity

level has decreased. He used to play golf four to five times a week and has not played for the past 2 weeks because he feels so bad. He says, "I guess this is what happens when you get old." You review his medications and find that his medications have gone unchanged for the past 2.5 years. He has dismissed his medications as the cause since they have not changed for years. Should you? Why or why not? What could be the problem?

CASE STUDY | *MR. HURTEIN*

Mr. Ima Hurtein, a 75-year-old Korean War veteran, recently had a fall while shoveling snow in his driveway. He is now experiencing a tremendous amount of hip pain. As his home health nurse, you advise him to go to urgent care, but he is stubborn and tells you he is fine. He asks you instead to go to the drug store to pick up a pain reliever for him.

His medical history includes high blood pressure, congestive heart failure with leg swelling, and heartburn. He currently takes metoprolol 25 mg twice daily, Lasix 20 mg twice daily, lisinopril 5 mg daily, aspirin 81 mg daily, and OTC Tums (calcium carbonate) as needed for heartburn.

1. What are some of your concerns with Mr. Hurtein's choice to self-medicate rather than go to the doctor?
2. Assuming Mr. Hurtein takes the analgesics as recommended on the OTC label, which OTC pain reliever from the drug store (Tylenol or ibuprofen) is preferred for him? Why?
3. It has been 2 weeks and Mr. Hurtein has taken ibuprofen 200 mg two tablets every 8 hours around the clock since the accident. He notices his heartburn is worsening, he has an upset stomach most days, and he is constipated. He has had to take his Tums more frequently. Is there another OTC product that may be better for his heartburn than Tums? Why?

REFERENCES

Altman, R. D., Hochberg, M. C., Moskowitz, R. W., & Schnitzer, T. J. (2000). Recommendations for the medical management of osteoarthritis of the hip and knee: 2000 update. *Arthritis & Rheumatology, 43,* 1905–1915.

Bent, S., Goldberg, H., Padula, A., & Avins, A.L. (2005). Spontaneous bleeding associated with ginkgo biloba: A case report and systematic review of literature. *Journal of General Internal Medicine, 20,* 657–661.

Berardi, R. R. (2002). Peptic ulcer disease. In J. T. Dipiro, R. L. Talbert, G. C. Yee, et al. (Eds.), *Pharmacotherapy: A pathophysiologic approach* (pp. 603–624). New York, NY: McGraw-Hill.

Borman, M. S. (2009). Organ-specific warnings: Internal analgesic, antipyretic, and antirheumatic drug products for over-the-counter human use. Final monograph. *Federal Register, 74,* 19835–19409.

Buscemi, N., Vandermeer, B., Pandya, R., Hooton, N., Tjosvold, G., Hartling, L., . . . Klassen, T. (2004). *Melatonin for treatment of sleep disorders. Summary, evidence report/technology assessment no. 108.* Rockville, MD: Agency for Healthcare Research and Quality.

Carrière, I., Fourrier-Reglat, A., Dartigues, J-F., Rouaud, O., Pasquier, F., Ritchie, K., . . . (2009). Drugs with anticholinergic properties, cognitive decline, and dementia in elderly general population. *Archives of Internal Medicine, 169*(14), 1317–1324.

Desai, J. C., Sanyal, S. M., Goo, T., Benson, A. A., Bodian, C. A., Miller, K. M. (2007). Primary prevention of adverse gastroduodenal effects from short-term use of non-steroidal anti-inflammatory drugs by omeprazole 20 mg in healthy subjects: A randomized, double blind, placebo controlled study. *Digestive Diseases and Sciences, 53,* 2059–2065

Ellis, J., & Mullan, J. (2009). Prescription medication borrowing and sharing: Risk factors and management. *Australian Family Physician, 30*(10), 816–819.

Fick, D. M, Cooper, J. W., Wade, W. E., Waller, J. L., Maclean, J. R., & Beers, M. H. (2003). Updating the Beers criteria for potentially inappropriate medication use in older adults. *Archives of Internal Medicine, 163,* 2716–2724.

Gallagher, P., & O'Mahony, D. (2008). STOPP (Screening tool of older persons' potentially inappropriate prescriptions): Application to acutely ill elderly patients and comparison with Beers' criteria. *Age and Ageing, 37,* 673–679.

Gisben, J. P., Gonzalez, L., Calvet, X., Roqué, M., Gabriel, R., & Pajares, J. M. (2001). Proton pump inhibitors versus H_2-antagonists: A meta-analysis of their efficacy in treating bleeding peptic ulcer. *Alimentary Pharmacology and Therapeutics, 15,* 917–926.

Glass, J. R., Sproule, B. A., Herrmann, N., & Busto, U. E. (2008). Effects of 2-week treatment with temazepam and diphenhydramine in elderly insomniacs: A randomized, placebo-controlled trial. *Journal of Clinical Pharmacology, 28,* 182–188.

Glass, J. R., Sproule, B. A., Herrmann, N., Streiner, D., & Busto, U. E. (2003). Acute pharmacological effects of temazepam, diphenhydramine, and valerian in healthy elderly subjects. *Journal of Clinical Psychopharmacology, 23,* 260–268.

Goldsworthy, R. C., Schwartz, N. C., & Mayhorn, C. B. (2008). Beyond abuse and exposure: Framing the impact of prescription-medication sharing. *American Journal of Public Health, 98,* 1115–1121.

Griffin, M. R., Yared, A., & Ray, W. A. (2000). Nonsteroidal anti-inflammatory drugs and acute renal failure in elderly persons. *American Journal of Epidemiology, 151,* 488–496.

Hamilton, H., Gallagher, P., & O'Mahony, D. (2009). Inappropriate prescribing and adverse drug events in older people. *BMC Geriatrics, 9,* 5.

Hawboldt, J. (2008). Adverse events associated with NSAIDs. *US Pharmacist, 33(12),* HS5–HS13.

Klepser, T. B., & Klepser, M. E. (1999). Unsafe and potentially safe herbal therapies. *American Journal* of *Health-System Pharmacy, 56,* 125–138.

Malfertheiner, P., Chan, F. K., & McColl, K. E. (2009). Peptic ulcer disease. *Lancet, 374,* 1449–1461.

Malone, D., & Bhandary, D. (2001). Factors associated with medication use among the elderly. *Academy for Health Services Research and Health Policy Meeting, 18,* 157.

Merck Manuals Online Medical Library. (2010). Retrieved September 15, 2010 from http://www.merckmanuals.com/professional/index.html

Moore, T. J., Cohen, M. R., & Furberg, C. D. (2007). Serious adverse drug events reported to the Food and Drug Administration, 1998-2005 *Archives of Internal Medicine, 167*(16), 1752–1759.

Nahin, R. L., Pecha, M., Welmerink, D. B., Sink, K., DeKosky, S. T., & Fitzpatrick, A. L. (2009). Concomitant use of prescription drugs and dietary supplements in ambulatory elderly people. *Journal of the American Geriatrics Society, 57,* 1197–1205.

National Sleep Foundation. (2008). *2008 Sleep in America poll.* Washington, DC: Author. Retrieved December 15, 2010, from http://www.sleepfoundation.org/sites/default/files/2008%20POLL%20SOF.PDF

Oborne, C. A., & Luzac, M. L. (2005). Over-the-counter medicine use prior to and during hospitalization. *The Annals of Pharmacotherapy, 39,* 268–273.

Oxman, A. D., Flottorp, S., Havelsrud, K., Fretheim, A., Odgaard-Jensen, J., Austvoll-Dahlgren, A., . . . Bjorvatn, B. (2007). A televised, web-based randomized trial of an herbal remedy (valerian) for insomnia. *Plos One, 17*(10), e1040.

Page, J., & Henry, D. (2000). Consumption of NSAIDs and the development of congestive heart failure in elderly patients: An underrecognized public health problem. *Archives of Internal Medicine, 160,* 777–784.

Peterson, A. M., Takiya, L., & Finley, R. (2003). Meta-analysis of trials of interventions to improve medication adherence. *American Journal* of *Health-System Pharmacy, 60,* 657–665.

Pope, N. D. (2009). Generic substitution of narrow therapeutic index drugs. *U.S. Pharmacist, 34*(6; Generic Drug Review Suppl.), 12–19.

Potentially harmful drugs in the elderly: Beers list and more. (2007). *Pharmacist's Letter/Prescriber's Letter, 23*(9), 230907. Retrieved December 15, 2010, from http://www.pharmacistsletter.com/(S(d5v5aw55o12014i4jhsksm3f))/pl/ArticleDD.aspx?rn=1&cs=&s=PL&pt=6&fpt=56&dd=230907&pb=PL#dd

Preskorn, S. H., Silkey, B., Shah, R., Neff, M., Jones, T. L., Choi, J., (2005). Complexity of medication use in the Veterans Affairs healthcare system: Part I: Outpatient use in relation to age and number of prescribers. *Journal of Psychiatric Practice, 11*(1), 5–15.

Qato, D. M, Alexander, C., Conti, R. M., Johnson, M., Schumm, P., & Lindau, S. T. (2008). Use of prescription and over-the-counter medications and dietary supplements among older adults in the United States. *Journal of the American Medical Association, 300,* 2876–2878.

Rathore, S. S., Curtis, J. P., Wang, Y., Bristow, M. R., & Krumholz, H. M. (2003). Association of serum digoxin concentration and outcomes in patients with heart failure. *Journal of the American Medical Association, 289,* 871–878.

Resnick, N. M., & Marcantonio, E. R. (1997). How should clinical care of the aged differ? *Lancet, 350,* 1157.

Richardson, G. S., Roehrs, T. A., Rosenthal, L., Koshorek, G., & Roth, T. (2002). Tolerance to daytime sedative effects of H_1 antihistamines. *Journal of Clinical Psychopharmacology, 22,* 511–515.

Roumie, C. L., & Griffin, M. R. (2004). Over-the-counter analgesics in older adults: A call for improved labeling and consumer education. *Drugs & Aging, 21,* 485–498.

Sateia, M. J., Doghramji, K., Huari, P. J., & Morin, C. M. (2000). Evaluation of chronic insomnia. An American Academy of Sleep Medicine review. *Sleep, 23,* 243–308.

Sawyer, P., Bodner, E. V., Ritchie, C. S., & Allman, R. M. (2006). Pain and pain medication use in community-dwelling older adults. *The American Journal of Geriatric Pharmacotherapy, 4,* 316–324.

Stumpf, J. L., Skyles, A. J., Alaniz, C., & Erikson, S. R. (2007). Knowledge of appropriate acetaminophen doses and potential toxicities in an adult clinic population. *The Journal of the American Pharmacists Association, 47*(1), 35–41.

Takeda Pharmaceutical Company Limited. (2010). *Rozerem prescribing information.* Retrieved December 10, 2010, from http://hcp.rozerem.com/

Tamblyn, R. M., McLeod, P. J., Abrahamowicz, M., & Laprise, R. (1996). Do too many cooks spoil the broth? Multiple physician involvement in medical management of elderly patients and potentially inappropriate drug combinations. *The Canadian Medical Association* Journal, *154,* 1177–1184.

Task Force for Compliance. (1993). *Noncompliance with medications: An economic tragedy with important implications for health care reform.* Baltimore, MD: Author.

Walston, J., Hadley, E. C., & Ferrucci, L. (2006). Research agenda for frailty in older adults: Toward a better understanding of physiology and etiology: Summary from the American Geriatrics Society/National Institute on Aging Research Conference on Frailty in Older Adults. *Journal of the American Geriatrics Society, 54*(6), 991–1001.

Watkins, P. B., Kaplowitz, N., Slattery, J. T., Colonese, C. R., Colucci, S. V., Stewart, P. W., . . . (2006). Aminotransferase elevations in healthy adults receiving 4 grams of acetaminophen daily: A randomized controlled trial. *Journal of the American Medical Association, 296,* 87–93.

Williams, D. B. (2002). Gastroesophageal reflux disease. In J. T. Dipiro, R. L. Talbert, G. C. Yee, et al.

(Eds.), *Pharmacotherapy: A pathophysiologic approach* (pp. 585–601). New York, NY: McGraw-Hill.

Wilt, T. J., Ishani, A., Stark, G., MacDonald, R., Lau, J., & Mulrow, C. (1998). Saw palmetto extracts for treatment of benign prostatic hyperplasia: A systematic review. *Journal of the American Medical Association, 280,* 1604–1609.

World Health Organization. (2010). *WHO's pain ladder.* Retrieved December 15, 2010, from http://www.who.int/cancer/palliative/painladder/en/index.html

Yudo, Y., & Kurihara, M. (1990). Clinical evaluation of diphenhydramine hydrochloride for the treatment of insomnia in psychiatric patients: A double-blind study. *Journal of Clinical Psychopharmacology, 30,* 1041–1048.

Zarowitz, B. J., Stebelsky, L. A., Muma, B. K., Romain, T. M., & Peterson, E. L. (2005). Reduction of high-risk polypharmacy drug combinations in patients in a managed care setting. *Pharmacotherapy, 25*(11), 1636–1645.

Unit III

Optimizing Economic and Social Well-Being

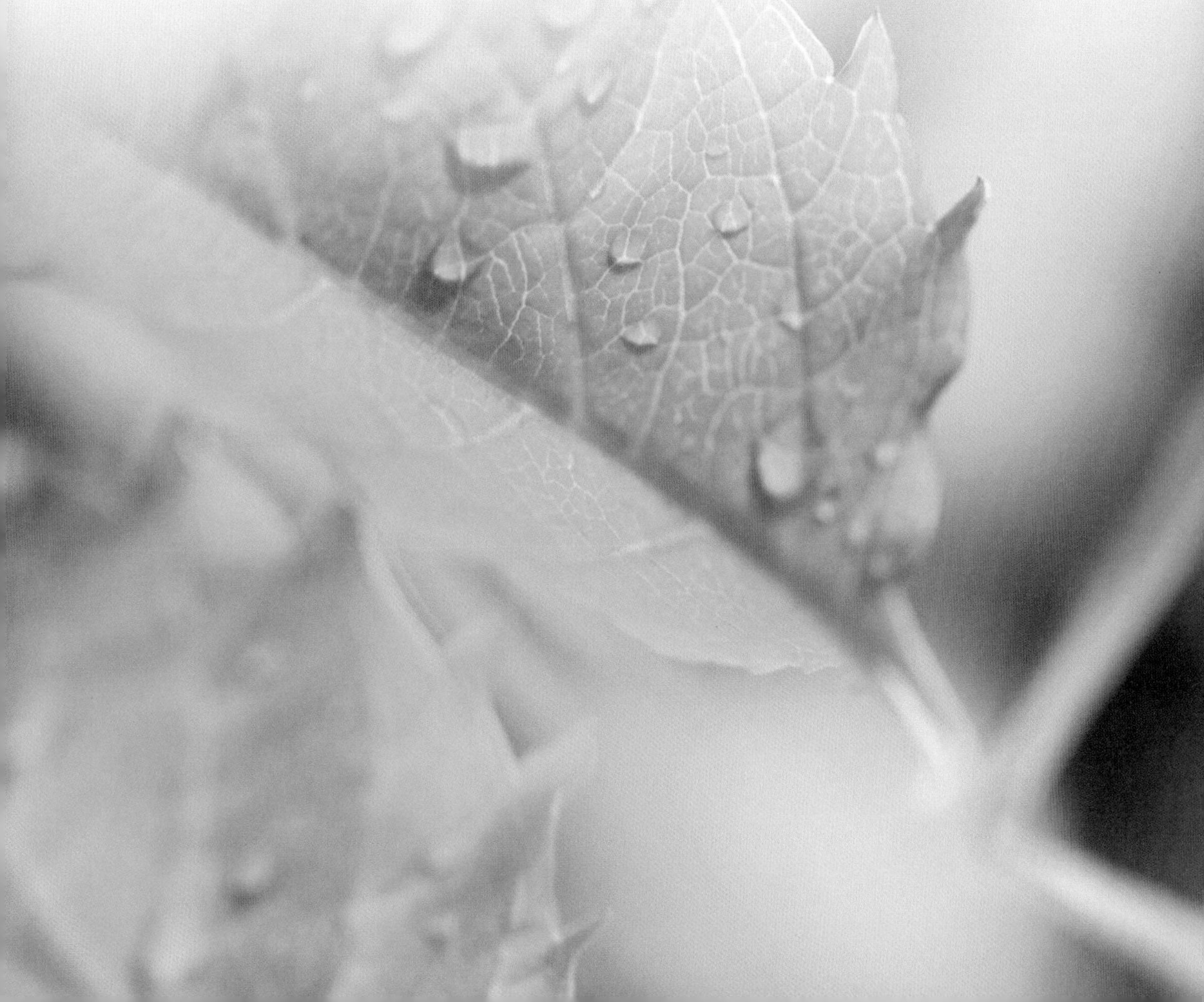

Chapter 16

Economic Considerations of Aging

Gloria Messick. Svare, PhD, LCSW, and Jeanne Wendel, PhD

LEARNING OBJECTIVES

- Describe recent changes in life expectancy, expected healthy life, and life with disability.
- Outline older adults' average income and assets.
- Review the components of Medicare, variations in Medicare coverage, and the relationship between the configuration of Medicare coverage and socioeconomic status.
- Summarize the web of interactions between socioeconomic status, health care utilization, and health.
- Discuss the implications of the web of interactions between socioeconomic status and health for nursing practice.

Do social and economic variables, such as gender and race, impact health? The answer to this question is clear: On average, women live longer than men, whites live longer than blacks, and individuals with more income and education live longer than individuals with less income and education. However, this straightforward answer raises a host of puzzling questions:

- *Why* do women, whites, and college graduates live longer than other people?
- The gender and race gaps have been shrinking. What steps can be taken to further reduce the gaps?
- Does analysis of the impact of these social and economic variables provide clues to help *all* people age successfully?

Research cannot currently answer these questions in detail. Nonetheless, it is important for nurses to understand the currently available evidence because nurses will deal with these issues when caring for patients from all levels of socioeconomic status. Understanding the relationships between socioeconomic status and health will provide nursing students with a framework for examining the factors that impact successful aging. This understanding will prepare students to target health care interventions to the real-world needs of their patients and to make appropriate referrals to social service resources, such as social workers (Box 16-1).

In this chapter, we analyze the web of interactions between socioeconomic status and health, to understand the factors that support and constrain successful aging. These three concepts—socioeconomic status, health economics, and successful aging—are fundamental to this chapter; hence, we provide definitions in Table 16-1, for convenient reference.

The health economist Michael Grossman laid the foundation for analysis of the impacts of personal, community, and health system inputs on health in his 1972 paper, *On the Concept of Health Capital and the Demand for Health.* Grossman argued that individual wellness activities, family income and education, community public health programs, and expert health care all contribute to health. On the other hand, factors such as risky behaviors, exposure to pollutants, and medical errors reduce health. Health economists have used this framework to understand the combination of factors that produced the dramatic 1900 to 2004 increase in life expectancy in the United States. A baby born in the United States in 1900 could expect

BOX 16-1 What Do Social Workers Do?

The unique perspective that social workers have is called *person-in-environment.* Social workers help people cope by assessing the strengths of the individual in the context of the environment. Coping can be increased through interventions that target the strengths of the individual through counseling. Coping can also be improved by adding supports to the environment through referrals to community resources. Common examples of referrals to social workers in hospital settings include these

- A patient is medically ready for discharge but has no food in the house.
- A patient is unable to purchase the medications prescribed at discharge.
- Family members disagree about whether to help the patient go home or to an assisted-living facility.

to live, on average, 47.3 years, while a baby born in the United States in 2004 could expect to live 77.8 years. The initial portion of this dramatic improvement was primarily generated by public health activities, including widespread access to sanitation, clean drinking water, and vaccinations. The economic standard of living (typically measured as gross domestic product [GDP] per capita) also increased dramatically during the 20th century, providing resources to support public health and health-care services, education, and nutrition. In addition, medical innovations such as antibiotics dramatically strengthened the quality of medical care.

This chapter examines the impacts of socioeconomic status on health and finds that it influences all three types of inputs into the production of health. Socioeconomic status affects:

- Personal decisions through its influence on health literacy, ability to navigate the health-care system, and health insurance literacy
- Community health issues such as risk of violence
- Financial access to health insurance and health care

The effects of socioeconomic status on health are complex and interrelated and complicated by the fact that health status also impacts socioeconomic status.

The effects of socioeconomic status on health are complex and interrelated. In addition, the

TABLE 16-1 Definitions of Key Concepts

Socioeconomic status	As defined by Hollingshead and Redlich (1958), socioeconomic status is a summary measure of a person's relative economic and social ranking that includes ■ Income ■ Education ■ Occupation
Health economics	Economics is more than analysis of costs and budgets. Economists work to understand the multitude of individual, family, work, retirement, leisure, and health decisions that shape our lives. These decisions reflect the interaction of individual goals and preferences with the reality of time, financial, and health constraints faced by all individuals. Health economists analyze the decisions recorded in large (several thousands) nationally representative samples of individuals and families to understand the relationships between social and economic variables and health.
Successful aging	As defined by Rowe and Kahn (1997), successful aging is the ability to maintain three behaviors or characteristics ■ Low risk of disease and disease-related disability ■ High mental and physical function ■ Active engagement in life

relationship between socioeconomic status and health is complicated by the fact that health status also impacts socioeconomic status, due to the impacts of health on decisions to work or retire. The chapter concludes by discussing the challenge posed by evidence that health and health care vary across geographic regions in ways that socioeconomic status does not explain. Three important topics provide the backdrop for analysis of the web of relationships between socioeconomic status and health for older adults:

- Life expectancy trends for older adults
- Income and assets of older adults
- Health insurance coverage for older adults

Information about these three topics is essential, prior to beginning our analysis of the relationship between socioeconomic status and health.

Trends

Increased Life Expectancy

The proportion of the U.S. population 65 and over is projected to grow from 12% in 2005 to 21% in 2050 (U.S. Census Bureau, 2004). This projected increase in the number of older adults reflects both the aging of the Baby Boomer generation and increased life expectancy. A person who reached the age of 65 in 1950 could expect to live another 13.9 years, whereas an individual who reached the age of 65 in 2005 could expect to live another 18.7 years (Fig. 1A). In addition, the U.S. Census Bureau projected that the percentage of older adults (over age 65) who are at least 85 years old will double from 12% of the older adult population in 2000 to 25% in 2050. This growth of the older adult population (and increasing average age within this population) will require careful thinking about strategies for providing health care and community support for older adults.

More Healthy Years

Increased longevity raises an important question: Are older adults enjoying additional healthy years, or are the additional years primarily marked by disability? This question is important for long-term care planning, Medicare budget planning, and individual retirement financial planning. The proportion of older adults reporting limitations in instrumental activities of daily living (IADLs), such as balancing a checkbook, has been decreasing since the mid-1980s, and the proportion reporting limitations of activities of daily living (ADLs), such as the ability to prepare a meal independently, has been decreasing since the mid-1990s (Cai & Lubitz, 2007).

Data from the years 1992 to 2002 show that life expectancy increased 0.5 years during that decade. A person who celebrated his or her 65th birthday in 2002 could expect to enjoy 0.8 *additional* years without IADL or ADL disabilities and 0.3 *fewer* years with any IADL or ADL disabilities, compared with a person who reached age 65 in 1992. Thus, we are not only living longer, but an increasing portion of our post-65 years are active and healthy, although it is important to note that these measures of IADLs and ADLs may not capture cognitive impairment.

The increasing proportion of active and healthy years reflects both increasing numbers of years before disabilities are reported and an increasing ability to recover from episodes of disability. And this good news is not limited to the young-old. Those who reach age 85 also experienced an increase in the expected number of active years and a decrease in the expected number of years with severe ADL disability. It is important for nursing students to note, however, that the reduction in disability reflects several types of changes in addition to improvements in medical care. One important change is technological advances such as direct deposits of Social Security checks and the advent of microwave ovens, which have reduced the physical tasks involved in activities such as handling finances and preparing meals.

Increased Diversity

Understanding the influence of demographic characteristics on health is also becoming increasingly important because the population of older adults is becoming increasingly racially and ethnically diverse. Although 69% of older adults are currently non-Hispanic white, this proportion is expected to decrease to 50% by 2050. The proportion of older adults who are Hispanic is expected to nearly double, from 13% to 24%. This trend may have significant effects on the socioeconomic status characteristics of the older adult population because older Hispanic adults currently have lower incomes, on average, than older non-Hispanic whites, and older Hispanics are less likely to have at least some college education and

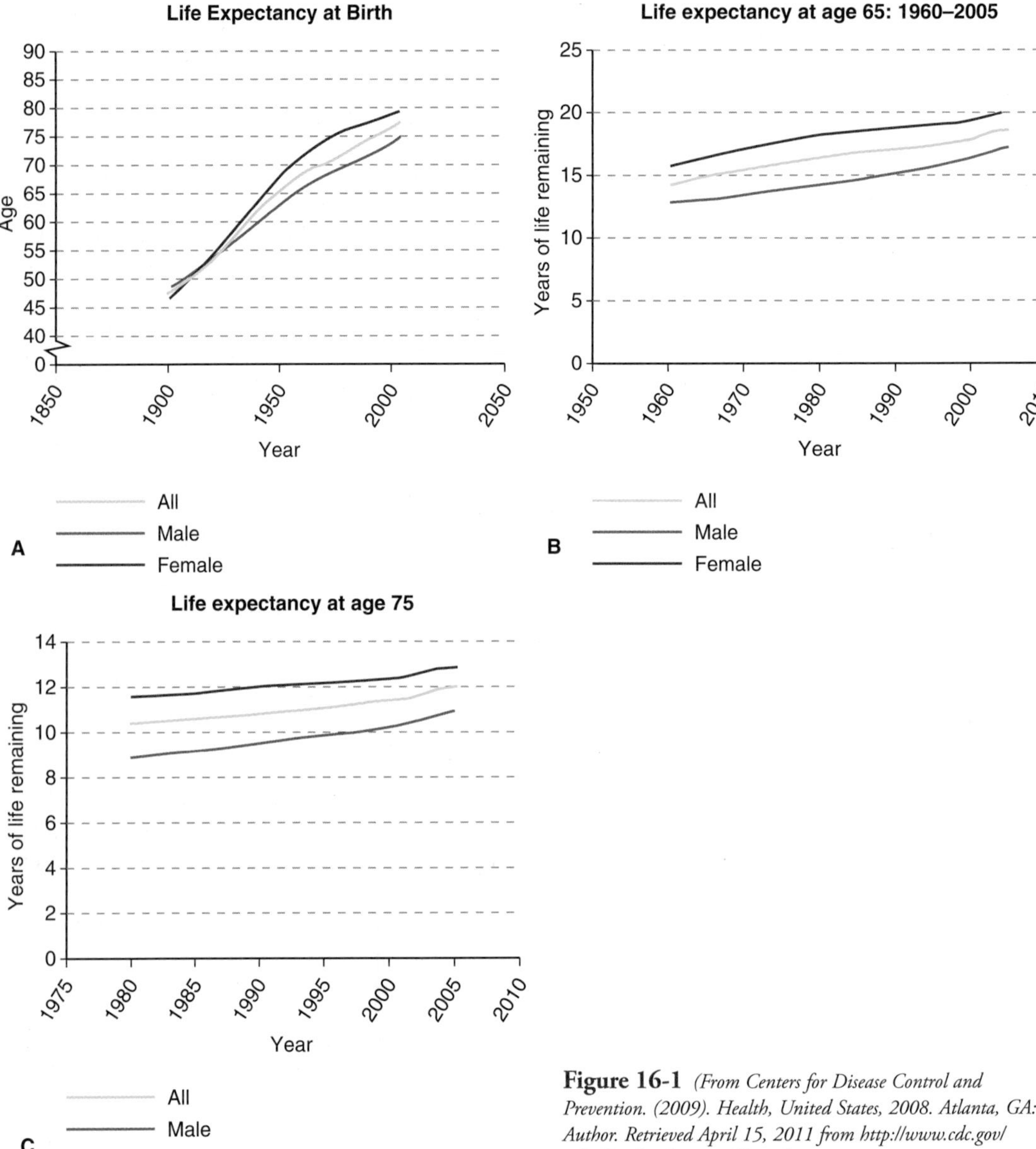

Figure 16-1 *(From Centers for Disease Control and Prevention. (2009). Health, United States, 2008. Atlanta, GA: Author. Retrieved April 15, 2011 from http://www.cdc.gov/nchs/data/hus/hus10.pdf#022)*

less likely to live alone than older non-Hispanic whites.

Income and Assets for Older Adults

As the expected number and health of years past age 65 increases, financial resources (income and assets) become an increasingly important topic. Further, when discussing income in older adulthood, it is important to understand that, although income decreases at retirement, many older adults supplement earnings with income from assets and money from selling assets.

Income

Older adults obtain income from four primary sources:

- Social Security
- Pensions and annuities
- Assets
- Earnings (McDonnell, 2007)

Social Security is the largest of these sources, accounting for 40% of income for older adults in 2005. Importantly, Social Security benefits are automatically adjusted for increases in the cost of living after a person begins receiving benefits. Social

Security payments are the sole source of income for 20% of older adults, although they account for less than half the income of two thirds of older adults (Hungerford, Rassette, Iams, & Koenig, 2001–2002). Earnings from employment and self-employment constituted the next-largest source of income in 2005, providing almost 25% of income for older adults. This may be expected to increase as the Social Security Administration adjusts the age at which people can begin receiving full retirement benefits. Income from assets, pensions, and annuities provided 33% of income for older adults in 2005 (McDonnell, 2007).

Over the quarter-century from 1976 to 2000, the poverty rate among older adults decreased from 15% to 10%. Consistent with this change, median real income (adjusted for inflation) increased 32% for the older population as a whole. Recent data indicate that:

- Median income for older adults was $15,407 in 2004.
- 80% of elderly households had annual incomes below $50,000 in 2002.
- Half of older adult households had nonhousing assets of $50,000 or less (Hungerford et al., 2001–2002).

It is important to note two issues related to this increase in real income. First, this increase has been uneven across ethnic and racial groups. From 1984 to 2000, real income increased 9% for older whites, compared with 36% for older blacks and only 5% for older Hispanics. Second, median income for older adults increased relative to the earnings of the working age population from 1976 to 1984, remained steady from 1984 to 1996, and declined slightly after 1996. One factor underlying this decline is the sensitivity of income from assets to changes in economic conditions. Asset income falls when interest rates fall, when stock market conditions decline, and when housing markets experience downturns (Hungerford et al., 2001–2002).

The increase in median real income allows older adults to consider an increased range of choices about living arrangements and use of time. The proportion of elderly women living with a nonspouse relative fell from 25% to 20%, and evidence indicates that increased real income was an important factor underlying this trend (Bethencourt & Ríos-Rull, 2009; Hungerford et al., 2001–2002).

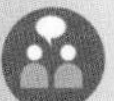

PERSONAL PERSPECTIVE
Opportunities of Aging

Judging by the 25th wedding anniversary photo hanging on the wall, Selig is as tall and handsome today at 83 as he was as a younger man. He is also as contemplative as he is robust, and that thoughtfulness is reflected in his response to the question: What are the special opportunities that come with aging?

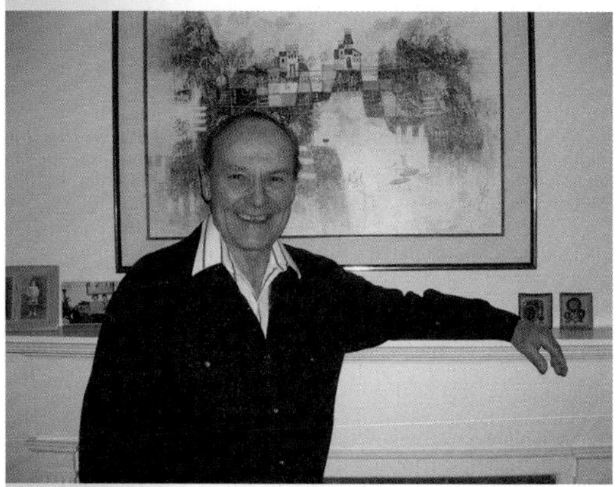

"The greatest opportunity is time," Selig offers after careful thought. "By that I mean, I'm unencumbered by the obligation of being a wage earner, concerned about taking care of the family. Not that that obligation ever stops. But it's time to sit back and say 'okay, those pressures have diminished by virtue of retirement from my previous life's obligations, so now I can spend more time with my wife, and spend more time with my children and grandchildren'. I have time to think about what I need to do to sustain my own life in a productive and meaningful way. My body needs to be challenged, and my mind needs to be challenged, because absent that I'll end up like a prune."

"So," he continues, "I need to spend time keeping my body fit and my mind fit. So I take classes at the university or the senior center and try to find friends who an engage in a way that stimulates each other's thinking about the issues that are of concern to both of us. I spend a lot more time thinking about the world around us and asking, how do I make it a little bit better than it is? How do I spend time doing things for others that utilize whatever inherent talents and capabilities I have?

"I have a lot of energy, and energy needs to be focused in a positive and constructive way. Since I feel so fortunate with my own life, I like to use that energy to have some meaning and utility for others." Selig has previously served as a hospice volunteer and today works as a greeter in a local hospital emergency room. He explains his interest: "In the emergency room, people come in under tension and anxiety, and if I can relieve that tension and anxiety and help make a positive outcome, I'd be happy with that."

"I'm still searching. I never want to stop searching," he sums up. "Just like I never want to stop learning and growing. I grow every day. I learn something from everybody. I learn from my kids. They're great teachers, my children. So I'm just really one happy contented fellow. But I don't want to stay contented. I want to push the envelope as far as I can."

About Selig Selig Danzig has shared his life with his wife Juliet for the past 57 years. They raised three sons and a daughter, and today Selig is all smiles when speaking of his four grandchildren. Selig worked for many years as a manager of human resources for General Electric Corp., taking an early retirement at age 53 to pursue other interests, including consulting, teaching, travel, and volunteer work. He is, in his own words "a political junkie." He needs to know what's going on in the world, to explore its problems and how they can be resolved. Selig shares that at one time he aspired to be a United States Senator so he could make a greater impact by influencing the world around him. Though that was not to be, it is evident that he has made a significant impact on both his family and his community.

Lorri B. Danzig, MS, CSL

Assets

The 2004 median level of assets (excluding Social Security and defined benefit pension payments) was $190,100 for households headed by those age 65 to 74 and $163,100 for household with older heads. Evidence also indicates that the composition of these assets changes with age. Although 80% of people ages 65 to 75 own a principle residence (and this residence constitutes an average of nearly 50% of the household's assets), the proportion of people over age 85 who own a principle residence drops to 60%. Similarly, most people ages 65 to 75 own vehicles, and the rate of vehicle ownership drops with increasing age. Among those age 90 and over, only 40% own vehicles (Coile & Milligan, 2009). The shift away from home ownership does not necessarily trigger a move out of the older adult's long-time residence. A second mortgage or a reverse mortgage could permit the individual to reduce the amount of equity invested in the home while continuing to live in the home.

The relationships between household finances and health are complex. Although income and assets impact older adults' ability to pay for health care and personal care services, health shocks also impact the older adults' financial decisions. Health shocks such as diagnoses of diabetes or heart disease increase the probability that an older adult will decide to retire. In addition, health shocks and death of a spouse are associated with decisions to sell assets such as residences and businesses. Thus, the rate at which older adults sell assets and adjust living arrangements is influenced by the pattern of health shocks that occur as they age. It is important for nurses to be aware of the interplay between health and household finances because stress, change in living or work arrangements, and the level of financial resources that are available can all impact health.

Insurance for Older Adults

Health insurance coverage provides a critical backdrop for understanding health care utilization by older adults and thus it is important for nurses to be aware of this information.

Medicare

Older adults enjoy near-universal single-payer health insurance coverage: Medicare is a federal program that provides health insurance for 97% of Americans age 65 or older. The program includes four components (Table 16-2). In 2004, Medicare paid 49% of health-care expenditures for beneficiaries age 65 and older, while individual out-of-pocket payments covered 15% of these expenditures (National Health Expenditure data, 2004). Medicaid and other public programs covered 18% of the expenditures, and private health insurance paid for 16% of the expenditures. Medicare beneficiaries incur out-of-pocket payments for:

- Monthly premiums for coverage for physician visits (Medicare Part B) and prescription drug coverage (Medicare Part D)
- Monthly premiums for Supplemental Insurance (Medicare Part C)
- Deductibles and copayments for services covered under Parts A (hospital care), B, and D
- Out-of-pocket payments for services, such as vision care, that are not covered by Medicare

TABLE 16-2 Components of the Medicare Program

TYPE OF CARE COVERED	MEDICARE PART
Hospital services	Part A
Physician visits	Part B
Supplemental insurance	Part C
Prescription drugs	Part D

Several strategies are available for obtaining insurance coverage for the portion of health care costs not paid by Medicare.

Employer-Sponsored Insurance

Some people are eligible for supplemental coverage as retirees, if their former employers offer this benefit. These Employer-Sponsored Supplemental Insurance plans, known as ESI plans, are similar to the health insurance plans offered to employees. These plans may cover such services as dental and vision care that are not covered by Medicare.

Medicaid

Low-income older adults may be eligible for Medicaid coverage through the Qualified Medicare Beneficiary or the Medically Needy programs. These people are known as *dual-eligibles* because they are eligible for coverage by both Medicare and Medicaid.

To qualify for the Medically Needy program, which was offered by 41 states as of 2000, a person must have high medical expenses and spend down to the Medically Needy income level.

Under the Qualified Medicare Beneficiary program, the state Medicaid program pays the Medicare part B premiums along with the coinsurance and deductibles. States may also provide full Medicaid benefits to adults over age 65 if their income falls below a state-established standard.

A 1990 federal law extended the income limit to participate in the Qualified Medicare Beneficiary program. Those covered by this law were designated *specified low-income Medicare beneficiaries.* States are required to pay Medicare part B premiums for these beneficiaries but not the coinsurance or deductibles.

Medicare beneficiaries who are not covered by either an ESI plan or Medicaid have two options: Medicare Advantage plans or Medigap coverage, to reduce the risk of incurring substantial costs for deductibles and copayments. Data from the *1996-1997 Community Tracking Study Household Survey* (Robert Wood Johnson Foundation, 1998) indicates that older adults view these options as substitutes: enrollment in Medicare Advantage plans is relatively high in geographic areas with high Medigap policy premiums.

Medigap

Those who are not eligible for retiree health benefits or Medicaid may elect to purchase a Medigap insurance plan, which is referred to as Medicare Part C. About 37% of Medicare beneficiaries purchase Medigap policies. Private companies sell 10 standard Medigap plans, which range from basic coverage to extensive coverage, as defined by federal law. These plans reduce individual out-of-pocket payments for the deductibles and copayments for Medicare Parts A and B.

Managed Care

Individuals may elect to enroll in a Medicare managed care plan (Medicare Advantage). The managed care plans cover the services that are included in Medicare Parts A and B, and some plans also include coverage of prescription drugs (McLaughlin, Chernew, & Taylor 2002). Participation in a managed care plan is optional, and it offers a trade-off: A person who enrolls in a Medicare Advantage plan obtains reduced out-of-pocket costs, including for prescription drugs (Box 16-2), in exchange for restrictions on provider choice.

Participation in a Medicare Advantage managed care plan is optional, and it offers reduced out-of-pocket costs, including for prescription drugs, in exchange for restrictions on provider choice.

BOX 16-2 Prescription Drug Coverage

Medicare Part D was implemented in 2006 to address the concern that prescription drugs account for an increasing portion of health-care expenditures. Older adults can obtain prescription drug cover by either enrolling in a Medicare Advantage managed care plan or purchasing a Medicare Part D plan. Participation in this program has exceeded initial expectations. Of older adults who did not have prescription drug coverage in 2004 (before implementation of Medicare Part D), more than 50% purchased plans. As a result, only 7% of Medicare beneficiaries lacked prescription drug coverage in 2006 (compared with 24% in 2004) (Levy & Weir, 2009).

Socioeconomic Status and Health

A recent study of socioeconomic status and diabetes provides insight into the multifaceted relationship between socioeconomic status and health and also the influence of socioeconomic status on successfully engaging patients in a helping relationship. This study of 3,000 men ages 25 to 70 included socioeconomic status information, lab test results that provided an objective measure of whether the person had diabetes, and self-reported information indicating whether the person had been diagnosed as diabetic. The study concluded that low socioeconomic status is a triple-threat:

- Those of lower socioeconomic status are more likely to be obese and more likely to have lab test results that indicate diabetes, compared with people of higher socioeconomic status.
- Those of lower socioeconomic status who have diabetes are more likely to be undiagnosed, compared with people of higher socioeconomic status who have diabetes.
- Those of lower socioeconomic status, with diagnosed diabetes, are less successful at implementing the instructions for at-home management of this condition, compared with people of higher socioeconomic status with diagnosed diabetes (Smith, 2007).

This study concludes that recent innovations in diabetes management can potentially strengthen health for those with diabetes, if the complex instructions can be implemented. Current technology, which requires adjusting insulin doses based on food intake and exercise, poses challenges for people with low education.

Two additional studies indicate that the influence of socioeconomic status on health is substantial and may accumulate over time. Bhattacharya and Lakdawalla (2002) analyzed data for a large sample (n = 13,000) of Medicare beneficiaries over age 65, and reached three conclusions:

- Lower income people have higher levels of health care utilization than higher-income people.
- Lower-income people use different types of care, compared with higher-income people. Specifically, lower income people are more likely to use home health care.
- Despite the higher levels of health care utilization, lower-income people have higher mortality rates.

These findings raise two important questions for health-care providers. The first is, "Does health status at age 65 have a lingering impact on health at older ages?" If so, strategies to support successful aging may require interventions at younger ages. For example, multivariate analysis of survey data (n = 14,000 people age 70 and older) showed that obesity is associated with greater functional limitation, after controlling for age, education, race, and disease conditions such as diabetes and hypertension (Himes, 2000). Because other work indicates that obesity at younger ages is associated with socioeconomic status, successful aging for those of low socioeconomic status may require interventions to address obesity issues in younger adults.

The second question is, "Do people with higher socioeconomic status make better use of the health care system?" Multivariate analysis of Medicare claims data for older adults indicates that higher-income households are more likely to have health care utilization that is consistent with evidence-based guidelines, compared with lower-income households, and that the gap has been widening over time (Skinner & Zhou, 2004). This evidence raises important issues about the influence of socioeconomic status on health literacy, health insurance literacy, and ability to navigate the health care system. Grossman's conceptual framework highlights the importance of proactive efforts by individuals and households; if low socioeconomic status is associated with gaps in these efforts, then it may be important to develop strategies to address these issues. Health economists provide two insights about this issue.

First, literacy issues encompass a broad range of topics. Analysis of older adults' understanding of health insurance and Medicare terminology showed that many older adults lack health insurance literacy and that literacy was positively correlated with education, income, and health status (McCormack, Bann, Uhrig, Berkman, & Rudd, 2009).

Second, health care utilization is significantly associated (n = 4,600) with beliefs about the value of medical care, history of health insurance coverage (which may impact ability to navigate the system), and self-reported ease of making an appointment—and many of these variables are associated with socioeconomic status. Higher-income people are more likely to believe in the efficacy of medical care, have experience with health insurance, report ease of making appointments, and self-report better memory and ability to make decisions (Kapur et al., 2004).

A second study reinforces the finding that literacy is only one of a complex set of factors that determine patient compliance with health-care advice. Sloan, Brown, Carlisle, Picone, and Lee (2004) analyzed patient compliance with advice that those with diabetes or age-related macular degeneration should have annual eye exams. Analysis of data for the years 1991–1999 (n = 21,000) indicates that the probability that a person will have the recommended eye exam is influenced by several factors in addition to the out-of-pocket cost of the exam. They included the perceived benefits of the exam (influenced by education, absence of dementia, and the likelihood that the exam would lead to useful treatment) and factors associated with the convenience of the visit.

In addition to the impacts on formal care discussed previously, socioeconomic status is associated with patterns of informal care that supplement formal health care. Older adults of lower socioeconomic status are more likely to live alone than those of higher socioeconomic status, and those with higher income are more likely to have a primary helper who is unpaid (LaPlante, Harrington, & Kang, 2002). This is an important finding because paid home health services are not the same as the services that are often provided by family members. Formal services often focus on one set of tasks, whereas family members tend to provide whatever services are needed, including cooking or providing emotional support and company. In addition, socioeconomic status also influences health through the stress of being poor over a long period of time. In an analysis of retrospective data collected from 1,167 older adults, researchers found that long-term financial stress was related to poor health outcomes, regardless of current financial status (Kahn & Pearlin, 2006). People who are aging with substantial mental or physical disabilities illustrate the complex interactions between individual choice and community factors at each level of socioeconomic status. Community factors, such as wheelchair accessibility, employment opportunities, and attitudes toward the disabled impact socioeconomic status, and socioeconomic status in turn impacts health (Minkler & Fadem, 2002).

The interactions among socioeconomic status, health-care utilization, and health are complex, and significant aspects of this relationship are not well understood. For example, substantial evidence documents wide variation in health care utilization and health across geographic areas—a variation that cannot be explained by differences in demographic characteristics across those areas. For example, a recent report, *Eight Americas: Documenting Mortality Disparities Across Race, Counties and Race-Counties in the U.S.* (Murray et al., 2006) concludes that white men living in the northern plains and the Dakotas have an average per capita income of $17,758 and an expected life of 76.2 years. White men in this geographic area live, on average, 4.2 years longer than white men living in Middle America, despite a substantial income disadvantage. White men living in Middle America have average per capita incomes of $24,640 and life expectancy of only 72 years.

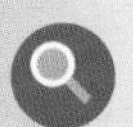

EVIDENCE FOR PRACTICE
End-of-Life Care: Regional Differences: Abstract

Purpose: To test whether regional variations in end-of-life treatment intensity were associated with regional differences in patient preferences for end-of-life care.

Methods: A dual-language (English/Spanish) survey was conducted from March to October 2005, either by mail or computer-assisted telephone questionnaire among a probability sample of 3,480 Medicare Part A- and/or B-eligible beneficiaries in the 20% denominator file, who were age 65 or older on July 1, 2003. Data collected included demographics, health status, and general preferences for medical care in the event the respondent had a serious illness and less than 1 year to live. End-of-life concerns and preferences were regressed on hospital referral region end-of-life spending, a validated measure of treatment intensity.

Results: A total of 2,515 Medicare beneficiaries completed the survey (65% response rate). In analyses adjusted for age, sex, race/ethnicity, education, financial strain, and health status, there were no differences by spending in concern about getting too little treatment (39.6% to 41.2%) or too much treatment (44.2% to 45.1%) at the end of life, preference for spending their last days in a hospital (8.4% to 8.5%), for potentially life-prolonging drugs that made them feel worse all the time (14.4% to 16.5%), for palliative drugs, even if they might be life-shortening (73.4% to 77.7%), for mechanical ventilation if it would extend their life by 1 month (21% to 21.4%) or by 1 week (11.7% to 12.1%).

Implications: Medicare beneficiaries generally prefer treatment focused on palliation rather than life extension. Differences in preferences are unlikely to explain regional variations in end-of-life spending.

Reference: Barnato, A. E., Herndon, M. B., Anthony, D., Gallagher, P.M., Skinner, J.S., Bynum, J.P.W., & Fisher, E.S. (2007). Are regional variations in end-of-life care intensity explained by patient preferences?: A study of the US Medicare population. *Medical Care, 45*(5), 386–393. doi 10.1097/01.mir.0000255248.79308.41

The Dartmouth Atlas Web site (http://www.dartmouthatlas.org) presents stark evidence that geography also influences the amounts and types of health care received by Medicare beneficiaries. For example, Medicare expenditures for inpatient care for severely ill patients during the last 2 years of life vary widely across states. These expenditures are substantially higher in California and New York, for example, than in Oregon or Wisconsin, and this difference cannot be explained by observable demographic or health status variables. This evidence, that health care practice patterns differ significantly across states and regions, has important implications for care of individual patients and for national health policy.

Thus, we close this section with the cautionary note that the complete connection between socioeconomic status, health, and health care utilization is not yet understood. Evidence about the importance of geography, for example, poses a conceptual challenge that is being investigated (Ong et al., 2009). However, current knowledge of the complex interactions between socioeconomic status and health—although incomplete—can facilitate conversations with patients at all socioeconomic levels. Nurses can use the Grossman framework to organize information about individual, community, and health care system factors, thereby supporting nuanced assessment of patient issues such as patient compliance, home-care support, and health literacy.

Implications for Nursing Practice

The multifaceted relationship between socioeconomic status and health has broad implications for nurses. Understanding the breadth of this relationship provides a basis for understanding patient behaviors and issues. For example, patients make personal decisions about their health care in the context of this complex web of interactions associated with socioeconomic status, much of which is not in the patient's control, such as the stress of living in chronic poverty or the patient's lack of access to health care as a young adult. Armed with increased awareness of the complexity of socioeconomic status, nurses can understand issues that may motivate patient behaviors and attitudes and use this understanding to build collaborative helping relationships with patients. These underlying issues can include problems with negotiating the health care system, lack of trust in medical personnel, and skepticism about the value of medical treatment.

The triple threat of low socioeconomic status for patients with diabetes provides a clear illustration. This research finds that patients with low socioeconomic status face:

- An increased likelihood of obesity
- Longer delays between onset and diagnosis of diabetes
- Lower rates of success at implementing instructions for at-home management (Smith, 2007)

Nurses may encounter many patients who fit this description. Older patients with a history of low socioeconomic status may arrive at a clinic or hospital setting with diabetes that has been undiagnosed and untreated. Once in treatment, some patients of low socioeconomic status miss appointments and appear unwilling to follow medical instructions, even after transportation and medical access issues are resolved. Nurses can use their knowledge of the factors related to low socioeconomic status to engage such patients in treatment. For example, nurses may need to assess a patient's ease in navigating the medical system, including making appointments and using telephone tree systems. If the patient is inexperienced in using the medical system, the nurse may refer the patient to a social worker or other health care advocate to increase the likelihood of understanding and follow through.

Some patients may appear unreceptive to education about diabetes, even when this information is given using the principles of health literacy. This may be due to negative perceptions of medical treatment or a lack of confidence in the benefits of following a complicated medical regimen. Patients are more likely to become engaged in treatment when their issues and concerns are addressed. Nurses who are attuned to a broad range of issues related to low socioeconomic status and health will be better prepared to respond as these issues arise.

Although the interactions between socioeconomic status and health are clearly important, our current understanding of the web of interactions between these two important variables is incomplete. This chapter provides an overview of current knowledge to help nurses evaluate specific issues that may be influencing patients and patient care plans as they assess patient health literacy, compliance, and home-care support and tailor nursing interventions to meet the individual needs of each patient.

KEY POINTS

- The relationship between health and socioeconomic status is strong. People with more income and higher education live longer than those with less income and education.
- The impacts of socioeconomic status on health are complex and interrelated, and the pathways of impact are often unknown.
- As a health economist, Michael Grossman provides a framework for looking at the web of interactions between socioeconomic status and health. Health is produced through inputs at three levels: personal, community, and health system. Factors such as community prevention programs contribute to health. Other factors, such as smoking, reduce health.
- Life expectancy has increased, and those additional years are healthy years, without severe impairment in activities of daily living or instrumental activities of daily living.
- Medicare provides health insurance for 97% of Americans age 65 and older.
- Medicare has four components. A person's coverage and out-of-pocket expenses depend on the configuration of Medicare coverage and socioeconomic status.
- The complexity of relationships between socioeconomic status and health is illustrated by a large study that used diabetes as an example to show that low socioeconomic status is a triple threat. People of low socioeconomic status are more likely to be obese and develop diabetes, more likely to have diabetes that is undiagnosed, and less successful at implementing at-home diabetes management.
- The impacts of health may accumulate over time. This is illustrated by a large study of Medicare beneficiaries over age 65, which found that lower-income people use more health care and different kinds of health care than higher-income people, yet those of lower income have higher mortality rates.
- Socioeconomic status impacts health literacy through a broad range of factors, including health insurance literacy, beliefs about the value of medical care, history of health insurance coverage (which may affect ability to navigate the health-care system), and self-reported memory and ability to make decisions.
- The pathways through which socioeconomic status impacts health-care utilization are complex. Studies have shown that people of high socioeconomic status are more likely to use informal (and probably more personal and responsive) care systems, that long-term financial stress is related to poor health outcomes, and that people with mental and physical disabilities are more likely to be poor, which affects health.

CRITICAL THINKING ACTIVITIES

1. Find out how many of the physicians in your area take Medicare and Medicaid patients.
   - Call local physicians. Ask whether it would be possible for a new patient with Medicare or Medicaid coverage to obtain an appointment.

- Call local physicians. Tell them you are a student. Ask the receptionist what proportion of their appointments they allot for Medicare patients? Are they accepting new Medicare patients?
- Go to http://www.Medicare.gov. Use "Search Tools" to find a doctor that takes Medicare in your area. Call one of the physicians listed and ask about the availability of new patient appointments.

2. Go to http://www.Medicare.gov. Read the information about Medicare plans, Medigap insurance options, and prescription drug plans. If you were preparing to make a decision to either enroll in a Medicare Advantage plan or purchase a Medigap plan, which option would you choose? Describe the rationale for your decision. If a patient asked about options for Medicare Part C, what would you advise?
3. Nurses may have opportunities to provide medication samples to patients who have limited income. The sample medications may be more effective in some cases but more expensive than older, generic medications, and the patient may not be able to continue with the newer medication. Pick one example of a situation in which health care providers choose between older generic and newer nongeneric drugs. Call a pharmacy to ask about typical copayments for the sample medication that is not generic and compare the cost to a generic counterpart.
4. Over the past 20 years the Dartmouth Atlas of Health Care Project has tracked Medicare spending, quality of care, and health outcomes across the United States. They have found some surprising results that suggest that the treatment a patient receives in one state differs significantly from treatment received in another state. Read one of the reports on their website: http://www.dartmouthatlas.org. Discuss the following questions:
   - According to this report, what accounts for the variation in practice patterns across the United States?
   - What implications does this evidence have for nursing care for individual patients?

CASE STUDY | *MR. SANDERS*

Mr. Sanders is a 72-year-old widower who has lived alone in a small apartment since his wife died 2 years ago. He has two grown children who call often, but they live at a distance. Six months ago, Mr. Sanders was diagnosed with diabetes. At that time the nurse provided comprehensive information about diabetes including instructions about diet, exercise, testing for insulin levels, and possible risks. Mr. Smith had been scheduled for a follow-up visit to check on his progress but missed that appointment.

1. Thinking of Grossman's framework of health production, what barriers related to socioeconomic status might get in the way of Mr. Sanders keeping his appointment at each level:
   - Individual factors, such as depression and social support
   - Community factors, such as the availability of safe transportation
   - Health care system factors, such as his wife navigating the medical system in the past
2. What factors might impact the patient's level of health literacy? How will this impact the patient's ability to implement self-care instructions? Does this impact the format in which these instructions are explained (and provided for repeated at-home reference)?
3. Was diabetes present, but undiagnosed, prior to the recent diagnosis? If so, does this signal lack of experience in using the health care system?
4. What referrals might the nurse consider? How might the referrals be made to increase the probability of their success?
5. What are the strengths in this case that the nurse can build on?
6. What is the next step in helping this patient obtain needed health care and manage his diabetes?

REFERENCES

Bethencourt, C., & Ríos-Rull, J. (2009). On the living arrangements of elderly widows. *International Review of Economics, 50*(3), 773–801.

Bhattacharya, J., & Lakdawalla, D. (2002). *Does Medicare benefit the poor? New answers to an old question* (NBER Working Paper #9280). Cambridge, MA: National Bureau of Economic Research. Retrieved December 8, 2010, from http://www.nber.org/papers/w9280

Cai, L., & Lubitz, J. (2007). Was there compression of disability for older Americans from 1992 to 2003? *Demography, 44*(3), 479–495.

Coile, C., & Milligan, K. (2009). How household portfolios evolve after retirement: The effect of aging and health shocks. *Review of Income and Wealth, 55*(2), 226–248.

Grossman, M. (1972). *On the concept of health capital and the demand for health.* Chicago, IL: University of Chicago Press.

Himes, C. L. (2000). Obesity, disease, and functional limitation in later life. *Demography, 37*(1), 73–82.

Hollingshead, A., & Redlich, F. (1958). *Social class and mental illness: A community study.* New York, NY: Wiley.

Hungerford, T., Rassette, M., Iams, H., & Koenig, M. (2001/2002). Trends in the economic status of the elderly, 1976-2000. *Social Security Bulletin, 64*(3), 12–22.

Kahn, J. R., & Pearlin, L. I. (2006). Financial strain over the life course and health among older adults. *Journal of Health & Social Behavior, 47*(1), 17–31.

Kapur, K., Rogowski, J. A., Freedman, V. A., Wickstrom, S. L., Adams, J. L., & Escarce, J. J. (2004). *Socioeconomic status and medical care expenditures in Medicare managed care* (NBER Working Paper #10757). Cambridge, MA: National Bureau of Economic Research. Retrieved December 10, 2010, from http://www.nber.org/papers/w10757

LaPlante, M. P., Harrington, C., & Kang, T. (2002). Estimating paid and unpaid hours of personal assistance services in activities of daily living provided to adults living at home. *Health Services Research, 37*(2), 397–415.

Levy, H., & Weir, D. (2009). *Take-Up of Medicare Part D: Results from the Health and Retirement Study* (NBER Working Paper 14692). Cambridge, MA: National Bureau of Economic Research. Retrieved December 10, 2010, from http://www.nber.org/papers/w14692

McCormack, L., Bann, C., Uhrig, J., Berkman, N., & Rudd, R. (2009). Health insurance literacy of older adults. *Journal of Consumer Affairs, 43*(2), 223–248.

McDonnell, K. (2007). Income of the elderly population age 65 and over, 2005. *Employee Benefit Research Institute Notes, 28*(5), 2–6.

McLaughlin, C. G., Chernew, M., & Taylor, E. F. (2002). Medigap premiums and Medicare HMO enrollment. *HSR: Health Services Research, 37*(6), 1445–1465.

Minkler, M., & Fadem, P. (2002). "Successful aging": A disability perspective. *Journal of Disability Policy Studies, 12*(4), 229–235.

Murray, C. J. L., Kulkarni, S., Michaud, C. K., Tomijima, N., Bulzacchelli, M. T., Landiorio, T. J., & Ezzati, M. (2006). Eight Americas: Investigating mortality disparities across races, counties, and race-counties in the United States. *PLOS Medicine, 3*(9), 1513–1524. Retrieved December 16, 2009, from http://www.plosmedicine.org

National Health Expenditure data. (2004). Retrieved from http://www.cms.gov/NationalHealthExpendData/04_National-HealthAccountsAgePHC.asp#TopOfPage

Ong, M. K., Mangione, C. M., Romano, P. S., Zhou, Q., Auerbach, A. D., Chun, A.,...Escarce, J.J. (2009). Looking forward, looking back. *Circulation: Cardiovascular Quality and Outcomes, 2,* 548–557, Retrieved from http://circoutcomes.ahajournals.org

Robert Wood Johnson Foundation. (1998). Community tracking study household survey, 1996-1997, and followback survey 1997-1998. Ann Arbor, MI: Center for Studying Health System Change. Retrieved December 10, 2010, from http://www.icpsr.umich.edu/icpsrweb/HMCA/studies/2524/detail

Rowe, J. W., & Kahn, R. L. (1997). Successful aging. *Gerontologist, 37*(4), 433–440.

Skinner, J., & Zhou, W. (2004). The measurement and evolution of health inequality: Evidence from the U.S. Medicare population (NBER Working Papers, #10842). National Bureau of Economic Research, http://www.nber.org/papers/w10842.pdf.

Sloan, F. A., Brown, D. S., Carlisle, E. S., Picone, G. A., & Lee, P. P. (2004). Monitoring visual status: Why patients do or do not comply with practice guidelines. *HSR: Health Services Research, 39*(5), 1429–1448.

Smith, J. P. (2007). *Diabetes and the rise of the SES health gradient* (NBER Working Papers, #12905).Retrieved December 10, 2010, from National Bureau of Economics Research, http://www.nber.org/papers/w12905.

U.S. Census Bureau. (2004, March). *U.S. interim projections by age, sex, race, and Hispanic origin: 2000-2050.* Retrieved December 16, 2009, from http://www.census.gov/popoulation/www/projections/usinterimproj/ Detailed Data Files

Chapter 17

Living Safely in the Environment

Diana DeBartolomeo Mager, DNP, RN-c

LEARNING OBJECTIVES

- Discuss aging in place, and list factors in the community environment that may help older adults to age in place safely.
- Discuss how transportation can positively or negatively affect an older adult's environment.
- Discuss the implications of employment versus retirement for older adults.
- Discuss ways that older adults can reduce the risk of victimization.
- Discuss ways in which the use of home-care services can help people live safely in their home environment.
- Describe factors that can contribute to unsafe medication management at home.
- Describe what a home-care nurse does during a home-care nursing visit.
- Explain how having an emergency preparedness plan for both in-home and community disasters can enhance safety for older adults.
- Describe the issue of homelessness in relation to older adults.

As people age, many of us like to surround ourselves with people and things that make us feel content and secure in our environments. Pets, possessions, gardens, hobbies, or something as simple as a day-to-day routine may help an older adult live comfortably in the community. However, as people grow older, they may also develop illnesses or diseases that compromise their health and contribute to frailty. When their ability to care for themselves safely at home diminishes, sometimes outside community services can supplement their care and create a safer and healthier environment to live in.

This chapter addresses the issues that affect how older adults can live safely in their environments. These issues include using the community as a resource, avoiding the risk of victimization, using transportation, employment, living at home with assistance, medication safety, preparing for emergencies at home and in the community, and homelessness.

Community

The Merriam-Webster online dictionary (http://www.merriam-webster.com) defines *community* as "an interacting population of various kinds of individuals in a common location." But achieving a community that meets that definition requires much more than might be apparent; indeed, other definitions assert that, to meet its function, a community must have qualities that make it livable. A more thorough definition is this: "A livable community is one that has affordable and appropriate housing, supportive community features and services, and adequate mobility options, which together facilitate personal independence and the engagement of residents in civic and social life" (Kochera, Straight, & Guterbock, 2005).

As people age, they may find it more difficult to function independently in their community. Yet despite the increasing difficulty, many older adults prefer to stay in their own home and their own community as they age, rather than moving into a long-term care facility or other type of senior housing. Most older adults in the United States own their homes, and many are long-time residents who contribute to their communities in positive ways (Alley, Liebig, Pynoos, Banerjee, & Choi, 2007). The idea of choosing to stay in one's own home and to modify the environment to compensate for disabilities is called *aging in place.* This phenomenon is becoming more sought after as the older adult population continues to grow (Bookman, 2008). By the year 2026, it is estimated that older adults will account for almost half of the increase in the total number of households in the United States, meaning there will be 2.4 million more older adult households than there are today (Crosby & Clark, 2008). However, as chronic illness and other disabilities may occur with increasing age, people will become less mobile and therefore less able to have their needs met while living independently. Economic resources may become scarce as people retire or become too frail to produce income, and immobility and lack of transportation can limit access to care, food, and social events. All of these factors contribute to limiting the ability of some people to meet their goal of aging in place.

Elder-friendly communities value and support older adults and include access to affordable transportation, housing, health care, safety, and social opportunities.

Community support and creating elder-friendly communities will be essential in order to allow older people to age in place (Alley et al., 2007). Elder-friendly communities value and support older adults and include access to affordable transportation, housing, health care, safety, and social opportunities (Alley et al., 2007). The U.S. government is working with local authorities to create a Public Service Agreement (PSA 17) that will address the level of satisfaction of older adults with their homes, neighborhoods, and services that are available to them. The overall goal of this movement is to remove barriers and promote independent living for older adults in the community (Crosby & Clark, 2008).

It is critical to assess a community based on whether it meets the needs of the people who live there (Box 17-1). Successful communities must also address the cultural, safety, and environmental needs of its citizens. As people age, they need easy access to places that we tend to take for granted: grocery stores, gas stations (for those who still drive), pharmacies, recreational places (movie theaters, libraries, parks), and medical providers for essential screenings, physical assessments, and sick and emergency visits. Within communities, there may be services available that are designed specifically to help support older adults as they age in place. Services may include transportation, meal delivery at reduced cost, availability of senior centers, adult day care, and other social programs in the community or at places of religious worship.

BOX 17-1 Assessing the Community

A number of resources are available to help older adults maintain their quality of life and their position as part of a community. One such resource is AARP, (formerly known as the American Association of Retired People), which is a nonprofit, nonpartisan, membership organization dedicated to improving the quality of life for people as they age (AARP, 2005). The AARP Web site has a link to a resource called the *Livable Communities: An Evaluation Guide.* The guide is written for older adults and encourages them to assess how easy it is to live in their communities. It helps readers evaluate safety, physical characteristics, and barriers in their communities. Topics are grouped into domains that include community services, drivability, health services, housing, mobility options, neighborhood safety, recreation and cultural activities, shopping, and walkability. The goal is to encourage older adults to focus on areas where potential changes in the community could make it more livable (AARP, 2005).

Some of the important aspects of a community in which older adults might age in place include the availability of other people willing to lend a hand, meal delivery, opportunities for social interaction, transportation, employment if needed, an appropriate urban or rural setting, and safety.

Access to Others

Not everyone is fortunate enough to have nearby support people who are willing and able to help a person who is elderly and perhaps living alone. The more support a person has, the more likely that he or she will be able to age in place with assistance from others. A combination of family members, neighbors, friends, church or synagogue members, town social workers, and perhaps private caregivers may all create a web of people that contribute to an older adult's success in staying in the community.

Meal Delivery

As people age, it may become more difficult for them to shop for groceries and then to actually cook themselves healthy meals. To help older adults to maintain a good diet and eat three meals a day, sometimes they need assistance with meal preparation. More than 200 programs exist across the

United States that offer meal delivery and other supportive services to older adults. One of the most well-known programs is called Meals on Wheels (http://www.mowaa.org). The program uses volunteers to deliver both hot and cold meals to older adults living in the community. Volunteers drop off the meals several times a week, often at a reduced cost or no charge, depending on the person's financial situation.

PERSONAL PERSPECTIVE
Preparing for Change

Juliet has just turned 80. She lives with her husband, Selig, in the large suburban two-story home that once sheltered their four children as well. Juliet is healthy and active, playing tennis and walking on a regular basis, and yet she recognizes that this is likely to change. "This has been on my mind for the last few years," she begins. "When I no longer can stay in my home, where will I go? I have two children in Boston and one in Connecticut, so which direction do I go?"

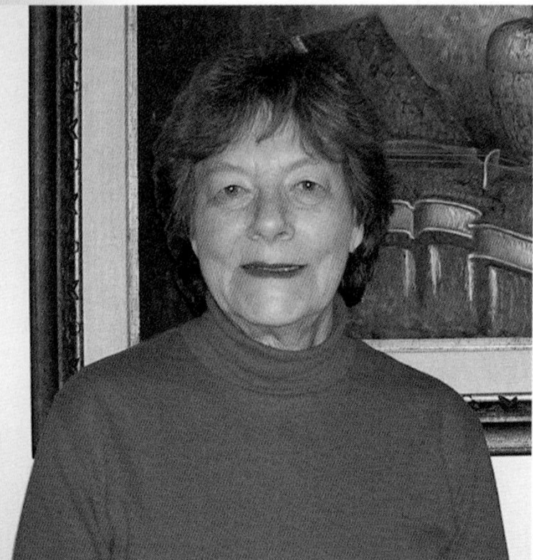

She pauses, then takes a step back. "Let me say this," she says, "I am in my home now and I hope I can die in my home. But we have steps. I hope I can manage the steps. We'll stay here as long as we can manage everything.

"There may be a final move, but I don't know where it will be. Will it be to assisted living? Will it be a nursing home? We go around and we look at different independent living places to see if this is for us. If we can afford it, do we really want to be in a place like this? We know that at this point we don't feel that way. We feel that if we went in there, because our minds aren't ready for it, that psychologically we would deteriorate, probably. I think I'll know when I might be ready for more help in my life and so I'm kind of trusting that feeling."

Juliet and her husband recently returned from a cruise, and memories of the vacation factored into her further comments. She said, "A realization came to me just this week. You know, one thing I really loved about the cruise was that all my meals were planned. I came in. I sat down like a lady. I had a menu, and I could choose from a variety of wonderful dishes. I didn't have to think about what to make for supper, what to make for lunch, shopping all the time. I'd never felt that way before. But all of a sudden I found it really wonderful. All of a sudden it feels a little like a burden to make all the meals. I'm not crazy about eating out. I'm not crazy about eating in any more, having to do it myself. I'm getting to the stage where I recognize that someday maybe I won't want to do the things in my house that I do right now, and I'll want someone else to do them for me. So what am I saying, really? That I'm thinking about it. That I know it will come. I'm not ready to say when, and I don't know where, but I'm definitely thinking about it."

About Juliet Originally a midwesterner, Juliet Danzig came east 57 years ago when she married her husband, Selig. She taught grade school until her children were born, and then she semiretired from teaching to pursue the full-time job of raising her four children. She continued to keep her teaching skills honed as a Sunday School teacher. After her children left the nest, Juliet went back to school and earned a master's degree in Counseling of the Elderly. She put her degree to good use running counseling groups for elders who were adjusting to the move from a private home to a senior housing community. Over the years, Juliet has undertaken many roles as a volunteer, including teaching English to Vietnamese and Russian immigrants and counseling clients of Planned Parenthood. Today she still volunteers, delivering meals to shut-ins through the Meals on Wheels program and reading to the blind. Juliet loves travel, bridge, entertaining, tennis, taking courses both at Elderhostel and in her community, and, she says with a big smile, "my family."

Lorri B. Danzig, MS, CSL

Socialization

One way for older adults to maintain social attachments is through the community's senior center or adult day care center. Basically, both are community-based centers where older adults can go to receive a number of different services and participate in various activities. Depending on the particular center, some are designed more for social interaction among older adults, and some provide a combination of social events and personal and/or medical care.

Senior and adult day care centers vary greatly in the types of activities and programs they offer, so it is important for those who are interested in joining to call their local center to see what is available. Services may include transportation to and from the center, supervision during the day, personal care and grooming, meal and snack provision (with dietary needs addressed), and structured activities (such as crafts, music, and exercise). Some centers are more like social clubs for older adults who are very independent and join merely to socialize at luncheons, join in card games, and attend various outings and trips. It is important to research the area first to ensure that a center provides not only the needed services but also quality care (National Adult Day Services Association, n.d.).

Researching the quality of senior centers is critical for success so that an older adult can attend and participate in a safe environment while perhaps their adult children attend work during the day. The National Institute of Senior Centers provides a valuable resource for older Americans by bringing together senior center professionals from around the country, helping to develop and expand senior centers nationwide. The Institute also works to improve the quality and services provided at local senior centers (National Council on Aging, n.d.). Similarly, the National Adult Day Services Association, which started in the 1970s, was formed to ensure the quality of such centers. It has developed operating standards and guidelines for local centers nationwide and provides education and training for managers and staff members who are running centers.

Just because people age, it does not mean that they don't want or need to socialize. Elder-friendly communities will have resources in place to meet the socialization needs of older adults. A good example of such a resource is a national program called the Lifelong Access to Libraries Initiative, which was launched by the nonprofit organization Libraries for the Future. The program is based on the idea that public libraries are well suited to meet the socialization needs of older adults and can be transformed into places that are convenient and helpful to aging community members who seek to learn, work, volunteer, attend lectures, and socialize (Schull, 2005). This is just one example of a unique way in which communities can meet the socialization needs of their older adults.

Transportation

Driving allows people to maintain independence and is often tied to quality of life (Owsley & McGwin, 2008). The availability of public transportation, such as buses, subways, and taxis, is not always widespread in the United States (Owsley & McGwin, 2008). Consequently, when older adults are forced to stop driving due to age-related problems, this loss of mobility may lead to isolation, depression, and other types of functional impairments (Wood, Anstey, Kerr, Lacherez, & Lord, 2008). Imagine not being able to just run out to the store when you need something, drive to a friend's house for dinner, or even get to the doctor's office when you are sick. Loss of driving can be devastating to someone who has always been independent and mobile.

However, driving and using other types of transportation in general can become much more difficult as people age. Driving requires a combination of visual, cognitive, and psychomotor skills that may become impaired with age (Wood et al., 2008). Older adults who have decreased mobility due to chronic illnesses and medication use are at risk for car accidents and traffic citations (Classen, Winter, & Lopez, 2009). More than 6,000 older adults were killed in automobile accidents in 2005, and it is estimated that those numbers will rise as the older adult population continues to grow (Classen et al., 2009).

Those who suffer from age-related macular degeneration may have severe visual impairment, which can limit the ability to pass the vision test for driving (Owsley & McGwin, 2008). Depending on the amount of visual loss, some people can still drive with this disease. There is no specific law about cessation of driving with macular degeneration. Many older adults tend to "self-regulate" their ability to drive and take their medical problems and vision into consideration when they decide whether or not they should be driving (Owsley & McGwin, 2008). People who are limited by vision loss can refer to the American Foundation for the Blind

(2010), which offers a number of suggestions and tips for alternatives to driving as vision fails. Their tips include using a white cane, using guide dogs, planning the route before leaving home, walking with another person, and gathering information about the mass transit possibilities in the area.

Limited vision, physical ailments, and economic limitations may all contribute to decreased mobility and an inability to drive or travel. The National Center on Senior Transportation is a rich resource for older adults and their caregivers as it provides links to public transportation options available to older adults by state (National Center on Senior Transportation, 2010). Their goal is to increase the options available so that older Americans may remain independent yet safe within their communities.

Employment

Since the late 1990s, participation in the labor force by people over age 65 has been increasing steadily and moving more toward full-time work rather than part-time (Bureau of Labor Statistics, 2008). The normal retirement age, according to the Social Security Administration, is based on the year of birth and ranges from age 65 to age 67 (Social Security Administration, 2009). However, many older adults cannot afford to leave the workforce at that age and are forced to continue working well past the normal retirement age for financial reasons (Wheeler & Guinta, 2009). In spite of the desire or need to continue to work, opportunities for older adults in the workforce are limited, which can cause economic hardships to those over retirement age who cannot afford to retire yet and cannot find work (Toder, Johnson, Mermin, & Lei, 2008).

Many factors beside financial need can influence the decision of whether or not one retires from the workforce. Some people continue working for continued health insurance coverage (beside Medicare), to socialize (Lee, Czaja, & Sharit, 2009), or to keep themselves active, stimulated, and busy. Some feel that once you retire, the next event is death, so they fear retirement and choose to continue working for as long as possible. Some people simply love to work and benefit from the feeling of usefulness it provides.

With so many older Americans working, some feel that, in the near future, society would benefit from marketing available job positions to this older population in order to hire them into the workforce. This could be helpful in areas where large numbers of people will soon be retiring, such as in hospitals and other health-care institutions (Runy, 2008). Others feel that new challenges will emerge as our current workforce ages. As advances in technology continue to soar, many older adults may not have had the experience of working with such rapidly changing equipment and so may need special training in order to be competitive within the workforce (Lee et al., 2009). Either way, older adults should not be forgotten when we think about opportunities for employment in the future.

Urban versus Rural Living

The word *urban* is an adjective that means "relating to, characteristic of, or constituting a city," while *rural* is defined as "of or relating to the country" (http://www.merriam-webster.com). Community resources may vary greatly in urban versus rural areas. Consider how difficult it would be if you lived in the country, there was only one health-care provider in the vicinity, that person's office was a 90-minute drive from your home, and you can no longer drive. What would you do if you had to be seen for an unexpected (or even planned) visit? Situations such as this may cause people in rural areas to avoid making trips to their health-care provider while trying instead to simply live with whatever health issues they have. It is easier in an urban area to find or hire transportation to get to where you need to go, providing you are fairly mobile.

Considering the livability of a community, if there are barriers to transportation and difficulties in obtaining services, livability and therefore quality of life may be limited in rural areas. One mission of the United States Department of Agriculture is to enhance the quality of life for rural Americans. This body has developed programs to promote self-sustaining community development in rural areas through a project called Rural Development (U.S. Department of Agriculture, 2010).

Rural Health Nursing

Rural health nursing includes a body of nurses who care for patients in rural settings. The Rural Nurse Organization, founded by rural health nurses in 1988, was developed to recognize, promote, and maintain rural health nursing. They represent a voice for rural nurses, and they advocate for continuing education and access to resources for rural nurses and quality care for rural citizens (Rural

Nurse Organization, n.d.). Nurses in a rural setting face a number of unique challenges because the needs of a rural setting are unique. For example, it may be difficult for nurses to find full-time nursing positions because there may not be a large enough population base to support more than a part-time nursing staff (Roberge, 2009). In addition, sometimes one advanced practice nurse is the only health care provider available for numerous people who need to be seen. Because other types of providers are not available (such as lab or x-ray technicians or radiologists), it may be difficult to have diagnostic testing done and evaluated for their patients (Roberge, 2009). Factors such as transportation, limited economic status, and limited health care providers can all affect accessibility to care for rural citizens, and especially for older adults.

Reducing the Risk of Victimization

Older adults living in the community, even in domestic settings (their own home or apartment), face many challenges, one being the risk of elder abuse. There are seven different types of elder abuse, including physical, sexual, and emotional abuse; financial exploitation; neglect; abandonment; and self-neglect (National Center on Elder Abuse, 1999). Many times these forms of abuse can be bestowed upon an older adult by a family member or a caregiver in the person's home. Much secrecy can occur as the older adult may fear the abuser or may not want to risk getting the person in legal trouble. Finding cuts and bruises while assessing an older adult may be a hint that abuse is occurring, especially when there are odd or unexplained reasons for how the injuries came to be. Many states mandate that certain professionals, such as health care providers or other adult care service providers, report suspected elder abuse. Each state has laws that address elder abuse along with particular agencies that receive and investigate any reports made. Usually the medical provider is notified, and, in addition, a report is made to the Adult Protective Services Association (http://www.apsnetwork.org/), as well as to law enforcement (National Center on Elder Abuse, 1997).

Although elder abuse is a tremendous concern, there are no official or standardized national statistics available to gain an understanding of exactly how large the problem is (National Center on Elder Abuse, 2005). Prevalence, or the total number of people who have experienced abuse over a given time, and incidence, or the number of new cases reported at a given time, are both difficult to assess. For example, in 1991, researchers suggested that 2.5 million people were victims of elder abuse, but this number was adjusted to "between 820,000 and 1,860,000" in 1996, when additional reporting data was collected (National Center on Elder Abuse, 1999). Such a wide range makes it difficult to assess the true magnitude of elder abuse. In attempting to track the incidence of elder abuse in the year 2000, states were asked to report the number of cases that had been reported in the most recent year where data were available. The total number of cases reported at that time was 472,813 (National Center on Elder Abuse, 2005), while in 2004, the number from a different source increased to 565,747 (National Center for Victims of Crime, 2008). Currently, national prevalence rates are vague, and they vary depending on how the sampling or surveying is done.

In general, studies have estimated that overall between 1 and 2 million older adults in the United States have been injured, exploited, or mistreated at some point in time, by someone they depend on, although some data suggest that only 1 in 14 incidents (excluding self-neglect) are ever reported to authorities (National Center on Elder Abuse, 2005). Reasons for the varied or unknown statistics regarding elder abuse include different definitions of what constitutes elder abuse, varied statistics among states, and lack of data collection on this topic (National Center on Elder Abuse, 2005). It is clear that elder abuse is an enormous problem in the United States regardless of the varying statistics available. The National Center on Elder Abuse, established in 1988 by the U.S. Administration on Aging, disseminates information about elder abuse to lay people and to professionals while also offering assistance and training on the topic to states and communities.

People living in the community can also experience other types of victimization beside physical harm. One reason older adults may fall prey to scam artists is that they were raised in a more trusting, safe environment than exists today (Gilbert, 2009), causing them to accept and believe what others tell them. In addition, cognitive changes, use of medications that may dull their thought processes, and use of complicated or complex terminology on paperwork may all contribute to the possibility of an older person becoming a victim of a scam (Gilbert, 2009).

Some examples of the types of events that can occur are listed in Box 17-2. People who set out to defraud older adults may do so by befriending them and then finding out ways to access bank accounts and legal documents or by convincing them to leave their property to them when they die. Telephone scams are commonly used to promise older adults money, prizes, or refunds if critical information is shared, such as bank account or credit card numbers. One way to avoid such calls is to register at the National Do Not Call Registry (https://www.donotcall.gov) or by calling a toll-free number available on the Stop Senior Scams website (http://www.stopseniorscams.org/). Educating the community about ways to avoid such victimization is essential for keeping older adults safe in their communities. Neighborhood watch organizations, church and religious groups, senior centers, and police departments can all work together to educate community members about avoiding scams and victimization (Table 17-1).

BOX 17-2 Examples of Victimization

- Identity theft
- Crime
- Online dangers
- Robbery and theft
- Financial abuse (loss of life savings, property, personal items)
- Medicare discount scams
- Prizes and sweepstakes scams
- Charity scams
- Counterfeit drug scams

From http://www.stopseniorscams.com and Gilbert, H. (2009). Protecting seniors from elder financial abuse & scams. Gilbert Guide Inc., Retrieved December 10, 2010, from http://www.caring.com/articles/protecting-seniors-from-elder-financial-abuse-scams

Living at Home with Assistance

Resources and Equipment

In 2008, only about 1.6 million, or 4.1% of people age 65 and older were living in institutions such as long-term care facilities (Administration on Aging, 2010). That means the remainder of people over age 65 were still living at home. With so many aging people living at home, it is probable that a large number of them will need some kind of assistance in the home as time goes on. About 7.2 million people received some type of personal assistance or care in their homes in 2000 (National Association for Home Care & Hospice,

TABLE 17-1 Tips for Avoiding Victimization

Walking or shopping	■ Stay alert. Avoid walking at night or in dark places. Avoid places where someone could hide. ■ Don't carry a purse. If you do, keep your keys and money in a pocket rather than in your purse. Don't put your name and address on your keys. ■ Don't dress in flashy clothes or wear obvious jewelry. ■ Ignore someone who bothers you. If confronted, scream loudly. If followed, run to a door or where people are.
Banking	■ Don't go to the bank at the same time each day. ■ Have checks deposited directly. ■ Step away from an ATM if someone comes behind you. ■ If approached by a robber, give up your money and don't resist.
Driving	■ Drive with your windows up and doors locked. ■ Keep your car in good condition and the gas tank at least half full. ■ Never pick up hitchhikers. ■ If the car breaks down, stay inside it. ■ If possible, always carry a cell phone.
Parking	■ If using a valet, give only the car key, not all keys. ■ Lock the car registration and garage door opener in the glove box.

Adapted from University of Nevada. (2000). *Reducing your risks of crime victimization in the community.* Cooperative Extension Fact Sheet 01-13. Reno, NV: Author. Retrieved December 5, 2010, from http://www.unce.unr.edu/publications/files/hn/2001/fs0113.pdf

2010). Rising health-care costs, lack of available family member caregivers (because they must work outside the home), and an increased need for home-care services (with declining numbers of home-care workers) all contribute to a concern for the rising number of people who will require health-care services in their homes over the next several decades (Bookman, 2008). In the United States in 2006, adults over age 60 made up about 17% of the population. By the year 2050, about 32% of the people in North America will be over age 60 (Bookman, 2008). Although being able to live in one's own home as one grows old is a wonderful and sought after situation, there are costs associated with having assistance in one's home.

Rising health-care costs, lack of available family and professional caregivers, and an increased need for home-care services all contribute to a concern for the rising number of people who will require health care services in their homes over the next several decades.

It is easy to think of the word *assistance* as physical help from another person. However, there are many resources and assistive devices that a person can use in the home to enhance safety and independence without requiring another person to be present. One factor than can influence the availability of these resources is money. Although some items may be paid for by medical insurance, Medicare (Title 18), or Medicaid (Title 19), many such products require out-of-pocket payment. For those who have financial stability, multiple insurance plans, monetary savings, or regular income, it may not be as difficult to obtain the products or services that are needed. However, in 2008, 3.7 million older adults in the United States were at or below the poverty level (DeNavas-Walt, Proctor, & Smith, 2009) and therefore may not have had the financial resources needed to gather the items needed to make an ideal and safe home environment. Poverty or lack of financial resources is always a factor to be considered when trying to make an appropriate plan of care for assisting an individual to promote a safe environment in the home.

Many types of equipment can be used as assistive devices. Before these items can be useful or helpful, however, the recipient must be willing and able to use them, and he or she must be able to pay for either renting or purchasing them. Assistive devices can be expensive, costing hundreds or thousands of dollars (such as hospital beds or automated chair lifts that go up a staircase [Fig. 17-1]), or they can cost just a few dollars (such as a simple device to help a person with arthritis pop the lid from a jar). Even when people have the money or resources to buy or rent equipment, sometimes it is difficult for them to accept this kind of help. It can be challenging to feel forced to rely on a piece of equipment, a cane, for example, in order to function. Some may feel self-conscious or embarrassed when using an assistive device, and some simply may be too proud to admit that they need help. There can be any number of reasons people may refuse to use such equipment.

Numerous items can be used as assistive devices. For example, people who are unsteady on their feet may use walkers, canes, crutches, or railings on the walls of their home to help prevent falls. Those who cannot stand or ambulate for long distances may need a battery-operated electric scooter or wheelchair to be mobile. Other items, such as a commode chair placed near a bed for toileting (Fig 17-2), a shower seat inside of a shower stall, or even a hospital bed can assist a person to be safely functional within the home. Devices are available to help people pull up their socks, pick up things that

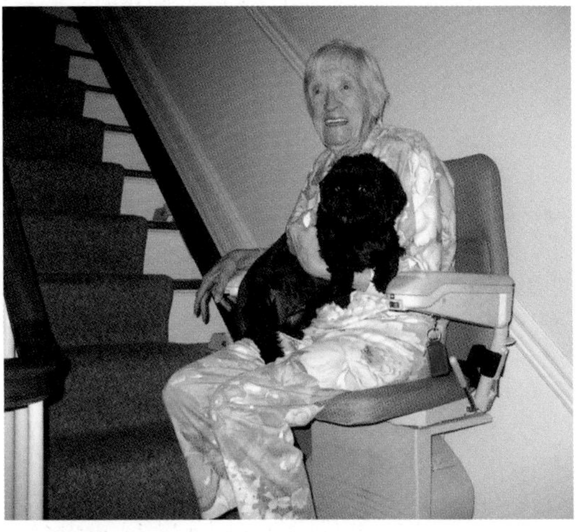

Figure 17-1 An automated chair can carry an older adult up the stairs.

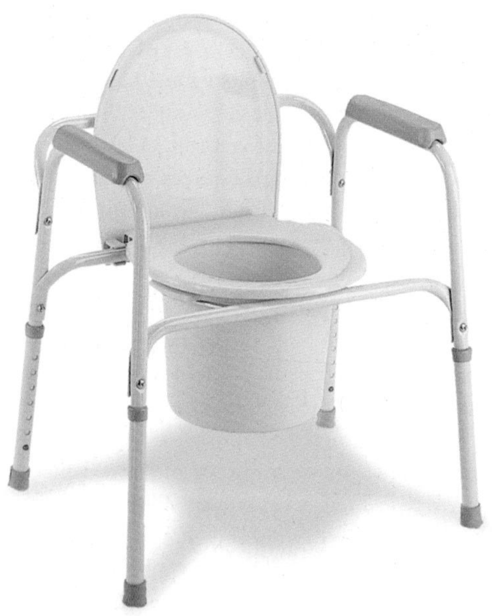

Figure 17-2 Commode chair.

they drop, and open jars or cans. (See Chapter 11.) Large lit magnifying glasses are made to assist those with visual deficits just as hearing aids are very common for the hearing impaired. Some community-dwelling older adults wear a wrist band or necklace with an emergency button to push in case they fall or become ill or injured. The device acts like an alarm system when activated, and the person is immediately called by the alarm company to see if he or she is alright. If the person does not respond, the emergency medical system or other contact people can be alerted and dispatched to the home as needed.

Safe Use of Medications

As people age and develop chronic illnesses, they typically need more medications. Recent statistics show that, on average, people ages 65 to 69 take almost 14 prescriptions each year, and those ages 80 to 84 average 18 prescriptions yearly (American Society of Consultant Pharmacists, 2010). Taking more than one prescribed drug at a time is known as polypharmacy, a common occurrence that puts older adults at increased risk of medication errors and adverse effects (Ellenbecker, Frazier, & Verney, 2004). Medication errors include such things as omitting doses, taking doses incorrectly, or taking medications without an order or at the wrong time of day (Ellenbecker et al., 2004). Very limited information is available in the literature regarding the types and numbers of medication errors that occur in the home setting (Mager & Madigan, 2010). However, personal observations in the context of delivering care in the home suggest that patients do in fact make mistakes when taking their medications.

Taking several different medications at different times of the day would be confusing for anyone. When vision is limited, it can become even more difficult to take medications correctly as many pills look alike, and sometimes the names on the bottles may look similar. In addition, it is sometimes easy to forget if medications were taken or not, so doses may be inadvertently omitted or taken twice. Sometimes older adults drop a pill and cannot retrieve it, and sometimes they choose to omit particular medications intentionally for any number of reasons.

There are a number of ways to help older adults avoid medication errors at home. Some people benefit from the use of a plastic medication box divided into the seven days of the week with an easy-to-open door for each set of morning, midday, afternoon, or evening pills (Fig. 17-3). Pills are removed from pill bottles and distributed into the pill box sections so that all pills for a given time of the day are available in one spot. The patient or his or her designee fills the box on a weekly basis. Boxes such as these can be used to help those who cannot open pill bottles or for those who have trouble remembering which pills to take out of which bottles.

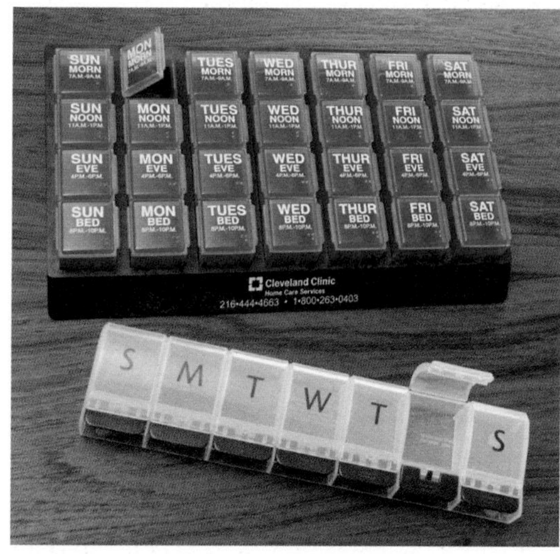

Figure 17-3 Examples of medication boxes to help older adults take their medications safely.

In addition to medication boxes, timers, beepers, and reminder systems are available to remind people when it is time to take their medications. Charts, signs, or notes can be made and left in a visible spot as reminders as well. Unfortunately, at times, all of the assistive devices, gadgets, pieces of equipment, and reminders in the world are not enough to ensure the safety of an older adult who lives alone or with a frail spouse. At such times, it may be helpful to refer the person to home-care services for help in the home.

Home-Care Services

I have been a home-care nurse for more than 18 years, and I have been in the grand homes of the rich and the electricity-deprived shacks of the poor. I have visited premature 3-week-old infants and centenarians, both healthy and dying. If I had to name the biggest difference between providing care in the home versus in the acute care setting, I would have to say that in a person's home, the nurse is an invited guest, and allowing entry into the home is totally up to the homeowner. The nurse and patient form a relationship that must consist of mutual respect and consideration to daily routines and "house rules," because the nurse is on the patient's "turf." I can remember when I worked in a hospital on a busy surgical unit and would prioritize my day based on medication schedules. I lived by the clock and would enter patient's rooms with medications, paying little attention to privacy, mealtimes, or routines. If there were visitors, I would respectfully interrupt to administer the medications. If a patient was finishing breakfast, I would move the tray a bit and offer the pills with some water. The medication schedule ruled my day because that was the only way to give the much needed medications in a timely, effective, and safe manner within the walls of the hospital.

In home care, walking into a patient's home with no regard to his or her scheduling requests or needs will get you fired from the case and thrown out of the house! One has to develop a rapport and a mutual understanding of what works for that particular patient and family in their home. And needs and requests vary greatly. You may be asked to come before breakfast, after breakfast, after the morning prayer service plays on television, after the nurse's aide leaves, through the side door, up the back stairs, or through basement to avoid the dog. And, of course, you may be asked not to come at all today!

Home-care services is a term that can mean any number of things given the situation at hand and the needs of the patient. Along with nurses, interdisciplinary professionals such as registered physical therapists, occupational and speech therapists, social workers, and dietitians can work with patients in their homes. Nonlicensed personnel such as home health aides can help with personal care and grooming, while companions and volunteers can help with household chores, driving to events, and socialization needs. Depending on funds and payment sources available, services may be in place for brief acute periods of time, or they may include full-time live-in help around the clock. The National Association for Home Care and Hospice has guidelines as to what constitutes a skilled visit that can be billed out to a third party payer such as Medicare Part B (T18) or Medicaid (T19) (National Association for Home Care and Hospice, n.d.-a). Services that do not meet the requirements for third-party billing may be offered at full or discounted private pay rates. See Table 17-2 for requirements to bill Medicare Part B and Medicaid for home-care visits.

The Home-Care Nursing Visit

In 2007, almost 3.4 million people received more than 110 million home-care visits from Medicare-certified home-care agencies (National Association for Home Care & Hospice, n.d.-b). That's a lot of people and a lot of visits! So, what happens during those visits?

Home-care visits from a visiting nurse are used to teach, assess, and evaluate patients in their homes. At times, the nurse is performing skilled nursing procedures, such as wound or intravenous care. Most home-care visits are used to assist the patient in becoming as independent as possible with his or her care in preparation for discharge from those services. In order to promote independence, the nurse is constantly using case management skills to assess the changing needs and desires of the patient and family, while incorporating their particular financial, social, and emotional needs into the plan of care.

Home-care nurses work collaboratively with a medical provider. Careful and thorough assessments must be made by the nurse and reported to the provider, while the nurse also often suggests an appropriate treatment plan for the individual in the home. Although some visits are more problem oriented (e.g., following up on a very high blood

TABLE 17-2 Requirements to Bill Medicare or Medicaid for Home-Care Visits

MEDICARE PART B (TITLE 18) VISITS	MEDICAID (TITLE 19) VISITS
Part-time or intermittent	Part-time or intermittent nursing services
Reasonable and medically necessary	Eligibility based on economic need by state
Skilled care (including nursing and physical, occupational, or speech therapy)	Skilled care as well as unskilled care, such as nursing assistant care
Nursing visits can be considered skilled for: ■ Observation and assessment of conditions ■ Management and evaluation of a plan of care ■ Teaching and/or training ■ Administration of medications ■ Skilled nursing procedures	
Ordered by a physician, and patient must be under the care of a physician	Ordered by a physician
Acute in nature	Can be chronic in nature
Patient must be homebound	Patient need not be confined to home

From Centers for Medicare and Medicaid Services. (2005). *Medicaid program - General information. Overview.* Retrieved December 7, 2010, from http://www.cms.gov/MedicaidGenInfo/ and Centers for Medicare and Medicaid Services Centers for Medicare and Medicaid Services. (updated 2009) *Medicare benefit policy manual. Chapter 7: Home health services.* Retrieved December 7, 2010, from http://www.cms.gov/manuals/Downloads/bp102c07.pdf

pressure or performing a dressing change to a draining wound), others require a general evaluation of the patient so that assessment is thorough and problems can immediately be reported to the health-care provider (e.g., assessing a patient newly discharged from the hospital who has a list of new medications, multiple medical problems, and many questions about their situation). The home-care nurse manages the patient's case and intervenes on behalf of the patient when his or her needs change. Visits can take on a life of their own when a nurse plans a visit to accomplish a particular goal (such as drawing blood), only to arrive and find that there is a new and more pressing problem (e.g., the patient has been vomiting for 2 days and is dehydrated and confused). In many cases, the newfound problem may become the priority of that visit, and other teaching and goals may need to be put off until another day.

Home-care nursing also differs from inpatient care because, in home care, a nurse can see the very life that the patient leads by stepping into his or her world for a brief time at each visit. To see patients in their own surroundings, dressed in their own clothes, with their belongings nearby and their favorite paintings on the wall allows a nurse to see the wholeness of the person, more than just seeing a patient in a bed with an unfortunate diagnosis. It forces us to see the individual as a person, rather than as a patient from the very minute we knock on their front door. We see family members baking cookies in the other room, trying to be cheerful while their loved one lies dying. We see pets walking over the bed covers as we take a blood pressure or try to do a sterile wound dressing. We deal with televisions blaring and neighbors popping in to visit bearing food or flowers. We hear family arguments, and we sometimes arrive to see a holiday meal being prepared as our ailing patient lies in a hospital bed in the dining room. By seeing this person embedded in his or her own life, we can try to work with patient and family to establish a plan of care that is relevant to their lifestyle. Sometimes all we can do is sit and hold patients' hands while they cry or mourn over the loss of their health or the stress of their situation ... and sometimes we cry with them. There is truly a special bond between a home-care nurse and his or her patients because we are invited into their lives when we get invited into their homes.

Safety

In addition to all of the physical, emotional, socioeconomic, and spiritual needs that may need to be addressed during home-care visits, the nurse is always thinking about overall patient safety at the same time. When we consider the issue of safety in the environment, we must think very broadly.

Numerous issues can affect the safety of the environment for an older adult, and numerous questions should be asked, including:

- Are there adequate resources for basic survival, such as heat, clean air, clean running water, food, and medications?
- Is the living environment safe from crime, abuse, and neglect?
- Is the patient mobile enough that, if left alone in the home, he or she could get out in case of an emergency, such as a fire?
- Are there electrical, plumbing, or carpentry issues that need to be resolved, such as poor lighting, unsafe wiring, leaking water, exposure to sewage, or broken floors, stairs, or handrails?
- Are there items in the home that create danger, such as loose wires, throw rugs, or clutter to trip over?
- Is the person at risk for falls?
- Are the necessary assistive devices available for the person, such as walkers, canes, crutches, wheelchairs, or a hospital bed?
- Is a person cognitively able to meet personal care needs, such as eating, toileting, taking medications, and knowing how to call for help when needed?

At times, people make decisions about their health that may not be the safest or the best for them. For example, they may decide they don't want to take a certain medication anymore, so they just stop taking it. Although this may be considered unsafe, patients have a right to make this choice as long as they are deemed competent and are alert and oriented. It is good nursing practice to make sure patients and families are educated about problems that could result from not taking a medication; however, it is ultimately up to the patient to make the decision. Choices like this become even more of a safety concern when the person is confused or disoriented and is actually unable to differentiate good judgments and decisions from poor ones. There are unsafe situations where a health care provider must report such findings to the provider, as well as to the local Adult Protective Services Association (http://www.apsnetwork.org/), so that a further assessment of safety can be made by that agency. Sometimes people are competent, but they simply make poor decisions about factors that could influence their health or safety in a negative way. In these complex situations, a home-care nurse may request an order from the provider to make a referral to another health care professional to assist in managing the challenging case.

Referrals

People who have multiple needs and whose care requires a considerable amount of case management may require the assistance of more than one type of professional (such as the home-care nurse) in the home. The nurse is usually the first one to see the patient and determine that other services will be needed. At that time, the nurse interacts with the patient, family, and physician or provider to discuss potential referral needs. Services may include physical, occupational, and speech therapy; social services; dietary services; and home health aide, companion, and/or housekeeping services. When a case is extremely complicated with many facets to the care, it helps the nurse to have a social service professional involved who can work with, counsel, and assist the family and patient with such topics as long-term care or end-of-life needs, filling out and filing paperwork for financial assistance, and connecting them with volunteers from the community or religious affiliations. Using collaboration among a team of professionals is not only beneficial to the family because all come with their own area of expertise, but it also helps the nurse to manage what can be a very complex and time-consuming situation. The main goal is the success of the patient's plan of care and safety and dignity for the patient.

Outcome and Assessment Information Set

The Centers for Medicare and Medicaid Services (CMS) is a federal agency that works in collaboration with the home-care industry to improve health outcomes for patients. CMS developed an assessment and documentation system that home-care agencies are required to utilize if they are billing Medicare for home-care services. The system is called OASIS, which stands for Outcome and Assessment Information Set. It is composed of numerous comprehensive assessment items to be used by home-care nurses during their visits (CMS, 2009, b). The purpose for using the OASIS assessment is to help document and measure patient outcomes to ensure quality improvement. Home-care agencies are required to keep OASIS data updated each time a patient is admitted, discharged, or has a change in status in the agency. Box 17-3 outlines types of assessments required for the OASIS document.

BOX 17-3 Areas of Assessment for OASIS

- Patient demographic information
- Payment source used for patient
- Patient history and diagnoses/conditions
- Therapies received at home and risk for hospitalization
- Sensory status
- Integumentary status (with detailed wound descriptions)
- Respiratory status
- Cardiac status
- Elimination status
- Neurological/emotional/behavioral status
- Functional status based on activities of daily living and instrumental activities of daily living
- Medications
- Care management (based on assistance needed with care)
- Therapy needs and plan of care
- Emergent care

From Centers for Medicare and Medicaid Services. (2009). OASIS user manuals. Washington, DC: Author. Retrieved December 7, 2010, from http://www.cms.gov/HomeHealthQualityInits/14_HHQIOASISUserManual.asp#TopOfPage

Preparing for Emergencies and Disasters

Avoiding Emergencies in the Home

Any number of emergencies can occur in the home, including medical emergencies, power outages, crimes, fire, and more. As difficult as it is to deal with emergencies for the average person, imagine how frightening and difficult it may be for those who are frail, ill, or immobile. As care providers, nurses must be able to assess how safe a person is in his or her home. Many situations may not look ideal or perfect, but if the person is generally safe and somewhat able to care for himself or herself and make appropriate decisions, then he or she is usually able to remain in the home in the community. The situation gets more complicated as frail health status, compromised cognitive status, or end-stage illnesses occur.

Sometimes family members choose to keep a sick or dying person at home and provide personal care themselves. This situation can create unique challenges that the caregiver may not think of at first. For example, if bedbound, the ailing person can never be left alone in the home because of the potential for fire or some other type of emergency. If no one were there to evacuate the immobilized person, it would surely end in disaster. Family members who commit to caring for bedbound or immobile loved ones at home may not realize the intensity of the time commitment needed to address such safety issues. Similarly, if a wheelchair is the only way a person can get around, it is imperative that one checks to see if the chair can fit through doorways and exits. If a person is housed upstairs and cannot ambulate down the stairs without assistance, then he or she cannot be left alone upstairs in case of a fire. People who are using oxygen at home must be aware of the danger of a power outage. Some cities will allow them to register on a priority list, so that if power goes out, restoration will be afforded to them first whenever possible. A back-up plan for such an event should be in place, such as availability of portable oxygen to use until power is restored.

Some basic steps can also be taken to help in certain types of medical emergencies. For example, a list of important phone numbers (health-care providers, police department, close family members, neighbors, poison control) should be kept in a visible consistent place (near the phone or on the refrigerator). A list of all medications and their doses, as well as a copy of a living will or other advance directives, should be present and visible in case emergency personnel enter the home and need to render immediate care, especially if the person is unresponsive.

Community Disasters

Being of an older age does not automatically make one more at risk when a community disaster occurs (Elmore & Brown, 2007). However, when natural disasters occur, older adults may be considered the most vulnerable population in the community setting for a number of reasons. Sensory changes such as decreased awareness of smell, touch, vision, and hearing, as well as potential changes in physical and mental health, chronic conditions, and socioeconomic disadvantages can all contribute to this vulnerability (Pekovic, Seff, & Rothman, 2007). In 2005, Louisiana suffered severe damage and loss of life from Hurricane Katrina. It is estimated that 74% of hurricane-related deaths were among those age 60 and older (Elmore & Brown, 2007). In normal situations, this older population may be able to maintain independence in the community, but when a disaster occurs, it is the sensory and physical changes that accompany aging that create danger for older adults (Pekovic et al., 2007). In addition, older adults may have unique behavioral and physical reactions to the trauma that occur during or after a disaster. They may withdraw and become isolated, and physical limitations may prevent them from leaving their home. Chronic illnesses, sleep disorders, and other physical symptoms may worsen during a time of trauma or stress (Pekovic et al., 2007). The severity of the trauma, as well as economic status, social support, cultural factors, and gender, can all influence how a person responds during or after an emergency (Elmore & Brown, 2007). For these varied physical and social factors, older adults living in the community need to plan ahead in case a disaster or an emergency occurs. Local, state, and federal agencies should be part of planning and practicing what to do if an emergency should occur. Planning should include coordination among both aging and nonaging service providers (Pekovic et al., 2007). Evacuation planning must be considered for older people living at home, as well as for those who are institutionalized (Willging, 2007).

Community-based disasters could include anything from human-made catastrophes, such as a war, a plane crash, or pillaging; to natural disasters, such as hurricanes, tornadoes, blizzards, heat waves, and floods; to medical epidemics, such as influenza or other contagious diseases. Massive or lengthy loss of electricity can result in hypothermia or hyperthermia, lack of clean water, and any number of other dangers related to being in a dark, cold, or hot environment for a long period of time.

A number of emergency preparedness resources are available for individuals and for communities, but preplanning is essential. As an example, the Stanford Geriatric Education Center has worked through their area American Red Cross to design an emergency preparedness pamphlet that citizens can fill out and share with their family and other community members (Stanford Geriatric Education Center, n.d.). The brochure includes a place to fill in emergency contacts both out of state and within the local or community area, and it provides a space to write out a plan for emergency meeting places.

Planning for emergencies also calls for getting a home prepared. Having blankets or sleeping bags and flashlights with extra batteries available can be helpful if electricity goes out. Storing a supply of nonperishable foods and bottled water also can be helpful in an emergency. Dates on these supplies should be checked periodically because even bottled water has a shelf-life. Cell phones are advisable for older adults in case telephone lines are down or power is out so they would have a way to communicate outside of the home if they are in danger. Also rescue services are available by pushing a button on a bracelet or necklace.

In some situations, evacuation is needed. Vehicles can now be equipped with global positioning systems (GPSs) to guide one on roads that are unknown. Services such as the American Automobile Association (AAA) are available to those who sign up as members and pay a yearly fee for services. If a vehicle breaks down, AAA can be called and will send service or a tow truck to the site as soon as possible. In addition, built-in or installed GPS services (such as "OnStar" or "Car Star") can track exactly where the car is so that, if the driver becomes lost, sick, or has an accident, operators can see exactly where the vehicle is and can send help.

Homelessness

A person who is homeless does not have a regular, adequate, night-time residence and instead uses a shelter, an institution that provides temporary residence, or a place not designed for or ordinarily used for sleeping (U.S. Department of Housing and Urban Development, n.d.). As people are living longer, it is projected that we will see more older adults over age 62 who are homeless (Mattessich, 2007). Older adults who find themselves homeless face a number of health issues and other challenges and barriers to access services.

According to one recent study done in Minnesota, homeless adults over age 55 faced a number of financial differences than younger adults who were homeless (Box 17-4) (Mattessich, 2007). In general, homeless older adults tend to have multiple

BOX 17-4 Differences Between Older and Younger Homeless Adults

- Older homeless adults are half as likely to be working for pay.
- Older homeless adults are more likely to receive income from General Assistance or Social Security.
- Older homeless adults tend to have higher monthly incomes.
- Older homeless adults are more likely to report chronic health conditions that limit daily activities.
- Older homeless adults have a greater overall level of physical and mental distress.

From Mattessich, P. (2007). The executive summary: Homeless older adults. St. Paul, MN: Amherst H. Wilder Foundation. Retrieved December 10, 2010, from http://execsum.blogspot.com/2007/12/homeless-older-adults.html

medical problems that may have gone untreated for many years (Health Resources and Services Administration, 2003). Lack of social support complicated by such medical conditions as dementia or depression can create a situation where the homeless older adult is not likely to follow up with appointments; therefore, it makes the task of securing housing very challenging (Health Resources and Services Administration, 2003). Other barriers to accessing services include lack of transportation, lengthy or difficult application processes (complicated by poor mobility), frail health, and physical or cognitive impairment. Additionally, shelter environments can be harsh for an older adult who may have multiple physical limitations and can also put them at greater risk of victimization (Health Resources and Services Administration, 2003).

It is difficult to get accurate numbers on how many older people in the United States are actually homeless. In 2010, the U.S. Department of Housing and Urban Development presented a report entitled, *The 2009 Annual Homeless Assessment Report to Congress,* which was based on estimated data encompassing 3 complete years of data. The report found that, on a single night in January, there were more than 643,000 sheltered and unsheltered homeless people nationwide (U.S. Department of Housing and Urban Development, 2010). The agency estimated that there were 43,450 sheltered homeless people over age 62 in 2008 and, thanks to the impending growth of the elderly American population, that number could grow to almost 60,000 in 2020 and more than 90,000 in 2050 (Sermons & Henry, 2010).

Although the number of homeless elderly may seem relatively small compared with the total homeless population, the trend is still quite concerning, particularly given the impending surge in the elderly population as Baby Boomers age. Not only are older adults considered a vulnerable population to begin with, but the effects of aging can put them at even a greater disadvantage than other homeless people (Dunn & Brown, 2008). For more on homelessness among the elderly, see the Homelessness Resource Center (http://www.nrchmi.samhsa.gov) and the National Coalition for the Homeless (http://www.nationalhomeless.org).

Conclusion

Older adults are a valued part of our society who have unique, multifaceted needs. Finding ways to incorporate older citizens into social and educational events, as well as into the workforce, will be a challenge as the number of older adults continues to rise. Creating safe and livable communities with rich resources for this population will be crucial to their being able to age in place.

KEY POINTS

- Livable communities are places where older adults can have a good quality of life and include such facets as community and health services, safe housing, recreational and cultural activities, and methods of transportation (AARP, 2005).
- Meal delivery, senior centers, and adult day care centers help older adults age in place.
- Older adults may suffer isolation as vision deteriorates and limits their ability to drive, given the limited public transportation options in some communities (Owsley & McGwin, 2008).
- Many older adults work past the general retirement age of 65 due to economic and socialization needs; however, job opportunities for older adults are limited (Wheeler & Guinta, 2009).
- Rural communities have unique needs, including health care accessibility and transportation (Rural Nurse Organization, n.d.).
- Victimization includes physical and sexual abuse and neglect, as well as falling prey to scams that cause loss of money, property, or other items. Older adults may be at risk for victimization because of their trusting nature (Gilbert, 2009).
- With the number of older adults living in the community increasing, the need for services in the home will increase as well over the next 15 to 20 years (Bookman, 2008).
- There are many ways to offer assistance to people living at home, including through the use of special equipment, home modifications, and in-home help.
- Financial resources via insurance, Medicare or Medicaid funding, and private pay may be used to receive the assistance people need, yet these resources can all be scarce.
- People who need the help of others in the home may be referred for home-care services, which could include nursing, home health aide (nursing assistant), therapist, and social service visits.

- Payment for home-care services can be via private pay, private insurance, Medicare Part B, or Medicaid if certain requirements are met.
- Home-care visits by a visiting nurse are used to observe and assess patients, teach and train, perform nursing skills, administer medications, and manage and evaluate a plan of care within the home-care setting (Centers for Medicare and Medicaid Services, [CMS] 2009, a).
- Evaluating an environment for safety includes assessing for dangers.
- The Outcome and Assessment Information Set is used in home care to help measure and document patient outcomes for the purposes of ensuring quality improvement (Centers for Medicare and Medicaid Services, 2009, b).
- Emergencies that occur in the home include medical emergencies, natural disasters, power outages, crime, and fire; well-made plans can help to avert disaster during an emergency.
- Older adults are at great risk during emergencies due to potential alterations in sensory organs, as well as changes in physical health and mobility (Pekovic et al., 2007).
- Emergency preparedness for community disasters includes planning ahead with evacuation routes, food and water storage, cell phones, and having a list of contact phone numbers available.
- Although only a relatively small number of older adults are reported as homeless in the United States, homelessness can have a greater impact on this vulnerable population (Dunn & Brown, 2008).

CRITICAL THINKING ACTIVITIES

You are a home-care nurse who is looking at your plan for visits the following day. You have seven patients to see tomorrow, and a huge snowstorm is expected to start during the night and continue through the day tomorrow.

1. What can you do to plan for this incoming storm?
2. What kinds of questions might you want to ask your patients in order to decide how critical a visit would be tomorrow?
3. What other question might you ask them in terms of their plan for being potentially snowed in for several days?

Your older adult patient is legally blind and no longer drives. She tells you that a kind person called her on the telephone and offered to drive her to wherever she needed to go for a small fee for gas. The person asked for the patient's credit card number so she could put gas in her car before coming to pick her up.

1. What would you say to your patient?
2. Is there someone you would report this incident to?

You are a public health nurse assigned to help out at a health fair by standing at the Emergency Preparedness table.

1. What kinds of information would you share with older adults as they approached the table to talk to you?
2. What are some questions you might ask them?

CASE STUDY | *MR. FRATINO*

You are a visiting nurse who gets assigned to go out and visit Mr. Fratino to give an insulin injection, although the referral form contains very little other information about the patient. You find out a bit more information when you arrive at the home: Mr. Fratino is a 92-year-old gentleman who lives alone. He has recently been on prednisone (a steroid) for an autoimmune disorder and, as a result, he has developed high blood glucose (a side effect of the prednisone). The physician has ordered daily insulin injections based on fasting blood glucose results that are to be taken three times a day.

1. What are some of the nursing interventions you may need to perform for Mr. Fratino?
2. How might this visit turn into a lengthy and complicated visit when it seemed so simple from the initial request for home-care services?

REFERENCES

AARP. (2005). *Livable communities: An evaluation guide.* Created by Arizona State University for the AARP Public Policy Institute. Retrieved December 1, 2010, from http://assets.aarp.org/rgcenter/il/d18311_communities.pdf

Administration on Aging. (2010) *A profile of older Americans.* Washington, DC: U.S. Department of Health and Human Services. Retrieved December 8, 2010, from http://www.aoa.gov/AoARoot/Aging_Statistics/Profile/2009/6.aspx

Alley, D., Liebig, P., Pynoos, J., Banerjee, T., & Choi, H. (2007). Creating elder-friendly communities: Preparation for an aging society. *Journal of Gerontological Social Work, 49*(1–2), 1–18.

American Foundation for the Blind. (2010). *Welcome to the AFB senior site.* Retrieved November 5, 2010, from http://www.afb.org/seniorsitehome.asp

American Society of Consultant Pharmacists. (2010). *ASCP fact sheet.* Alexandria, VA: Author. Retrieved December 8, 2010, from http://www.ascp.com/articles/about-ascp/ascp-fact-sheet

Bookman, A. (2008). Innovative models of aging in place: Transforming our communities for an aging population. *Community, Work & Family, 11*(4), 419–438.

Bureau of Labor Statistics. (2008). *Older workers.* Washington, DC: U.S. Department of Labor. Retrieved December 9, 2010, from http://www.bls.gov/spotlight/2008/older_workers/

Centers for Medicare and Medicaid Services. (2005). *Medicaid program - General information. Overview.* Retrieved December 7, 2010, from http://www.cms.gov/MedicaidGenInfo/

Centers for Medicare and Medicaid Services. (updated 2009a). *Medicare benefit policy manual. Chapter 7: Home health services.* Retrieved December 7, 2010, from http://www.cms.gov/manuals/Downloads/bp102c07.pdf

Centers for Medicare and Medicaid Services. (2009b). *OASIS user manuals.* Washington, DC: Author. Retrieved December 7, 2010, from http://www.cms.gov/HomeHealthQualityInits/14_HHQIOASISUserManual.asp#TopOfPage

Classen, S., Winter, S., & Lopez, E. (2009). Meta-synthesis of qualitative studies on older driver safety and mobility. *Occupation, Participation & Health, 29*(1), 24–31.

Crosby, G., & Clark, A. (2008). A place to live. *Housing, Care & Support, 11*(4), 20–23.

DeNavas-Walt, C., Proctor, B., & Smith, J. (2009). *Income, poverty, and health insurance coverage in the United States: 2008.* Washington, DC: U.S. Department of Commerce, U.S. Census Bureau, Current Population Reports, P60-236. Retrieved December 6, 2010, from http://www.census.gov/prod/2009pubs/p60-236.pdf

Dunn, J., & Brown, L. (2008). Homeless older adults: Aging without a place. *Geriaction, 26*(3), 5–11.

Ellenbecker, C., Frazier, S., & Verney, S. (2004). Nurses' observations and experiences of problems and adverse effects of medication management in home care. *Geriatric Nursing, 25*(3), 164–170.

Elmore, D., & Brown, L. (2007). Emergency preparedness and response: Health and social policy implications for older adults. *Generations, 31*(4), 66–74.

Gilbert, H. (2009). *Protecting seniors from elder financial abuse & scams.* Gilbert Guide Inc., Retrieved December 10, 2010, from http://www.caring.com/articles/protecting-seniors-from-elder-financial-abuse-scams

Health Resources and Services Administration. (2003). *Homeless and elderly: Understanding the special health care needs of elderly persons who are homeless.* Washington, DC: U.S. Department of Health and Human Services. Retrieved December 3, 2010, from http://bphc.hrsa.gov/policiesregulations/policies/pdfs/pal200303.pdf

Kochera, A., Straight, A., & Guterbock, T. (2005). *Beyond 50.05: A report to the nation on livable communities: Creating an environment for successful again.* Washington DC: AARP Public Policy Institute.

Lee, C. C., Czaja, S., & Sharit, J. (2009). Training older workers for technology-based employment. *Educational Gerontology, 35*(1), 15–30.

Mager, D., & Madigan, E. (2010). Medication use among older adults in a home care setting. *Home Healthcare Nurse, 28*(1), 14–21.

Mattessich, P. (2007). *The executive summary: Homeless older adults.* St. Paul, MN: Amherst H. Wilder Foundation. Retrieved December 10, 2010, from http://execsum.blogspot.com/2007/12/homeless-older-adults.html

National Adult Day Services Association. (n.d.). *Adult day services: A smart choice.* Retrieved November 5, 2010, from http://www.nadsa.org/

National Association for Home Care and Hospice. (n.d.-a). *Back to basics: Medicare's coverage of home health services.* Retrieved December 8, 2010, from http://www.nahc.org/Meetings/Pol/09/Handouts/401.pdf

National Association for Home Care and Hospice. (n.d.-b). *Medicare Part A & Part B from the health care information system: Home health agency national state summary for calendar year 2007.* Retrieved December 8, 2010, from http://www.nahc.org/Facts/HHHCIS2006.pdf

National Association for Home Care and Hospice. (2010). *Basic statistics about home care.* Retrieved December 8, 2010, from http://www.nahc.org/facts/10HC_Stats.pdf

National Center for Victims of Crime. (2008). *Elder abuse.* Washington, DC: Author. Retrieved December 15, 2010, from http://www.ncvc.org/ncvc/main.aspx?dbName=DocumentViewer&DocumentID=32350

National Center on Elder Abuse. (1997): *Reporting of elder abuse in domestic settings. Elder abuse information series No. 3.* Washington, DC: Author. Retrieved December 5, 2010, from http://www.ncea.aoa.gov/ncearoot/main_site/pdf/basics/fact3.pdf

National Center on Elder Abuse. (1999). *Types of elder abuse in domestic settings. Elder abuse information series No. 1.* Washington, DC: Author. Retrieved December 5, 2010, from http://www.ncea.aoa.gov/ncearoot/main_site/pdf/basics/fact1.pdf

National Center on Elder Abuse. (2005). *Fact sheet: Elder abuse and prevalence and incidence.* Washington, DC: Author. Retrieved December 5, 2010, from http://www.ncea.aoa.gov/Main_Site/pdf/publication/FinalStatistics050331.pdf

National Center on Senior Transportation. (2010). *For older adults/caregivers.* Retrieved November 5, 2010, from http://seniortransportation.easterseals.com/site/PageServer?pagename=NCST2_older

National Council on Aging. (n.d.). *National Institute of Senior Centers.* Retrieved December 5, 2010, from http://

www.ncoa.org/strengthening-community-organizations/senior-centers/nisc/

Owsley, C., & McGwin, G. (2008). Driving and age related macular degeneration. *Journal of Visual Impairment and Blindness, 102*(10), 621–635.

Pekovic, V., Seff, L., & Rothman, M. (2007). Planning for and responding to special needs of elders in natural disasters. *Generations ProQuest Nursing & Allied Health Source, 31*(4), 37–41.

Roberge, C. (2009, Spring). Who stays in rural nursing practice? An international review of the literature on factors influencing rural nurse retention. *Online Journal of Rural Nursing and Health Care, 9*(1)82-93.

Runy, L. A. (2008). The aging workforce. *Pulse, 45*(2), 12.

Rural Nurse Organization. (n.d.). *Welcome.* Retrieved November 19, 2010, from http://www.rno.org

Schull, D. (2005). A new look at lifelong access: Innovative projects tap the interests and skills of a growing population of active, older adults. *American Libraries, 36*(8), 42–44.

Sermons, M. W., & Henry, M. (2010). *Demographic of homeless series: The rising elderly population.* Washington, DC: National Alliance to End Homelessness. Retrieved December 6, 2010, from www.endhomelessness.org/files/2698_file_Aging_Report.pdf

Social Security Administration. (2009). *Normal retirement age.* Retrieved on November 5, 2010, from http://www.ssa.gov/oact/progdata/nra.html

Stanford Geriatric Education Center. (n.d.) *My emergency contact plan.* Retrieved December 9, 2010, from http://sgec.stanford.edu/pdf-word/emergency.pdf

Toder, E., Johnson, R. W., Mermin, G. B., & Lei, S. (2008). *Capitalizing on the economic value of older adults work: An Urban Institute roundtable.* Washington, DC: Urban Institute.

U.S. Department of Agriculture. (2010). *About Rural Development.* Retrieved November 9, 2010 from http://www.rurdev.usda.gov/Home.html

U.S. Department of Housing and Urban Development. (n.d.). *Federal definition of homeless.* Washington, DC: Author. Retrieved December 2, 2010, from http://portal.hud.gov/portal/page/portal/HUD/topics/homelessness/definition

U.S. Department of Housing and Urban Development. (2010). *The 2009 annual homeless assessment report to Congress.* Washington, DC: Author. Retrieved December 3, 2010, from http://www.huduser.org/Publications/pdf/2009_homeless_508.pdf

University of Nevada. (2000). *Reducing your risks of crime victimization in the community.* Cooperative Extension Fact Sheet 01-13. Reno, NV: Author. Retrieved December 5, 2010, from http://www.unce.unr.edu/publications/files/hn/2001/fs0113.pdf

Wheeler, D., & Giunta, N. (2009). Promoting productive aging. *Health and Social Work, 34*(3), 237.

Willging, P. (2007). When it comes to public health, seniors really are different. *Nursing Homes: Long Term Care Management, 56*(9), 14–18.

Wood, J., Anstey, K., Kerr, G., Lacherez, P., & Lord, S. (2008). A multidomain approach for predicting older driver safety under in-traffic road conditions. *Journal of the American Geriatric Society, 56*(6), 986–993.

Chapter 18

Legal Considerations

Mary Toole, JD

LEARNING OBJECTIVES

- Explain the importance of advance directives.
- Detail the difference between legal capacity and medical capacity.
- Recognize that it is possible to preserve assets for spouses, disabled children, and other family members even when an older adult needs long-term care.
- Outline the many challenges in remaining at home for older adults.
- Understand the financial risks for older adults.

Advance Directives

In 1990, the U.S. Congress passed legislation, called the Patient Self-Determination Act, that requires health-care facilities to inform patients that they have a right to refuse treatments, including resuscitation, and to appoint a person of their choosing to make health-care decisions for them if they cannot. The documents used to convey these choices are called advance directives, and they include a living will, power of attorney for health care, and do-not-resuscitate order (Robert Wood Johnson Foundation, 2002). These directives are created in advance of disability or death and may specify the person's wishes, appoint a representative to carry out the person's wishes, or both. Advance directives take effect when a person is no longer able to make those choices.

Completing advance directives in a time of good health—thinking ahead about a time when you might not be in good health—means, in essence, that you can still make choices about your life and your possessions, even when you physically cannot. For example, imagine that you have no advance directives and are in a car crash that results in permanent brain injury, leaving you unable to work, pay your own bills, or make decisions about how or where you will live. Now think about having those decisions made for you by the person you trust most in your life and, conversely, think about having those decisions made for you by a complete stranger or by the relative you would least want to be in control of your life. Planning in advance for incapacity is one of the most important things you can do to ensure that your life, in the event of incapacity, is a life you would choose.

There are three categories of advance directives: health-care directives, financial powers of attorney, and estate planning documents such as wills and trusts. The health-care directives and financial powers of attorney are for use during a person's life, while the estate planning documents take effect after the person's death, ensuring that the person's estate is distributed to those the decedent wanted to benefit, whether family, friends, or charities.

Health-Care Directives

Health-care directives include a living will, a durable power of attorney for health care, and a do-not-resuscitate order. The requirements and forms used for these directives can vary by state. There has been some effort to create a uniform document for use across the United States, but both the form that is used and the formalities for execution, such as how many witnesses and whether notarization is required, continues to vary. State-specific forms can be downloaded from the internet (Caring Connections, n.d.).

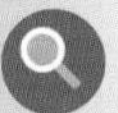

EVIDENCE FOR PRACTICE
Advance Directives

Purpose: To study healthy older adults to determine what prompts an individual to write advance directives.

Sample: Participants were eight Caucasians (three men and five women) who already had advance directives and were in good health. They were ages 60 to 77. All had an undergraduate degree, and five had advanced degrees.

Methods: Personal interviews were conducted with each participant and analyzed for data. Significant statements were identified as family influences, quality of life concerns, and pragmatic concerns.

Results: No one influence emerged as the reason for having advance directive; all were impacted by the three basic influences considered. Many life experiences lead people to prepare advanced directives, such as seeing a family member suffer a long death, wanting some control over end-of-life decisions, or a conversation with an attorney.

Implications: Nurses can have a significant impact on their patients' decisions to prepare advance directives. Given the nature and frequency of the nurse-patient relationship, a dialogue about advance directives could lead to a patient having them.

Reference: Crisp, D. H. (2007) Healthy older adults' execution of advance directives: A qualitative study of decision making. *Journal of Nursing Law, 11,* 4.10.

Living Will

Living wills were the first efforts to allow people to make choices about their own health care in advance of illness. Living wills were declarations of intent and stated end-of-life preferences. Usually they were straightforward and stated whether someone wanted to be kept alive by extraordinary measures and describe what comfort measures were desired; they did not address specific illnesses or situations.

The national nonprofit agency, Aging with Dignity, distributes a living will form that is valid in much of the United States. The form is called Five Wishes, and although it is written in simple language, it raises very specific questions about quality of life and the very personal choices that may have to be made in the event of serious illness (Aging with Dignity, 2010).

Durable Power of Attorney for Health Care

The limited scope of living wills resulted in the development of additional forms, which include the ability to appoint a health-care proxy. In many situations, a person might experience illness or injury that makes him or her unable to make health-care decisions. For that reason, medical powers of attorney or advance health-care directives were added to living wills. In some states, two documents are used, a living will and a durable power of attorney for health care, while in other states a single form is used that addresses all medical decisions that might have to be made in one document. An advance health-care directive can name someone to act on an individual's behalf if he or she cannot speak for himself or herself, include preferences about selection of medical provider, indicate wishes about organ donation, address end-of-life decisions, and contain burial wishes.

Naturally, the selection of an agent is one of the most important decisions in advance health-care directives. A successor should be chosen as well, in case the first person selected is unable or unwilling to help. Another consideration when appointing an agent for a health-care directive is to make sure the named agent is willing to not only serve, but will also honor the wishes of the individual and not substitute his or her own judgment. As a practical matter, it is wise for a person who has signed a health-care directive to let other family members know who has been appointed and that all family members should respect his or her wishes. Advance medical directives may not be honored by health professionals if family members disagree with each other and offer different instructions, even when there is a valid document naming only one person as agent.

Advance medical directives may not be honored by health professionals if family members disagree with each other and offer different instructions, even when there is a valid document naming only one person as agent.

Do-Not-Resuscitate Order

A patient's wish not to be resuscitated in the event of cardiac or respiratory arrest would appear on the living will. Usually, however, health-care facilities have their own do-not-resuscitate (DNR) forms and signage that should also be completed. Although the living will might indeed specify such a wish, the staff on the floor would be more likely to call a code, if needed, than to search the patient's chart for his or her living will.

Out-of-hospital DNR orders are valid in most states and can be given to emergency medical personnel to prevent an unwanted resuscitation. Advance directives are designed to communicate the type of care patients want when they cannot speak for themselves, and to appoint someone to make treatment decisions on their behalf.

Financial Powers of Attorney

In a financial power of attorney, a person specifies who will manage his or her money and property if he or she is alive but unable to manage them himself or herself. The first aspect of the financial power of attorney is when it goes into effect, in other words, what triggers it. For example, perhaps the person specifies that it will go into effect if the primary doctor deems him or her unable to handle his or her own funds. Or perhaps two separate doctors must reach this conclusion before the document takes effect. An alternative is to have the power of attorney take effect the moment it is signed.

The person signing a power of attorney is called the *principal,* and the person named to assist if needed is called either the *agent* or *attorney in fact.* If the power of attorney is effective upon signing, it should not be delivered to the named agent until, and if, it is ever needed. Documents can be as broad as allowing the agent to handle all of the person's affairs or very narrow and used for limited purposes, such as selling a house. The principal loses no power after signing the power of attorney; doing so simply authorizes someone else to act on his or her behalf.

The word *durable* is almost always used in conjunction with powers of attorney. A durable power of attorney is one that continues to have effect after any disability. It includes specific language that states if the individual was competent when signing, the power of attorney is still good, after any incapacity. The vast majority of powers of attorney are durable, although, on occasion, a power of attorney for a limited purpose might not be durable.

When selecting someone to act as an agent, it is best for the individual to pick the person who will do the best job and not worry about hurting another person's feelings because he or she was not chosen. If an individual is injured or incapacitated by illness, he or she will need someone with his or her best interests in mind but who is also capable of dealing with money and property. It is always wise to name someone to act as a successor to the first person selected as an agent. The reason for this is the individual trusts someone, he or she probably spends some time with that person, and the possible car accident that injured the principal may also have rendered the first named agent incapable.

Spouses often assume that the marital relationship will allow them to transact financial business for their spouse. That is not true. If an asset is owned only in the name of one spouse, such as a retirement account or insurance policy, no one can make changes in that investment unless they either are the agent on a power of attorney or have been court appointed to act on behalf of an incapacitated individual.

It is possible to change or revoke a power of attorney as long as the individual remains competent. It may turn out that the agent the individual thought he or she could trust the most is not trustworthy or may subsequently suffer from incapacity. If that occurs, the individual can revoke the power of attorney and create a new one.

Powers of attorney vary in different states; some states have mandatory forms while others do not require any specific terms. Also, some states require only that they be notarized and others require that there be witnesses as well as a notary public. When moving to a new state it is not always necessary to have a new power of attorney drafted, but it is important to check with an attorney to make sure the old power of attorney is valid in the new location.

In the absence of advance directives such as a financial power of attorney and a health-care directive, there may be no one who can act on a person's behalf in an emergency. That can result in expensive court costs for family or friends who have to petition a court to become the decision maker. If needed, a guardian will be appointed to make medical decisions, and a conservator will be appointed to make financial decisions. Some states aggregate both roles into one person usually known as the guardian.

In the absence of advance directives such as a financial power of attorney and a health-care directive, there may be no one who can act on a person's behalf in an emergency.

Many states have laws describing who has priority to serve as a guardian or conservator in the absence of health-care directives and powers of attorney. Those people are family members, but not always domestic partners. A couple could live together for years in a committed relationship but be shut out of decision making at a critical moment if there are no advance directives. Depending on the family dynamics and attitude toward the domestic partner, the domestic partner could not only be denied a role in the decision-making process but not even permitted to visit. Moreover, if one member of the couple owns the home and the other member of the couple does not have power of attorney, the family can force the non-owner partner to move from the home. In the event of disability and incapacitation, advance directives can prevent consequences that neither partner intended nor desired.

Medical and Legal Incapacity

Under the law, an adult or emancipated minor is deemed to have capacity until a court decides otherwise. In the absence of a court determination, an adult is able to manage financial affairs, decide where and how to live, and make medical decisions, even if the actions taken are bad. If there are periods of lucidity, then an adult will be allowed to make his or her own decisions, even if he or she forgets what occurred later, unless a court determines otherwise.

Medical or clinical incapacity is determined by a doctor who assesses a person's ability to understand his or her medical condition, the types and risks of treatment options available, and how to communicate about the decision. A doctor may decide that a patient is incapacitated to make a medical decision and ask the agent specified in the health-care directive to make the decision. If the patient objects, either to the agent's decision or even the agent's involvement, the doctor may become liable.

The differing definitions of medical incapacity and legal incapacity can, and do, collide. For example, an elderly woman who had a poor relationship with her family, drank heavily, and lived an isolated life fell and broke her hip. She was informed by her doctor that surgery was required and would in all likelihood be successful. She was also told if she did not have the surgery, she would never walk again. She refused the surgery. When the doctor asked the woman's son to assent to the surgery in her stead, the son refused and contacted an attorney. It was the attorney's assessment that the woman did have capacity and that a petition filed in the probate court for guardianship would fail because the evidence would not lead to the conclusion that the woman was legally incapacitated. The woman was able to speak clearly and consistently about her fear of surgery and preference to never walk again rather than face surgery. Although she was abrasive and eccentric, she did not meet the legal definition for a finding of incapacity.

At the same time, however, the hospital ethics board became concerned about the woman's decision-making capacity and a call was made to the state's adult protective agency, which has the power to seek guardianship on behalf of the state when a person is incapacitated and is at risk. The state agency also concluded the woman had capacity. As the days passed, the woman began to change her mind and, on occasion, would agree to the surgery. When she assented to the surgery, the doctors involved (by now, several had become involved) would agree that the woman had capacity and prepare her for surgery. As the surgery was about to occur, she would refuse the surgery and the doctors would conclude the woman lacked capacity.

The point is that for legal purposes, a court never adjudicated the woman unable to make decisions, and she was allowed to make a bad decision. The medical community felt the correct decision was so clear that her decision not to have surgery must mean incapacity. After about 2 weeks, the elderly woman did consent to the surgery, which was successful.

In the practice of elder law, it is common to have to assess capacity; however, there are no clear standards on how that assessment should be made. Some lawyers ask questions to determine if the client knows who his or her family members are and remembers where they live; the type and value of assets; and can state his or her wishes clearly, at least in the moment. Other lawyers may turn to doctors for an opinion.

Planning to Pay for Long-Term Care

Long-term care takes several forms: care by a spouse or other family member, private care managers and caregivers, agency care managers and caregivers, residential care facilities, and long-term care facilities. States differ on the manner in which caregivers and long-term care facilities are licensed and funded. All states in the United States, however, offer some type of publicly funded long-term care.

Planning in advance of any illness, injury, or incapacity is one of the most important steps anyone can take to ensure he or she gets the kind of care he or she needs, when he or she needs it, and where he or she wants it when the time comes. A large component of advance planning is determining how to pay for necessary care. At this writing, in 2010, long-term care facilities can cost $8,000 a month or more, and residential care facilities are not far behind. Most people cannot afford to pay such an expense for very long.

Many, if not most, older adults deny they will ever need long-term care, particularly in a nursing home setting. Common comments are, "My family has never needed nursing home care. We just die at home." Many say, "My family will take care of me if I need care; they promised." Sadly, there are certain kinds of illness that cannot be treated in the home by family or even professional homecare providers. Sometimes the only place to receive the needed care is in a residential facility or nursing home.

Long-Term Care Insurance

One option for paying for long-term care is to purchase insurance. Again, how the insurance companies are regulated and what products they are able to sell depends on the laws of the state in which the policy is purchased.

Long-term care insurance can pay for home care, residential care, day care, respite care, and nursing home care. Some policies will permit family members to be paid for care provided by them. A huge advantage of long-term care insurance is the flexibility it offers the person needing care. Some institutional settings refuse to accept public funding because the rate paid is set by a governmental entity and not the facility. A facility generally sets its private rate higher than the publicly funded rate, so a patient paying privately is a more desirable resident.

The disadvantage of long-term care insurance is primarily the cost. Premiums for long-term care insurance are based on choices that the insured makes at the time the policy is purchased and the age of the purchaser. Whenever someone decides to purchase long-term care insurance, he or she needs to work with a long-term care insurance expert who will take the time to explain how choices impact the premium and the levels of care that will be covered.

States, through their insurance commissions, regulate long-term care insurance and often offer free educational materials. Also, the National Association of Insurance Commissioners (2009) has published *A Shopper's Guide to Long-Term Care Insurance.*

Medicare

Many people assume that Medicare will pay for long-term care. Medicare is an entitlement program available to elderly, disabled, and a few other categories of people (The Public Health and Welfare, 42 U.S.C. Sections 1395 - 1395ccc). It has no asset or income tests, and eligibility is based on these categories and not financial criteria. Medicare is divided into parts:

- Part A pays for hospital care.
- Part B pays for traditional health insurance coverage, such as doctor bills.
- Part C operates like a health maintenance organization or preferred provided organization.
- Part D is prescription coverage.

Medicare is a complex program and provides extensive health coverage, but what it does not do is provide extensive coverage for long-term care.

The rule that applies to most people is that Medicare will pay for a maximum of 100 days in a facility, only after 3 nights in a hospital for the same condition for which the patient will receive treatment in the nursing home, and the patient must continue to improve during that time. Medicare pays for the first 20 days in full, but the patient must pay a copayment for days 21 through 100. Most people buy additional insurance to cover this gap. In fact, this supplemental insurance is known as a *Medigap policy.* Twelve different standardized Medigap policies are available (Plan A through Plan L). All are highly regulated by federal law. Information about Medigap policies can be obtained from http://www.medicare.gov/medigap/default.asp.

Medicare will pay for some long-term care in the home. That home care is available if the patient is homebound but the care is not around the clock.

Medicaid

Medicaid is a federal and state program, funded in large part by federal funds, but states make a contribution for a percentage of the expenses (The Public Health and Welfare, 42 U.S.C. Sections 1396 et. seq). Therefore, states opt in or out of certain options, and Medicaid is different in every state. Medicaid is also known by different names in different states; for example, in California, Medicaid is called Medi-Cal; in Maine, is it known as MaineCare.

Medicaid eligibility is based on both categorical and financial eligibility. Categorical eligibility is the category that the applicant or recipient falls into, such as aged (over age 65), blind, or disabled. Financial eligibility is based on income and assets because Medicaid is a needs tested social welfare program. Medicaid is intended to provide health insurance to low-income people, but many middle income people are also eligible for Medicaid because the costs of nursing homes and other long-term care are so high that most people cannot afford to pay for them without Medicaid.

When someone needs long-term care and files an application, he or she files the application with the state agency charged with making the determination of eligibility for Medicaid. Some states require a medical assessment to determine whether a person actually has a medical or mental condition that cannot be met in a community setting before determining financial eligibility for a facility. If a medical assessment is required, it includes a review of all nursing needs, how much help is needed with activities of daily living, and a cognitive assessment on the risk of dangerous behaviors, such as combative behavior.

Financial eligibility is assessed in two ways. One is a review of current assets to ensure the only assets the applicant owns are ones he or she is allowed to keep. These can include a home as long as he or she intends to return home, although how the person demonstrates that intent and the length of time that the exemption lasts varies widely among the states. A person can also own limited life insurance, liquid assets of less than $10,000 (sometimes as little as $2,000), a prepaid funeral within limits, sometimes a car, personal possessions, and sometimes income-producing property. The second is a review of financial transactions in the past, to ensure nothing was given away that could have been used to pay for care. At the time of application, if there are nonexempt assets, which are assets the person cannot keep, these will have to be spent down to reach eligibility.

In 1988, the U.S. Congress passed legislation to protect a spouse from becoming impoverished if his or her spouse enters a nursing home (The Public Health and Welfare, 42 U.S.C. Sections 1396r-5). This law protects the spouse's assets, which include additional liquid assets with amounts that change in most years. In 2010, the maximum amount that a spouse can keep is $109,540, while some states use formulas that result in less than that amount. The spouse also can keep his or her own limited life insurance, a prepaid funeral within limits, a vehicle, personal possessions, and income-producing property. That law is referred to as *spousal impoverishment* even though its intent is to protect the spouse at home from becoming impoverished. The spouse in the nursing home is known as the *institutionalized spouse,* while the spouse who is healthy enough to remain at home is known as the *community spouse.*

Federal law also makes some provisions to help minor children or adult disabled children of a recipient of Medicaid. Certain assets can be transferred to those children, either in a trust or outright, without any adverse impact on the applicant.

This second component of determining financial eligibility for long-term Medicaid is called the *look-back period.* Before 2006, the period typically was 3 years. Since then, states have been converting to a 5-year look-back period. When someone applies for long-term Medicaid, the applicant must bring in all monthly financial records regarding assets for the entire look-back period. Assets include, but are not limited to, bank accounts, certificates of deposit, stocks, bonds, insurance policies, pensions, retirement accounts, and annuities, as well as hard assets such as real property. The state determines if the applicant or the applicant's spouse gave away any asset for less than fair market value during the look-back period. If the state finds that a transfer occurred without fair compensation, then the applicant is denied eligibility for a period of months. Spouses can give money and property to each other without any ineligibility.

The ineligibility period for Medicaid commences when the applicant is in a nursing home and otherwise eligible for Medicaid. The consequences of this law can be particularly harsh when a transfer was made, not for the purposes of obtaining Medicaid, but perhaps to help a child who was getting a divorce or going through some other personal crisis. The applicant may have given the child $20,000 to get through a difficult time, never imagining he or she would need nursing home care. There is a provision under the law that allows the state to waive the transfer penalty if a transfer was made for a purpose other than obtaining Medicaid; however, the states are not known to grant such waivers very often.

Challenges to Remaining at Home

It can become very difficult for those on fixed retirement incomes to remain in their homes. Increased costs for property taxes, insurance, and utilities may make the primary residence unaffordable. Many people retire with limited fixed incomes and small amounts of savings. They may own a home (which may still have a mortgage) and have income from Social Security, a vehicle, and personal possessions. Yet the ongoing expenses include increasing costs for virtually everything and, although the person may wish to remain at home, he or she may be unable to do ordinary maintenance and have to hire help for mowing or small repairs.

Public Benefits

Public benefits programs are available from federal, state, and local communities and can help seniors remain in their homes. Public benefit programs have complex eligibility rules based on income and assets, and older adults simply may not have heard of them. Some of those programs include property tax rebate programs (which refund property taxes), programs to pay Medicare premiums for those with lower incomes, fuel assistance programs for low-income adults, veteran's benefits (which can include a payment to help with costs of care), food stamps, and subsidized housing.

The National Council on Aging maintains a Web site (http://www.benefitscheckup.org) that has a short questionnaire to help determine programs that may be available to help. Also, Area Agencies on Aging offer advocacy and support programs.

Reverse Mortgage

Another avenue to allow an older adult to remain at home is a reverse mortgage. With a reverse mortgage, the homeowner takes out money against the equity value in the home. The money can come in three ways: a lump sum, a monthly payment, or a combination of the two. Although there can be great value to a reverse mortgage because it may keep someone at home, the mortgage will deplete the equity in the home, diminishing the amount that will be left for heirs and reducing the cash that the homeowners receive if they decide to sell their home at some later point. There are both good and bad points about reverse mortgages, but they can be very effective in the right situations.

Scams and Financial Exploitation

Another risk for seniors is the vast array of scams that target them. The Federal Bureau of Investigation (FBI) at their website, http://www.fbi.gov, describes five reasons older adults are good targets for scams:

- Older adults tend to have some kind of nest egg.
- People of that generation grew up in polite and trusting times.
- Older adults are less likely to report a bad situation, either because they do not know where to report it or are too embarrassed to report it.
- They make poor witnesses because they have not paid attention to all of the details.
- Older adults are prone to try some of the promised magical health products because they are more likely to have those illnesses.

Many scams are flagrant, yet the perpetrator often succeeds and is not caught. For example, in one case of which I am aware, a woman in her early 90s lived alone. She received phone calls promising millions of dollars in cash winnings as long as she paid some up-front expenses, which would be refunded later. She received calls early in the morning, before 7 a.m., and was told to go her bank and given instructions to wire money quickly before her opportunity would expire. She was also warned not to discuss the situation with her family as the money would be a "wonderful surprise for her family." She sent nearly $20,000 before a bank employee suggested to her son, who also had an account at the same bank, that he should speak with his mother about some large transactions. The case was referred to the FBI but, to date, no one has been prosecuted and no money has been refunded.

Another case involved a man, also living alone, with some early signs of dementia, who responded to letters advising him that he had won money but needed to mail amounts of money, in cash, to an offshore location in order to receive the money. He repeatedly sent cash ranging from $20 to several hundred dollars. He did not keep the secret from his family but proudly told them of his winnings. It took some time and more money before he was convinced that he would not receive any money in return.

Perhaps worse than scams is financial exploitation of an older person by a friend, neighbor, or family member. The National Center on Elder Abuse notes there is no way to determine how many elders are financially exploited. There is no national clearinghouse for reporting elder abuse, and it is believed that the number of reports is dramatically understated. It is thought that only 1 in every 25 cases of financial exploitation are reported and there may be as many as 5 million older adults financially abused every year.

Forms of financial exploitation include but are not limited to forging signatures on checks, feeling undue duress to change a will or transfer property to the perpetrator, abuse of a power of attorney, the taking of money or personal possessions, abuse of jointly held bank accounts, and the charging of excessive amounts for services. Elders often are reluctant to report exploitation because of embarrassment, not knowing where to report it, and a reluctance to take legal action particularly against a family member.

In order to combat elder abuse and exploitation, many states have laws requiring certain professionals to report any suspected abuse or financial exploitation to Adult Protective Services. The list of mandatory reporters can include physicians, caregivers, other medical professionals, and social workers. When a report is made to Adult Protective Services, the agency opens an investigation to determine if there is a basis for the report and can bring significant powers to bear to intervene and protect the senior.

The 2004 Survey of Adult Protective Services on abuse of adults age 60 and over concluded that 20.8% of abuse of elders is some form of financial exploitation and the study also found that between the years 2000 and 2004, abuse of adults over age 60 increased by 20%.

KEY POINTS

- Planning in advance of incapacity is something all adults should do because waiting until it is too late can lead to unwanted consequences and high financial costs.
- Medical and legal capacity differ and can lead to conflicts between the two disciplines. Because there is not always a clear resolution to the conflict, a clear understanding of the differing perspectives is necessary.
- Ability to pay for long-term care can determine the quality of long-term care. Consumers should make themselves aware of the available options and also understand the options may change as policies and laws change. Assumptions about how long-term care is funded are common and often wrong.
- Publicly funded programs for such things as health care, fuel assistance, property tax rebates, and other necessities can help keep seniors in their homes.
- Elderly people are at increasing risk of financial exploitation or of becoming the victims of scams due to factors relating not only to age, but the different times in which they were raised.

CRITICAL THINKING ACTIVITIES

1. Argue the position that legal capacity is more reasonable as an approach to incapacity and then argue the medical model makes more sense. If you were incapacitated, would you want the protections that the legal model provides by making a presumption of capacity or would you rather have a doctor who is attuned to your mental status make the judgment? Does it make sense to have a judge, who may never have met you, rule on your capacity even with all the evidence before him or her?
2. The costs of providing long-term care through public funding are enormous. Yet the government allows some assets to be preserved for a spouse in the community. Is this good social policy? Should spouses be allowed to keep a home and other assets and then be able to leave them for heirs as the law currently allowed or should a lien be placed on the assets the spouse is allowed to keep so that the government gets paid back after the death of the second spouse?
3. Given the costs for health care paid through government funding, should that care be rationed? Should those who have the resources to pay privately receive a different higher level of care in reward for planning to pay for their own care?

CASE STUDY | *ARTHUR SMITH*

Arthur Smith is an 84-year-old bachelor who lived for many years with his sister, who has recently died. Although Mr. Smith is a lawyer, he has no advance directives and harbors an irrational fear that if he signs advance directives, something bad will happen to him. He is mentally very capable but secretive about his assets and income.

Mr. Smith inherits his sister's house and can continue to live there, except that he has never cooked or cleaned for himself. He has two living siblings, but they are both older than he and not able to help with his daily needs or his finances. Other living relatives include several nieces and nephews, two of whom are local, but those two have never gotten along with each other and refuse to work together to help Mr. Smith, each suspecting the other of trying to get Mr. Smith's money.

While out with his dog one day, Mr. Smith falls and breaks his hip in the backyard, which is not visible from the street. He is unable to move and remains in the yard for many hours before a neighbor hears his calls for help. Mr. Smith is taken to the hospital and then to a rehabilitation facility.

Upon discharge, he returns home, and you are his visiting nurse. His niece, Judy, becomes very attentive to his needs and runs errands for him, helps him cook and clean, and drives him to the doctor. You notice that whenever Judy visits, items disappear from the house. Crystal vases are missing from the shelves, and silverware and china are missing from the kitchen. You also notice that, as time goes by, that Mr. Smith's bank statements, checkbooks, and personal papers are no longer stacked neatly in his desk but instead are in a messy pile in the spare room.

Mr. Smith continues to refuse to sign advance directives. His nephew, Mike, visits infrequently but seems truly concerned about his uncle, and you do not notice things missing or papers out of place after visits from Mike. Mike is trying very hard to get his uncle to enter a facility, while Judy is totally opposed to that. Mr. Smith wants to remain at home. He continues to be unsteady on his feet and should use his walker, but he forgets to use it and falls frequently. Mr. Smith talks with you about his situation and values your opinion.

1. What steps should Mr. Smith take to protect himself?
2. Would it be appropriate for you to raise concerns about Judy? If so, whom would you feel it is appropriate to contact?
3. What steps would you take if you thought Mr. Smith was not physically safe?

REFERENCES

Aging with Dignity. (2010). *Five wishes.* Tallahassee, FL: Author. Retrieved December 12, 2010, from http://www.agingwithdignity.org/five-wishes.php

Caring Connections. (n.d.).*Download your state's advance directives.* Alexandria, VA: National Hospice and Palliative Care Organization. Retrieved December 12, 2010, from http://www.caringinfo.org/stateaddownload

Crisp, D. H. (2007) Healthy older adults' execution of advance directives: A qualitative study of decision making. *Journal of Nursing Law, 11*(4), 180–190.

National Association of Insurance Commissioners. (2009). *A shopper's guide to long-term care insurance.* Washington, DC: Author. Retrieved December 10, 2010, from http://www.ltcfeds.com/documents/files/naic_shoppers_guide.pdf

Robert Wood Johnson Foundation. (2002). *Means to a better end: A report on dying in America today.* Washington DC: Author. Retrieved December 10, 2010, from http://www.rwjf.org/files/publications/other/meansbetterend.pdf

Chapter 19

Older Adults as Caregivers and Care Recipients

Priscilla M. Koop, PhD, RN

LEARNING OBJECTIVES

- Define family caregiving.
- Describe the characteristics of family caregivers of older adults.
- Discuss the challenges and rewards of caregiving.
- Describe the characteristics of the recipients of family caregivers.
- List key support services available to support caregivers.
- Explain the nurse's role in supporting caregivers.

"If (the) health care system was a plant, family caregivers would be its roots—fragile, vital and invisible. The part we see—branches, leaves and flowers—is the apparatus of doctors, nurses, clinics, labs and hospitals. But the "visible" health care system has always been supplemented by the invisible support of home caregivers. We rely more heavily on those caregivers with every passing year. We do very little to provide them with support, recognition or respite." (Cameron, 2003, p. 4).

Family caregiving is defined as unpaid assistance and support for family members, friends, or neighbors who are disabled, frail (due to old age), or living with a long-term health problem. This assistance and support may be occasional or constant and may last for a short time or for months or years (Adamson & Donovan, 2005; Family Caregiver Alliance, 2006). Family caregivers help with feeding, bathing, toileting, and medications; shop for groceries; do housework and yard work; and offer myriad other forms of assistance. This work is unpaid and not always freely chosen. Caregiving can be both difficult and rewarding, and its effects on the health and well-being of both the caregiver and care recipient can be experienced for many years.

It has been estimated that family caregivers provide 75% of the care received by those with chronic illnesses or disabilities (Family Caregiver Alliance, 2009). The demand for caregivers continues to increase, and most of us will, at some point in our lives, provide unpaid care for a family member, friend, or neighbor (George, 2001). As nurses, we encounter family caregivers in many sectors of the health care system—anywhere where there are patients with chronic illnesses, long-term disabilities, or frail old age. We and other members of the health care system need to recognize these caregivers as our partners in health care. We also need to recognize that caregivers themselves need care and support.

In this chapter, we examine who today's caregivers tend to be, what they do, how they are challenged and rewarded by this work, what the threats are to their own health, and how we can help them. What nurses do to help homebound patients and their caregivers matters a great deal—to the patient, the caregivers, and the health-care system.

Characteristics of Caregivers

Caregiving is still largely the domain of women, who make up about two thirds of caregivers in the United States (National Alliance for Caregiving, 2009). The care these women provide may be invisible to society, to health care professionals, and even to themselves, especially if they see their care as an extension of their family roles. Whether men or women provide care, their caregiving involves similar tasks and may take substantial amounts of time, especially if the person is a sole caregiver with no other family members available to provide help. Typically, caregivers of older adults provide an average of 20 hours of care per week (about 3 hours daily), and the trajectory of caregiving is months to years, with no vacation, sick time, or days off. The tasks of caregiving can range from monitoring and emotional support to personal tasks such as bathing, toileting, and feeding. Caregiving also may include administering medications; changing dressings; providing wound care; and monitoring blood glucose levels, blood pressure, weight, and so on. Most caregivers perform these activities with minimal training or support.

Average Age

The average age of caregivers in the United States ranges from 43 to 51, but this average is somewhat misleading because it includes caregivers of parents, caregivers of spouses, and caregivers of children and adolescents, many of whom are fairly young. More than half the caregivers in the United States are age 50 or older (National Alliance for Caregiving, 2009), and a significant number are in their 60s and 70s.

Older caregivers are likely to be looking after their spouses or siblings, although a small proportion (about 1 in 12) is caring for children under age 18 who have physical or mental disabilities (Decima Research, 2002). (Childcare and other forms of helping that older adults provide to their children's families to support working parents are not included in this tally.)

The largest group of caregivers is looking after a parent, typically a mother. Many caregivers who are Baby Boomers look after both parents and minor children and are sometimes referred to as the *sandwich generation.* Neighbors, friends, and colleagues also provide care but usually as part of a caregiving network that involves relatives and family members.

Family Culture

Variations in cultural values affect the perceptions family caregivers have of their caregiving roles. In cultures oriented toward extended families, attitudes toward family caregiving tend to be more favorable, and caregivers in these cultures tend to perceive themselves as being less burdened by caregiving compared with family caregivers from a culture oriented toward the nuclear family. The ethnicity of family caregivers roughly follows that of the population, despite the many variations in cultural values about aging and caring for vulnerable family members.

Proximity

Typically, ill older adults are looked after by someone who lives with or near them. North Americans are highly mobile, however, and extended family members often live considerable distances from each other. This can result in ill older adults without nearby family to help out. It is important to remember that distant family can and do participate in caregiving, in the form of monitoring and providing emotional support. This form of caring is vital and often sufficient for many older adults who are relatively independent.

For those whose care needs are greater and who require hands-on care, caregivers (especially daughters) may temporarily move in with parents to provide needed care. Alternatively, parents who need assistance may move closer to children in order to receive care. Such moves can be disruptive to the normal routines of the ill person, caregiver, or both—causing tension in the relationship. Whether the caregiver moves to be closer to the care recipient, or the care recipient moves to be closer to the caregiver, the person who moves leaves behind a social network for the duration of the move. Although the Internet and telephones allow social engagement to some extent, casual encounters are lost at a time when they are badly needed. As a result, such moves need to be considered carefully.

Employment Status

More than half of adult child caregivers of older adults are employed at least part-time. As care needs increase, caregiving can have major disruptive effects on paid employment. Caregivers report shortening their work hours, using their own sick leave and vacation time to provide care, and being interrupted and distracted at work because of caregiving responsibilities. Employers vary in their support of caregivers, and many caregivers report taking early retirement or moving from full- to part-time work. These changes can have significant financial consequences and may put family caregivers at risk for lost benefits, including pensions. A serious long-term financial risk is for reduced income in the caregiver's own senior years.

If caregivers must give up jobs or reduce full-time to part-time jobs, caregiving can be very costly, both in the short- and long-term. Finding another job when caregiving is complete can be difficult, especially if the caregiving was lengthy. Plus, in addition to possible lost pensions and other benefits, out-of-pocket costs may be significant. Even in Canada, where the national health insurance program (commonly called Medicare) covers doctor appointments, hospital stays, and some home care and long-term care, it does not cover extended in-home nursing care, nonprescription medications, transportation costs, or complementary and alternative medicine, such as chiropractic and massage therapy. Prescription medications may not be fully covered, and medical equipment must be purchased or rented.

Talking about caregivers and care receivers as though they were different people, although convenient, is not fully accurate.

Givers and Receivers

Many older adult caregivers have chronic illnesses of their own. In fact, among older couples, both people are likely to have one or more chronic illnesses, each taking care of the other in different ways. Thus, talking about caregivers and care receivers as though they were different people, although convenient, is not fully accurate. Couples who are both caregivers and care receivers have an increased level of vulnerability in that, if one member of the couple is hospitalized, is placed in long-term care, or dies, the other member will lose the independence previously supported by the absent partner's caregiving. While they live together, they look after each other, but when one partner is absent, the other may prove more vulnerable than might have been apparent.

Strains and Benefits of Caregiving and Care Receiving

Caregiving—and care receiving—comes with a variety of challenges and rewards, all of which need to be taken into account when planning nursing support and interventions (Box 19-1). As a general rule, nurses need to support caregivers so they can reap the rewards of caregiving, meet its challenges, and avoid the problems that threaten their well-being.

Sleep

Sleeping patterns change as a person ages, although it isn't entirely clear how much these changes are from aging itself and how much from the chronic illnesses that may accompany aging (Buckley & Schatzberg, 2005). Whatever the reason, changes in sleeping patterns affect not only the ill person but the person's partner, who often is the caregiver. Patients with Alzheimer's disease, for instance, commonly have changes in diurnal rhythms that result in night-time wandering. Patients with chronic obstructive pulmonary disease have trouble breathing when recumbent. This affects their sleep and may increase their anxiety during the night. In both cases and many others, caregivers may feel that they need to sleep with "one eye open" in order to keep the patient safe.

When you think of the multitude of decisions a caregiver must make in any given day and the effect of disrupted sleep on cognitive status, the disrupted sleep becomes a legitimate concern for nurses who support older adults and their family caregivers. Research on disrupted sleep in family caregivers is

BOX 19-1 Benefits of Caregiving

Until recently, the focus of caregiving research has been on the strains of caregiving. More recently, however, research has begun looking at its benefits. For instance, one qualitative study of bereaved cancer caregivers found that caregivers were happy with their experience of caregiving overall. Bereaved caregivers said they believed that they had accomplished something very valuable in the process of giving care. The participants in this study discovered that, as difficult as caregiving was, they had strengths that were previously unknown.

Strang, V. R., Koop, P. M., & Peden, J. (2002). The experience of respite during home-based family caregiving for persons with advanced cancer. Journal of Palliative Care, 18(2), 97–104.

in early stages, and little is known yet about the long-term health effects of accumulated sleep disruptions in caregivers.

Respite and Leisure

There is growing evidence that caregiving interferes with leisure activities, particularly for women (Gahagan, Loppie, Rehman, MacLellan, & Side, 2007), and the lack of leisure activities is thought to account for a portion of the negative health effects of caregiving for some older adults. Respite has been defined as "taking a break" from the emotional and physical demands of caregiving. The rationale is that taking a break from caregiving will help the caregiver reduce stress, rejuvenate, and resume caregiving feeling more rested and able to continue providing care in the home. As a result, the care recipient will be able to remain in the community for a longer time.

Obtaining respite may mean admitting the care recipient to an adult day-care program or other care setting for safe care while the caregiver pursues recreation and opportunities for socialization. Alternatively, a paid care provider may come into the home to stay with the care recipient for a few hours while the caregiver runs errands, meets with friends, or simply rests.

Respite services are a welcome relief for many caregivers. For others, though, these services are not what they need. In our research on caregiving at the end of life, caregivers reported that they wanted respite from the caregiving role without separation from the person for whom they were caring (Strang, Koop, & Peden, 2002). What caregivers and care recipients want is to be together, not as caregiver and care recipient but as people who care *about* each other. They want to be in relationship simply as mother and daughter, for example, or husband and wife. For these caregivers, it is hard to get the break that meets their needs. Sometimes their needs can be met quite simply—by watching a favorite television show together, listening to music, snuggling together in bed—and this time of togetherness can rejuvenate both caregiver and care recipient. Leisure activities that involve care recipients, if they are meaningful, can facilitate caregiver well-being as well.

It is easy, in the busyness of caregiving, to forget to take time to simply be together. Nurses can help family caregivers remember to take care of their relationship and thus take care of themselves and not get caught up in the caregiving tasks.

PERSONAL PERSPECTIVE
Talking about Losses

"If we could only go back 10 years and things could be the way they were," says Gertrude, age 93. "Everything was wonderful. And now it's not as wonderful because I'm more tied down with Ed. I don't like to leave him."

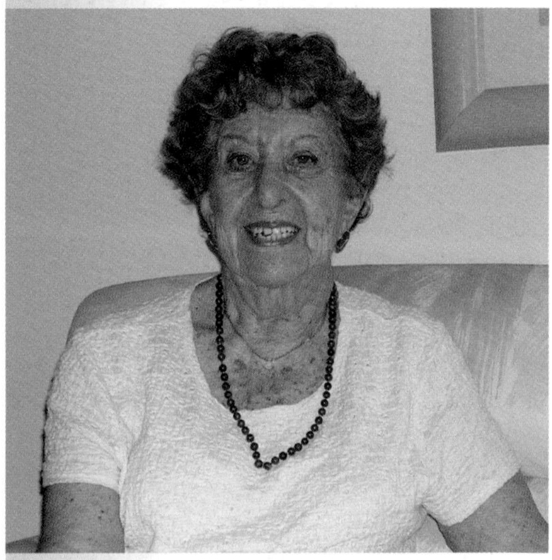

Ed, Gertrude's husband of 68 years, cannot walk unaided. "There's lot's to do in the building, and there are a lot of nice people here, but it's a different life for me than I had up to two years ago," Gertrude continues. "I've lost my car, my independence, being able to just go and do what I want all the time, because everything is governed by leaving Ed. I leave him for two hours or three hours at the most to go have lunch, do errands, go shopping with friends. But now I have to depend on them to take me.

Gertrude acknowledges that Ed's losses have impacted her a great deal because: "He has trouble just getting up from the chair, and he'll call, 'Gertrude,' and I have to come and take my two hands and lift him up. And then he'll get into the bathroom. And then, 'Gertrude,' and I have to go in there and help him get up. So, I'm really on call all the time. During the night, if I hear him get up, I jump up because I'm afraid he'll fall getting up and going into the bathroom. So it's not easy like it used to be. But I keep consoling myself that I'm one of the very few lucky people who still have my husband, and I'm very grateful for that."

Gertrude and Ed lived in Florida for many years before making the move up north to an assisted-living complex. "We had a big beautiful villa," she explains, "and we enjoyed it to the fullest for as long as we could. But it reached a point when Ed started having trouble getting around, the place was big, and for him just to come from the bedroom into the kitchen, out to the porch, entailed a lot of moving around. So we decided to put our place up on the market. And then instead of buying another place, we rented an adorable place that I just loved. It was small but had everything we needed. We enjoyed that because he was still able to get around. We played cards, we took courses at Florida Atlantic University, [attended] a concert series, and went to dinner three times a week. We had a great time, and then all of a sudden there was a complete change in our lifestyle, because we decided to move back up here, because I needed help with Ed. I'm glad we came up here. I mean, for this time in our life I think it's the right place. I've just got to learn to be happy this way."

About Gertrude Gertrude Lerman speaks lovingly of her daughter, two grandchildren, and two great grandchildren and, with sigh of sadness, of her son who died while still a young man. Family has always been central in her life. Before her two children were born, she had a career as a dental hygienist. Afterward she devoted herself full-time to raising her family. Only much later did she work again as a dental hygienist, this time as a volunteer on a kibbutz in Israel for 2 months each year. Gertrude's greatest love is travel. She once read a story in *Reader's Digest* about a widow who, on a trip to Hawaii, kept repeating, "Oh, Charlie would have loved this," and she was determined that Ed would never voice the same sentiment. So began their many years of world travel, which produced a wealth of rich memories that she treasures to this day.

Lorri B. Danzig, MS, CSL

Relationships between Caregivers and Care Receivers

What happens to relationships when the family bond is supplanted by the caregiver/care receiver bond? Boundaries need to shift. Caregiving commonly involves a different kind of physical intimacy than may have been present in the original relationship. Think of bathing, giving an enema, or inserting a suppository—all common caregiving tasks. Even for spouses, these kinds of activities differ from the intimacy they once shared. How do these caregiving activities affect the relationship? How can we help spouses, or parents and children, incorporate these changes into their relationships while enjoying the original bonds that they once had? Our respite research suggests that caregivers achieve respite by engaging in shared activities with their care recipients in order to maintain their bonds. Nurses can help by reminding caregivers to take care of their relationships.

PERSONAL PERSPECTIVE
The Challenges of Caregiving

It's been many years since Joe, age 89, and Lillian, age 90, shared the responsibility of caregiving for their two children. Now, after 66 years of marriage, Joe has assumed the role of primary caregiver to Lillian. It is not the tasks of daily living but the emotional component of caregiving that they find most challenging. "Caregiving," Joe says, "is sometimes one of the conflicts Lillian and I have. And I imagine that other people in this situation do, too. Sometimes I will tend to run her life, and tell her what to do, and she naturally resents some of that and can be disturbed by it. I think we've learned a great deal about each other and how to deal with that sort of thing, yet it's still one of the major problems of getting along together."

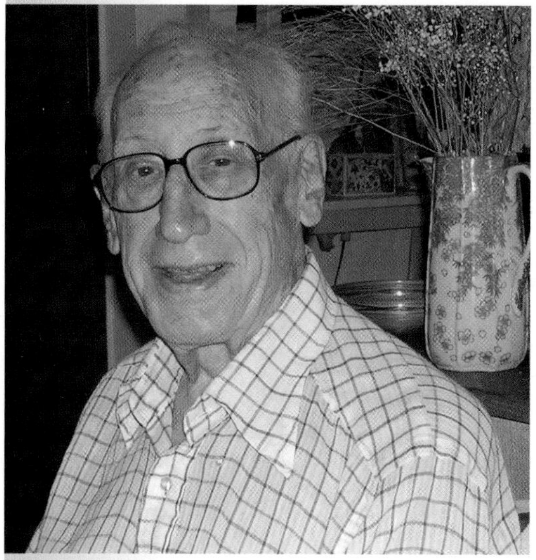

"How do I remind her to take her medications without treating her like a child?" Joe wonders. "How do I let her assume as much responsibility as she can? With a child you have that parent-child relationship. It's much easier to say, 'This is what I want you to do.' I know she doesn't want to be a burden on me, and I don't want to look at her as a burden. Treating her like a child can cause humiliation and embarrassment, especially if it's in front of someone else. These things can be difficult at times." Yet despite the difficulties, Joe says there are rewards to caregiving as well, "in the sense of learning more about yourself, when to bite your tongue and so on." Joe meets the emotional challenges by taking care to retain the intimacy that has always been there between them. "We still have expressions of love that we use," he shares. "We kiss each other good night. We try in some way to maintain a meaningful relationship."

About Joe and Lillian Joseph Dimow is a World War II veteran. A self-taught toolmaker, Joe continued his tool making after the war and worked as the manager of a machine shop. At an early age, Joe became interested in radical politics, an interests that is reflected in his lifelong involvement in political campaigns and active participation in the antiwar and antiracism movements. To this day, he keeps up with his community and political interests and continues to sit on the Editorial Advisory Board of *Jewish Currents,* a progressive magazine dedicated to social and economic justice and participation in Jewish life through Yiddish culture. Joe's wife, Lillian, worked as a bookkeeper during the early years of their marriage and then, for many years, taught arts and crafts to adults in senior centers and children in public schools throughout New Haven, her Connecticut hometown.

Lorri B. Danzig, MS, CSL

Sense of Home

As care has moved out of institutions back into the community, a home in which an ill older adult is receiving care can sometimes start to look quite institutional. Hospital beds, commodes, and grab bars are needed for safe care, but they change the appearance of home for many people (Williams, 2002). How does all this equipment affect the sense of home? And how is the sense of home restored when the frail or ill person moves into long-term care or dies? Caregivers report needing to renovate or redecorate the rooms in which caregiving once took place in order to restore their sense of home.

Decision Making

Two difficult decision-making points take place over the caregiving trajectory. The first one occurs when an older adult no longer has the ability to manage without assistance. Decisions have to be made regarding where caregiving will take place and who will provide care. The second major decision-making point occurs when caregiving needs exceed the abilities of family caregivers. At this point, decisions have to be made regarding placement. The options available depend on the care needs and prognosis of the care recipient.

For care recipients expected to live less than 6 months, a hospice or palliative care unit may be available. In Canada, the 6-month stipulation generally limits admission to care recipients with cancer, amyotrophic lateral sclerosis, and degenerative neuromuscular disorders. Specialized dementia units are available to care recipients with an established diagnosis of dementia who need to be in a protected environment.

For other care recipients, assisted living or long-term care may be more appropriate, depending on the degree of disability. These decisions are complex and fraught with implications and emotions for both caregivers and recipients. Waiting lists can be lengthy for some settings, and costs vary with setting.

Ending the Caregiving Role

You might imagine that, when a person needs care, family members would sit down together and determine how much care will be needed and who among family members, friends, and neighbors would be willing to provide it. In fact, this explicit joint decision-making process rarely happens. Instead, family caregivers tend to fall into the caregiving role. When asked why they do it, caregivers typically say they see caregiving as a family responsibility, that they choose to provide the care, or that no one else is available (Decima Research, 2002).

It is difficult, once a family member has become the caregiver, to extricate herself or himself from the role.

This falling into caregiving has some long-term consequences. It is difficult, once a family member has become the caregiver, to extricate herself or himself from the role. Stajduhar and Davies (2005) found that caregivers often did not feel they had a choice of whether or not to become caregivers, and they felt unable to stop providing care.

For many caregivers of older adults, the only way to stop caregiving is for the ill person to be admitted to long-term care or a hospital. This decision is difficult and fraught with emotional distress (Strang, Koop, Dupuis-Blanchard, Nordstrom, & Thompson, 2006). And often, because of limited space in long-term care or assisted-living centers, caregivers must continue to provide care even after they have decided to place their family member on a waiting list for placement.

Life after Placement

Even after the older adult is placed in assisted living or a long-term care facility, caregiving does not end. Keating, Fast, Dosman, and Eales (2001) found that even in continuing care, family members provide about 30% of the care required. Often, significant negotiation must happen between family and paid care staff in the setting to which the care recipient has been admitted.

Support Services for Caregivers

Information

It seems that caregivers cannot get enough information. They want to know about the care recipient's illness. They want to understand what is wrong and how it will change over time. They want to know what to expect in the future. They want to know the significance of new symptoms and what to do in response. As nurses, one of our responsibilities is to anticipate what information caregivers will need to do their jobs and then to give that information to caregivers in a timely fashion and at a level that they can understand. In our interviews of family caregivers (Koop & Strang, 2003), they most valued the nurses who were skilled at helping them anticipate changes in the care recipient's well-being and helping them learn what to do in response.

Equipment

It's amazing, really, how little caregivers ask for in order to do their jobs. Besides information, caregivers want to have the basic equipment they need to keep their loved ones safe. This includes grab bars, commodes, and bed pans. There are shops and Internet sites, of course, where people can buy wheelchairs, walkers, commodes—whatever they need. But not all caregivers can afford to purchase equipment, nor is it always cost-effective to do so. In Canada, the Canadian Red Cross—home-care agencies and organizations whose mandate is support for older adults or caregivers—have equipment to lend or rent. Caregivers need to know what their options are and how to get what they need. Nurses need to be aware of local sources of basic equipment for providing care in the home.

Navigating the Agency Maze

The health care system is sometimes referred to as an agency maze—a term that highlights what patients and caregivers experience as they try to determine what services are available and how to obtain them when they need them. The health-care system is amazingly complex. Some services require a referral from a physician. Others are directly accessible. Then there is the matter of payment. Which services require a doctor's order? Which services are covered by insurance? Which services must be paid for out of pocket? Are subsidies available? How does one qualify?

Finding necessary information demands a great deal of time, energy, and persistence on the part of caregivers. The role of nurse navigator has been developed in a number of health care institutions to assist patients and their caregivers in finding their way through the agency maze to resources that will help them manage their health challenges. In the United States, each town has a designated municipal agent who is knowledgeable about community resources for aging individuals. Social workers and home health nurses also can be helpful in working through the agency maze.

In-Home Care

In Canada, access to prepaid home care is a mandate of every provincial and territorial health care plan. (Canada's health-care plan is delivered by the 10 provinces and 3 territories of Canada. This health care is entirely funded by Canadian taxpayers.) However, the specific home-care services provided vary across provinces and territories. Generally, home care involves personal care workers who assist with instrumental activities of daily living, visits by nurses (in person or telephone monitoring, including telehealth), and homemaking. Other types of assistance are also available, although less common, and include physiotherapy, respite, occupational therapy, or social workers (Decima Research, 2002). In the United States, more than 40% of home care is funded by Medicare (National Association for Home Care & Hospice, 2010), and more than half of home-care receivers are adults over age 65 years.

Home-care services have been found to allow older adults to remain in their own communities as they age (Chen & Thompson, 2010). To help increase this possibility, a movement called "aging in place" is developing in cities across North America. It focuses on allowing older adults to remain in their own homes. In this initiative, people age along with their neighbors until a large proportion of the residents in the community are considered older adults. This phenomenon is referred to as a Naturally Occurring Retirement Community (NORC). (See http://www.seniorresource.com/ageinpl.htm#norc for further information.) Such initiatives aim to keep older adults in their communities, which evolve into senior-friendly places as their residents age.

Respite Care

Many hospices and long-term care settings make a small number of beds available for respite care. For many caregivers and patients, these services are welcome. However, as discussed earlier, some caregivers are ambivalent about using respite services (de la Cuesta-Benjumea, 2010). A broad range of respite services is recommended in order to meet the needs of caregivers and care recipients. For caregivers whose sleep is disrupted, for instance, a night-time respite may allow the caregiver to get much needed sleep. What is critical is that respite services are oriented to meet the needs of care receivers and caregivers.

Support Groups

Caregiver support groups exist both online and in many communities. In these forums, caregivers get support from peers—people who are on a similar journey and can understand their experiences. The Canadian Caregiver Coalition, for instance, provides links to provincial and local chapters of caregiver associations (http://www.ccc-ccan.ca).

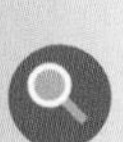

EVIDENCE FOR PRACTICE
Supporting Caregiver Self-Care

Purpose: To describe the development of an intervention, *Self-Care Talk,* and evaluate pilot testing of the intervention with caregivers of older adults.

Sample: 6 spouse caregivers of persons with dementia.

Methods: Advanced-practice nurses delivered the *Self-Care Talk* interventions to caregivers by telephone. Sessions focused on practicing healthy habits, building self-esteem, focusing on the positive, avoiding role overload, communicating, and building meaning.

Results: Research participants reported their understanding of the session content and their intentions to practice improved self-care.

Implications: Nurses can help family caregivers take care of their own well-being while providing care to a family member.

Reference: Teel, C. S., & Leenerts, M. H. (2005). Developing and testing a self-care intervention for older adults in caregiving roles. *Nursing Research, 54,* 193–201.

Residential Care Options

Senior Living Communities

These communities typically provide senior-friendly housing along with health promotion activities. These communities aim to promote independent living for older adults and aging in place. On-site health care providers may be able to offer support to older adult caregivers and care receivers, thus reducing the burdens on older adult caregivers.

Assisted Living

Assisted living typically involves the provision of housing and health care support for older adults who need assistance with activities of daily living. In these settings, care receivers are likely to get more support than is generally available through home care. Meals and housekeeping typically are provided, and assistance with bathing and medication management is available for those who need it. In assisted-living environments, older adults live in lockable apartments or rooms furnished with their own belongings. Older adult caregivers and care recipients can live together in assisted-living units and get help with caregiving requirements, thus significantly reducing the burden on caregivers.

Long-Term Care

Long-term care is considerably more institutional than assisted living and includes specialized dementia units. Older adults who need long-term care typically have chronic illnesses and disabilities requiring more care than their families can provide. Within long-term care, paid staff provide assistance with activities of daily living, administer medications, and provide any other needed health care to residents. Family and friends are encouraged to visit with residents (care receivers) and become involved in care provision.

Neglect and Mistreatment in Caregiving

It is a sad fact of life that neglect and abuse are a part of the lives of some older adults, whether they are caregivers or care recipients. It is difficult to get a clear picture of the incidence of elder abuse and neglect, in part because the definitions of abuse and neglect vary. However, a recent study of community-dwelling older adults in Chicago found that 113 of 9,318 respondents (1.2%) had been reported to social agencies for suspected abuse (Dong et al., 2009). Another study reported a range of elder abuse of up to 18.4% (Yaffe, Wolfson, Lithwick & Weiss, 2008).

Part of the nature of abuse is the isolation of victims. Dixon and colleagues (2010) conducted a large study of older adults to explore their understanding and experiences of abuse and neglect. Typically, abuse is experienced at the hands of family members or paid care workers and includes multiple categories of abuse, including psychological (intimidation, belittling, insulting), financial (stealing, fraudulent attainment of power of attorney), sexual (sexual talk/touching or intercourse against the person's will), and physical abuse (slapping, kicking, inappropriate restraint) and neglect (consistently withholding necessities of life).

Abuse and neglect of older adults typically takes place in private settings and therefore may not be detected. Nurses need to be aware of the signs of abuse and neglect. A history of family violence and caregivers who seem overwhelmed or particularly controlling are warning flags. In addition, care recipients who are particularly withdrawn or make poor eye contact; are malnourished; or have hygiene issues, cuts, bruises, or inappropriate clothing need further assessment. If further assessment strongly suggests abuse or neglect, the nurse should report the situation to Adult Protective Services in the United States.

Keep in mind that, although abuse usually is perpetrated on care receivers by caregivers, it also may occur in the other direction. Care receivers who are emotionally labile, mentally ill, or experiencing delusions may strike out at or otherwise abuse their caregivers.

Transition Planning

It is important, especially as Baby Boomers age, that we develop plans for ourselves as we grow older. Patty Randall, a Canadian who struggled with the care of her parents, advocates that we plan for our own eventual care needs (see http://www.longtermcarecanada.com/index.html). On the other hand, successful aging experts urge us to focus on remaining fit, healthy, and disease-free into old age. As individuals and as a society, we would be well served by taking time to consider the future, the possible demands on our family members, particularly spouses and children, and the wide range of living and health care options available to older adults.

KEY POINTS

- Family caregiving is defined as unpaid assistance and support for family members and others who are disabled, frail, or ill.
- The typical caregiver is an employed middle-aged woman looking after a parent or an older woman looking after her spouse. Time spent caregiving is approximately 20 hours weekly and lasts many months to years at a time.
- Caregivers and care recipients are sometimes the same people—older couples who look after each other.
- The decision to place the care recipient in long-term care is emotionally difficult for caregivers, and caregiving continues in long-term care.
- In general, caregivers are happy to provide care, but stresses such as sleep disruption and lack of leisure activity can result in poor health.
- Caregivers need information on how to provide excellent care, equipment, and assistance with navigating the health care system.
- Caregivers and care recipients are at risk for elder abuse.
- Various services are available to support caregivers, including home care, respite care, and support groups.
- Residential care options include senior living communities, assisted living, and long-term care.
- Middle-aged adults are encouraged to engage in transition planning well in advance of needing care.

CRITICAL THINKING ACTIVITIES

1. Imagine yourself as a frail, older person. Where are you? Where would you like to be? Who helps you manage your life so that you can be where you would like to be?
2. What characteristics do you think make for a good family caregiver? How does one acquire those characteristics?
3. Think about your family. How would your family make decisions with or about a frail or ill family member? What are the advantages and disadvantages of this decision-making method? How would you want the decisions to be made if you were the frail or ill person?

CASE STUDY | *JAMES THICKE*

You are a home-care nurse on the regional palliative home-care team and have just admitted James Thicke to your caseload. Mr. Thicke, age 73, has a stage 4 gastric adenocarcinoma that was diagnosed 6 weeks ago. He had surgery in which the tumor was resected and sent for biopsy. Distant metastases have been discovered, and Mr. Thicke has been admitted for palliative care. His prognosis is estimated at "weeks to months," and he spends most of his day in bed, getting up only for meals and going to the toilet. He has minimal discomfort, which surprises and pleases him. He would prefer to die at home but is worried about his wife's ability to manage. Until he became ill, Mr. Thicke was his wife's primary caregiver.

Mrs. Thicke, age 68, has severe osteoarthritis in both hips and is awaiting total hip replacement. She wonders how she will manage to look after Mr. Thicke, particularly as his care needs increase. She also wonders how they will manage when she undergoes surgery and rehabilitation. She wonders if she should postpone her surgery, but she is in considerable pain and has been waiting for the surgery for several months already.

1. What is your assessment of this situation? What additional information do you need? Think about other family members, organizations that the Thickes may belong to, and friends and neighbors.
2. How will you advise Mrs. Thicke?
3. What supports are needed to allow Mr. Thicke to remain at home for as long as possible?

REFERENCES

Adamson, J., & Donovan, J. (2005). Normal disruption: South Asian and African/Caribbean relatives caring for an older family member in the UK. *Social Science & Medicine, 60*(1), 37–48.

Buckley, T. M., & Schatzberg, A. F. (2005). Aging and the role of the HPA axis and rhythm in sleep and memory-consolidation. *American Journal of Geriatric Psychiatry, 13*(5), 344–352.

Cameron, S. L. (2003). *This day is for me: Caring for caregivers.* Montreal: The J.W. McConnell Family Foundation.

Chen, Y-M., & Thompson, E. A. (2010). Understanding factors that influence success of home- and community-based services in keeping older adults in community settings. *Journal of Aging and Health, 22,* 267–291.

de la Cuesta-Benjumea, C. (2010). The legitimacy of rest: Conditions for the relief of burden in advanced dementia care-giving. *Journal of Advanced Nursing, 66,* 988–998.

Decima Research. (2002). *National profile of family caregivers in Canada – 2002. Final Report.* Ottawa: Health Canada. Retrieved December 5, 2010, from http://www.hc-sc.gc.ca/hcs-sss/alt_formats/hpb-dgps/pdf/pubs/2002-caregiv-interven/2002-caregiv-interven-eng.pdf

Dixon, J., Manthorpe, J., Biggs, S., Mowlam, A., Tennant, R., Tinker, A., . . . (2010). Defining elder mistreatment: Reflections on the United Kingdom Study of Abuse and Neglect of Older People. *Ageing and Society, 30,* 403–420.

Dong, X. W., Simon, M., Mendes de Leon, C., Fulmer, T., Beck, T., Hebert, L., . . . Evans, D. (2009). Elder self-neglect and abuse and mortality risk in a community-dwelling population. *Journal of the American Medical Association, 302*(5), 517–526.

Family Caregiver Alliance. (2006). *Caregiver assessment: Principles, guidelines and strategies for change.* Report from a National Consensus Development Conference (Vol. I). San Francisco: Author.

Family Caregiver Alliance. (2009). *Caregiving: A universal occupation.* Retrieved December 8, 2010, from http://www.caregiver.org/caregiver/jsp/content_node.jsp?nodeid=2313

Gahagan, J, Loppie, C., Rehman, L., MacLellan, M., & Side, K. (2007). Far as I get is the clothesline: The impact of leisure on women's health and unpaid caregiving experiences in Nova Scotia, Canada. *Health Care for Women International, 28,* 47–68.

George, M. (2001). *It could be you: A report on the chances of becoming a carer.* Retrieved December 5, 2010, from http://www.carersuk.org/Professionals/ResearchLibrary/Profileofcaring/1207223744

Keating, N., Fast, J., Dosman, D., & Eales, J. (2001). Services provided by informal and formal caregivers to seniors in residential continuing care. *Canadian Journal on Aging, 20*(1), 23–45.

Koop, P. M., & Strang, V. R. (2003). The bereavement experience following home-based family caregiving for persons with advanced cancer. *Clinical Nursing Research, 12*(2), 127–144.

National Alliance for Caregiving. (2009). *Caregiving in the U.S. A focused look at the ethnicity of those caring for someone age 50 or older.* Retrieved from http://assets.aarp.org/rgcenter/il/caregiving_09_es50.pdf

National Association for Home Care & Hospice. (2010). *Basic statistics about home care.* Washington, DC: Author. Retrieved December 2, 2010, from http://www.nahc.org/facts/10HC_Stats.pdf

Stajduhar, K. I., & Davies, B. (2005). Variations in and factors influencing family members' decisions for palliative home care. *Palliative Medicine, 19,* 21–32.

Strang, V., Koop, P. M., Dupuis-Blanchard, S., Nordstrom, M., & Thompson, B. (2006). Family caregivers and transition to long-term care. *Clinical Nursing Research, 15,* 27–45.

Strang, V. R., Koop, P. M., & Peden, J. (2002). The experience of respite during home-based family caregiving for persons with advanced cancer. *Journal of Palliative Care, 18*(2), 97–104.

Williams, A. (2002). Changing geographies of care: Employing the concept of therapeutic landscapes as a framework in examining home space. *Social Science & Medicine, 55,* 141-154.

Yaffe, M. J., Wolfson, C., Lithwick, M., & Weiss, D. (2008). Development and validation of a tool to improve physician identification of elder abuse: The Elder Abuse Suspicion Index (EASI). *Journal of Elder Abuse & Neglect, 20,* 276–300.

The chapter author wishes to thank Dr. Marge deJong-Berg for the opening quote and Dr. Jean Lange for thoughtful and helpful comments on an earlier draft of this chapter.

Chapter 20

Relating to Older Adults in a Culturally Diverse World

Jean W. Lange, PhD, RN, FAAN, and Denise Miner-Williams, PhD, RN

LEARNING OBJECTIVES

- Examine how personal sociocultural origins influence attitudes toward individuals from different backgrounds.
- Discuss demographic trends regarding diversity in the United States.
- Apply theories of sociocultural competence to nursing practice.
- Distinguish sociocultural sensitivity from sociocultural competence.
- Explain how standards and competencies for socioculturally competent care affect nursing practice.
- Explore strategies to improve the sociocultural sensitivity among health care providers and organizations.
- Discuss components of a culturally appropriate ethnogeriatric assessment.
- Recognize culturally appropriate verbal and nonverbal communication skills.
- Discuss the situations in which interpreters should be used.
- List criteria for qualified interpreters.
- Describe the process and use of translation/back-translation to achieve better conceptual equivalence of materials and assessment tools.
- Evaluate the credibility of health-related information sources designed for professionals and lay persons.

The Diversity Challenge

Most U.S. residents or their ancestors originally came from another country. Although some have lived here for many generations, others came more recently and bring the traditions and values from their home country. Most of the nearly 300 million people living in the United States today originated from Europe. Each of these countries has a unique culture. Today, however, most immigrants come from non-European nations such as Latin and South America, the Caribbean islands, Asia, the Middle East, or Africa.

Cultural patterns are often handed down from older to younger family members, so even those who no longer identify with their country of ancestry still retain some of that culture's practices and beliefs. Consider how your family celebrates special holidays. Is this different from how some of your friends celebrate? Are these differences related to different ancestral origins?

Older adults living in the United States are becoming increasingly diverse. (See Fig. 3-2 in Chapter 3.) Often, general statistics about Asian, African-American, Hispanic, and American Indian populations underestimate the true extent of ethnic and racial diversity because these broad categories contain many different cultures. For example, a Hispanic person may originate from Spain, Latin America, or the Caribbean. Similarly, the ancestors of those categorized as non-Hispanic whites brought unique traditions from many different countries, such as Italy, Ireland, England, and Russia. Traditions, values, and life patterns are often handed down and preserved through many generations. Cultural heritage influences our ideas, behaviors, preferences, and expectations despite the fact that many Americans have lived in the United States for generations. Table 20-1 illustrates the percentages of Americans originating from various countries.

People also differ according to gender roles, geographic residence, family composition, sexual or religious preferences, educational level, and socioeconomic status, to name a few. The sociocultural context in which we live and grow helps to shape us, including how we maintain health and manage illness. Imagine how the following three situations might influence the health outcomes of these individuals:

- An African-American grandfather with hypertension may fear visiting a clinic because of the distrust he developed while a participant in the Tuskegee trials.
- A Puerto Rican woman with chest pain worries about falsely alarming her family by revisiting the emergency departments where her symptoms were attributed to anxiety.
- A Vietnamese man may not question his physician out of respect for the physician's authority.

TABLE 20-1 U.S. Legal Permanent Residents by Country of Birth, 2009

COUNTRY OF BIRTH	NUMBER	PERCENT
Mexico	164,920	14.6
China	64,238	5.7
Philippines	60,029	5.3
India	57,304	5.1
Dominican Republic	49,414	4.4
Cuba	38,954	3.4
Vietnam	29,234	2.6
Colombia	27,849	2.5
South Korea	25,859	2.3
Haiti	24,280	2.1
Jamaica	21,783	1.9
Pakistan	21,555	1.9
El Salvador	19,909	1.8
Iran	18,553	1.6
Peru	16,957	1.5
Bangladesh	16,651	1.5
Canada	16,140	1.4
United Kingdom	15,748	1.4
Ethiopia	15,462	1.4
Nigeria	15,253	1.3
All other countries	410,726	36.3
Total	**1,130,818**	**100.0**

From U.S. Department of Homeland Security. (2010). *U.S. legal permanent residents: 2009.* Washington, DC: Office of Immigration Statistics. Retrieved December 6, 2010, from http://www.dhs.gov/xlibrary/assets/statistics/publications/lpr_fr_2009.pdf

Nurses care for patients of all backgrounds. Understanding the perspective of an older adult whose values and beliefs differ from your own can present opportunities and challenges. The challenge of not understanding a person's sociocultural perspective presents an opportunity to learn about that culture and ensure that the care you provide is sensitive to that patient's values, beliefs, and traditions. For example, one may assume that a patient who nods and asks no questions during a teaching session fully understands what is said, but the health-care professional may be misinterpreting those cues.

Misunderstandings due to sociocultural differences can result in failed communication and poor patient outcomes. According to data from the National Center for Minority Health and Health Disparities (2003), minorities and those who are socioeconomically disadvantaged are more likely to experience health disparities. Older adults who have limited incomes or who cannot read, write, or speak English are particularly vulnerable.

Healthy People 2020 is a national initiative that sets goals to improve the nation's health over the next decade (U.S. Department of Health and Human Services, 2005). Its goals underscore the importance of health care workers acquiring the necessary knowledge and skills to effectively communicate with patients from diverse backgrounds. This means being willing to learn about the values, beliefs, and expectations of patients who think and perhaps act differently from ourselves.

Cultural Diversity and Patient Outcomes

Believing that the ideas and beliefs of others are as valid as one's own is a challenge for many people. The tendency to believe that our perspective is right or is more correct than another person's is known as ethnocentrism. Studies show that ethnocentrism is common among health care workers (Institute of Medicine, 2002). Such beliefs may lead to care planning that fails to consider patients' values or resources and that is therefore not followed.

The tendency to believe that our perspective is right or is more correct than another person's is known as ethnocentrism. Studies show that ethnocentrism is common among health care workers.

Just as the failure to value patient differences can lead to nonadherence and poor outcomes, assuming that all members of a sociocultural group have the same beliefs can be problematic. Strong opinions or stereotypes about people, whether good or bad, are a form of bias that influences how we act and communicate with one another. Clues to personal biases can be subtle and are often revealed in our behavior. Consider the following examples:

- A nursing assistant who dons a gown, mask, and gloves when caring for a homeless person who is not on precautions may be perceived as judgmental by the patient.
- A medical doctor who refuses to speak with a native healer who has treated his patient's asthma for many years may be viewed by the patient as devaluing the patient's belief system.
- A nurse who fails to acknowledge the family visitors of a hospitalized older adult may be viewed by the patient and family as disrespectful.

Behaviors like these can compromise trust and undermine the patient-provider relationship. Biases among health-care professionals can also lead to care inequity. In a review of more than 100 studies, the Institute of Medicine (2002) reported that "minorities are less likely than whites to receive needed services, including clinically necessary procedures ... [for] cancer, cardiovascular disease, HIV/AIDS, diabetes, mental illness, and ... routine treatments for common health problems" (pp. 1–2). Neither patient attitude nor lack of evidence about treatment efficacy accounted for the discrepancy. They concluded that bias plays a significant role in treatment decisions, stating that "even well-intentioned whites who are not overtly biased and who do not *believe* that they are prejudiced typically demonstrate unconscious, implicit negative racial attitudes and stereotypes" (p. 4). This is of particular concern because the vast majority of nurses and physicians (80% and 76%, respectively) in the United States are non-Hispanic and white (U.S. Department of Labor, 2008). The disparity in health care is reflected in the perceived health quality of older adults according to race and ethnicity (Fig. 20-1).

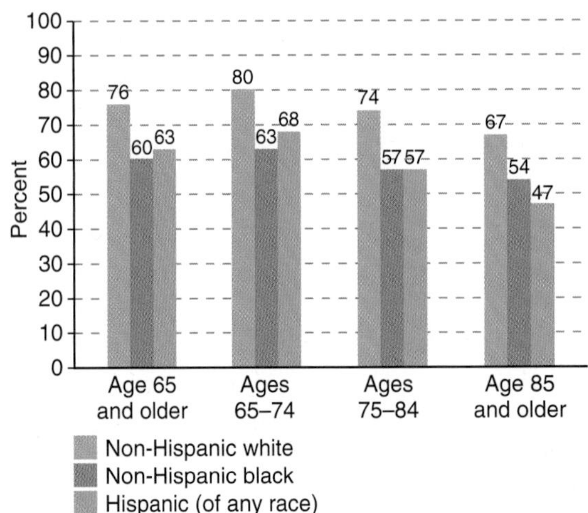

Figure 20-1 *(From Federal Interagency Forum on Aging-Related Statistics. Older Americans 2008: Key indicators of well-being. Washington, DC: Author. Retrieved November 30, 2010, from http://www.aoa.gov/agingstatsdotnet/Main_Site/Data/2008_Documents/Health_Status.aspx)*

Bias is also evident in how participants are recruited for research. Many studies exclude frail older adults, the poor, non–English-speaking, or illiterate persons from their samples. Excluding a particular group from a research study is known as selection bias. The consequences of selection bias are that the results of such studies may not hold true for people like those excluded. Only those similar to participants in the study can benefit from the results; thus, advances in health care do not necessarily apply to all. It is important when translating research into practice to carefully consider whether the participants accurately represent the patients you care for.

The Call for Education

Numerous groups—including the Institute of Medicine, Office of Minority Health, and World Health Organization—have called for the inclusion of cross-cultural training in the education of health-care professionals (Kreitzer, Kligler, & Meeker, 2009; U.S. Department of Health & Human Services, 2007; World Health Organization, 2008). The Office of Minority Health, a division of the U.S. Department of Health and Human Services, issued standards for health-care organizations and individuals to ensure that the services they provide are culturally and linguistically accessible (Office of Minority Health, 2001). The standards address provision of care, literacy, language, and resources needed in the organization (Table 20-2). Culturally and linguistically appropriate services (called CLAS Standards) are incorporated into the evaluation criteria used by most health-care accrediting agencies.

Nurses have a central role in ensuring that provision of care is consistent with patient values and preferences. A spokesperson for the U.S. Department of Health and Human Services (2007) noted that "nurses are in a unique position to bridge the health-care gap by providing culturally competent care [because they] spend more time in direct patient care than any other group of health professionals" (p. 1). Nursing leaders assert that cultural competency involves shaping attitudes, developing good communication skills, and acquiring knowledge

TABLE 20-2 National Standards of Culturally and Linguistically Appropriate Service (CLAS)

CULTURALLY COMPETENT CARE	
Standard 1	Health-care organizations should ensure that patients/consumers receive from all staff member's effective, understandable, and respectful care that is provided in a manner compatible with their cultural health beliefs and practices and preferred language.
Standard 2	Health-care organizations should implement strategies to recruit, retain, and promote at all levels of the organization a diverse staff and leadership that are representative of the demographic characteristics of the service area.
Standard 3	Health-care organizations should ensure that staff at all levels and across all disciplines receive ongoing education and training in culturally and linguistically appropriate service delivery.
Language Access Services	
Standard 4	Health-care organizations must offer and provide language assistance services, including bilingual staff and interpreter services, at no cost to each patient/consumer with limited English proficiency at all points of contact, in a timely manner during all hours of operation.
Standard 5	Health-care organizations must provide to patients/consumers in their preferred language both verbal offers and written notices informing them of their right to receive language assistance services.
Standard 6	Health-care organizations must assure the competence of language assistance provided to limited English proficient patients/consumers by interpreters and bilingual staff. Family and friends should not be used to provide interpretation services (except on request by the patient/consumer).

Continued

TABLE 20-2 National Standards of Culturally and Linguistically Appropriate Service (CLAS)—cont'd

CULTURALLY COMPETENT CARE	
Standard 7	Health-care organizations must make available easily understood patient-related materials and post signage in the languages of the commonly encountered groups and/or groups represented in the service area.
Organizational Supports for Cultural Competence	
Standard 8	Health-care organizations should develop, implement, and promote a written strategic plan that outlines clear goals, policies, operational plans, and management accountability/oversight mechanisms to provide culturally and linguistically appropriate services.
Standard 9	Health-care organizations should conduct initial and ongoing organizational self-assessments of CLAS-related activities and are encouraged to integrate cultural and linguistic competence-related measures into their internal audits, performance improvement programs, patient satisfaction assessments, and outcomes-based evaluations.
Standard 10	Health-care organizations should ensure that data on the individual patient's/consumer's race, ethnicity, and spoken and written language are collected in health records, integrated into the organization's management information systems, and periodically updated.
Standard 11	Health-care organizations should maintain a current demographic, cultural, and epidemiological profile of the community, as well as a needs assessment to accurately plan for and implement services that respond to the cultural and linguistic characteristics of the service area.
Standard 12	Health-care organizations should develop participatory, collaborative partnerships with communities and utilize a variety of formal and informal mechanisms to facilitate community and patient/consumer involvement in designing and implementing CLAS-related activities.
Standard 13	Health-care organizations should ensure that conflict and grievance resolution processes are culturally and linguistically sensitive and capable of identifying, preventing, and resolving cross-cultural conflicts or complaints by patients/consumers.
Standard 14	Health-care organizations are encouraged to regularly make available to the public information about their progress and successful innovations in implementing the CLAS standards and to provide public notice in their communities about the availability of this information.

From Office of Minority Health. (2001). *National standards for culturally and linguistically appropriate services in health care: Final report.* Washington, DC: U.S. Department of Health and Human Services. Retrieved December 5, 2010, from http://minorityhealth.hhs.gov/assets/pdf/checked/finalreport.pdf

about other sociocultural groups. The authors of *Essentials of Baccalaureate Nursing Education for Professional Nursing Practice* affirm that the "multicultural healthcare environment" in which nurses practice requires the capability to give "culturally appropriate care" (American Association of Colleges of Nursing, 2008, p. 6). A second document, *Cultural Competency in Baccalaureate Nursing Education,* further delineates the cultural competencies desired of all baccalaureate nurse graduates:

- Apply knowledge of social and cultural factors that affect nursing and health care across multiple contexts.
- Use relevant data sources and best evidence in providing culturally competent care.
- Promote achievement of safe and quality outcomes of care for diverse populations.

- Advocate for social justice, including commitment to the health of vulnerable populations and the elimination of health disparities.
- Participate in continuous cultural competence development (American Association of Colleges of Nursing, 2009, pp. 3–7).

These five competencies provide a framework for preparing graduate nurses who respect diversity and can effectively integrate patients' sociocultural preferences into their nursing practice.

As implied in these competencies, acquiring the capacity to deliver culturally competent care is an ongoing process of development that requires being open to learning about another person's reality and experience. Competency is therefore a higher goal than merely being sensitive to differences (Marks, Reed, Colby, & Ibrahim, 2004). Betancourt, Green, and Carrillo (2002) emphasized that cultural competence means providing care "to patients with diverse values, beliefs, and behaviors, [and] tailoring delivery of care to meet patients' social, cultural, and linguistic needs. The ultimate goal is a health-care system and workforce that can deliver the highest quality of care to every patient, regardless of race, ethnicity, cultural background, or English proficiency" (p. v, 2). Culturally competent care improves patient-provider communication, patients' satisfaction and willingness to commit to their treatment plan, and patient outcomes.

Moving Beyond a Single Viewpoint

Many authors have written extensively about the need to consider sociocultural factors in order to plan care that is consistent with patients' beliefs and preferences. One of the most frequently cited theories in nursing is the Culture Care Diversity and Universality theory developed by Leininger (1995). This holistic theory defines culture as multidimensional. It includes the "learned, shared, and transmitted values, beliefs, norms, and life-way practices of a particular group that guides thinking, decisions, and actions in patterned ways" (Leininger, 1995, pp. 9–10). Traditions that are handed down from generation to generation may include language, art forms, dietary practices, sick-role behavior, gender roles, family interactions, holiday rituals, body language, sense of time, and personal space needs. All of these dimensions can provide clues to an older adult's beliefs, life patterns, and treatment preferences.

We all have traditions, values, and experiences that shape our opinions. How then do we move beyond our own viewpoint toward understanding the perspectives of others? Camphina-Bacote (1999, 2003) proposes that becoming culturally competent is a process that requires commitment. Camphina-Bacote developed a model for attaining competence that includes five ingredients: awareness, skills, knowledge, encounters, and desire.

The first step of the process involves developing the *awareness* or sensitivity that the beliefs of others are valid and may differ from our own. Camphina-Bacote (1999) describes cultural awareness as a "... deliberate, cognitive process in which health-care providers become appreciative and sensitive to the values, beliefs, life-ways, practices, and problem solving strategies of [patients'] cultures" (p. 204). Part of becoming aware requires that health providers take a close look at their own sociocultural heritage and values, as well as their biases and stereotypes about others.

Acquiring skills—such as being able to communicate effectively with people from diverse groups and conducting a thorough assessment that is sensitive to patients' sociocultural context—is critical to developing cultural competence. Providers need *knowledge* about the sociocultural groups they work with in order to understand the patient perspectives and respect patient preferences. A disadvantage of learning solely through secondary sources is that individual differences exist among members of a group and predominant beliefs and practices of a group can change over time. Learning from secondary sources cannot equal the deeper understanding that is gained through real-life *encounters* with those from other sociocultural groups. Camphina-Bacote (2003) also pointed out that providers must be willing to engage in the process of becoming culturally competent. This *desire* is a critical factor that is individually determined.

Examining your own sociocultural heritage is a starting point from which to gain insight into your values and beliefs. Box 20-1 lists a number of good questions to ask yourself. Sharing answers to these questions with a friend or colleague may help you to discover similarities and differences, as well as to uncover some beliefs that may be less apparent to you. Tools developed to aid health professionals in cultural self-assessment may also be useful (Coffman, Shellman, & Bernal, 2004; Smith, 1998; also see the resource section of the CD-ROM accompanying this text).

BOX 20-1 Discovering Your Cultural Heritage

- Where did my ancestors come from?
- Do I identify with a specific ethnic group?
- What beliefs, attitudes, values, and traditions does my family have?
- What holidays are important to us, and how do we celebrate them?
- Are there special foods we enjoy?
- What about my culture am I proud of?
- What are the gender roles in my culture?
- Do men and women have similar roles and responsibilities or are there gender-specific expectations?
- How do religion and my economic background affect my beliefs?
- How are decisions about health care made in my family?
- How does my family respond when someone becomes ill?
- What rituals do we have when someone dies?
- What contact have I had with persons from different sociocultural backgrounds? What were these experiences like?
- Have I ever felt uncomfortable when around a group of people that were different from me? What was that experience like?
- What messages did I receive from my family about people from different cultures than my own?
- What beliefs do I hold about people from sociocultural groups that are different from my own (e.g., racial, ethnic, religious, disables, lower socioeconomic status, age, gender, sexual orientation)?
- What are my personal challenges to working effectively with people from other sociocultural groups?

Building Knowledge

Understanding the perspective of another sociocultural group requires knowledge about the patterns, historical context, and beliefs held by that group. Several authors assert that lack of provider knowledge is the real barrier to culturally sensitive health care, not the actual presence of sociocultural differences (Tripp-Reimer, Choi, Kelley, & Enslein, 2001). This underscores the importance of accessing resources that can help you to better understand your patient's needs and preferences. Written guides that summarize the beliefs and practices of different sociocultural groups, although never completely true for everyone in a group, can often provide useful general insights (D'Avanzo, 2007).

Numerous resources are available to support the sociocultural education of nurses working with older adults. A national center for ethnogeriatrics is located at Stanford University's Geriatric Education Center. Ethnogeriatrics is the study of older adults from the perspective of various sociocultural groups. Online resources designed for all health-care professionals are available free on their Web site (Yeo, 2000). Of particular interest is the 18-module Ethnogeriatric Curriculum designed to "educate health-care professionals [about] cultural issues associated with aging and health" (http://sgec.stanford.edu) and the diversity modules that discuss health beliefs and recommen dations for communicating with 15 cultures, 11 religions, and 8 American immigrant cohorts. A second Web-based program that contains video-based case studies was specifically designed for nurses (Office of Minority Health, 2007). The program, *Culturally Competent Nursing Care: A Cornerstone of Caring,* contains three modules based on the CLAS Standards and is available through the U.S. Department of Health and Human Services Office of Minority Health (http://www.thinkculturalhealth.org). The goals of the program are to help nurses integrate cultural competency awareness, knowledge, and skills to effectively treat increasingly diverse patient populations. Several reference books designed for health-care providers are also available that contain profiles of the traditional behaviors and beliefs of selected sociocultural groups (D'Avanzo, 2007; Galanti, 2008; Giger & Davidhizar, 2007; Kirkwood, 2005; Ray, 2010; Rundle, Carvalho, & Robinson, 2002; Spector, 2008).

In addition to learning through secondary sources such as the Internet or printed materials, spending time in a sociocultural context other than one's own furthers the insight practitioners can gain about diverse groups. In clinical experiences, one can express an interest in the beliefs and traditions of patients who come from different sociocultural backgrounds. One excellent way to engage an older adult in sharing life stories is through the use of a guided life review, in which the person reflects on his or her life history. Haight (1988) suggested a series of questions one might use to stimulate this discussion. Study abroad opportunities are also an excellent way to learn about another culture.

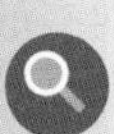

EVIDENCE FOR PRACTICE
Reminiscence Education Programs

Purpose: The purpose of this pilot study was to test the effects of a reminiscence education program on BSN students' cultural self-efficacy in caring for older adults.

Sample: Sixty-four senior baccalaureate nursing students in a community health practicum at a northeastern U.S. university participated. The typical subject was 25 years old (range 20 to 57), Caucasian (84.4%), and female (96.9%).

Methods: A two-group quasi-experimental design was used to test the effectiveness of a 2-hour reminiscence education program followed by a 13-week experience using reminiscence with older adults in their homes or at senior centers. Two clinical groups in a community health course participated. Students were not randomly assigned to the treatment or control group. The eldercare cultural self-efficacy scale (ECSES) was used with student self-perceptions about their confidence in caring for older adults from Caucasian, Hispanic, black, and Asian origins. The ECSES is a 28-item Likert-type scale measuring four dimensions: assessing for lifestyle and social patterns, determining cultural health practices, determining cultural beliefs, and dealing with grief and the losses associated with aging. Participants completed the scale as a pretest at the end of junior year, before the intervention, immediately after the intervention, and 30 days later.

Results: An independent t-test revealed no significant differences between the two groups with respect to prior cultural experiences. Students receiving the reminiscence education program had significantly higher levels of eldercare cultural self-efficacy ($F[1, 62] = 5.34$, $p = 0.024$) than those in the control group who did not receive the intervention until after the study was completed. Students with increased cultural exposure had significantly higher ECSES scores.

Implications: Reminiscence education programs during clinical practica may increase nursing students' confidence in caring for older adults from other sociocultural backgrounds.

Reference: Shellman, J. (2007). The effects of a reminiscence education program on baccalaureate nursing students' cultural self-efficacy in caring for elders. *Nurse Education Today, 27*(1), 43–51.

Culturally Sensitive Practice

Assessment Skills

"Cultural skill is the ability to collect relevant cultural data regarding [patients'] health histories and presenting problems, as well as accurately performing a culturally specific physical assessment" (Camphina-Bacote, 1999, p. 204). Knowledge about sociocultural differences helps nurses tailor assessments and communications to a patient's beliefs and values. Respecting patient preferences also promotes trusting relationships that can yield more complete information about patients' needs. Conducting informed, individual assessments is critical to avoiding the stereotypical assumption that all members of a sociocultural group hold similar values and traditions.

One important reason for variations among group members is the process of acculturation. This is the extent to which a person from one sociocultural background adopts the beliefs, patterns, and practices of a new or host culture. It can affect the extent to which sociocultural traditions are maintained or abandoned in favor of the predominant patterns in the host culture. For example, an older adult of Italian heritage whose ancestors have lived in the United States for three generations may have very different expectations regarding gender roles than a grandparent who moved to the United States as a teenager. It is important to remember that, although profiles of sociocultural groups can be useful, an older adult's views do not necessarily reflect the traditions associated with his or her heritage.

It is important to remember that, although profiles of sociocultural groups can be useful, an older adult's views do not necessarily reflect the traditions associated with his or her heritage.

Cultural assessment typically includes questions about primary spoken and written language, food preferences, support systems and resources, patterns of decision making, spiritual and end-of-life preferences, health beliefs and expectations, and use of native medicine or healers (Narayan, 2003). It is also important to consider the impact that living through major historical events (e.g., economic depression, major wars, experiences of discrimination, forced tribal relocation, immigration trends) may have on an older adult's perspective. Responses to these questions can provide insight that informs the development of a more realistic treatment plan. Learning how to ask questions that provide insight into how patients' cultural heritage may influence their care is an important nursing skill. Sociocultural assessment tools can help frame questions that are comprehensive and not offensive. The Sociocultural Assessment tool in the *Core Curriculum in Ethnogeriatrics* is tailored to older adults (Table 20-3).

Communication Skills

Basic knowledge about sociocultural groups can help you to communicate more effectively with patients, gather more complete information, develop care that is more realistic, and produce better patient outcomes (Betancourt, Green, Carrillo, & Park, 2005). For example, after learning that traditional Laotian culture practices *Cao gio* (dermabrasion by coin rubbing with oils, usually over the ribs and spine) as a healing technique, you may be less likely to assume that the red marks on your patient are suggestive of elder abuse. Instead, you decide to inquire about what treatment measures the family has already tried. In another context, knowing that an older veteran is homeless helps the nurse understand why he or she may bring bags of seemingly unnecessary personal belongings into the emergency department. Instead of locating a family member to remove the

TABLE 20-3 Sociocultural Assessment

Background	■ What is your family ancestry?
	■ With what ethnic or social groups do you identify?
	■ Acculturation indicators:
	  ■ How long have you or your ancestors lived in this country?
	  ■ What language do you prefer to speak? Write?
	  ■ What is the highest grade you completed in school?
	  ■ How comfortable are you with understanding written and spoken English?

Physical examination	■ Cross gender physical examinations are unacceptable in many cultures. Ask for preference of presence of other family members during physical exam. ■ Throughout the assessment, inform elder of procedures and ask for permission to examine different areas of the body. ■ Note evidence of elder abuse or neglect (hygiene, malnutrition, bruises, burns, patterned scarring) ■ Assess preference for amount and type of information communicated to the elder and family members. ■ Recognize terms used in different cultures to express symptoms (e.g., "air heavy" or "air not right" may mean dyspnea for some Native American elders [Kramer, 1996]; "heavy heart" may indicate depression among Chinese)
Cognitive and affective status	■ Dementia and depression are considered mental illness in some cultures and highly stigmatized. In others, dementia is seen as a normal part of aging.
Functional status	■ Activities of daily living ■ Instrumental activities of daily living
Home assessment	■ Living patterns: Who lives in the home, relationship to elder, and length of time in the home? ■ Support from those living with the elder ■ Safety, comfort, and adaptation of the home to elder's health status ■ Economic stability and adequacy

TABLE 20-3 Sociocultural Assessment—cont'd

Family assessment	■ Composition and structure ■ Kinship patterns: expectations of and for family members (e.g., for elder care). Stereotypes that ethnic families "take care of their own" can be very misleading because some elders from ethnic backgrounds are not part of strong family networks and are vulnerable to loneliness and isolation. ■ Decision making: In many cultures, there is not the assumption of patient autonomy in decision making as there is the U.S. ethical paradigm, and the family is assumed to be the decision maker about health care. ■ Spokesperson ■ Gender sex-role allocation ■ Support from family members
Community and neighborhood assessment	■ Overall features of the community and neighborhood (e.g., involvement of ethnic elders in community planning, use of space) ■ Population characteristics (e.g., ethnic community, length of time in community, proportion of elders, children, and adults in population, intergenerational relations, status of elders) ■ Environmental and safety conditions (e.g., topography, sidewalks, pavement, air and water quality, crime rate) ■ Services available and used by elder and their family (e.g., allopathic, folk and alternative health practitioners, social services, religious, shopping [such as food, clothing, banking], educational, transportation, recreational and elder services [such as senior center]) ■ Support from neighborhood and community members
End-of-life preferences (when appropriate)	■ Preparation for death including availability of advance directives. Because talking about death is considered inappropriate in some cultures (e.g., Chinese, Navajo), the issue should be approached carefully and sensitively, and only in the context of an established trusting relationship. A possible introduction after several visits might be, "In case something happens to you and you are not able to make decisions about your care, we need to know what your preferences are." ■ Preference for hospital or home end-of-life care ■ Death rituals for care of the body and mourning behaviors during and after death ■ Attitudes about organ donation and autopsy
Patient/family perspectives	■ What do you think caused your problem? ■ Why do you think it started when it did? ■ What do you think your sickness does to your body? How does it work? ■ How severe is your sickness? ■ How long do you think it will last? ■ What are the main problems your sickness has caused you? ■ Do you know others who have had this problem? How did they treat it? ■ Do you think there is any way to prevent this problem in the future?

Continued

TABLE 20-3 Sociocultural Assessment—cont'd

Intervention-specific data	■ What are you and/or your family doing for this problem? What kinds of medicines, home remedies, or other treatments have you tried for this sickness? Have they helped? ■ What type of treatment do you think you should receive from me? ■ Elicit cultural-specific content as needed for specific interventions. For example, if dietary recommendations are being made, elicit data about food preferences and practices; if discharge planning is necessary, elicit information regarding family care patterns, resources, and residential preferences. ■ Is there any other information that might help us design a treatment plan? ■ How should family be involved? (e.g., family structure, roles, and dynamics, as well as life style and living arrangement need to be identified). ■ How should family members treat one who has this condition/problem? ■ Does anyone else need to be consulted?
Expected outcomes	■ What are individual/family expectations for quality care? ■ What are the most important results you hope to receive from this treatment? ■ What is the best outcome from family/individual perspective? ■ What is the worst outcome from family/individual perspective?

Adapted from Tripp-Reimer T., et al. (2000). In G. Yeo (Ed.), Module four. Culturally appropriate geriatric care: Assessment. *Core curriculum in ethnogeriatrics.* Stanford, CA: Stanford University. Retrieved November 7, 2010 from http://www.stanford.edu/group/ethnoger/index.html

belongings, the nurse can find space to secure the patient's property.

Learning how to communicate effectively with patients who hold different values can be challenging. Teal and Street (2009) proposed that having a repertoire of communication skills, being sensitive to verbal and nonverbal patient cues, and being willing to adapt care practices and treatment to be consistent with patient values, beliefs, and preferences are essential to culturally competent communication. Examples of how one might adapt in response to sociocultural differences include reframing health assessment questions to be inoffensive and more understandable to an older adult, respecting social distance norms, and respecting cultural norms regarding the use of touch, gestures, or eye contact.

To communicate effectively, nurses should understand that patient-provider differences in basic values such as role expectations or beliefs about managing illness can lead to misunderstandings and mistrust that can undermine care (Eiser & Ellis, 2007). Using basic interpersonal skills, such as actively listening to patient concerns and perspectives and respecting patients' sociocultural identity in a nonjudgmental way, portrays interest in the patient as an individual and can help to prevent misunderstandings. Other strategies that convey respect include using the patient's title (e.g., Mr., Mrs., Dr.) and surname rather than their first name (unless given permission by the patient). Greetings such as *honey, dear,* or *sweetheart* are depersonalizing and should be avoided.

Spending a few minutes getting to know your patient before proceeding to ask more formal questions about their illness, conducting a physical exam, or performing a procedure gives the patient time to feel more comfortable with you. Studies have shown that patients feel respected when they do not feel rushed and when healthcare providers take the time to explain and answer questions (Shapiro, Hollingshead, & Morrison, 2002). Learning key words of a foreign language and consulting with trained interpreters or providers who are more familiar with a patient's culture can also improve communication. Additional communication tips are summarized in Box 20-2.

BOX 20-2 Strategies for Communicating Effectively with Older Adults from Diverse Sociocultural Backgrounds

- When greeting a family, address older persons first.
- When meeting for first time, introduce yourself by name and position.
- Use surname and title, not first names when greeting an older adult unless permission is granted to use a more personal form of address (i.e., first name or nickname).
- Include older adults when discussing their care with significant others. Do not speak about older adults as if they are not present.
- Use trained interpreters when a patient and provider do not speak the same language.
- Speak at a pace that is comfortable for the patient.
- Recognize that eye contact, use of touch, the meaning of body language, emotional expression, and physical space needs can vary among cultures.
- Be authentic. Share your lack of knowledge about their culture.
- Use language that is culturally sensitive.
- Find out what the patient knows about his or her health problems and treatments and whether this information is congruent with dominant or traditional health care systems.
- Do not make assumptions; ask if you don't know or understand.
- Respect the patient's values, beliefs, and practices, even if different or you don't agree.
- Show respect for the patient's support people; they may also make the decisions.
- Make a concerted effort to obtain the patient's trust; however, it may come slowly or not at all.

Adapted from Tripp-Reimer T., et al. (2000). In G. Yeo (Ed.), Module four: Culturally appropriate geriatric care: Assessment. Core Curriculum in Ethnogeriatrics. Stanford, CA: Stanford University (retrieved from http://www.stanford.edu/group/ethnoger/index.html) and S. Phillips. (2007). Transition to professional nursing: Culture and cultural competence. Florida International University (retrieved November 7, 2010 from http://chua2.fiu.edu/faculty/phillips/NUR3055/TransCulture.htm)

The Role of Health Literacy

Health literacy is the ability to obtain, process, and understand health information and services in order to effectively care for oneself (Nielsen-Bohlman, Panzer, & Kindig, 2004). It involves basic literacy skills, such as the ability to read, write, and do basic mathematical computations. Making healthy lifestyle choices, knowing when and how to seek medical care, and taking steps to prevent disease require that people be able to understand and apply health information. With the vast amount of information accessible through media and online sources, deciding what information is relevant and accurate poses a significant challenge for many people. The ability to understand and evaluate the credibility of health information is critical to making informed decisions about one's health (Box 20-3).

Health literacy can directly affect health outcomes and the cost of care (Cutilli, 2007; Howard, Sentell, & Gazmararian, 2006). Persons with limited health literacy:

- Are more likely to have chronic conditions
- Have less knowledge about their health care issues
- Have poorer health status, average 6% more hospital visits, and remain in the hospital nearly 2 days longer than adults with higher health literacy (National Patient Safety Foundation, n.d.)
- Are likely to use health services more frequently and incur higher costs (Department of Health & Human Services, n.d.).

It is estimated that as a result of these and other health outcomes, low health literacy in the United States costs between $106 and $238 billion annually (Vernon, Trujillo, Rosenbaum, & De.Buono, 2006).

Health Literacy and Older Adults

In 2003, a major project was undertaken by the National Center for Education Statistics to assess

BOX 20-3 Facts about Health Literacy

- Reports estimate that the health of 90 million people in the United States is at risk because of low health literacy skills (Mason, Leavitt, & Chaffee, 2007).
- Almost half of all Americans are estimated to have trouble understanding health information and acting upon it (Nielsen-Bohlman, Panzer, & Kindig, 2004).
- Ethnic minorities are disproportionately affected, but most people with limited health literacy are within the largest segment of the U.S. population: white, native-born, Americans (Vernon, Trujillo, Rosenbaum, & De.Buono, 2006).
- The estimated annual cost of limited health literacy ranges from $106 billion to $238 billion (Vernon, Trujillo, Rosenbaum, & De.Buono, 2006).

the status of adult literacy in the United States (Kutner, Greenberg, Jin, & Paulsen, 2006). Based on the findings, four performance levels were created to describe health literacy: below basic, basic, intermediate, and proficient. These ratings were based on a person's reading level, ability to comprehend health-related documents, and numerical skills (Fig. 20-2). According to the authors, an intermediate rating is the minimum level needed to adequately address one's health-care needs.

Although the literacy rate is increasing as the Baby Boomers age, a disproportionate number of older adults are at a basic or below-basic level of proficiency (Kutner et al., 2006). More than half of adults between ages 65 and 74 have insufficient skills to accurately interpret health care information. This percentage increases among Americans over age 75, of whom 70 percent do not have the reading, writing, and numerical skills needed to fully understand health information (Fig. 20-3). Uninsured persons and Medicare or Medicaid recipients tend to have lower proficiency levels than those with private insurance.

Proficiency level also relates to educational attainment, which varies among racial and ethnic groups. For example, Hispanic adults are least likely to have completed high school (Fig. 20-4) and most likely to have basic or below basic literacy levels. Proficiency level often affects how adults prefer to access health information. Adults with basic or below basic capability tend to access health information from radio and television, while adults in the intermediate or proficient range are more likely to use printed sources of information. Lack of computer

Percentage of People Age 50 and Older in Each Health Literacy Performance Level, by Age Group, 2003

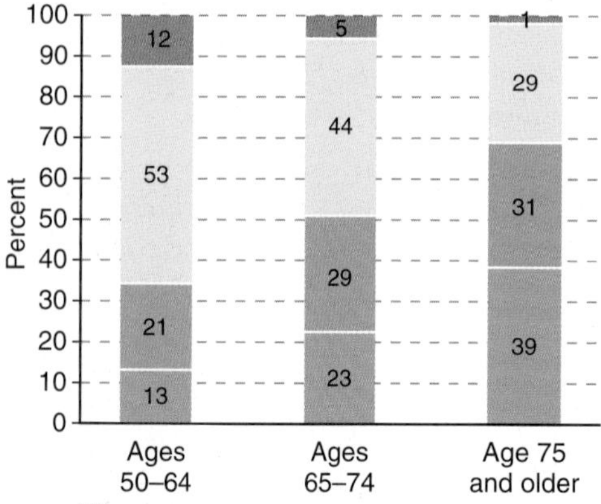

Proficient: Find the definition of a medical term in a complex health document.

Intermediate: Determine a healthy weight range using a body mass index chart.

Basic: Understand a one-page article about a health condition.

Below Basic: Circle the date of a medical appointment on a hospital appointment slip.

Note: Health literacy is the ability to locate and understand health-related information and services and requires skills represented in the three general components—prose, document, and quantitative literacy. Tasks used to measure health literacy were organized around three domains of health and health care information and services—clinical, prevention, and navigation of the health care system—and mapped to the performance levels (proficient, intermediate, basic, and below basic) based on their level of difficulty.
Reference population: These data refer to people residing in households or prisons.
Source: U.S. Department of Education, National Center for Education Statistics, National Assessment of Adult Literacy.

Figure 20-2 *(From Federal Interagency Forum on Aging-Related Statistics. Older Americans 2008: Key indicators of well-being. Washington, DC: Author. Retrieved November 30, 2010, from http://www.aoa.gov/agingstatsdotnet/Main_Site/Data/2008_Documents/Special_Feature.aspx)*

Percentage of People Age 65 and Older in Each Literacy Performance Level, by Literacy Component, 1992 and 2003

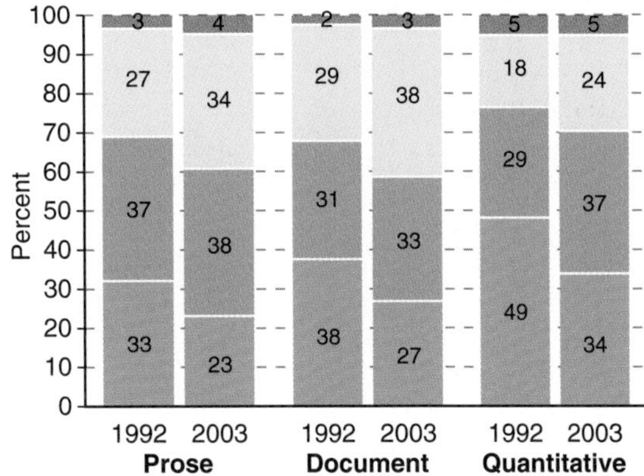

Proficient: Read complex material and draw sophisticated inferences.

Intermediate: Read moderately complex text and draw simple inferences.

Basic: Read simple words in common text.

Below Basic: No more than the most simple and concrete reading skills.

Note: Literacy is measured using three different components: prose literacy is the ability to search, comprehend, and use information from continuous texts (e.g., reading a newspaper); document literacy is the ability to search, comprehend, and use information from noncontinuous text (e.g., bus schedules); and quantitative literacy is the ability to identify and perform computations using numbers embedded in printed materials (e.g., calculating numbers in tax forms).
Reference population: These data refer to people residing in households or prisons.
Source: U.S. Department of Education, National Center for Education Statistics, National Assessment of Adult Literacy.

Figure 20-3 *(From Federal Interagency Forum on Aging-Related Statistics. Older Americans 2008: Key indicators of well-being. Washington, DC: Author. Retrieved November 30, 2010, from http://www.agingstats.gov/agingstatsdotnet/Main_Site/Data/2008_Documents/Special_Feature.aspx)*

skills or access among older adults may limit online information resources.

Providing information in ways that patients can access and understand can profoundly influence their health. In particular, older adults are more prone to chronic illnesses, and effective management requires understanding the disease process, as well as its treatment. Individualizing information delivery to meet older patients' needs shows respect and empowers them to make knowledgeable decisions. Understanding the rationale for treatment recommendations also increases the likelihood of adherence to a lifestyle that will minimize complications of chronic illness and contribute to an older adult's well-being.

Optimizing Health Literacy

Ensuring that all patients, regardless of literacy level, have access to information needed to make good decisions about their health is a shared responsibility (Gazmararian & Parker, 2005; Kessels, 2003). Most patients forget 40% to 80% of what their physician tells them as soon as they leave the office (Kessels, 2003). Patients can improve understanding of their health needs by bringing family members to visits, asking questions, and having the desire to learn and the motivation to take the necessary steps to maximize their well-being.

Most patients forget 40% to 80% of what their physician tells them as soon as they leave the office.

Providers facilitate health literacy by using good communication skills to assess patients' reading ability; preferred spoken and written language;

Educational Attainment of the Population Age 65 and Older, by Race and Hispanic Origin, 2007

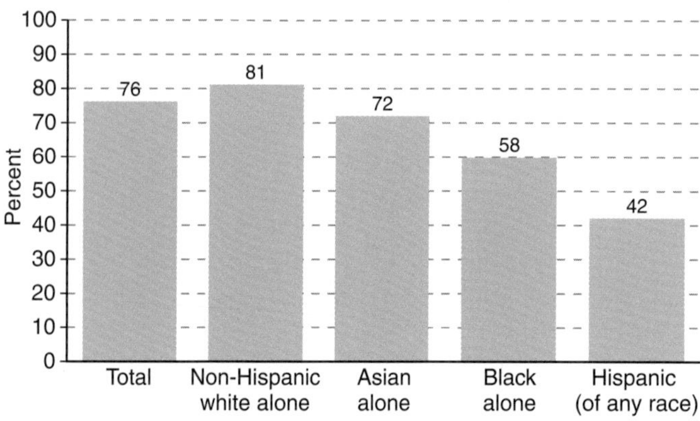

Note: The term *non-Hispanic white alone* is used to refer to people who reported being white and no other race and who are not Hispanic. The term *black alone* is used to refer to people who reported being black or African American and no other race, and the term *Asian alone* is used to refer to people who reported only Asian as their race. The use of single-race populations in this report does not imply that this is the preferred method of presenting or analyzing data. The U.S. Census Bureau uses a variety of approaches.
Reference population: These data refer to the civilian noninstitutionalized population.
Source: U.S. Census Bureau, Current Population Survey, Annual Social and Economic Supplement.

Figure 20-4 *(From Federal Interagency Forum on Aging-Related Statistics. Older Americans 2008: Key indicators of well-being. Washington, DC: Author. Retrieved November 30, 2010, from http://www.agingstats.gov/agingstatsdotnet/Main_Site/Data/2008_Documents/Population.aspx)*

limitations in vision, hearing, or cognition; and readiness to receive information. The Newest Vital Sign is a bilingual (English and Spanish) screening tool that identifies patients at risk for low health literacy (Weiss et al., 2005). It can be administered in a clinical setting in about 3 minutes by showing the patient a nutrition label and asking a set of questions about its interpretation. Scoring provides an indication of the patient's proficiency and can guide providers in selecting appropriate teaching materials and strategies. Supplementary printed, verbal, or audiovisual materials should be consistent with the patient's capacity to comprehend.

Health care systems also have a role to play in promoting health literacy. Consider the following: How easy are activities such as making appointments, navigating the physical space, and accessing support services in the agency? The availability of multilingual signage, literature designed for varied educational levels, and easy access to bilingual providers and receptionists improve the "user-friendliness" of a health care facility and enhance health literacy among consumers. System processes such as electronic medical records that facilitate care coordination across disciplines can improve communication and the confusion associated with multiple providers (Table 20-4).

The Nurse's Role in Promoting Health Literacy

Nurses play an important role in health literacy by helping patients apply their literacy skills in the context of health care (Weiss, 2005). For example, nurses help older adults comprehend appointment slips and prescriptions, interpret ingredients on nutrition labels or over-the-counter drugs, understand preventive care, and complete medical forms. Nurses also advocate for health literacy by helping patients interpret information from lay sources such as newspapers, magazines, and websites and assess the accuracy and credibility of such sources.

Understanding involves careful planning regarding the setting, method of communication, and materials selected to reinforce health teaching. The environment should minimize distractions to facilitate the older adult's ability to focus on the discussion. Including a family member may be helpful if the older adult has memory loss or cognitive impairment. Adapt all teaching to address sensory losses such as speaking toward an ear with better hearing, using larger font sizes (14 points or larger) in printed materials, and making sure that older adults are wearing their eyeglasses or hearing aids during teaching. Encourage patients to interrupt as questions occur

TABLE 20-4 Issues in Health Literacy

The patient	■ General literacy (i.e., skills in prose, document, and quantitative literacy as defined by the Adult National Literacy Survey (Kirsch, Jungeblut, Jenkins, & Kolstad, 1993) ■ Communication skills ■ Media/computer skills ■ Motivation to receive information ■ Beliefs that are open to acceptance of health information ■ Perceived relevance ■ Freedom from impairment (or assistance of surrogate) ■ Cultural beliefs
The health care provider	■ Two-way communication skills ■ Positive, accepting attitude versus being judgmental ■ Ability to assess the learning state of the patient ■ Cultural competence
The system	■ User-friendliness ■ The vast number of medications available, with their complexity of instruction and interactions ■ The increased requirement for self-care ■ Fragmentation of health care ■ Insurance policies and other required forms

and offer writing materials for note taking. Conveying that you value the patient's needs above completing the task is important and requires that you plan enough time to allow for questions and to actively listen to each patient's concerns.

Style of communication can affect how well the patient comprehends information. To help patients understand your explanations, use plain language and avoid the use of acronyms such as "CT scan." Be aware of words with multiple meanings that may confuse patients (e.g., gait/gate, dressing, and stool). Emphasizing positive behaviors (e.g., "Try to eat natural foods without added salt.") is often more motivating than cautioning about behaviors to avoid (e.g., "Don't eat salty foods."). Providing a context and interpreting the meaning of health tests and assessment numbers also facilitates understanding. For instance, you might say, "Your blood pressure is 180 over 110. The normal is closer to 120 over 80, so your blood pressure is high."

If you assess that an older adult has limited health literacy skills, give concise explanations using words with fewer syllables and supplement with audiovisual materials or pictures. Using multiple methods of communication (e.g., oral, written, and media-based materials) enhances understanding and retention of information. Because health information can be intimidating for people of all educational levels, patient education materials should target less than a ninth-grade reading level. For many patients, a lower reading level is needed. Formulas to assess the reading levels of your materials are available online and in most word processing software (University of California, Davis, 2010).

Elderly and low-literate patients may benefit if you speak more slowly and in shorter sentences that emphasize key words. Research indicates that more information is recalled by older patients when this communication style is used (McGuire, Morian, Codding, & Smyer, 2000). For some patients however, this exaggerated manner of speaking may seem condescending and disrespectful, so it is important to assess patient's needs on an individual basis.

Because many people are embarrassed to admit that they do not understand information (Parikh, Parker, Nurss, Baker, & Williams, 1996), patients may be reluctant to ask questions (Baker et al., 1996). When health providers convey a nonjudgmental attitude, patients are more likely to reveal sensitive information, such as a language barrier or an inability to read. In the case of language barriers, trained interpreters should be used.

A common but sometimes inaccurate assumption is that well-educated patients understand health information. Cutilli (2007) noted that proficiency in health literacy is typically lower than education level may imply. Many factors, including stress and anxiety, can restrict the ability to absorb new information. In one study, 30% of well-educated, affluent participants had poor comprehension of written health care information, and only 50% could accurately answer questions on a Medicaid application (Benson & Forman, 2002).

Many older adults are well informed about their health issues and present with questions or opinions about their treatment. They also may ask for guidance about finding good sources of information. It is important to convey criteria that help patients distinguish credible information from sources that are less reliable or trustworthy. The following questions can help patients judge the quality of information by evaluating its source:

1. *Who is putting out the information?* If it is written or issued by an authoritative source (e.g., government, university, or professional organization), it is typically trustworthy.
2. *Is there a listing of the names and credentials of those responsible for the content?* Contact information by phone or e-mail allows questions about the background of those responsible for the information and its origin.
3. *Does the source indicate that the material has been evaluated by experts?* Information written by reporters without a health-care background may not be accurate, so it is important to know whether the content was reviewed by a provider with expertise in the topic.
4. *Does the source indicate when it was last reviewed or updated?* Particularly with online sources, undated material may no longer be current.

The ultimate goal of health literacy is for patients to obtain, process, and understand health information and to effectively care for themselves. One effective way to evaluate comprehension is the teach-back method, which suggests that rather than simply asking whether the patient understands, providers should ask patients to explain what was learned. An example of this approach is the *Ask Me 3* system recommended by the National Patient Safety Foundation (n.d.).

1. What is my main problem?
2. What do I need to do?
3. Why is it important for me to do this?

Nurses teach older adults every day and are well positioned to promote health literacy among the aging population. In addition to providing care, nurses can advocate for health literacy in organizations that serve older adults in residential, acute, home, and community care environments. Many providers are not proficient in dealing with or even aware of the concept of health literacy. For a simple way to start remedying that problem, consider introducing the *Ask Me 3* approach in your organization. You can also promote health literacy by interviewing patients to assess your organization's user-friendliness or start a community effort designed to raise awareness about health literacy.

Conclusion

Culture is best understood in its broadest context, embracing not only ethnicities but any group that shares a set of beliefs, practices, or attitudes. This could include people who live in rural areas, people whose identity revolves around motorcycles, people who are homeless, and people who are aged. The possibilities are essentially endless. Cultural competence in health care is ultimately about equity. It involves patients having equal access to quality care that is patient centered and nondiscriminatory. Cultural competence requires providers to communicate effectively in words, actions, and written materials the information needed for patients to care for themselves. More importantly, care must be planned in a way that is consistent with patients' values, preferences, and resources. It is about recognizing and valuing each patient as a unique and important person deserving the best nursing care you can give.

KEY POINTS

- Sociocultural heritage helps to shape our ideas, behaviors, preferences, and expectations.
- Understanding the sociocultural perspective of older adults enables nurses to give care that respects patient values, beliefs, and traditions.
- Misunderstandings due to sociocultural differences can result in failed communication and poor patient outcomes.
- Older adult minorities with limited incomes or who are illiterate or cannot speak English are more likely to experience health disparities.
- Ethnocentrism and stereotyping among health care workers can lead to mistrust, biased decision making, and treatment plans that are inconsistent with a patient's preferences.
- Evidence shows that the majority of health-care workers unconsciously exhibit biased behavior.
- Selection bias is a problem in research studies that exclude certain socioeconomic groups because

the results cannot be applied to individuals like those excluded.

- The Culturally and Linguistically Appropriate Services Standards define the care services and literacy and language resources needed within an organization.
- Nurses have a central role in ensuring that the provision of care is cultural competent and consistent with patient values and preferences.
- Cultural competency involves shaping attitudes, developing good communication skills, and acquiring knowledge about other sociocultural groups.
- Acquiring the capacity to deliver culturally competent care is an ongoing process of development that requires being open to learning about another person's reality and experience.
- Cultural competence means providing care "to patients with diverse values, beliefs and behaviors, [and] tailoring delivery of care to meet patients' social, cultural, and linguistic needs (Betancourt, Green, & Carrillo, 2002, p. v, 2).
- Leininger's (1995) theory, Culture Care Diversity and Universality, includes language, art forms, dietary practices, sick role behavior, gender roles, family interactions, holiday rituals, body language, sense of time, and personal space needs as elements of one's culture.
- Camphina-Bacote (1999, 2003) describes cultural competence as a five-stage process: self-awareness, acquiring skills and knowledge about other cultures, seeking encounters with diverse individuals, and having the desire to acquire cultural competence.
- Insight about the perspectives and preferences of other sociocultural groups can help nurses to provide more culturally sensitive care.
- Conducting informed, individual assessments is critical to avoiding the stereotypical assumption that all members of a sociocultural group hold similar values and traditions.
- Acculturation can affect the extent to which sociocultural traditions are retained or abandoned.
- Sociocultural assessment includes questions about primary spoken and written language, food preferences, support systems and resources, patterns of decision making, spiritual and end-of-life preferences, health beliefs and expectations, use of native medicine or healers, and important historical events or experiences that impact an individual.
- Culturally sensitive communication involves being sensitive to verbal and nonverbal patient cues, actively listening, being nonjudgmental, respecting norms regarding social distance and the use of touch or gestures, and willingness to adapt care practices and treatment to be consistent with patient preferences.
- Taking time, showing interest, greeting patients by title and surname, and using trained interpreters demonstrate respect and enhance the effectiveness of nurse-patient communication.
- Health literacy, or the ability to obtain, process, and understand health information and services in order to effectively care for oneself, is an important issue in today's health care environment. Understanding and addressing health literacy is critical to patient education.
- Each time a person interacts with a health care provider, he or she should be able to answer the *Ask Me 3* questions: What is my main problem? Why do I need it? Why is it important for me to do this?"

CRITICAL THINKING ACTIVITIES

1. Consider the questions in Box 20-1. Choose a partner and discuss your responses to these cultural self-assessment questions. Compare similarities with and differences from your partner. Can you identify any stereotypes or biases?
2. Complete the "Cultural Competence Health Practitioner Assessment" and write a brief summary of what insights you gained from this experience. (Available at the National Center for Cultural Competency, Georgetown University: http://www11.georgetown.edu/research/gucchd/nccc/features/CCHPA.html).
3. Visit the EthnoMed websites at Stanford Geriatric Education Center (http://geriatrics.stanford.edu/ethnomed/) or University of Washington (http://ethnomed.org). Choose a socioethnic group to research. Create a class Web page and post a summary of what you learned about the group you selected.
4. Watch the movie *Crash* (Haggis, 2005). Discuss how cultural differences were evident. What were the consequences? How might the outcome have been improved?
5. Interview an elderly person from an ethnic background other than your own about his or her cultural beliefs and practices.
6. Attend a festival held by a culture that is different from your own. Notice the foods, events, dress, and music. What insights did you gain about this culture from your experience?

CASE STUDY | *MRS. ELDRIDGE*

Mrs. Eldridge, an 80-year-old African-American woman, has been widowed for 3 months. She has a degenerative neurological condition and cannot cook for herself any more. She also has trouble with balance. Mrs. Eldridge's husband used to take care of her and prepare their meals, but now that he is gone, her family is unable to provide the level of care that Mrs. Eldridge needs. After discussing the situation with her brother, Mrs. Eldridge's daughter has asked the physician to suggest a good long-term care facility. After contacting the facility, her daughter was pleased to learn that there was an opening. The family selected some of Mrs. Eldridge's belongings and moved her into the facility, where she shares a room with a woman who does not speak English. After 1 month, the staff contacts Mrs. Eldridge's daughter to report that Mrs. Eldridge refuses to participate in activities or to eat her meals in the dining room with the other residents. When the social worker inquires about Mrs. Eldridge's refusal to join the other residents in activities, Mrs. Eldridge quietly replies that she is uncomfortable joining activities because she feels "out of place."

1. Give some reasons why this resident might be feeling out of place in the facility.
2. What could the facility do to increase this resident's comfort level?
3. What kinds of culturally specific questions would have been important to ask Mrs. Eldridge and her family before she entered the long-term care facility?

REFERENCES

American Association of Colleges of Nursing. (2008). *The essentials of baccalaureate education for professional nursing practice.* Washington, DC: Author.

American Association of Colleges of Nursing. (2009). *Cultural competency in baccalaureate nursing education.* Washington, DC: Author.

Baker, D., Parker, M., Williams, M., Pitkin, K., Parikh, N. S., Coates, W., . . . (1996). The health care experience of patients with low literacy. *Archives of Family Medicine, 5*(6), 329–334.

Benson, J. G., & Forman, W. B. (2002). Comprehension of written health care information in an affluent geriatric retirement community: Use of the test of functional health literacy. *Gerontology, 48*(2), 93–97.

Betancourt, J. R., Green, A. R., & Carrillo, J. E. (2002). *Cultural competence in health care: Emerging framework and practical approaches.* New York, NY: The Commonwealth Fund.

Betancourt, J. R., Green, A. R., Carrillo, J. E., & Park, E. R. (2005). Cultural competence and health care disparities: Key perspectives and trends. *Health Affairs (Millwood), 24,* 499–505.

Camphina-Bacote, J. A. (1999). Model and instrument for addressing cultural competence in health care. *Journal of Nursing Education 38,* 203–207.

Camphina-Bacote, J. A. (2003). The process of cultural competence in the delivery of health care services: A culturally competent model of care. *Journal of Transcultural Nursing, 13*(3), 181–184.

Coffman, M. J., Shellman, J., & Bernal, H. (2004). An integrative review of American nurses' perceived cultural self-efficacy. *Journal of Nursing Scholarship, 36,* 180–185.

Cutilli, C. C. (2007). Health literacy in geriatric patients: An integrative review of the literature. *Orthopaedic Nursing, 26*(1), 43–48.

D'Avanzo, C. E. (2007). *Pocket guide to cultural health assessment* (4th ed.). St. Louis, MO: Mosby.

Eiser, A. R., & Ellis, G. (2007). Viewpoint: Cultural competence and the African American experience with health care: The case for specific content in cross-cultural education. *Academic Medicine, 82*(2), 176–183.

Galanti, G. (2008). *Caring for patients from different cultures* (4th ed.). Philadelphia, PA: University of Pennsylvania Press.

Gazmararian, J. A., & Parker, R. M. (2005). Overview of health literacy in health care. In J. G. Schwartzberg, J. B. VanGeest, & C. C. Wang (Eds.), *Understanding health literacy* (p. 253). Chicago, IL: American Medical Association Press.

Giger, J. N., & Davidhizar, R. E. (2007). *Transcultural nursing: Assessment and intervention.* St. Louis, MO: Mosby.

Haggis, P. (2005). *Crash.* Los Angeles, CA: Bob Yari Productions.

Haight, B. (1988). The therapeutic role of a structured life review process in homebound elderly subjects. *The Journals of Gerontology, 43*(2), 40–44.

Howard, D. H., Sentell, T., & Gazmararian, J. A. (2006). Impact of health literacy on socioeconomic and racial differences in health in an elderly population. *Journal of General Internal Medicine, 21*(8), 857–861.

Institute of Medicine. (2002). *Unequal treatment: What healthcare providers need to know about racial and ethnic disparities in health-care.* Washington, DC: National Academy Press.

Kessels, R. (2003). Patients' memory for medical information. *Journal of the Royal Society of Medicine, 96,* 219–222.

Kirkwood, N. A. (2005). *A hospital handbook on multiculturalism and religion.* Harrisburgh, PA: Morehouse.

Kirsch, I., Jungeblut, A., Jenkins, L., & Kolstad, A. (1993). *Adult literacy in America: A first look at the results of the national adult literacy survey.* Washington, DC: National Center for Education Statistics.

Kreitzer, M. J., Kligler, B., & Meeker, W.C. (2009). *Health professions education and integrative health care.* Washington, DC: Institute of Medicine.

Kutner, M., Greenberg, E., Jin, Y., & Paulsen, C. (2006). *The health literacy of America's adults: Results from the 2003 national assessment of adult literacy (NCES 2006–483).* Washington, DC: U.S. Department of Education National Center for Education Statistics.

Leininger, M. (1995). *Transcultural nursing: Concepts, theories, research and practice.* Blacklick, OH: McGraw-Hill.

Marks, J. P., Reed, W., Colby, K., & Ibrahim, S. A. (2004). A culturally competent approach to cancer news and education in an inner city community: Focus group findings. *Journal* of *Health Communication, 9*(2), 143–157.

Mason, D. J., Leavitt, J. K., & Chaffee, M. W. (2007). *Policy & politics in nursing and health care* (5th ed.). Philadelphia, PA: Elsevier Health Sciences.

McGuire, L. C., Morian, A., Codding, R., & Smyer, M. A. (2000). Older adults' memory for medical information: Influence of elderspeak and note taking. *International Journal of Rehabilitation and Health, 5*(2), 117–128.

Narayan, M. C. (2003). Cultural assessment and care planning. *Home Healthcare Nurse, 21*(9), 611–620.

National Center for Minority Health and Health Disparities. (2003). *Vision and mission.* Retrieved November 16, 2010, from http://ncmhd.nih.gov/about_ncmhd/mission.asp

National Patient Safety Foundation. (n.d.). *Ask Me 3.* Retrieved November 30, 2010, from http://www.npsf.org/askme3/

Nielsen-Bohlman, L., Panzer, A., & Kindig, D. (2004). *Health literacy: A prescription to end confusion.* Washington, DC: National Academy Press.

Office of Minority Health. (2001). *National standards for culturally and linguistically appropriate services in health care: Final report.* Washington, DC: U.S. Department of Health and Human Resources. Retrieved December 4, 2010, from http://minorityhealth.hhs.gov/assets/pdf/checked/finalreport.pdf

Office of Minority Health. (2007). *Culturally competent nursing care: A cornerstone of caring.* Retrieved November 20, 2010, from https://ccnm.thinkculturalhealth.org/

Parikh, N., Parker, R., Nurss, J., Baker, D., & Williams, M. (1996). Shame and health literacy: The unspoken connection. *Patient Education* and *Counseling, 27*(1), 33–39.

Ray, M. A. (2010). *Transcultural caring dynamics in nursing and health care.* Philadelphia, PA: Davis.

Rundle, A., Carvalho, M., & Robinson, M. (2002). *Cultural competence in health care: A practical guide.* San Francisco, CA: Jossey-Bass.

Shapiro, J., Hollingshead, J., & Morrison, E. H. (2002). Primary care resident, faculty, and patient views of barriers to cultural competence, and the skills needed to overcome them. *Medical Education, 36,* 749–759.

Shellman, J. (2007). The effects of a reminiscence education program on baccalaureate nursing students' cultural self-efficacy in caring for elders. *Nurse Education Today, 27*(1), 43–51.

Smith, L. S. (1998). Cultural competence for nurses: Canonical correlation of two culture scales. *Journal of Cultural Diversity, 5*(4), 120–126.

Spector, R. E. (2008). *Cultural diversity in health and illness* (7th ed.). Upper Saddle River, NJ: Prentice-Hall.

Teal, C. R., & Street, R. L. (2009). Critical elements of culturally competent communication in the medical encounter: A review and model. *Social Science & Medicine, 68*(3), 533–543.

Tripp-Reimer, T., Choi, E., Kelley, L. S., & Enslein, J. C. (2001). Cultural barriers to care: Inverting the problem. *Diabetes Spectrum, 14,* 13–22.

University of California, Davis, Health System. (2010). *Guidelines for preparing patient education handouts.* Retrieved December 5, 2010, from http://www.ucdmc.ucdavis.edu/cne/health_education/guide.html

U.S. Department of Health and Human Services. (n.d.). *Quick guide to health literacy.* Retrieved December 1, 2010, from http://www.health.gov/communication/literacy/quickguide/

U.S. Department of Health and Human Services. (2005). *Healthy People 2010/2020.* Retrieved December 6, 2010, from http://www.healthypeople.gov/2020/default.aspx

U.S. Department of Health and Human Services. (2007, April 6). *OMH to help nurses provide culturally competent care.* Office of Minority Health. Retrieved December 7, 2010, from http://www.omhrc.gov/templates/content.aspx?ID=5017

U.S. Department of Labor. (2008). *U.S. labor force characteristics by race and ethnicity, 2007.* Washington, DC: Author.

Vernon, J., Trujillo, A., Rosenbaum, S., & De.Buono, B. (2006). *Low health literacy: Implications for national health policy.* Washington, DC: George Washington University. Retrieved December 3, 2010, from http://www.gwumc.edu/sphhs/departments/healthpolicy/CHPR/downloads/LowHealthLiteracyReport10_4_07.pdf

Weiss, B. D. (2005). Epidemiology of low health literacy. In J. G. Schwartzberg, J. B. VanGeest, & C. C. Wang (Eds.), *Understanding health literacy* (p. 253). Chicago, IL: American Medical Association Press.

Weiss, B. D., Mays, M. Z., Martz, W., Castro, K. M., DeWalt, D. A., Pignone, M. P., . . . Hale, F. A. (2005). Quick assessment of literacy in primary care: The newest vital sign. *Annals of Family Medicine, 3*(6), 514–522.

World Health Organization. (2008). *Global standards for the initial education of professional nurses and midwives.* Geneva, Switzerland: Author.

Yeo, G. (2000). *Core curriculum in ethnogeriatrics.* Palo Alto, CA: Stanford Geriatric Education Center.

Chapter 21

Lesbian, Gay, Bisexual, and Transgender Older Adults

Patricia Burbank, DNSc, RN

LEARNING OBJECTIVES

- Discuss the demographics of lesbian, gay, bisexual, and transgender (LGBT) older adults in the aging population.
- Identify sources of discrimination that limit access to health care for LGBT elders.
- Describe health issues facing LGBT individuals as they age.
- Propose strategies to promote an accepting environment and improve delivery of health care to LGBT elders.

Lesbian, gay, bisexual, and transgender (LGBT) older adults are among the most invisible of all Americans. Stigma and fear of discrimination cause many LGBT older adults to hide their identity. This is emotionally costly and often results in LGBT elders limiting visits to health care providers, selectively choosing social activities, and experiencing denial of partner rights in health care and disenfranchised grief. In addition, health care providers and the public in general lack awareness of LGBT issues. All of these factors contribute to the increased risk of health problems and increased vulnerability of LGBT older adults. This chapter describes the older LGBT population, discusses issues of discrimination, and gives an overview of health issues facing these groups of older adults. Strategies for health care professionals to improve health care and promote an open, accepting environment for LGBT older adults are also discussed.

Because many older LGBT people hide their identities, it is difficult to determine the size of the population; however, estimates range from 1.75 to 3.5 million lesbians, gays, and bisexuals (or about 10% of the older adult population) in the United States. The number of transgender individuals (referring to those with all forms of biological sex and gender variations) is more difficult to identify, with numbers ranging from 0.25% to 1% of the U.S. population (Human Rights Campaign, 2010). It should be noted that transgender people are of all sexual orientations. Bisexuals have been estimated at 1.8% of men and 2.8% of women (Cahill, n.d.).

Using the term LGBT may seem to imply that lesbian, gay, bisexual, and transgender people are one group or population. In reality, there is great diversity across these four groups, and great diversity within each group. Another level of diversity is added with age, as the older adult population in general is very heterogeneous, making the older population of LGBT people especially diverse. Additionally, this is a difficult population to study. Although researchers have attempted to more accurately sample the LGBT population, sampling bias continues to exist and caution must be used in interpreting the results (Burbank & Burkholder, 2007).

Using the term LGBT may seem to imply that lesbian, gay,

bisexual, and transgender people are one group or population. In reality, there is great diversity across these four groups, and great diversity within each group.

Demographically, the LGBT older adult population differs from the heterosexual population in several ways, including education, income, and the proportion in committed relationships, living alone, and having children. Although there is little research on the experiences of gay, lesbian, bisexual, and transgender individuals who are members of racial minority groups (Brotman, Ryan, & Cormier, 2003), there is evidence that samples of LGB people are as racially diverse as heterosexual samples (Cahill, South, & Spade, 2000). Table 21-1 summarizes important characteristics of LGBT older adults.

Health Issues

Discrimination and Homophobia

Among LGBT older adults, heterosexism, homophobia, and ageism are part of the fabric of life. Many in this population are marginalized in multiple ways. About three-quarters of this group are women and may experience sexism and racism among those identifying with communities of color. Discrimination within one's own ethnic community is not uncommon as different ethnic groups have varying degrees of tolerance for same-sex relationships. By becoming or remaining closeted, LGBT elders can eliminate one of the major categories of bias, but not without negative effects on their mental health. Most of today's older adults grew up during an era in which homosexuality was considered a mental illness, and some may have directly experienced aversive techniques to change sexual orientation (Haldeman, 1994). The experience of "coming out" into a homophobic, transphobic culture that has a number of physical, mental, and psychological consequences, no matter one's position in the life span. Homophobia and fear of discrimination affects all aspects of health and health care and poses a major public health risk for LGBT people (O'Hanlan, Cajab, Schatz, Lock, & Nemrow, 1997). The need to stay hidden to prevent discrimination is an important coping strategy for many older LGBT adults and may serve to

TABLE 21-1 Snapshot of LGBT Population

CHARACTERISTIC	PERCENT OR COMPARISION WITH HETEROSEXUAL POPULATION
Education	■ More gays and lesbians have baccalaureate and graduate degrees
Income	■ Gay men tend to earn less ■ Lesbians earn the same or slightly more ■ Transgender experience more poverty and wage discrimination
Partnered	■ Higher percentage of lesbians ■ Lower percentage of older gay men
Formerly in a heterosexual marriage	■ 42% of lesbians ■ 33% of gay men
Have biologic children	■ 30% of lesbians ■ 15% of gay men ■ Increasing among younger lesbians and gay men
Home ownership	■ 61% own their own homes ■ Most live in urban areas
Live alone	■ LGBT seniors twice as likely to live alone
Loneliness	■ No differences
Relationships with family	■ Older LGBTs report close relationships with parents, siblings, and children
Friends	■ Most common sources of support ■ Have become families of choice
Caregivers	■ 27% of LGBT seniors reported they did not know who would take care of them if they needed care

Burbank & Burkholder, 2007; Burbank & Manning, 2005. Note: These statistics reflect studies with sample limitations, so they should be viewed as approximate.

silence them about health concerns (Cook-Daniels, 1997; Harrison & Silenzio, 1996; Rosenfeld, 1999; Schatz & O'Hanlan, 1994).

Physical Health Issues

Lesbians are at higher risk for certain health problems not because of their sexual orientation but because of important risk factors that are more prevalent in this group, such as smoking, obesity, and alcohol use (Box 21-1) (Solarz, 1999). Other risk factors more prevalent in lesbians are nulliparity (never having given birth) and fewer screening exams of all kinds (Denenburg, 1995; Haynes, 1995). Studies have, in general, supported the hypothesis that lesbian and bisexual women are at higher risk for breast cancer (Dibble, Roberts, & Nussey, 2004) and for ovarian cancer (likely due to fewer pregnancies and lower use of birth control pills; Dibble, Roberts, Robertson, & Paul, 2002). Given that lung cancer is the number one cause of cancer death in women and that numerous studies suggest that lesbian and bisexual women are more likely to smoke, it appears that these women may be at differential risk for this form of cancer. Cardiovascular disease is the number one killer of women in North America, including lesbians (Ulstad, 1999). The actual risk of coronary artery disease is unknown among older lesbians; however, some sources do indicate that they are at higher risk because of increased smoking and body weight (Case et al., 2004).

Gay and bisexual men are also at higher risk for cardiovascular disease and some cancers for many of the same reasons (Box 21-2). Gay (but not bisexual) men have been more likely to smoke than their heterosexual counterparts (Tang et al., 2004), increasing their risk for lung cancer (Peterkin & Risdon, 2003). The rates of smoking among adolescents in the gay and bisexual male population continue to be higher than for their heterosexual counterparts (D'Augelli, 2004; Rosario, Schrimshaw, & Hunter, 2004), indicating that the increased risk for cardiovascular disease and cancer will likely continue. Gay and bisexual men are at higher risk for HIV and other sexually transmitted diseases (STDs) such as hepatitis. It seems that older gay men may have more difficulty changing to safer sex practices and may not use condoms with every sexual encounter (Linsk, 1997).

Much less is known about health issues related to transgender adults, as there is little research on older transgender adults (Berreth, 2003). It appears that substance abuse rates among transgender individuals are much higher than the norm (Leslie, Perina, & Maqueda, 2001). Additionally, rates of HIV infection are higher. There also appears to be significant risk of physical violence and harassment toward transgender individuals. Also, little is known about the long-term effects of the hormone use and surgeries associated with sexual reassignment. After sexual reassignment has taken place, health concerns associated with the previous sex remain (e.g., men who undergo male-to-female reassignment still need to have prostate exams; Berreth, 2003).

BOX 21-1 Priority Areas for Assessment of Older Lesbians

- Cardiovascular disease
- Cancers, especially breast, ovarian, and lung
- Decreased participation in screening exams
- Anxiety
- Substance abuse
- Domestic violence
- Discrimination and homophobia
- Disenfranchised grief
- Unmet spiritual needs

BOX 21-2 Priority Areas for Assessment of Older Gay Men

- Cardiovascular disease
- Cancers, especially lung
- HIV/AIDS
- Decreased participation in screening exams
- Depression and anxiety
- Substance abuse
- Domestic violence
- Discrimination and homophobia
- Ageism
- Disenfranchised grief
- Unmet spiritual needs

Mental and Spiritual Health Issues

Research suggests that most older gays and lesbians are well-adjusted with high levels of self-acceptance (Brown, Sarosy, Cook, & Quarto, 1997; Ehrenberg, 1996; Friend, 1991). The term *crisis competence* refers to a person's ability to successfully manage challenges and crises, based on previously developed coping skills. Many LGBT older adults age with a sense of crisis competence that they have developed in response to earlier stress and life crises around homophobia and discrimination, losses of loved ones from the AIDS epidemic, and experiences with the blurring of gender role responsibilities throughout life (Cahill, South, & Spade, 2000; Friend, 1991).

Studies also report that LGBT adults are at increased risk for anxiety, mood, and substance use disorders and for suicidal thoughts and plans (Gilman et al., 2001). Cochran and Mays (2000) found that gay men were more likely than other men to experience major depression and panic attack syndromes. Both gays and lesbians were more likely than heterosexuals to have used mental health services in the year prior to interview. A recent study by Hatzenbuehler, McLaughlin, Keyes, and Hasin (2010) found a significant increase in the prevalence of mood disorders, generalized anxiety disorders, and alcohol use disorders among lesbians, gays, and bisexuals after states banned gay marriage. The greatest increase, more than 200%, was seen in generalized anxiety disorder.

Gay men may experience "accelerated aging" or perceive themselves as being old at an earlier age than their chronological age (Baron & Cramer, 2000), with these feelings beginning as early as age 30 (Berger, 1982). Lesbians, on the other hand, seemed to have advantages over heterosexual women in that youthful appearance may not be as important in intimate relationships. Lesbians also tend to have more support from a wider intergenerational circle of family and friends than gay men (Baron & Cramer, 2000).

An important issue among transgender individuals is the effect of their changing lives on family relationships, in which family ties may have been severed due to the stress of the transition (Berreth, 2003). Midence and Hargreaves (1997) found that, in general, poor social support and negative family reactions predicted postsurgery psychopathology. It was also noted that the rates of suicide attempts, completed suicides, depression, and substance use were high especially before surgery (Dean et al., 2000).

Substance Abuse, Violence, and Domestic Violence

Although there are limitations with studies on the LGBT population, and a paucity of literature on substance abuse among LGBT older adults, it seems apparent that drug and alcohol abuse among the LGBT population is significantly higher. Lesbians seem to have higher rates of alcoholism, while gay men have more alcoholism and drug use than their heterosexual counterparts (Cochran & Mays, 2000; Hughes & Wilsnack, 1997; U.S. Department of Health & Human Services, 2001; Woody et al. 1999). Substance abuse problems are also prevalent in the transgender population, with alcohol abuse rates ranging from 27.1% to 33% (Valentine, 1998; Xavier, 2000).

Domestic violence is also an issue in the LGBT community. Evidence suggests that it occurs at about the same rate in lesbian and gay relationships as in heterosexual relationships, with some form of abuse occurring in about one of every four relationships. Incidents of domestic violence, domestic violence–related fatalities, and incidents among many race and ethnicity categories were reported to be increasing. Reports of domestic violence also increased among those with disabilities (Elliot, 1996; National Coalition on Anti-violence Programs, 2009). Lombardi, Wilchins, Priesing, and Malouf (2001) found that about 25% of the respondents reported violence against them, while over 50% reported either physical violence or harassment. Older transgender people are also at risk of being victimized in the health care system as dependency increases and they become unable to care for themselves.

Loss and Grief

Losses are an inherent part of the lives of all older adults, and LGBT older adults are no different. What is different is that often, in same-sex relationships, the most significant loss, the loss of a life partner, is often not recognized, validated, or valued. The heterosexual who loses a spouse is expected to grieve and usually receives open and caring support from a wide circle of friends and family and the culture at large. Depending on the degree of disclosure and acceptance of the older LGBT person's relationship, the remaining partner may be left to grieve alone. This has been called *disenfranchised grief* by Doka (1989) and may result in complicated mourning. Additionally, this generation of older gay men has lived through multiple losses of many friends from AIDS, sometimes resulting in chronic sorrow.

Because in most states, same-sex couples cannot legally marry, they are excluded from spousal rights. This may have a serious impact in health care settings, on health care decision making, and in settlement of the estate after the death of a partner.

Spiritual Issues

Spirituality is very important to older gays and lesbians. In a 2005 study, more than 90% of older gays and lesbians surveyed reported being raised with a religious affiliation, although 65.5% currently had no religious affiliation. The majority indicated that spirituality was very important to them, however (Burbank & Manning, 2005). Homophobia from organized religious groups can cause LGBT people to stop going to religious services because of the hostile treatment they have received (Finnegan & McNally, 2002).

Health Care Strategies

Despite an increase in the acceptance of homosexuality over the past two decades, fear of stigma and discrimination continues to impact the daily lives of LGBT individuals, particularly older adults. Dean et al. (2000), in their review of the health status of LGBT individuals, suggested that stigma continues to be a major factor in health care provision to those in this group. Gay men and lesbians tend to visit doctors less often and may postpone treatment longer than heterosexuals (Carroll, 1999; Harrison & Silenzio, 1996). This is presumably due, at least in part, to a health care system perceived to be homophobic (Klitzman & Greenberg, 2002; Peterkin & Risdon, 2003).

Cultural Competence

Health care providers exhibit a wide variety of responses to caring for LGBT older adults, ranging from acceptance and tolerance to ignorance and hostility. Discrimination on the part of health care professionals and perception of bias by LGBT individuals have been identified as barriers to care, leading to a decrease in care sought and quality of care obtained (Millman, 1993). To change this environment, providers need to become culturally competent in the care of LGBT older adults by learning about and understanding the complexities of the lives of LGBT individuals. This can be achieved through education and consciousness raising (by service providers) to explore their own attitudes toward LGBT people.

Cultural competence is "the ability to provide effective and helpful services to people from varied cultures and communities in a respectful and informed manner" (Finnegan & McNally, 2002, p. 67). Although cultural diversity commonly refers to different ethnic and racial groups, it also includes differences of many kinds including those related to sexual orientation and age. There is much debate over what constitutes gay culture; however, there is no question that many LGBT people experience a way of life that is considered a culture (Wright, Shelton, Browning, Orduna, & Wong 2001). As discussed previously, diversity within the LGBT community is great; thus, health care providers must be careful to avoid stereotyping when considering the cultural characteristics of the LGBT population.

EVIDENCE FOR PRACTICE

Old Age Meaning, Support Networks, and Delivery Services of Gay Men and Lesbians 60 Years and Older

Purpose: To explore the meaning of being old among gay men and lesbian Puerto Ricans and their perceived needs and support networks.

Methods: This sequential explanatory design was guided by the theory of social constructionism.

Sample: A convenience sample of 43 gay or lesbian Puerto Rican and Spanish-speaking individuals age 60 or older (17 female and 26 male) participated. Six of the participants also completed a second phase of individual interviews.

Results: Participants experienced aging as a positive process associated with gains rather than losses. Partners, friends, and family were important sources of social support. Participants expressed that their needs related to growing old were not unlike those of heterosexual elders but that they sometimes experienced discrimination that posed barriers to accessing needed services.

Implications: Policies, care provision, and services must be nondiscriminatory and sensitive to the needs of older adults, regardless of sexual orientation.

Reference: Santiago O., & Astrid E. (2009). Old age meaning, support networks, and delivery services of gay men and lesbians 60 years and older. *Dissertation Abstracts International, A: The Humanities and Social Sciences, vol. 70, no. 07,* 2732, ISSN 0419-4209.

Communicating with LGBT Elders

Most health care professionals, when asked, report having cared for very few, if any, older LGBT patients. One study reports "After a period of silence, one of the social workers [respondent] said 'I remember a man I think was gay ... he never exactly came out to me ... but then I never really asked him about it' (Quam, 1997, p. xv). This is a common experience in heterosexist health care environments, in which providers generally assume everyone is heterosexual and do not ask questions to refute that assumption. These typical responses seem to reflect a "don't ask, don't tell" approach to patient interaction that has the effect of reinforcing silence and invisibility. Providers may assume everyone, including the older person, is more comfortable not discussing sexual orientation, or they may think that it does not matter because sexual orientation is not central to the health care issue being addressed. The person's own nondisclosure to health care professionals may indeed contribute to this. The discomfort that health professionals may feel discussing issues of sexual orientation, along with the older LGBT person's decision to remain invisible to protect against discrimination (or from their own discomfort dealing with the issue), reinforces a vicious cycle of oppression (Brotman, Ryan, & Cormier, 2003).

Further complicating open communication with LGBT elders is the issue of labeling and language used to describe themselves and their partners. For instance, older women who would be considered lesbians by current definition rarely use terms such as lesbian, dyke, queer, or homosexual (Simkin, 1998). Older lesbians and gay men often say they are single or divorced when asked about marital status, or they may say they live with a close friend, housemate, or even a sister or brother (Box 21-3). Even those who would like to report being married to their partner often cannot because the laws in most states forbid them from marrying.

Older gays and lesbians may acknowledge loving relationships with another of the same sex but still not identify as lesbian or gay. These elders may be deeply offended when others, even younger gays or lesbians, apply labels to them (Deevey, 1990). For these reasons, communication with elders about their sexual orientation must be done cautiously and with sensitivity. It is essential that providers listen carefully to how each patient describes his or her living situation or partner status. The provider should then follow the patient's example, using words that are consistent with the patient's own description (Burbank, Burkholder, & Fournier, 2007).

BOX 21-3 Assessing Partnerships

The first place in the health care system where an older LGBT person may encounter difficulty is completing the intake form in the health care provider's office. Typically, questions about marital status list four options: single, married, divorced or separated, and widowed. Often no option is available for identifying a same-sex or long-term partnership, nor is there a way to describe nontraditional living situations.

In addition to adding such an option to assessment forms to more accurately reflect LGBT realities, you could consider asking such open-ended questions as, "Who is most important to you? Who lives with you?" If the response is that they live alone, then a follow-up question might be "Have you always lived alone?" This will give clues as to whether the patient could be experiencing the recent loss of a partner (Burbank, Burkholder, & Fournier, 2007).

A Welcoming Environment

The Gay and Lesbian Medical Association (2006) has developed guidelines for creating a safe clinical environment for lesbian, gay, bisexual, transgender, and intersex patients (see reference list for the Web address). This guideline includes sample recommended questions for LGBT-sensitive intake forms and recommendations for successful communication. It includes questions about HIV and STDs that are also relevant for older LGBT adults.

Comprehensive guidelines specific to changing long-term care settings to be welcoming of LGBT older adults can be found in *Diversity our Strength: LGBT Tool Kit* (Toronto Long-Term Care Homes & Services, 2008). The Transgender Aging Network (http://www.forge-forward.org/tan/index.php) is a resource for transgender older adults and their significant others, families, and friends and also assists health care organizations to make programs more transgender friendly by providing consultation services and onsite training. An excellent curriculum guide useful for educating health professionals about general and mental health issues of older LGBT adults has been developed by Prairielands Addiction Technology Transfer Center (n.d.).

Creating a welcoming environment for LGBT patients is essential and should begin in the waiting room. Posters or pictures depicting older gay and lesbian adults and indicating that this is a facility that welcomes LGBT patients can be hung on the wall. Written materials listing community resources for LGBT elders can also be made available in the waiting room for patients to read. An additional benefit of including such reading material is that other patients and office staff may increase their awareness about the needs of LGBT older adults as well (Burbank, Burkholder, & Fournier, 2007).

Health Policy

Because many LGBT older adults are hidden, their issues and concerns are not typically reflected in health care policy. These elders "lose the critical potential for empowerment and the ability to participate in the design of services and policies that may improve their access to appropriate health care" (Dean et al., 2000, p. 28). The *Healthy People 2010* document (the primary document that drives public health research funding and outlines the principle concerns of focus for the decade) included very few references to sexual orientation and none related to LGBT older adults. In response, the Gay and Lesbian Medical Association, along with a variety of experts in LGBT health, composed a document to serve as a companion to the *Healthy People 2010* document (Gay and Lesbian Medical Association, 2001). In the new proposed *Healthy People 2020,* sexual orientation is included as an important factor requiring particular attention to achieve health equity and eliminate health disparities.

Another publication, *Outing Age 2010,* issued by the National Gay and Lesbian Task Force Policy Institute, outlines policy issues affecting the lives of LGBT elders and makes several recommendations (Grant, 2009). Major recommendations (abbreviated) include:

- Add questions on sexual orientation and gender identity in all research surveys.
- Designate LGBT elders as a "vulnerable senior constituency and identity."
- Enforce state and local employment nondiscrimination laws.
- Enforce and pass laws banning discrimination on the basis of age, sexual orientation, and gender identity.
- Reframe and expand the definition of family to recognize same-sex relationships and LGBT family kinship structures in the designation of federal benefits such as Social Security, Medicaid, and Veterans benefits.
- Ensure access to LGBT-affirming health care for people of all ages.
- Amend the federal Family and Medical Leave Act to cover LGBT caregivers and their family and friends regardless of whether they are related by blood or marriage.

These recommendations can be accomplished through a combination of policy reform, education, research, and advocacy. Exciting new research and policy initiatives are also underway with the work of special organizations and committees such as the Committee on Lesbian, Gay, Bisexual, and Transgender Health Issues and Research Gaps and Opportunities at the Institute of Medicine. The Committee will conduct a review and prepare a report assessing the state of the science on the health status of LGBT populations, identify research gaps and opportunities related to LGBT health, and outline a research agenda that will assist the National Institute of Health in enhancing its research efforts in this area.

Conclusion

At the heart of the increased vulnerability of LGBT older adults is the stigma and bias associated with their sexual orientation. This stigma and bias has resulted in discrimination against LGBT people by society in general, including the health care system. Fortunately, the potential exists for taking action on a number of levels (individual, organizational, and policy) to provide an environment where LGBT elders have the same privileges and rights as other Americans. When this happens, vulnerability will decrease. For this to occur, interventions across levels are necessary.

Change must take place at the individual level among the LGBT elders themselves; recognizing the effects of internalized homophobia would be an important step toward taking a more proactive stand on mental and physical health care needs. The LGBT community in general must continue to advocate for the health of all LGBT individuals, including those who are older.

Health-care providers need to assess their own attitudes around sexual orientation and actively seek ways to improve awareness of the physical, psychological, and mental health needs of LGBT people. They also need to better understand the impact of heterosexism on the state of health of their LGBT patients.

Researchers must work to provide reliable and valid research that minimizes sampling bias when studying LGBT people, especially older adults. Services that meet the general physical and mental health needs of the entire LGBT population are necessary.

Finally, advocacy at the policy level needs to include the voices of LGBT elders. Gains made here at the policy level will do much to counter the legacy of heterosexism and its effects on the lives of older LGBT adults. Through reduced discrimination and improved quality of care, the LGBT elder population can become less vulnerable and experience healthy aging.

KEY POINTS

- Stigma, fear of discrimination, and lack of awareness about LGBT issues increase the risk of health problems among this aging population.
- Sampling bias continues to exist in most studies.
- LGBT older adults experience discrimination on several levels: heterosexism, homophobia, and ageism that may negatively affect their mental health.
- The prevalence of nulliparity, smoking, obesity, alcohol abuse, and unprotected sex among LGBT individuals increases their risk for related diseases.
- LGBT people are at greater risk for substance abuse, anxiety, and mood disorders.
- Lesbians tend to have stronger social supports than gay or bisexual men.
- The significance of losing a partner is underrecognized by society and may lead to complicated or unresolved grieving.
- Lack of spousal rights can pose barriers to visitation rights, health care decision making, and settlement of the estate after the death a partner.
- Religious homophobia may prevent LGBT people from accessing spiritual sources of support.
- Stigma continues to be a major factor in health care provision to LGBT adults, leading to fewer visits and delayed treatment.
- Providers need to explore their attitudes toward LGBT people and become more culturally competent by learning about the complexities of LGBT lives.
- Providers generally assume everyone is heterosexual and do not ask questions to refute that assumption.
- Labels can be offensive; therefore, assessment of sexual orientation and significant others must be done cautiously and with sensitivity.
- Environments inclusive of pictures representing diverse lifestyles and written materials with resources for LGBT individuals convey a message of acceptance.
- The National Gay and Lesbian Task Force has made numerous recommendations to reduce political discrimination.

CRITICAL THINKING ACTIVITIES

1. Examine legislation in your state regarding gay and lesbian marriage. How do these policies affect individual rights to a partner's Social Security or pension, taxation status, property inheritance, and participation in health care decision making?
2. Watch the video, *Beauty before Age* (Terra Nova Films, Inc.). Discuss how aging is viewed in the gay male community. How are these views similar or different from other groups in society?
3. Contact your campus student services or local Area Agency on Aging to learn what is currently being done to address LGBT issues in your community and what resources are available.

CASE STUDY | *ELEANOR JONES*

Eleanor Jones, age 85, is a patient of yours on the oncology unit where you work. She is recovering from pneumonia following her last round of chemotherapy for Stage IV lung cancer. On her admission history, she has reported her marital status as single and stated she lives in her own home. When planning for her discharge, it is discovered that Ms. Jones lives with her friend, Ms. Smith, who is available to help care for her when she returns home. They have lived together for 56 years and have no other family nearby.

1. Is it important for the health care system to recognize and label Ms. Jones and Ms. Smith's lesbian relationship? Why or why not?
2. What kinds of support do Ms. Jones and Ms. Smith need as they enter this difficult phase of life together?
3. How might you help to support each of them as Ms. Jones' illness progresses?

REFERENCES

Baron, A., & Cramer, D.W. (2000). Potential counseling concerns of aging lesbian, gay, and bisexual clients. In R. M. Perez, K. A. DeBord, & K.A . Bieschke (Eds.), *Handbook of counseling and psychotherapy with lesbian, gay and bisexual clients,* pp. 207-223. Washington: American Psychological Association.

Berger, R. M. (1982). The unseen minority: Older gays and lesbians. *Social Work, 27*(3), 236–242.

Berreth, M. (2003). Nursing care of transgendered older adults: Implications from the literature. *Journal of Gerontological Nursing, 29*(7), 44–49.

Brotman, S., Ryan, B., & Cormier, R. (2003). The health and social service needs of gay and lesbian elders and their families in Canada. *Gerontologist, 43*(2), 192–202.

Brown, L. B., Sarosy, S. G., Cook, T. C., & Quarto, J. G. (1997). *Gay men and aging.* New York, NY: Garland.

Burbank, P., & Burkholder, G. (2007). Health issues of lesbian, gay, bisexual, and transgender older adults. In P. M. Burbank (Ed.), *Vulnerable older adults: Issues and strategies* (pp. 149–175). New York, NY: Springer.

Burbank, P., Burkholder, G., & Fournier. (2007). Health care strategies for lesbian, gay, bisexual, and transgender older adults. In P. M. Burbank (Ed.), *Vulnerable older adults: Issues and strategies* (pp. 177–205). New York, NY: Springer.

Burbank, P., & Manning, C. (2005). *Meet the older neighbors: Report of the SAGE/ RI survey of lesbian, gay, bisexual and transgender older adults in Rhode Island.* Providence, RI: SAGE/RI.

Cahill, S. (n.d.). Bisexuality: Dispelling the myths. National Gay and Lesbian Task Force. Retrieved November 30, 2010, from http://www.thetaskforce.org/downloads/reports/BisexualityDispellingtheMyths.pdf

Cahill, S., South, K., & Spade, J. (2000). *Outing age: Public policy issues affecting gay, lesbian, bisexual, and transgender elders.* New York, NY: The National Gay and Lesbian Task Force Policy Institute.

Carroll, N. (1999). Optimal gynecologic and obstetric care for lesbians. *Obstetrics & Gynecology, 93*(4), 611–613.

Case, P., Austin, B., Hunter, D. J., Manson, J. E., Malspeis, S., Willett, W. C., . . . (2004). Sexual orientation, health risk factors, and physical functioning in the Nurses' Health Study II. *Journal of Women's Health, 13*(9), 1033–1047.

Cochran, S. D., & Mays, V. M. (2000) Relation between psychiatric syndromes and behaviorally defined sexual orientation in a sample of the U.S. population. *American Journal of Epidemiology, 151*(5), 516–523.

Cook-Daniels, L. (1997). Lesbian, gay male, bisexual, and trangendered elders: Elder abuse and neglect issues. *Journal of Elder Abuse & Neglect, 9*(2), 35–50.

D'Augelli, A. R. (2004). High tobacco use among lesbian, gay, and bisexual youth: Mounting evidence about a hidden population's health risk behavior. *Archives of Pediatrics & Adolescent Medicine, 158*(4), 309–310.

Dean, L., Meyer, I. H., Robinson, K., Sell, R. L., Sember, R., Silenzio, V. M. B., . . . Tierney, R. (2000). Lesbian, gay, bisexual, and transgender health: Findings and concerns. *Journal of the Gay and Lesbian Medical Association, 4*(3), 102–151.

Deevey, S. (1990). Older lesbian women: An invisible minority. *Journal of Gerontological Nursing, 16*(5), 35–37.

Denenberg, R. (1995). Report on lesbian health. *Womens Health Issues, 5*(2), 81–91.

Dibble, S. L., Roberts, S. A., & Nussey, B. (2004). Comparing breast cancer risk between lesbians and their heterosexual sisters. *Womens Health Issues, 14*(2), 60–68.

Dibble. S. L., Roberts, S. A., Robertson, P. A., & Paul, S. M. (2002). Risk factors for ovarian cancer: Lesbian and heterosexual women. *Oncology Nursing Forum, 29*(1), E1–E7.

Doka, K. (1989). *Disenfranchised grief: Recognizing hidden sorrow.* Lexington, MA: Lexington Books.

Ehrenberg, M. (1996). Aging and mental health: Issues in the gay and lesbian community. In C. J. Alexander (Ed.), *Gay and lesbian mental health: A sourcebook for practitioners* (pp. 189–209). Binghamton, NY: The Haworth Press.

Elliott, P. (Ed.). (1996). *Confronting lesbian battering.* St. Paul, MN: Minnesota Coalition for Battered Women.

Finnegan, D. G., & McNally, E. B. (2002). *Counseling lesbian, gay, bisexual, and transgender substance abusers.* New York, NY: Haworth.

Friend, R. A. (1991). Older lesbian and gay people: A theory of successful aging. *J Homosexual, 20*(3–4), 99–118.

Gay and Lesbian Medical Association. (2001). *Healthy People 2010 companion document for lesbian, gay, bisexual, and transgender (LGBT) health.* San Francisco, CA: Author. Retrieved December 9, 2010, from http://www.glma.org/index.cfm?fuseaction=document.showDocumentByID&DocumentID=30&d:\CFusionMX7\verity\Data\dummy.txt

Gay and Lesbian Medical Association. (2006). *Guidelines for care of lesbian, gay, bisexual, and transgender patients.* Retrieved November 31, 2010, from http://glma.org/index.cfm?fuseaction=document.showDocumentByID&DocumentID=16&d:\CFusionMX7\verity\Data\dummy.txt

Gilman, S. E., Cochran, S. D., Mays, V. M., Hughes, M., Ostrow, D., & Kessler, R. C. (2001). Risk of psychiatric disorders among individuals reporting same-sex sexual partners in the National Comorbidity Survey, *American Journal of Public Health, 9*(6), 933–939.

Grant, J. M. (2009.) *Outing age 2010: Public policy issues affecting lesbian, gay, bisexual, and transgender elders.* Washington, DC: National Gay and Lesbian Task Force Policy Institute. Retrieved November 30, 2010, from http://www.thetaskforce.org/downloads/reports/reports/outingage_final.pdf

Haldeman, D. C. (1994). The practice and ethics of sexual orientation conversion therapy. *Journal of Consulting and Clinical Psychology, 62*(2), 221–227.

Harrison, A. E., & Silenzio, V. M. B. (1996). Comprehensive care of lesbian and gay patients and families. *Primary Care: Models of Ambulatory Care, 23*(1), 31–46.

Hatzenbuehler, M. L., McLaughlin, K. A., Keyes, K. M., & Hasin, D. S. (2010). The impact of institutional discrimination on psychiatric disorders in lesbian, gay, and bisexual populations: A prospective study. *American Journal of Public Health, 100*(3), 452–459.

Haynes, A. (1995). Cancer among special populations: Women, ethnic minorities, and the poor. *Environmental Health Perspectives, 103*(8), 319–320.

Human Rights Campaign. (2010). Transgender population and number of transgender employees. Retrieved November 30, 2010, from http://www.hrc.org/issues/9598.htm#_ednref6

Hughes, T. L., & Wilsnack, S. C. (1997). Use of alcohol among lesbians: Research and clinical implications. *American Journal of Orthopsychiatry, 67*(1), 20–36.

Klitzman, R. L., & Greenberg, J. D. (2002). Patterns of communication between gay and lesbian patients and their health care providers. *Journal of Homosexuality, 42*(4), 65–75.

Leslie, D. R., Perina, B. A., & Maqueda, M. C. (2001). Clinical issues with transgender individuals. In *A provider's introduction to substance abuse treatment for lesbian, gay, bisexual, and transgender individuals* (pp. 91–97). Rockville, MD: U.S. Department of Heath and Human Services, Center for Substance Abuse Treatment. DHHS Publication No. (SMA) 01-3498. Retrieved November 28, 2010, from http://www.nalgap.org/PDF/Resources/ProvidersGuide-SAMSHA.pdf

Linsk, N. L. (1997). Experience of old gay and bisexual men living with HIV/AIDS. *Journal of Gay, Lesbian, & Bisexual Identity, 2,* 285–308.

Lombardi, E. L., Wilchins, R. A., Priesing, D., & Malouf, D. (2001). Gender violence: Transgender experiences with violence and discrimination. *Journal of Homosexuality, 42*(1), 89–101.

Midence, K., & Hargreaves, I. (1997). Psychosocial adjustment in male to female transsexuals: A review of the research evidence. *Journal of Psychology, 131*(6), 602–614.

Millman, M. (1993). *Access to health care in America.* Washington, DC: National Academy Press.

National Coalition on Anti-violence Programs. (2009). *Lesbian, gay, bisexual, transgender and queer domestic violence in the United States in 2008.* Retrieved on April 1, 2010 from www.avp.org

O'Hanlan, K., Cajab, R. B., Schatz, B., Lock, J., & Nemrow, P. (1997). A review of the medical consequences of homophobia with suggestions for resolution. *Journal of the Gay and Lesbian Medical Association, 1*(1), 25–40.

Peterkin, A., & Risdon, C. (2003). *Caring for lesbian and gay people: A clinical guide.* Toronto: University of Toronto.

Prairielands Addiction Technology Transfer Center. (n.d.) *A provider's introduction to substance abuse treatment for lesbian, gay, bisexual, and transgender individuals.* University of Iowa. Based on U.S. Department of Health & Human Services Publication No. (SMA) 01-3498. Retrieved November 28, 2010, from http://www.nalgap.org/PDF/Resources/TrainerGuide1stEd.pdf

Quam, J. K. (Ed.). (1997). *Social services for senior gay men and lesbians.* Binghamton, NY: Harrington Park Press.

Rosario, M., Schrimshaw, E.W., & Hunter, J. (2004). Ethnic/racial differences in the coming-out process of lesbian, gay, and bisexual youths: A comparison of sexual identity development over time. *Cultural Diversity and Ethnic Minority Psychology, 10,* 215–228.

Rosenfeld, D. (1999). Identity work among lesbian and gay elderly. *Journal of Aging Studies, 13*(2), 121–145.

Schatz, B. & O'Hanlan, K. (1994). *Anti-gay discrimination in medicine: Results of a national survey of lesbian, gay and bisexual physicians.* San Francisco, CA: American Association of Physicians for Human Rights.

Simkin, R. (1998). Not all patients are straight. *Journal of the American Medical Association, 159*(54), 370–375.

Solarz, A. L. (Ed.). (1999). *Lesbian health: Current assessment and directions for the future* (pp. 70–105). Washington, DC: National Academy Press, Institute of Medicine.

Tang, H., Greenwood, G. L., Cowling, D. W., Lloyd, J. C., Roeseler, A. G., & Bal, D. G. (2004). Cigarette smoking among lesbians, gays, and bisexuals: How serious a problem? (United States). *Cancer Causes and Control, 15*(8), 797–803.

Toronto Long-Term Care Homes & Services. (2008). *Diversity our Strength: LGBT Tool Kit.* Retrieved December 1, 2010, from http://www.toronto.ca/ltc/pdf/lgbt_toolkit_2008.pdf

Ulstad, V. K. (1999). Coronary health issues for lesbians. *Journal of the Gay and Lesbian Medical Association, 3*(2), 59–67.

U.S. Department of Health and Human Services, Substance Abuse and Mental Health Services Administration. (2001). *A provider's introduction to substance abuse treatment for lesbian, gay, bisexual, and transgender individuals.* DHHS Publication No. (SMA) 01-3498. Retrieved November 28, 2010, from http://www.nalgap.org/PDF/Resources/Providers Guide-SAMSHA.pdf

Valentine, D. (1998). *Gender identity project: Report on intake statistics, 1989 – April 1997.* New York, NY: Lesbian and Gay Community Services Center.

Woody, G. E., Donnell, D., Seage, G.R., Metzger, D., Marmor, M., Koblin, B. A., . . . Judson, F. N. (1999). Non-injection substance use correlates with risky sex among men having sex with men: Data from HIVNET. *Drug and Alcohol Dependence, 53*(3), 197–205.

Wright, E., Shelton, C., Browning, M., Orduna, J. M. G., & Wong, F. Y. (2001). Cultural issues in working with LGBT individuals. In *A provider's introduction to substance abuse treatment for lesbian, gay, bisexual, and transgender individuals* (pp. 91–97). Rockville, MD: U.S. Department of Heath and Human Services, Center for Substance Abuse Treatment. DHHS Publication No. (SMA) 01-3498. Retrieved November 28, 2010, from http://www.nalgap.org/PDF/Resources/ProvidersGuide-SAMSHA.pdf

Xavier, J. M. (2000). *The Washington, D.C. transgender needs assessment survey: Final report for phase two.* Washington, DC: Administration for HIV/AIDS of the District of Columbia Government. Retrieved November 18, 2010, from http://www.gender.org/resources/dge/gea01011.pdf

Unit IV

Optimizing Mental Well-Being and Spiritual Fulfillment

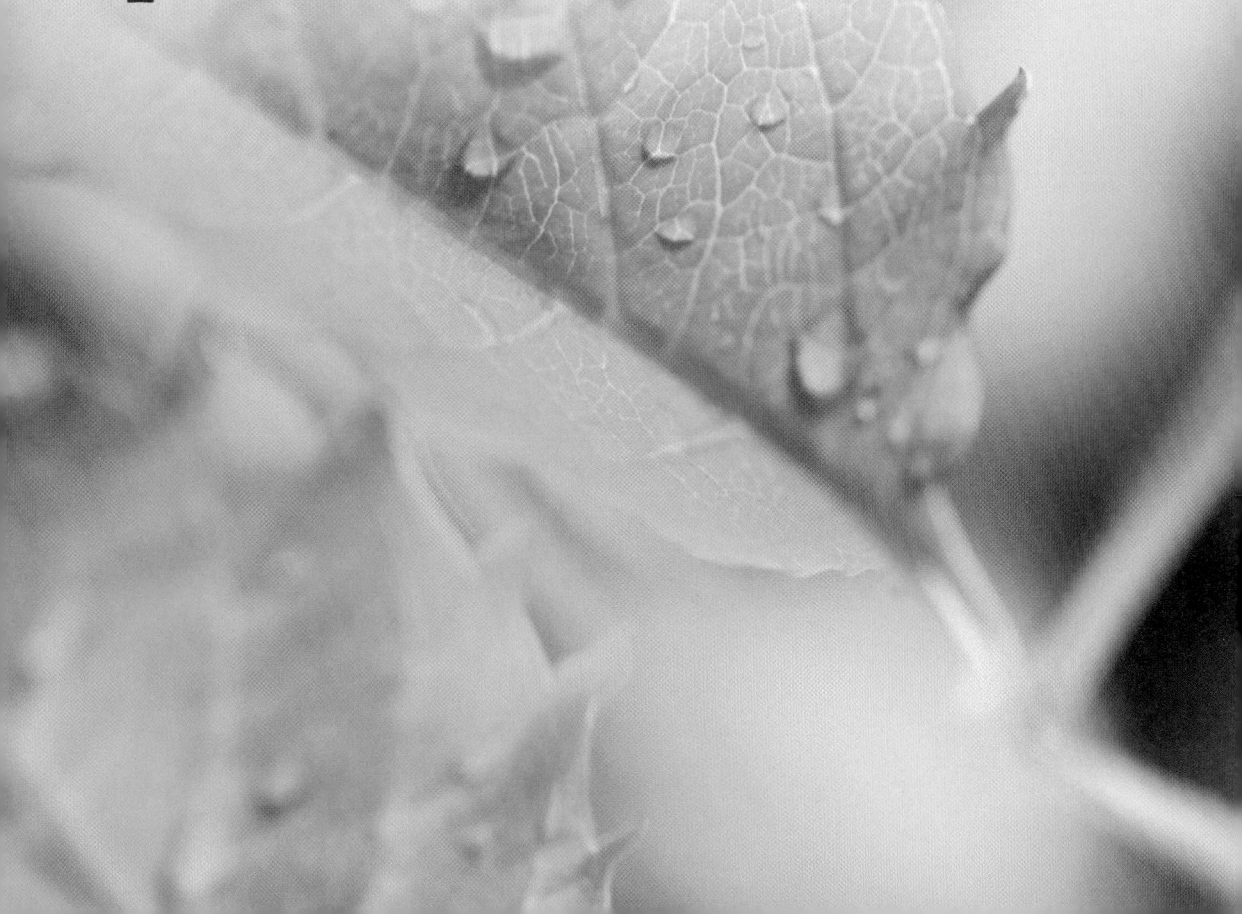

Chapter 22

Challenges to Mental Wellness

Roni Lang, LCSW

LEARNING OBJECTIVES

- Outline influences on mental health and emotional wellness in older adults.
- Describe the unique psychosocial challenges of later life, including grief and loss.
- Identify the most common mental disorders in older adults.
- Describe the similarities and differences in depression, delirium, and dementia.
- Develop strategies to diagnose and treat common mental health disorders in older adults.
- List specific assessment tools for mental health in older adults.
- Provide patient education about mental health issues to older adults.
- Describe mental health challenges specific to veterans of the armed forces.

Keeping Emotionally Fit

Emotional Wellness Late in Life

Pessimism about being healthy, happy, and emotionally sound in one's later years is widespread. It is assumed that depression, disease, unhappiness, and dementia are synonymous with aging. However, current research dispels this faulty notion (Singh & Misra, 2009). Mental wellness in late life is not an oxymoron. This is not to say that older age has no real hardships or challenges, but rather that these do not automatically lead to mental illness. Health care professionals, older adults themselves, and their families need to recognize it is both possible and likely to reach one's eighth or ninth decade and be happy and emotionally fit.

With the increasing longevity over the past two decades and the aging of 77 million Baby Boomers, there has been increased interest and focus on healthy and successful aging both in scholarly literature and in books written for a wider audience (Hill, 2006, 2008; Valliant, 2002; Weil, 2005). The goal of adding life to one's years instead of just adding years to one's life is a common theme in the literature on well-being in late life. Older adults wish for a good mental and emotional life as much as they wish for a good physical life, as has been outlined in other chapters.

PERSONAL PERSPECTIVE
Staying Connected

Beverly, an 83-year-old widow, feels strongly about the importance of staying connected. "I try to be involved with people as much as I can," she explains. "I find that that's a very helpful thing at this point in life, as our friends pass on or move to another state. Isolation is the worst thing people can do to themselves. I try to stay connected with people by telephoning. For example, I have some nieces and nephews that I wasn't in touch with very frequently, but in the last couple of years I call them periodically, and they call me, which is very nice. It's just a matter of feeling that you're part of the ongoing world."

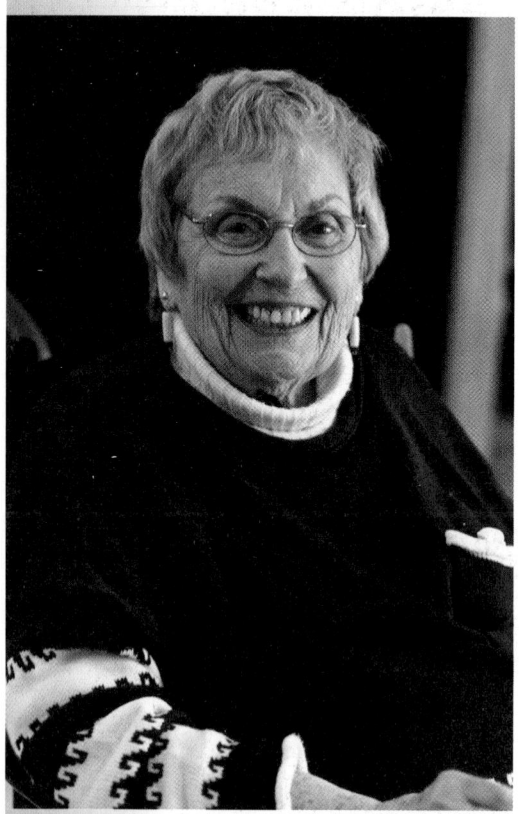

Beverly also stays connected through reaching out to her community. "I volunteered for several groups in my synagogue. I just said yes to everything for awhile. Eventually I found that some groups were not appropriate for me, but I am still involved with several groups that I find very positive and enriching. One is involved in reaching out to other people in the community. It's called the Caring Committee, and I find being involved in it very positive."

A few years ago, Beverly became reinvolved in an organization with which she has had a long affiliation. "The meetings," she says, "present a situation where there is a lot of interaction between people of all backgrounds and all ages. It reminds me that I have a lot to offer and that other people have a lot to offer, and I can learn from the older people and from the younger people, and that your age doesn't have to stop you from going on. I've made special friends both at synagogue and in this other organization, and it's been very enriching. It helps me feel alive and part of this world, and I don't feel isolated and alone, which is what I felt initially."

About Beverly Beverly Hochman was married to her beloved Eli for 54 years. They raised two children together, and today she has one grandson and is in close touch with the entire family. Beverly and Eli grew as a couple through their participation in Marriage Encounter. Beverly has long been active in an organization that offers help and support to families affected by alcoholism. She was on the Board of Jewish Alcoholics, Chemically Dependent Persons, and Significant Others, a program of the Jewish Board of Family and Children's Services. She is also active in, and has served on the Board of, the Gold Card Club, a community group that provides activities for seniors who still reside and pay taxes in the school district. Today, she is active in her synagogue's Caring Committee and Social Action Committee, and she participates in other community work as well.

Lorri B. Danzig, MS, CSL

Health care professionals need to focus as much on mental wellness and psychological resilience in aging as on prevention of physical disease and the physical elements of successful aging. If we can understand what makes for a comfortable and satisfying late life, we can help others with emotional challenges learn resilience and improve coping skills, as well as be encouraged to actively treat mental illness. Learning about those who survive the vicissitudes of a long life and continue to feel "happy and well rather than sad and sick" (Valliant, 2002) can be instrumental both to professionals who work with older adults and to the general public.

The good news about aging and mental health, according to recent research, is that older people commonly are happier than younger people (Kisley, Wood, & Burrows, 2007). It is surprising but true that older adults are among the most stable and mentally healthy of all the age groups and, despite discomforting ailments, personal loss through the deaths of loved ones and friends, retirement, changes in living situations, and limited finances, most older adults experience a remarkably high level of subjective well-being (Carstensen, 2009) and meet life with confidence and good humor. This has been called the *paradox of well-being* (Herschbach, 2002). Even with the phase-of-life challenges people experience in old age, older adults generally feel good about themselves and their situations and show no decline in happiness ratings across the older adult years (Whitbourne, 2008). Older adults can apply their lifetime experience in dealing with problems to the difficulties that come up in later life. In addition, the good news is that even troubled childhoods and setbacks in earlier adult life do not necessarily lead to emotional troubles in later life. The paradox of life is that the past may predict but never determines old age, meaning that "life can be disturbingly wonderful" (Vaillant, 2002).

Psychologic Late Life Development

We spend one-quarter of our lives growing up and three-quarters growing old, according to Bromley (1966), yet much of the psychologic literature on human development focuses on the first 20 years of life. Erik Erickson was one of the first developmental psychologists to extend the study of adult development into adulthood and old age (Erikson, 1963). He proposed eight stages from birth to death. The first six stages focus on development up to early adulthood. He addresses issues of adulthood and maturity in his last two stages, which, given the life expectancy of Americans today, can encompass as many as 50 years of a person's life. Erikson believed that each stage of life brings a psychosocial crisis with a set of two possible resolutions, one adaptive and one maladaptive. Outcomes in one stage influence the next stage but do not completely determine outcomes in the next; deficits can be overcome at crucial turning points in life. Erikson's theory allows us to view adult development as building on the successes of earlier challenges, so that trust, autonomy, initiative, industry, identity, and intimacy are the positive resolutions of the developmental stages from infancy to adulthood.

In middle adulthood (ages 35 to 55 or 65), the ego development challenge is generativity versus stagnation. Generativity means being occupied with meaningful work and issues surrounding family life. The significant task is to have concern over the young and toward making the world a better place. If this stage is not navigated successfully, the individual can become stagnant and self-absorbed. The final life crisis described by Erikson is integrity versus despair, which entails facing the ending of life, accepting one's successes and failures, and viewing one's life with satisfaction and contentment. The ego quality that emerges from a positive resolution is wisdom, which Erikson (1982) defines as a kind of "informed and detached concern with life itself in the face of death itself" (p. 61). The negative resolution of this stage of life leads to a sense of despair, manifesting itself in depression, fear of death, and a sense that life is too short.

Today, most psychologists accept the idea that human development is a lifelong process in which each period of life influences what occurred before and will influence what is to come. One model that looks at how older adults cope when taxed by the challenges of later life is known as the Selective Optimization with Compensation theory (Baltes & Baltes, 1993). It focuses on successful aging and adaptation. According to this model, successful aging calls for making the most of strengths and compensating for losses. People need to *select* activities that meet their functional, cognitive, and emotional capabilities. This may include a restriction of the variety of activities but not a withdrawal from pursuits. People also need to *optimize* their strengths and abilities as well as available resources while engaging in life pursuits. *Compensation* means that people adapt to their functional or cognitive losses. This may include the use of adaptive devices (glasses, hearing aids, walkers, canes, wheelchairs) and cognitive strategies to maximize their abilities.

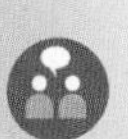

PERSONAL PERSPECTIVE

A Merry Heart Is Good Medicine

"I want to share with you how I managed to arrive at my 102nd birthday with my health and marbles intact," says Izzy Warshaw, "and how I guarded and cared for this marvelous body and kept it in repair for so many years. To some, the golden years are peaceful retirement years or a time of pain and uncertainty. For me, I have so much 'work' to do that I can't catch up. I read books, magazines, and newspapers. I write a column for our residence newsletter and articles for newspapers. I write e-mails to an increasing list of far-away friends. I do chores outdoors for myself and others, preparing food for my breakfast and lunch, and filing and classifying news clippings for history. These activities require time, and the time flies without boredom. Doctors tell us that more energy is consumed in boredom, restlessness, and unhappiness than can be consumed on the most taxing job."

"Back in the mid 30s, when I had some disastrous business difficulty, I suffered from boils. The doctor to whom I went to have them lanced told me, 'You don't get boils and ulcers from what you eat. You get them from what's eating you.' That started me on the job of controlling my attitude in crises. About being happy, Abraham Lincoln once said, 'You can be as happy as you make up your mind to be.' And so I made up my mind to be happy."

"I like to smile and laugh. I like to listen to and tell jokes. I have a file of jokes and humorous stories that I've saved for years. My personal library has a three-foot shelf of humor by many humorists and comedians—all of which I have read and enjoyed. A person does not find life monotonous that is filled with humor. You have to get the happiness habit."

"I could go on with many more examples of how to live happier and longer. Instead, I'll offer a quotation from the Book of Proverbs: *A merry heart is a good medicine.*"

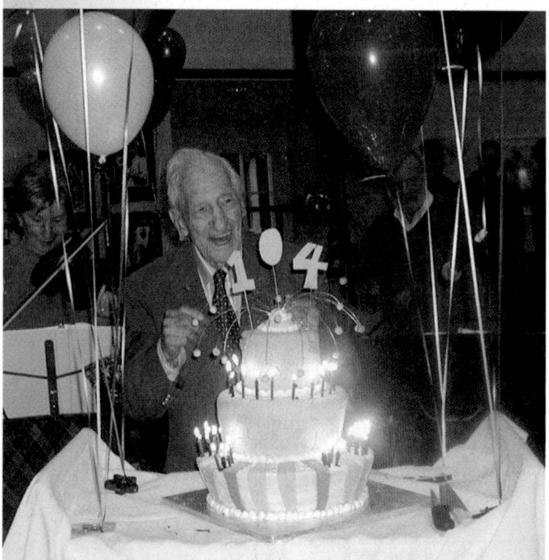

About Izzy Isidore Warshaw lived until a few months shy of his 106th birthday. He spent the last 8 years of his life living at a senior living facility and was a source of inspiration to his family, friends, fellow residents, and residence staff. Izzy worked out three times weekly and taught physical fitness and exercise classes at his residence. He was physically active and intellectually engaged, regularly attending his college reunions. He learned to use a computer at age 95 and kept up communication with his family and friends using e-mail, phone calls, and visits. Izzy attributed his longevity to his busy schedule. He wrote in one of his newsletter articles, "Some people think that creativeness and pleasures thin down and fade away with advancing age. There is a common assumption that 'aging' means that all activities cease. Not so! De-accelerate? Yes! But Cease? ... No!"

The field of psychology has had a long history of focusing on the negative, and little to say about goodness, happiness, and contentment (Seligman & Csikszentmihalyi, 2000). By paying more attention to those who demonstrate healthy aging and psychologic resilience, we are better prepared to help older adults manage personal shortcomings, cope with loss or illness, and achieve personal potentials. Aging happily and well is under at least some personal control and can lead to good physical and mental health even in late life (Vaillant, 2002). There are real challenges such as physical ailments, limited finances, and personal losses, but most older Americans are remarkably tough and meet life with confidence and good humor.

In his book *Aging Well,* author George Vaillant (2002) suggests that making the right choices before age 50 can increase the likelihood of good physical and mental health into the 70s, 80s, and beyond (Box 22-1). He stresses the importance of a good marriage and healing relationships, humor, optimism, the ability to love and be loved, and the capacity for gratitude and forgiveness. Valliant discusses the importance of adult developmental tasks and mature and adaptive coping styles essential to aging well. Adaptive coping in late life means being able to give to others when capable, receiving gratefully from others when needed, being greedy enough to develop one's own self, and having the ability to turn lemons into lemonade rather than turning molehills into mountains. He concludes that the paradox of life is that the past may predict but never determines old age: "life can be disturbingly wonderful."

BOX 22-1 Predictors of Aging Well

- Not being a smoker or stopping young
- Adaptive coping style and development of mature defenses
- Ability to change with time
- Absence of alcohol abuse
- Stable marriage or intimate relationship by age 50
- Some exercise
- Maintaining a healthy weight
- Years of education, intellectual curiosity, and lifelong learning
- Embracing social connectedness
- Accepting limitations with humor and dignity

Adapted from Vaillant, G. S. (2002). Aging well: Surprising guideposts to a happier life from the landmark Harvard study of adult development. Boston, MA: Little, Brown.

Keeping Cognitively Fit

Memory problems in old age are the subject of endless jokes and substantial worry, especially for those in midlife who are approaching their later years. Because there are so many myths and stereotypes, it is important to separate facts from fears. Impairment in cognitive function, although statistically more common in late life, should not be considered a natural or inevitable consequence of aging. It is important for health care professionals to be able to distinguish "normal" changes in cognition that occur over the life course from diseases and disorders. Longitudinal and cross-sectional studies of normal changes in intellectual functioning across the life span have helped address some of these issues (Belleville et al., 2006; Rowe & Kahn, 1998; Salthouse, 1996, 2010; Schaie & Willis, 2005). Normal age-related change in older adults are summarized in the following:

- Substantial changes in intellectual functioning occur only in late life, usually not before the 80s.
- Some primary mental abilities (verbal ability, spatial orientation, inductive reasoning, numeric ability, verbal memory, and perceptual speed) decline with age, but no particular ability declines for every person.
- Most older adults show a decline in at least one ability by age 60, but no one declines in all abilities.
- Individuals are likely to maintain the abilities central to their life experience (in other words, an accountant is likely to maintain math skills).
- Adult intelligence is multidirectional in that some aspects improve while others decline during adulthood.
- The major age-related change is cognitive slowing.
- Even well-documented changes, such as a slower reaction time in older adults, may not be enough to interfere with everyday life.
- Mental abilities may be modified under certain conditions. In this case, training in memory and reasoning may improve an older adult's performance and enhance feelings of efficacy.
- Older adults often have trouble thinking of the right word to use when speaking, but greater experience in communication provides compensation.
- The capacity for creativity and wisdom can expand in later life, but not all older people are wise.

Preventing Cognitive Decline

According to a Met Life study (Met Life Foundation, 2006), the greatest health fear of older adults is of developing Alzheimer disease. Jokes about a "senior moment" are cause for serious concern among many middle-aged adults (Kleinfield, 2002). This is understandable given the grim portrayal of Alzheimer disease in the media. Many older adults have also witnessed the ravages of this disease in family members or friends. No wonder there is a growing market for dietary supplements, memory rejuvenators, and "brain gyms" promising improved memory and robust cognitive functioning.

Brain gyms offer brain fitness using computer software and training to improve memory function and cognitive skills. Participants in these workshops say the exercises keep their brains sharp, but scientific evidence is unclear (Greene, 2009), and these programs may be preying on the public's fear of Alzheimer disease (Benson 2007; Fernandez, 2008; Hafner, 2008; Quinn 2009).

Is it possible to maintain good cognitive function and prevent dementia? For many or most, yes. Recommendations made by clinicians to maintain physical well-being also contribute to cognitive wellness. They include regular exercise, maintaining a healthy diet, managing stress, getting adequate and restful sleep, and not smoking. In addition, predictors of good mental function in old age include a strong social support system and emotional resilience or the ability to handle change and challenge in life (Rowe & Kahn, 1998). This is similar to Vaillant's findings on emotional wellness. Shaie and Willis (2005) add the importance of engaging in stimulating intellectual activities and a flexible personality by midlife.

Despite age-related declines in memory, speed, and word retrieval, older adults are able to learn and apply new knowledge. Patient education is a valuable part of the nurse's relationship with patients and their families and caregivers, and improved health literacy has been linked to better health outcomes. However, nurses may need to tailor patient education to an older adult's learning style (Box 22-2). Additional basic health and wellness information for older adults can be found at http://NIHSeniorHealth.gov.

Defining Psychologic Well-Being Late in Life

Well-being is based not just on the absence of disease. Characteristics of a good old age (or, as Valliant says, being happy and well) include an active engagement

BOX 22-2 Patient Education and Older Adults

Nurses may need to tailor patient education to an older adults' learning style. Here are some suggestions to enhance communication between patients and family caregivers and health care professionals.

- Use plan language and don't use medical lingo or technical jargon
- Be clear and simple in your explanation
- Allow sufficient time for the older patient to process new information
- Don't defer to younger family members, speak to the older adult directly
- Provide a respectful and supportive environment for learning
- Repeat as needed
- Speak slowly and distinctly (not necessarily louder)
- Face-to-face communication will make the communication more meaningful
- Select written educational materials are well organized and designed
- Utilizing good examples may help patients take specific action
- If possible, use repetition or rehearsal to promote learning

Adapted in part from Centers for Disease Control and Prevention. (2009). Improving health literacy for older adults. Atlanta: U.S. Department of Health and Human Services. Retrieved December 17, 2010, from http://www.cdc.gov/healthmarketing/healthliteracy/reports/olderadults.pdf

in life, good coping skills, positive social relationships, optimism, and a zest for life. Mental wellness includes environmental mastery, self-acceptance, personal growth, and purpose in life (Qualls, 2002), as well as the capacity to thrive rather than just survive (Butler, 1975). Given the challenges and changes experienced by older adults, mental health in later life must also include the ability to make positive adaptations to the limitations of aging (Blazer, 2006) and the ability to regulate emotion and emotional intelligence. The National Institute on Aging Healthy Brain Workshop suggests that emotional health requires both emotional regulation and emotional intelligence (National Institutes of Health, n.d.). Emotional regulation is the ability to influence which emotions a person has and how these emotions are experienced and expressed. Emotional intelligence is the ability to perceive and express emotion, understand emotions expressed by others, and use emotional knowledge to enhance well-being.

In summary, what determines psychologic well-being in late life is a function of multiple factors. It can spring from a lifetime of good functioning, resourcefulness, strong social supports, meaningful engagement in social activities, psychologic hardiness and resilience, and relative physical health. Psychologic health also may be achieved through appropriate identification and successful treatment of psychiatric problems at any point in life.

Surviving Loss

Everyone faces problems, difficulties, and struggles that present challenges to their emotional well-being and quality of life. These can include such phase-of-life issues as choosing a career, choosing a mate, growing a family, and coping with relocation, retirement, and loss of loved ones. Other difficulties may include dealing with disappointments, regrets, failure, and problems in interpersonal relationships.

Although older people struggle with these issues and problems, the most pervasive emotional issue for most older adults is loss. Losses specific to older adults include retirement, failing health, the end of driving, relocation from living independently to living in an assisted facility or long-term care facility, and experiencing multiple deaths, including those of pets, friends, siblings, and spouse. The loss of a spouse after many years of marriage is one of life's most stressful events (Whitbourne, 2008).

Most older adults survive these challenges without developing a mental illness, but sadness and grief can cause much distress. It is important for health care professionals to understand the experience of loss and grief so as to not to underestimate its impact on the emotional life of older adults and to identify those who may need more support than just an acknowledgment of the loss or a sympathy note (Box 22-3).

Grief, Bereavement, and Mourning

Grief is the natural response to losing someone important. Bereavement is the state or condition caused by loss through death. Mourning is the way we express our grief. Mourning practices differ by religion and culture. For example, Catholics commonly have a wake or vigil before burial. In the Jewish tradition, the deceased is buried as soon as possible, usually the day after death, and the immediate family then observes a 7-day mourning period called sitting shiva. Those of many cultures observe a mourning period, wear dark clothes, and say prayers for the dead. Ideally, mourning periods and rituals allow the full expression of grief and provide the support of family and friends.

BOX 22-3 Describing Grief

Listening to the words of the bereaved can enhance our understanding of the experience.

"Nobody ever told me grief felt so much like fear ... there is an invisible blanket between the world and me," wrote C. S. Lewis after the death of his wife to cancer (Lewis, 1961).

"Life changes fast, life changes in the instant." So starts Joan Didion's memoir, *The Year of Magical Thinking,* which documents how Didion coped after her husband died of a sudden heart attack (Didion, 2005).

Jane Brody, journalist at the *New York Times,* recently wrote about the death of her husband after a long illness, describing the experience as "anguish within ... welled like a dam ready to burst ... It is not that I will miss my husband's company ... there are also practical issues that serve as daily reminders of his absence. Who will open the jar that defies my efforts, close a stuck window, hold the ladder while I change a light bulb ... or take the wheel when I'm too sleepy to drive?" (Brody, 2010).

The Experience of Grief

Grieving is a personal experience and may be experienced and expressed in many different ways. People who are grieving may have intense feelings and describe the experience as being "sick with grief." However, although grief is an emotionally painful experience, it is not the same as clinical depression. Solomon (2001) described grief as "depression in proportion to circumstances" and depression as "grief out of proportion to circumstances." Physical symptoms include crying, sighing, disrupted sleep, fatigue, loss of appetite, and physical complaints, such as headaches and other aches and pains. The stress of grieving may weaken the immune system over time, resulting in episodes of illness. For a person with chronic illness, grief may worsen the illness (Bonifas, 2008). Grief may involve a fierce tangle of emotions, such as sorrow, hurt, anger, resentment, numbness, loneliness, bitterness, guilt, confusion, and yearning. Cognitive reactions include denial, disbelief, disorganization, difficulty with decision making, and a sense that the deceased person remains present. All these reactions are normal and expected and do not indicate mental illness.

For most people, grief follows a vague process that moves, eventually, toward something that could be called resolution. Worden (2001) views grief as an active process in which a person must acknowledge the reality of a loss, work through the emotional pain and turmoil, adjust to an environment in which the deceased is missing, loosen ties to the deceased, and reengage in the social network. Rando (1984) describes a three-tier process of loss:

- **Avoidance,** which includes shock, denial, disbelief, confusion, and disorganization, followed by
- **Confrontation,** which is a highly emotional state of intense grief and acutely felt psychologic reactions, followed by
- **Reestablishment,** which includes a gradual decline of grief and the beginning of reentry to one's life.

Grief may begin before a loss, and it may not always progress readily after a loss (Box 22-4). Some people may become stuck in prolonged grief, or grief may evolve into depression. Symptoms of pathologic grief may include intense grief lasting more than 2 years after the death, continued social withdrawal, prolonged feelings of helplessness, exaggerated anger or guilt, low self-esteem, and suicidal ideation. This level of continued grief may require professional psychologic treatment (Hospice Education Institute, n.d.).

Health care professionals can help grieving patients by learning about the phases of grief and

BOX 22-4 Types of Grief

- *Anticipatory grief.* The grief that occurs when there is opportunity to anticipate the death of a loved one. Anticipatory grief is experienced from the perspective of the dying individual and those who care for him or her. The focus of anticipatory grief includes the past that was had, shared, and will never be regained; the present and ongoing experience of loss as capabilities diminish; and the future with thoughts of the actual death. Feelings of loss and loneliness and thoughts about events that will never be shared also (Rando, 1986).
- *Ambiguous loss.* Frequently present in family members caring for patients with Alzheimer disease. Caregivers provide care for a person perceived as physically present but psychologically absent, leaving no possibility of closure. The type and nature of ambiguous losses change with each stage of the disease (Boss, n.d.).
- *Complicated grief.* This is a chronic prolonged grief, excessive in duration, with no satisfactory conclusion. It may involve a delayed grief reaction where emotion is "inhibited, suppressed or postponed." Exaggerated grief occurs when feelings of fear, hopelessness, and depression become so excessive they interfere with daily function of the bereaved.

helping the bereaved understand the process. As a health care professional, you may send a note expressing sympathy, or say, "I'm sorry," when you see a grieving person. Do not respond to a person's grief with platitudes, such as, "It was God's will" or "He's in a better place now." Listen to the person to understand, not to respond. Remember that grief is an individual process. No two people navigate the stages of grief in the same manner. Accept that grieving takes time. Usually, 1 year is required, and 2 years may be required (Cavanaugh & Blanchare-Fields, 2006). Encourage good health maintenance, healthy habits, self-care, nutrition, rest, and exercise. Learn about bereavement support groups in your community so that you can provide a list of resources to grieving patients. Be attentive for evidence of depression, and encourage professional help when needed.

Common Mental Disorders in Later Life

We began this chapter by looking at the relative psychologic strength and resilience of older adults. Indeed, except for dementias, older adults have a lower prevalence of mental health disorders than younger adults (American Psychological Association, 2004). Mental health problems such as depression and anxiety are not a normal part of aging and, when they occur, should be diagnosed and treated.

Despite this picture of relatively good mental health, however, unrecognized and untreated mental disorders among older adults are a growing public health concern. Mental illness rates in older adults range from 15% to 25%, with expected increases expected by 2030 (Administration on Aging, 2001; Jeste et al., 1999). Through population growth alone, by 2030 the number of people over age 65 with mental illness will equal or exceed the number of such people in all other age groups (Bartels & Smyer, 2002). However, only one third of community-dwelling older adults who need mental health services actually receive care (Bartels & Smyer, 2002). Primary care physicians are most likely to identify, diagnose, and treat mental illness in older adults because few older adults make use of specialty mental health services (Kaplan, Adamek, & Calderon, 1999; Klap, Unroe, & Unutzer, 2003). Older adults' underutilization of mental health services is attributed to the following factors:

- Social stigma of mental illness, particularly among older adults
- Ageism among those in the helping professions (Freud himself [1976] considered people over age 50 unable to change and not good candidates for psychoanalysis.)
- A limited understanding of psychotherapy among older adults
- Limited reimbursement by health insurance, particularly Medicare, for mental health services
- Inadequate numbers of trained mental health professionals specializing in geriatric medicine, geriatric psychiatry, nursing, pharmacy, and social work (Institute of Medicine, 2008)
- Lack of culturally sensitive mental health programs (O'Conner, Koeske, & Brown, 2009)
- Failure of primary care providers to identify emotional problems and refer for treatment (Table 22-1)
- Persistence of the YAVIS syndrome (Schofield, 1964), which is a personal bias for patients who are **Y**oung, **A**ttractive, **V**erbal, **I**ntelligent, and **S**uccessful—to which some add another S for those who make a **S**peedy recovery.

Given the transitions and losses associated with aging, it should come as no surprise that older adults are at risk for a wide range of mental health problems, including anxiety disorders, substance abuse, and posttraumatic stress disorder. Some of the most common mental health conditions among older adults are depression, dementia, and delirium. These conditions are not mutually exclusive and may present in similar ways in older adults, which can present a major challenge in diagnosis and treatment (Arnold, 2004). Further, these syndromes are complex and multifaceted in older adults, and they are commonly unrecognized and untreated (Bonifas, 2008), preventing the treatment that could reduce distress and improve quality of life.

Depression

An ever-growing number of high-profile people are revealing and describing their experiences of depression (Box 22-5). However, although progress is being made in removing the stigma of mental illness, many older adults still have negative attitudes about mental health issues. They may be reluctant to seek treatment, or they may stop treatment prematurely. As a group, older African-Americans may have a higher level of internalized stigma than older white adults (O'Conner, Koeske, & Brown, 2009).

Symptoms of depression can include sadness, hopelessness, helplessness, low self-worth, feeling that there is no use, and having a sense that nothing has any meaning. In addition to being an emotionally brutal experience, depression can have dire

TABLE 22-1 Diagnosing Mental Illness

The *Diagnostic and Statistical Manual of Mental Disorders* (*DSM*) contains the official classifications of mental disorders with symptom-based definitions of mental disorders and syndromes that impair functioning and cause personal distress. The manual is organized to provide a biopsychosocial profile of the patient using a five-level system, with each level called an axis, as shown below. The *DSM* is not specific to older adults.

Axis I	■ Clinical disorders, including major mental disorders ■ Developmental and learning disabilities
Axis II	■ Pervasive maladaptive personality patterns or personality disorders ■ Mental retardation
Axis III	■ General medical problems, including acute medical conditions and physical disorders
Axis IV	■ Psychosocial problems ■ Environmental problems
Axis V	■ Global Assessment of Functioning, which is a numeric scale (0 to 100) used by mental health clinicians to rate the social, occupational, and psychologic functioning of adults

Adapted from American Psychiatric Association. (2000). *Diagnostic and statistical manual of mental health disorders* (4th ed., text rev.). Washington, DC: Author.

BOX 22-5 Describing Depression

Winston Churchill called his bouts of major depression his "Black dog," and Abraham Lincoln suffered from such serious depressive episodes that his White House staff used to hide his guns. Sigmund Freud, Nathaniel Hawthorne, the astronaut Edwin ("Buzz") Aldrin, and Robert Young all suffered from depression. We are getting used to hearing celebrities disclose publicly their difficulties with depression. Here are just a few of the celebrities who have spoken freely about their depression: Brooke Shields, Jim Carrey, Lorraine Bracco, Dick Clark, Sting, Elton John, and Art Buchwald. Two more descriptions appear below from writer William Styron and journalist Mike Wallace.

"Depression is a disorder of mood, so mysteriously painful and elusive in the way it becomes known to the self ... as to verge close to being beyond description. It thus remains incomprehensible to those who have not experienced it in its extreme mode, although the gloom, "the blues" which people go through occasionally ... give many individuals a hint of the illness in its catastrophic form" (Styron, 1990, p. 7).

"Depression takes over your life .... It's painful ... you don't eat .... you don't sleep. Your self-esteem drops to zero, and you're trying to hide it, which makes it more difficult" (Wallace, 2006).

consequences. Depression in older adults is a serious illness and carries with it a risk of morbidity and mortality. In fact, older Americans with the most severe depression are nearly twice as likely to die during a given period than nondepressed patients. That puts severe depression on the same mortality risk level as cancer, heart disease, hypertension, and emphysema (Schultz et al., 2000; Unitzer, Patrick, Marmon, Simon, & Katon, 2002). According to Geerlings, Beekman, Deeg, Twisk, and Van Tilburg (2002), the mortality effect of depression is a function of both the length of time the person is depressed and the severity of symptoms. A recent study linked increased mortality in patients with cerebrovascular disease and depression. It is believed that poor outcomes with depression may be related to direct biologic effects of the disease and the neurovegetative symptoms of depression may deter compliance with medical care (Lavretzky et al., 2010).

Depressed older adults are also at a higher risk of suicide. Although they comprise only 12.6% of the U.S. population, people over age 65 accounted for 16% of suicide deaths in 2004. The suicide rate is highest in elderly white men, and 75% of older patients who commit suicide saw their primary care physician within the preceding month (Birrer & Venuri, 2004; National Institute of Mental Health, 2003). Rosenberg, Mielke, Xue, and Carlson (2010) report increasing evidence that a depressive episode late in life may be a prodromal marker for development of dementia. Rosenberg's research suggests that depression doubles the risk of significant cognitive impairment.

Prevalence

Prevalence estimates of major depression vary widely, with lower rates of major depression among community elderly and progressively higher rates in medically ill older adults in home care, acute hospitalization, and institutional settings. Major depression occurs in 1% to 3% of the general elderly population with another 8% to 16% having clinically significant depressive symptoms (Cole & Dedukuri, 2003). The prevalence of depression in primary care setting is 17% to 37% and, of those, 30% have major depression with a recurrence rate of 40% (Birrer & Venuri, 2004). In long-term care settings, depression is found in one third of residents or more (Wagenaar et al., 2003). Despite these astounding statistics, depression in the long-term care setting is often unrecognized and untreated. In a study by Teresi, Abrams, Holmes, Ramirez, and Eimicke (2001), only 37% to 45% of cases eventually diagnosed by a psychiatrist had been recognized by the staff.

Clearly, we may not be capturing the "full range of depressive phenomena that have clinical significance in late life" (Bruce, 2010), possibly in part because epidemiologic studies use criteria for major depression. However, even mild or moderate levels of depression yield poorer physical, mental, and social function, poorer attitudes toward aging, and a reduced sense of personal mastery, self-efficacy, optimism, and resilience (Vahia et al., 2010). Therefore, it is important to identify older adults who have mild or subsyndromal depression because of their increased risk of poor health outcomes.

Identifying Depression and Its Risk Factors

Older adults who have depression may never see a mental health professional. This is why nurses and primary care physicians need to know what to look for and what to say to patients, particularly older patients (Unitzer, Katon, et al., 2002). Family physicians may fail to recognize 30% to 50% of patients with major depressive episodes (Thibault & Steiner, 2004). Especially in older adults, emotional disorders may not be immediately evidenced for a number of reasons, including the brief time generally spend in an office visit, the reluctance of many older adults to identify depression or a mood problem, and the differing symptom picture for older as opposed to younger adults.

The *Diagnostic and Statistical Manual of Mental Disorders* (*DSM*) describes depression as a syndrome of persistent symptoms present for at least 2 weeks and representing a change from previous functioning. The *DSM* gives nine criteria for a diagnosis of depression:

- Depressed mood
- Diminished interest in pleasurable activities
- Weight loss (and loss of appetite) or weight gain
- Sleep disturbance (either sleeping too much or too little)
- Psychomotor agitation or retardation
- Fatigue or lack of energy
- Guilt and feelings of worthlessness
- Loss of concentration and difficulty making decisions
- Recurrent thoughts of death (not just fear of dying) and suicidal ideation

The presence of at least five of these criteria, occurring nearly every day during the 2-week period, indicates a diagnosis of depression (American Psychiatric Association, 2000).

As with other medical problems, depression exists on a continuum. Some patients present with minor depression, which involves the symptoms listed previously but fewer and with less impairment in function. Minor depression is more common in the elderly than major depression and can be precipitated by routine stressors (Birrer & Venuri, 2004).

Risk factors for depression among older adults living in the community include:

- Chronic physical health conditions
- Disability
- A new medical illness
- Sleep disturbance
- A history of depression
- Being female
- Being single or divorced
- Loneliness
- Brain disease
- Alcohol abuse
- Abuse of certain medications
- Stressful life events, such as the death of a loved one
- Poor social supports (Birrer & Venuri, 2004; Cole & Dendukuri, 2003; Singh & Misra, 2009).

Older adults are more likely to have medical comorbidities, making diagnosis and treatment of depression more complex. Certain medical conditions themselves present with depression including certain cancers, heart disease, Parkinson disease, cognitive disorders, and thyroid disorders, to name a few (Blazer, 2003; Lebowitz, 1997). Medications associated with depressed mood include cardiovascular drugs, antiparkinsonians, antipsychotics, anticonvulsants, several anti-infective drugs, and hormones. This is not an exhaustive list (Birrer & Venuri, 2004).

Older adults don't always fit the typical picture of depression and may have fewer symptoms than younger patients, so they may not meet the criteria for major depression despite significant impairment in mood, function, and quality of life. They may deny feeling sad or depressed. The symptom picture for older adults is likely to be one of somatic complaints without underlying medical etiology, or disproportionate complaints of discomfort or concern. Physical symptoms, such as arthritis pain, gastrointestinal complaints, or headaches that have worsened, are often the predominant complaints in the older person with depression. Existing medical issues may confound the diagnostic picture, and the patient may be dismissed as a chronic complainer and the depression not identified in the primary care setting (Billig, 1993).

Clearly, it is important to tease out existing or new-onset medical issues in older adults and appropriately treat them. It is also essential to identify and treat depression. Other symptoms particular to late-life depression are feelings of hopelessness, helplessness, pervasive worry and anxiety, fretfulness, irritability, low motivation, lack of energy, and decreased interest in personal care. Older adults may not express frank suicidal thoughts but instead express a nihilism about life by saying things like, "People live too long," or "I wish I just wouldn't wake up tomorrow."

Given the complexity of late-life depression issues, older adults' reluctance to discuss emotional problems, and the variable presentation, health-care professionals should make use of a variety of screening tools to identify depression. Formal screening can improve identification and outcomes. Two well-established valid and reliable screening tools are the Geriatric Depression Scale–Short Form (Yesavage, Brink, Rose, Lum, Huang, Adey, & Leirer, 1983) and the PHQ 9, which is a nine-item depression scale (Pfizer, 2009). Both tools can be completed by the patient or administered by a nurse or physician. Both are available online (see professional resources). There are a number of easy to use screening tools to assist the physician in identifying depression in the primary care setting.

Another easy-to-use tool is the Whooley Depression Screen (Whooley, Avins, Miranda, & Browner, 1997), in which the clinician asks the patient two questions:

- During the past month have you often been bothered by feeling down, depressed, or hopeless?
- During the past month have you often been bothered by little interest or pleasure in doing things?

Simply asking, "Do you often feel sad or depressed?" is a relatively sensitive way to identify depression. Although it lacks specificity, it does provide a good place to start (Sherman, 2001). A five-item version of the geriatric depression focuses on questions of life satisfaction, feelings of boredom, helplessness, worthlessness, and preferring to stay home rather than going out and doing things (Hoyl et al., 1999). It is important to remember that all these tools are for screening and are not diagnostic. Patients who screen positive may need further evaluation by a mental health professional with expertise in geriatrics.

Treatment

When older adults get treatment for depression, it usually comes from their primary care physician. Older patients at risk for depression are mostly likely to be seen in primary care settings, not in clinical subspecialties such as geriatric psychiatry. Primary care is the logical setting for the identification of mood problems in the elderly (Scogin & Shah, 2006). Indicators for depression (fatigue, functional decline, cognitive issues) are routinely assessed in primary care, and markers for clinically significant depression can be identified. This should support the need for routine screening of depression in primary care, according to Lyness, Yu, Tang, Tu, and Conwell (2009). However, in a study reported in the Journal of the American Geriatric Society, older adults' mental health issues get short shrift with physicians. According to Tai-Seale, McGuire, Colenda, Rosen, and Cook (2007), mental health issues were addressed in only 22% of visits and a typical mental health discussion lasted about 2 minutes. Health care professionals working in primary care need to ask about current symptoms of depression, as well as past depressive symptoms in their older patients.

Clinical depression does not go away on its own, but effective treatment options are available, and older adults can be successfully treated in most cases. Commonly used antidepressants include

- Selective serotonin reuptake inhibitors, including sertraline, fluoxetine, paroxetine, citalopram, and escitalopram
- Serotonin-norepinephrine reuptake inhibitors, including venlafaxine and duloxetine
- Other antidepressants, such as bupropion and mirtazapine

Less common treatments include monoamine oxidase inhibitors, tricyclic antidepressants, and, for refractory or psychotic depression, electroconvulsive therapy.

Psychotherapy, either alone or with drug therapy, is also effective in treating depression. A variety of psychotherapy models are adaptable to older adults. The most effective treatments with older adults are cognitive behavioral therapy, interpersonal therapy, and problem solving therapy. *Cognitive behavioral therapy* focuses on modifying thought patterns and altering emotional states that contribute to the onset and perpetuation of emotional distress. This model has been shown to be effective in treating late life depression (Blazer, 2003; Rowe & Rapaport, 2006; Snowden, Steinman, & Frederick, 2008). *Problem-solving therapy* helps older adults deal with phase-of-life issues such as daily stresses, managing chronic illness, and living on a fixed income. The focus of this treatment is to help the person solve problems effectively through active problem-solving skills such as seeking information and asserting oneself. The goal is to help the older person become better able to deal with the environment and the challenges of life (Alexopoulos, Raue, & Areán, 2003; Areán, Hegel, Vannoy, Fan, & Unuzter, 2008). *Interpersonal therapy* was initially designed as a time-limited treatment for midlife depression. It focuses on grief, role disputes, role transitions, and interpersonal deficits. This form of treatment may be especially meaningful for older patients dealing with bereavement and other losses, role changes, social isolation, and helplessness associated with late-life depression. Interpersonal therapy looks at the person's relationship with other people and identifies patterns that may have triggered depression or may be contributing to it. The therapist works toward increasing the patient's awareness of the link between mood and relationships. This form of therapy is effective alone and with drug therapy with older adults.

Relieving loneliness through volunteer work or group programs can help relieve symptoms of depression (Singh & Misra, 2009). Physical activity and exercise is also helpful, and short-term group-based physical exercise programs can help as well. Self-help guides stress the need to get out in the world, connect with others, participate in enjoyable activities, volunteer, learn a new skill, take care of a pet, exercise, eat a healthy diet, and learn a new skill as ways to combat depression.

Dementia

Dementia is a clinical syndrome characterized by a chronic and progressive loss of intellectual function severe enough to interfere with everyday life (Table 22-2). It presents as a constellation of symptoms caused by diseases of the brain, including Alzheimer's disease, stroke, Parkinson's disease, and others (Gellis, McClive-Reed, & McCracken, 2008; Lichtenberg, Murman, & Mellow, 2003). It involves both memory impairment and disturbance in at least one other area of cognition:

- Aphasia (language disturbance)
- Apraxia (difficulty carrying out motor activities despite intact motor function)
- Agnosia (failure to recognize objects despite intact sensory function)
- Disturbance in executive function (planning, organizing, sequencing, abstracting) (American Psychiatric Association, 2000)

The prevalence of dementia increases with age and affects 37.4% of those age 90 and older (Plassman, 2007). Many of us may someday be in the position of being diagnosed with a dementia. We should begin our study of dementia by thinking about how we would want to be treated. Certainly we want dignity and respect.

Alzheimer's Disease

Alzheimer's disease is the most common cause of dementia and accounts for an estimated 60% to 80% of dementia cases. An estimated 5.3 million Americans have Alzheimer's disease, and this number is expected to rise as the Baby Boom generation ages (Alzheimer's Association, 2010a). Thirteen percent of people age 65 or older currently have Alzheimer's disease. If no cure is found, the number of Americans who develop Alzheimer's disease is likely to grow significantly and only underscores the need for additional research so that prevention and treatment can become a reality.

Twenty years ago, people with dementia were rarely diagnosed at early stages, and the diagnosis of Alzheimer's disease often waited till symptoms were significant enough to clearly impact daily function. Early expertise focused on the design and treatment of special care units, adult day care programs, and educational programs. It has only been in the past 10 years that researchers, clinicians, and people with Alzheimer's themselves have looked more closely at the experience of dementia at its earliest stages and have advocated for earlier diagnosis, increased scientific research into new treatments,

TABLE 22-2 Common Types of Dementia

Alzheimer's disease	Most common type characterized by insidious onset and progressive decline in cognition and frequently accompanied by behavioral and mood difficulties.
Vascular dementia (also known as multi-infarct or post-stroke dementia)	Second leading cause of dementia. Develops more quickly, usually with abrupt onset with step-wise decline. Usually presents with other neurological symptoms. Associated with strokes and transient ischemic attacks. Patient more likely to be aware of cognitive deficits. Depression common. Thirty percent of patients with Alzheimer's disease also have vascular disease.
Frontotemporal lobe dementia	Involves damage to brain cells in frontal lobe. Major symptoms are personality changes, apathy, lack of inhibition, obsessiveness, and loss of judgment.
Parkinson's disease	Disease presents with tremors, shuffling gait, postural instability, and speech problems. Dementia symptoms begin later in the disease process.
Lewy body dementia	Pattern of decline similar to Alzheimer's disease, with the addition of impaired alertness, prominent drowsiness, visual hallucinations, and parkinsonian-like movement symptoms. It should be noted that these patients are particularly sensitive to antipsychotic medication, so this medication should not be used.
Normal pressure hydrocephalus	Caused by buildup of fluid in the brain. Symptoms include mental decline, difficulty walking, and urinary incontinence. Can sometimes be corrected with surgical placement of shunt in the brain to drain excess fluid.
Wernicke-Korsakoff syndrome	The most common cause is alcoholism. Presents with confusion and permanent gaps in memory and new learning. Individuals have a tendency to "confabulate" or make up information they can't remember. May also present with muscle weakness and lack of coordination.

TIA, transient ischemic attack.
Adapted from Lang, R. (2003). *Dementia handout for family caregivers.* Center for Healthy Aging, Greenwich (CT) Hospital.

and more support services at this stage of the disease. Perhaps the first public disclosure of a diagnosis of Alzheimer's disease was by former president Ronald Reagan (1994). In an open letter to the American public, former President Reagan said that, by revealing his own diagnosis, he hoped to promote greater awareness and a clearer understanding of the condition.

Alzheimer's disease and other dementias tap into Americans' deepest fears. A MetLife Foundation Alzheimer's Survey called *What America Thinks* found that Americans fear getting Alzheimer's disease more than heart disease, stroke, or diabetes (Met Life Foundation, 2006). However, nearly 9 of 10 have taken no steps to prepare for this illness. The study also found that more than one third of Americans have a family member or friend who has Alzheimer's disease, and 3 out of 5 are concerned that they may someday have to provide for or care for someone with the mind-robbing disease.

Diagnosis Alzheimer's disease is a progressive, chronic, irreversible, organic brain disorder. It is not a mental illness, but it does cause psychiatric symptoms and much emotional distress for patients, families, and caregivers. The most prominent symptom is gradual and progressive deterioration of memory. Other capacities—such as judgment, higher level organizational skills, verbal abilities, problem solving and abstract thinking—are also affected. Behavioral and personality changes may make caring for the person difficult.

Alzheimer's disease usually starts insidiously with subtle symptoms that may be attributed to normal memory loss. However, it is progressive, with different people progressing at different rates. There may be no visible signs of Alzheimer's early in the disease, and the person may look well. As the disease progresses, however, all aspects of independent function decline, and the person is forced to depend on others. The exact cause of the disease is unknown, and there is no cure, although ongoing research is very active and there are treatments for many common symptoms. Medication and care management strategies are often effective in treating the behavioral problems associated with Alzheimer's disease (Lang, 1999).

There is no test for diagnosing Alzheimer's disease in a living person. Instead, it is diagnosed clinically by its symptom picture and by reports from family members. Although diagnosis cannot be made with 100% certainty, geriatric specialists have become better able to diagnose the disease by understanding its presentation and course, ruling out other causes, and listening to the history of the disease as presented by the patient and the family or significant others. A dementia work-up should include:

- Blood studies to rule out thyroid problems and vitamin B_{12} deficiency
- Cranial imaging consisting of either a magnetic resonance imaging (MRI) or computed tomography (CT) scan of the brain
- Other tests as directed by history and physical exam
- Good history and input from family
- Mental status testing

Things to rule out before a diagnosis of Alzheimer's disease include drug interactions; emotional problems (such as depression, severe anxiety, or psychosis); metabolic and endocrine problems; sensory loss (hearing and visual); poor nutritional status; brain tumors; infections; alcohol or other substance abuse; and vascular issues (such as stroke or transient ischemic attack).

Signs and Symptoms Signs and symptoms of Alzheimer's disease include:

- Memory loss that disrupts daily life
- Challenges in planning or solving problems
- Difficulty completing familiar tasks at home, at work, or at leisure
- Confusion with time and place
- Trouble understanding visual images and spatial relationships
- New problems with speaking or writing words
- Misplacing things and losing the ability to retrace steps
- Decreased or poor judgment
- Withdrawal from work or social activities
- Changes in mood and personality (Alzheimer's Association, 2010b).

Course of the Disease Although the course of Alzheimer's is variable and patients experience symptoms to different degrees, experts have documented stages of progression on the basis of common patterns. Barry Reisberg, MD, developed a staging scale that helps define the decline of patients with Alzheimer's disease (Alzheimer's Association, 2007). They include the following:

1. **No cognitive impairment.** No memory problems are experienced by the patient, and none are evident to a health professional conducting an interview.
2. **Very mild cognitive decline.** Patients feel they have memory problems, but these problems are not evident to family, friends, or a health professional performing a medical examination.
3. **Mild cognitive decline.** Memory deficits are noticed by family and friends and may be detected by a health professional. Some people may be diagnosed at this stage.
4. **Moderate cognitive decline.** Memory deficits can be clearly detected by a health professional. Patients may have decreased memory of recent events or personal history and a decreased ability to perform mental arithmetic or complex tasks. Emotionally, there may be a flattening of affect and withdrawal from challenging situations. This stage is considered mild or early-stage Alzheimer's disease.
5. **Moderately severe cognitive decline.** Patients have major gaps in memory, including trouble with their address and telephone number. At this point, patients may be disoriented about time and dates and can no longer manage without assistance. They usually know their own name and those of spouse and children. This stage is considered moderate or mid-stage Alzheimer's disease.
6. **Severe cognitive decline.** Patients lose more awareness of recent events and may sometimes forget the name of a spouse or caregiver. Sleep is often disturbed, and personality and emotional changes may occur, which may include delusional behavior, paranoia, anxiety, and repetitive actions. This stage is considered moderately severe or mid-stage Alzheimer's disease.
7. **Very severe cognitive decline.** Patients lose the ability to speak, they may lose basic psychomotor skills, and they need assistance with all activities

of daily living. This stage is considered severe or late-stage Alzheimer's disease.

When speaking with patients, family members, and other caregivers, it may be helpful to describe Alzheimer's disease in three stages, as outlined by Lisa Gwyther (2001):

The **first stage,** or mild Alzheimer's disease, can last 2 to 4 years and is characterized by loss of memory for recent events; difficulty with attention; inability to perform simple tasks; repetitious questions; word-finding problems; emotional changes; lack of spontaneity; loss of initiative and sense of humor; and emotional changes, such as depression, irritability, and frustration with deficits.

The **second stage,** or moderate Alzheimer's disease, is the longest stage and can last 2 to 10 years after diagnosis. At this stage, the family is aware of the disease, and symptoms are more pronounced. Common symptoms and changes include increasing memory loss and confusion; shorter attention span; obvious deficits in memory, retention, and recall; tendency to forget appointments and socially significant events; tendency to forget to initiate or complete normal routines; repetitiousness; tendency to lose items and claim they are stolen; disorientation to time; inappropriate social behaviors; tendency to be suspicious, irritable, fidgety, teary, or silly; increased dependence on significant others; social isolation; problems recognizing close friends and family; problems with reading, writing, and simple math; decreased ability to use language; and psychotic symptoms, such as paranoia, delusions, hallucinations, and behavioral problems. By the end of this stage, most people need full-time supervision.

The **third stage** can last 1 to 3 years. During this stage, families face decisions about placement in a long-term care facility or full-time help in the home because the patient needs total physical care. This is the end stage of Alzheimer's and the disease debilitates the body with the likelihood of infections. In this final stage, patients do not look at themselves in the mirror, have little capacity for self-care, lose the capacity for language, are unable to perform purposeful movements, may become mute and unresponsive, and may have seizures.

Behavioral Disturbance in Dementias

Alzheimer's disease and other dementias affect not only cognition but also behavior and mood, causing much disability, misery, and hardship for patient, family, and other caregivers. The range of difficulties includes a wide spectrum of symptoms including affective (depression, anxiety, agitation, apathy, and mania), psychotic (delusion and hallucinations), sleep-wake cycle disturbances, and behavioral (agitation, aggression, verbal disruption, impulsivity) (Tampi, 2010). These behavioral disturbances in patients with dementia affect up to 95% over the course of the illness (Gellis, McClive-Reed, & McCracken, 2008). The impact of behavioral problems includes significant caregiver distress and burnout, need for nursing home placement, and admission to emergency departments and acute care hospitals and adds to the direct and indirect costs of care (Tampi, 2010). Antidepressants are used for depressed mood and irritability, such as citalopram, fluoxetine, paroxetine, sertraline, and trazodone. Anxiolytics such as lorazepam and oxazepam are used to target anxiety, restlessness, verbal behavior, and resistance (Tampi, 2010).

There are no Food and Drug Administration (FDA)-approved medications for treating agitation in dementia, so when they are used, they are used "off label." When managing acutely agitated behavior, physicians tend to favor newer atypical drugs, such as aripiprazole, olanzapine, quetiapine, and Risperdal (Tampi, 2010). In April 2005, the FDA issued an advisory and black box warning that elderly patients taking atypical antipsychotics for dementia had an increased risk of stroke and death. According to Dorsey, Rabbini, Gallagher, Conti, and Alexander (2010), there has been a decrease in the use of these medications and more emphasis on behavioral and environmental interventions. Behavioral interventions for families, other caregivers, and staff at facilities that care for people with dementia include psychoeducation about the disease process, training staff in the care of these patients with a focus on communication skills, and use of cognitive stimulation to increase goal activities and therapeutic activities.

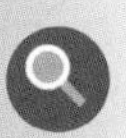

EVIDENCE FOR PRACTICE
Psychotropic Drugs and Dementia

Purpose: To examine the relationship between different types of psychotropic medication and specific cognitive functions in older people with dementia.

Sample: 206 adults over age 70 and diagnosed with mild to moderate dementia were recruited from 28 nursing homes in the Netherlands. Most (180) were women. The average age was 85.

Methods: Neuropsychological tests for memory (direct recall, delayed recall, and delayed recognition) and executive/attentional function were administered to each participant by trained research assistants who were blinded to the study's design. Use of prescribed psychotropic medications (sedatives, antidepressants, and antipsychotics) were extracted from their medical records. Test results were compared between users and nonusers of psychotropic medications.

Results: Psychotropic users were less educated and had more symptoms of depression and anxiety than nonusers. After controlling for these three variables, the results showed that patients taking psychotropic drugs, particularly those who used antipsychotics, had significantly lower performance on neuropsychological tests of executive/attentional functioning than nonusers. There were no significant differences with respect to memory.

Implications: Although there appears to be an association between antipsychotic drug use and impairment in executive/attentional functioning in these older institutionalized adults with dementia, this study did not account for length of psychotropic drug use, and depression was measured using a scale that has not yet been validated in this population. Longitudinal studies are necessary to further clarify this relationship.

Reference: Eggermont, L. H. P., de Vries, K., & Scherder, E. J. A. (2009). Psychotropic medication use and cognition in institutionalized older adults with mild to moderate dementia. *International Psychogeriatrics, 21*(2), 286–294.

Disclosing a Dementia Diagnosis

It is generally assumed that people have the right to be told the truth about their medical conditions, but when it comes to Alzheimer's disease, many health care practitioners are reluctant to disclose the diagnosis because they fear a catastrophic reaction. Recent research does not bear this out, however, and disclosure may indeed offer some relief by providing the person with an explanation of symptoms and treatment options (Carpenter et al., 2008; Sullivan & O'Conor, 2001). Murna Downs, Chair in Dementia Studies and Head of the Bradford Dementia Group at Bradford University, U.K., writes that the reason for disclosure includes a "person's right to know ... and put their personal and financial affairs in order ... and to become involved in planning future care needs" (Downs, 1999; Downs, Clibbens, Rae, Cook, & Woods, 2002). Another reason for disclosure is the importance of maintaining the patient's sense of autonomy (Post, 1995). Clearly, disclosing a diagnosis of dementia should be handled sensitively and individualized to the person's needs and support system. Referral for psychological support may be in order. A diagnosis early on may provide access to clinical trials while the person has the capacity for decision making. There is also a greater range of services available for those at the early stage of Alzheimer's disease, including early-stage support groups and access to psychotherapy. There is even a website designed solely for people with dementia, the Dementia Advocacy and Support Network International, founded in 2000 and available at http://dasninternational.org/. Their mission is to "promote respect and dignity for persons with dementia; provide a forum for the exchange of information; encourage support mechanisms such as local groups, counseling groups, and Internet linkages; advocate for services for people with dementia; and assist people to connect with their local Alzheimer's Association."

There is much information and guidance available on coping with Alzheimer's disease for patients and family caregivers in the form of Internet sites, guides, and books. (See resources for patients and family members.) As a clinician who has worked with those who have Alzheimer's disease and their families, my belief is that something can be done to improve the quality of life for those with this disease. We need to look at and change factors that cause excess disability and think creatively about how we can improve existing resources and design new, more effective treatments, programs, and interventions for those diagnosed, family members who are also affected, and professionals who choose to work with this population.

Impact on the Family

"A chronic illness places a heavy burden on families. It may mean a lot of work or financial sacrifices. It may mean accepting the fact that someone you love will never be the same again. It may mean that responsibilities and relationships within the family will change" (Mace & Rabins, 2006). Alzheimer's disease is not a one-generation disease, and the person with the disease is not the only victim. The disease can take an immense toll on a family's emotional life. Frequently, the burden of care falls on a spouse. It is important to note that caregiving experienced as stressful and burdensome causes psychiatric morbidity and puts the caregiver at higher risk of poor health outcomes. Whether a family can rally to the challenge of Alzheimer's or become overwhelmed by the challenges is complicated. Not all families handle it gracefully. The range of emotions family members express include feelings of sadness, an overwhelming sense of responsibility, resentment, helplessness, despair, hopelessness, tension, stress, denial, frustration, anger, guilt, fear, and embarrassment. The family's sense of unity and ability to solve problems and come together is often sorely tested when faced with a dementing disease (Lang, 2003). Given these facts, health care professionals need to assess the psychosocial and medical condition of caregivers, not just those with dementia.

Delirium

Delirium is a global disorder of attention and cognition common in hospitalized older patients (Rathier & McElhaney, 2005). It is characterized by acute onset, disturbed consciousness, impaired cognition, acute confusion, fluctuating levels of consciousness, and an identifiable underlying medical cause (Box 22-6). Delirium is the most acute condition of the three Ds and is a true medical emergency. Delirium may be underrecognized by physicians and nurses due to its fluctuating nature, overlap with dementia, lack of formal assessment, underrecognition of the deleterious consequences, and failure to realize the diagnostic importance (Inouye, 2006). It is usually reversible but is associated with increased morbidity and mortality, increased hospital costs, and long-term functional and cognitive impairment (Tullman, Mion, Fletcher, & Foreman, 2008).

Many factors can cause delirium, and the syndrome involves the complex interaction of a "vulnerable patient ... and exposure to precipitating factors" (Inouye, 2006; Inouye & Charpentier, 1996). Predisposing risk factors for delirium include age, dementia, impaired functional status, sensory impairment, pain, poor nutritional status, and coexisting medical conditions (Tullman et al., 2008). Precipitating causes include an underlying acute medical condition, head injury, abnormal blood glucose level, adverse reaction to prescribed medication, dehydration, malnutrition, polypharmacy, severe pain, high fever, and abrupt discontinuation of drug and alcohol abuse. Delirium indicators include acute change in mental status, presence of medical illness, visual hallucinations, fluctuating levels of consciousness, acute onset of psychiatric symptoms without history of psychiatric illness, or an acute onset of a new or different psychiatric symptoms with a previous history of psychiatric illness. The common denominator is an abrupt change in mental status over hours to days rather than a slow, insidious onset. In the hospital or long-term care setting, health care providers must become adept at identifying delirium so that the underlying medical cause can be treated and the behavioral symptoms managed (Gleason, 2003). Delirium if treated may resolve in a few hours to a few days or persists for weeks to months (Tullman et al., 2008). Rates of delirium are highest among hospitalized older adults. Delirium affects 10% to 30% of hospitalized patients with medical illness, 25% of hospitalized patients with cancer, more than 50% of postoperative patients, and 70% to 80% in the intensive care unit (ICU). It may be present in up to 60% of nursing home residents older than age 75 at any time. The 1-year mortality rate is 35% to 40%. The prevalence of delirium superimposed on dementia ranges from 22% to 89% in hospitalized and community populations age 65 and older and is likely to be overlooked in that context with behavioral problems attributed to dementia (Bonifas, 2008). It is also common in the emergency department because that is the likely starting point for admission of a confused elderly patient.

BOX 22-6 Criteria for Delirium

- Disturbance of consciousness (reduced clarity of awareness of the environment) with reduced ability to focus, sustain, or shift attention
- A change in cognition (such as memory deficit, disorientation, language disturbance) or the development of a perceptual disturbance that is not better accounted for by a preexisting established or evolving dementia
- Disturbance that develops over a short period of time (usually hours to days) and tends to fluctuate during the course of the day
- Evidence from the history, physical examination, or laboratory findings that the disturbance is caused by direct physiological consequences of a general medical condition

Adapted from American Psychiatric Association. (2000). Diagnostic and statistical manual of mental health disorders (4th ed., text rev.). Washington, DC: Author.

Diagnosis

An acute altered mental status is a frightening experience, and the impact is profound, causing much emotional distress for patients and their families. Patients with delirium are likely to have complicated and extended hospital stays, increased morbidity and mortality, and increased risk for institutionalization and cause greater caregiver burden (Inouye, 2000). Accurate identification initiates appropriate treatment. The Confusion Assessment Method (CAM) (Inouye, 2003; Inouye et al., 1990) was designed to provide a standardized method for quick and accurate identification of delirium for nonpsychiatrically trained clinicians. It has been found to be an easy-to-administer, a valid, and a reliable tool for screening for delirium (Waszynski, 2007). It provides an algorithm to assess four key clinical criteria: acute onset and fluctuating course, inattention, disorganized thinking, and altered level of consciousness. The longer version provides a more comprehensive instrument to screen for clinical features and correlates with *DSM IV* features.

Management of patients with delirium includes assessment and treatment of the underlying cause and ensuring the patient's safety from behavioral symptoms. It is important to get a good history of the problem from a family member or caregiver. Current clinical guidelines focus on detection and management of delirium (American Psychiatric Association, 2000; Inouye et al., 1999). Aside from treating the underlying medical cause of the delirium, both pharmacological options and environmental and behavioral interventions are essential to treat the behavioral manifestations. When patients present with an acute change in mental status, a cognitive assessment and evaluation of delirium should be initiated, and when a delirium is confirmed appropriate treatment guidelines should be followed (American Psychiatric Association, 2000; 2003).

Anxiety

Although occasional anxiety is a normal response to stress, excessive or persistent worry and anxiety may indicate an anxiety disorder. Anxiety disorders include:

- Generalized anxiety disorder
- Obsessive-compulsive disorder
- Panic disorder
- Posttraumatic stress disorder
- Social anxiety disorder (National Institute of Mental Health, 2010)

Older adults are as likely to have anxiety as young adults, particularly in response to a traumatic event, such as falling (Anxiety Disorders Association of America, 2010). Many older adults with persistent anxiety had the same problem when they were younger.

The most common anxiety disorder among older adults may be generalized anxiety disorder, in which the person has persistent, excessive, unrealistic worry about ordinary things (Anxiety Disorders Association of America, 2010). People with this disorder tend to expect the worst, even with no reason.

Like other mental health issues, anxiety may cause different signs and symptoms in older adults than it does in younger adults. Further, symptoms may mimic other health problems. Anxiety may be particularly difficult to diagnose in an older adult with dementia. Older adults with anxiety may have headaches, back pain, or tachycardia. To assess for possible anxiety, consider asking whether the patient knows what prompts the symptoms, whether the person is worrying about a particular thing, and whether the person has trouble letting go of worrisome thoughts. If the symptoms could indicate a different diagnosis, such as chest pain, tachycardia, or insomnia, ask the person what he or she was thinking or doing when the symptom started.

Treatment for anxiety may involve reduced doses of anxiolytic drugs, possible psychotherapy, or both (NIH Senior Health, 2010).

Substance Abuse

Health care professionals should never assume that a person is too old to have a substance abuse problem. Although more professional attention has focused on substance abuse in younger age groups, older adults are not immune to the complex problems associated with this issue. Alcohol use problems are the most prevalent substance abuse issues among older adults, but misuse of psychoactive medication, over-the-counter medication, and the use of illicit drugs also causes problems among older people (Blow, Oslin, & Barry, 2002). Substance abuse problems among older adults are frequently overlooked, undetected, underestimated, and untreated by health care professionals and a growing health problem among those age 60 and older.

Alcohol abuse in the elderly is common and associated with increased morbidity and mortality. The numbers affected are likely to increase along with the older population, necessitating a need for improved identification and treatment. Abuse of alcohol puts older adults at increased risk for injury and falls, sleeping problems, multiple medical problems, stroke, nutritional problems, worsening of memory issues, dementia, and depression. The psychosocial toll includes depression, anxiety, impaired relationships, feelings of shame, and social isolation. Health care professionals need education in the detection of alcohol abuse so that they can increase the incidence of assistance to individuals with alcohol problems. Substance abuse problems in the elderly, if identified, can be effectively treated, reducing medical comorbidity and improving psychological function.

The criteria for substance abuse as defined in the *DSM-IV R* include a "maladaptive pattern of substance use manifested by recurrent and significant adverse consequences related to repeated use of substance ... having occurred repeatedly during a 12-month period." Substance dependence has the added criteria of "tolerance, withdrawal, increased consumption of substances over a longer period of time, the use of substances despite knowledge of its recurrent physical and psychological impact, and consuming larger amounts of the substance over a longer period than was intended, leading to clinically significant impairment or distress" in multiple areas of functioning (American Psychiatric Association, 2000).

Alcohol and Prescription Drugs

Alcohol and prescription drug misuse affects up to 17% of people 60 and older (Blow, 1998). Rates specific to drinking vary across studies; 15% of men and 12% of women over age 60 seen in primary care settings drank more than National Institute on Alcohol and Alcoholism (NIAAA) recommended limits (Adams, Barry, & Fleming, 1996). Higher rates of at-risk drinking have been consistently found across all medical settings—inpatient, primary care, and other health care settings over the general community (Adams, 1993). Substance abuse is projected to increase as the Baby Boomers enter old age. In a study of projected drug use by Baby Boomers, it was reported that by 2020 there will be a substantial increase in the amount of illicit drug use among the elders (Colliver et al., 2006). One study estimates that the number of adults over 50 with substance abuse problems will double from 1999 to 2020 Gfroerer, Penne, Pemberton, & Folsom, 2008). Prevalence rates often underestimate the problem because of a tendency to underestimate drug use among older adults (Blow, Berry, Fuller & Booth, 2008)). Alcohol is the leading substance misused by the elderly followed by misuse of prescription medication (Ross, n.d.). The prevalence of alcohol abuse in the elderly is likely to be underestimated because of underdetection. With the elderly less likely to disclose a history of excessive alcohol use coupled with health care professionals with limited knowledge about abuse, the prevalence is likely to be underestimated.

Drinking guidelines for healthy adults that are age 65 years or older are no more than seven drinks per week or 3 drinks on any given day. Older women are more sensitive than men to the effects of alcohol. A standard drink is defined as 12 ounces of beer, one shot (1.5 ounces) of hard liquor, 5 ounces of wine, or 4 ounces of sherry, liqueur, or aperitif. Older adults need lower limits of alcohol intake because alcohol sensitivity increases with age, less body mass and fat increases circulating alcohol, and less efficient liver metabolism and polypharmacy may increase the effects of alcohol (National Institute on Aging, 2008).

Risk Factors for Alcohol Abuse Older adults can present with a life-long pattern of drinking and have been alcoholic all their life, and now they are elderly. Known as early-onset alcoholism, these individuals are likely to have had a family history of alcohol and more legal and occupational difficulties related to their pattern of excess drinking (Schuckit & Pastor, 1979). Medically, they are more likely to present with alcohol-related medical illnesses such as cirrhosis, organic brain syndrome, and comorbid psychiatric disorders (Liberto & Oslin, 1995). As they age, these individuals may continue heavy drinking patterns that were established earlier in life and may not realize that they are not able to consume the same amount of alcohol as when they were younger without adverse effects (Naegle, 2008).

Late-onset alcohol abuse refers to those who develop problem drinking for the first time in late life. It may arise insidiously with older adults in response to the stressors of late life including loneliness, lack of social supports, losses, relocation, diminished mobility and independence, health problems, chronic pain, and declining economic resources (Bartels & Smyer, 2002). It can be triggered rather abruptly by a stressful life event.

Late-onset drinkers generally have fewer medical problems related to alcohol consumption and are more amenable and compliant, but, on the other hand, their use/abuse of alcohol is more likely to be missed by health care professionals (Liberto & Oslin, 1995). Substance abuse can coexist with a range of psychiatric conditions including depression, anxiety disorders, and cognitive impairment. However, depression, loneliness, and lack of social support were the most frequently identified precipitants to both early-onset and late-onset alcohol abuse (Schonfeld & Dupree, 1991), and alcohol may be used to reduce psychological, emotional, or physical stress (Menninger, 2002). Co-occurring psychiatric conditions represent both a risk factor and a complication of substance abuse in older adults (Bartels & Smyer, 2002). Special considerations with the elderly are important because tolerance to alcohol decreases with age related to decreased body mass, slower alcohol pharmacokinetics, and the use of many medications that can affect alcohol metabolism.

Illicit Drug Use

Little research is available on the extent of illicit substance use in older adults, but it is generally accepted that the current cohort of adults age 65 and older is less likely to use illicit drugs than younger adults are. As reported in a recent National Survey on Drug Use and Health, illicit use of such substances as marijuana, heroin, or cocaine is rare in the elderly with only 1.2% of elderly reporting any illicit drug use (U.S. Department of Health and Human Services, 2009). The report goes on to project that high rates of lifetime drug use among the Baby Boomers suggests that the number of older adults using drugs will increase in the next 20 years. So we may see a different pattern of substance abuse with the incidence of abuse expected to increase rapidly and dramatically (Patterson & Jeste, 1999). Because elders are not exempt from alcohol or other substance abuse problems, health care professionals must develop an increased awareness and provide routine screening to identify at-risk substance abusing older adults. Substance abuse specialists must develop prevention and additional treatment services that meet the needs of older adults (U.S. Department of Health and Human Services, 2009).

Psychoactive Drugs

The inappropriate use of prescribed drugs, especially psychoactive ones, is a more common substance abuse problem with older adults. People age 65 and older consume more prescribed and over-the-counter drugs than any other age group. Older adults represent 12.4% of the U.S. population but receive 25% to 30% of the prescription medication (John A. Hartford Institute for Geriatric Nursing, 2001). The average use for those age 65 and older in the ambulatory setting is two to four prescription drugs and one to four over-the-counter medications (Qato, Alexander, Conti, Johnson, Schumm, & Lindau, 2008). A sizable share of prescriptions for older adults are psychoactive, mood-changing drugs that have the potential for misuse, abuse, or dependency (Blow, 1998). The most likely prescription drugs abused by the elderly are tranquilizers and sleeping pills. These drugs are prescribed for anxiety and insomnia.

Signs and Symptoms Because older adults who abuse alcohol and illicit drugs or who are addicted to medication rarely admit it, clinicians should be aware of medical and behavioral signs and symptoms related to such abuse (Box 22-7).

Barriers to Identification and Treatment

Older adults who need treatment for substance abuse might not get it for varied reasons. Alcohol and other substance abuse problems hide under the

BOX 22-7 Cues to Possible Substance Abuse

Signs and symptoms that may relate to substance abuse in an older adult may include

- Anxiety (possibly from tolerance or withdrawal)
- Memory loss
- Depressed mood
- Agitation
- Disorientation
- Poor hygiene
- Falls
- Poor nutrition
- Changes in blood pressure
- Pain in the upper abdomen
- Fatigue
- Confusion
- Sleep disturbance
- Appetite and weight loss
- Weakness
- Family problems

Adapted from Blow, F. C., Oslin, D. W., & Barry, K. L. (2002). Misuse and abuse of alcohol, illicit drugs, and psychoactive medication among older people. Generations, XXVI(1), 50-54. Retrieved December 17, 2010, from http://www.asaging.org/publications/dbase/GEN/GEN.26_1.Blow.pdf

radar of health professionals. As with other mental health problems, there is stigma around this issue. Older adults rarely self-identify or seek treatment. They may hide their substance abuse problems. They may have a "go it alone" attitude. Living alone, limiting their drinking to evenings, avoiding drinking and driving, and not opening up a conversation about their alcohol intake make detection difficult. If retired, there are no associated work-related problems. Family may not live nearby, so there is no one to notice. Family members, especially adult children, may feel ashamed and not choose to address the problem. Even if adult children suspect a parent is drinking too much, they may believe that "it can't hurt him or her at this age" (Wolin, Bennett, & Jacobs, 2003). Family members may think, "at his/her age there is nothing you can do about it," or " a little nightcap helps him sleep."

Health care professionals may be slow to spot a substance abuse problem due to multiple medical comorbidities that appear more prominent, and clinicians may carry their own ageism and biases about treating older adults with alcohol abuse (Blow, 1998). Additionally, health care professionals may have limited time due to short encounters with patients and be unaware of age-sensitive screening tools. Thus, patient, family, and professional issues can lead to misdiagnosis and lack of appropriate assessment, monitoring, and treatment of substance abuse disorders in the elderly.

Screening and Treating

The Hartford Institute for Geriatric Nursing recommends the use of the Short Michigan Alcoholism Screening Instrument-Geriatric version (SMAST-G) (Naegle, 2007). The goal of screening is to identify an "at-risk" individual drinking at levels linked with negative outcomes for physical and mental health problems.

Another common screen for alcohol abuse is the CAGE questionnaire, which consists of just four questions to ask the patient:

- Have you ever felt you should **C**ut down on your drinking?
- Have people **A**nnoyed you by criticizing your drinking?
- Have you ever felt **G**uilty about your drinking?
- Have you ever needed an **E**ye opener drink first thing in the morning to steady your nerves or to get rid of a hangover?

Madeline Naegle (2008) writes that the goal for clinicians working with patients with excessive drinking is "to explore further interventions that might reduce the harmful effects of alcohol consumption (p. 54)." She goes on to report that *brief intervention* with an "empathic, nonjudgmental health education approach that provides information, offers choices for making change, emphasizes the patient's autonomy and responsibility and communicates the belief that the patient is capable of changing his or her behavior" has been shown to be effective (p. 54). The Hartford Foundation *Try This* Series has many resources for nurses including videos on how to administer the SMAST-G. A brief intervention for nurses put forth by Dyehouse, Howe, and Ball (1996) utilizes the FRAMES model. This acronym stands for:

1. **F**eedback information to patients about current health problems or potential problems associated with their level of consumption.
2. **R**esponsible choice; how to respond to the information provided to the patients is their choice.
3. **A**dvice must be clear about drinking their amounts and recommended moderate levels of drinking.
4. **M**enu of choices is provided by the nurse to the patient/client regarding future drinking behaviors.
5. **E**mpathy is essential to the exchange. Offer information based on scientific evidence, acknowledge the difficulty of change, and avoid confrontation.
6. **S**elf-efficacy of the individual is supported and the nurse helps patient explore options for change.

It is most important to remember that treatment for older adults with substance problems can have positive outcomes. Older adults can benefit from alcohol treatment programs and age-integrated programs. The goal of identifying and treating alcohol and drug problems in older adults is to prevent morbidity (functional, physical, and psychiatric), as well as open the door to improved quality of life and enriched social relationships. Treatments for alcohol and drug abuse in the elderly can be highly effective. Knowing that current elders are not exempt from alcohol or other substance abuse problems and that the projected incidence of abuse is likely to increase, it is imperative for all health care professionals who work with the elderly to be provided with education about substance abuse and learn about appropriate interventions and treatment resources.

Tobacco

According to the Centers for Disease Control and Prevention (CDC) (2010), cigarette smoking is the leading cause of preventable death in the United States, including in older adults. Despite the antismoking messages in the media and reduced advertisements for tobacco, the prevalence of tobacco use in older adults is still significant. The CDC reports that for people over age 65, 9.3% use tobacco. For those ages 45 to 64 the prevalence rate is 22%. Older adults are more likely to have a longer history of tobacco use and to be chronic smokers.

The medical consequences of tobacco use include lung, heart, vascular, and oral problems and an increased risk of cancer. These serious physical illnesses are almost always accompanied by a reduced quality of life that comes with poor health and reduced functional capacity. The Centers for Disease Control and Prevention (2009) reports that 70% of smokers want to quit and 40% of smokers try to quit each year.

The U.S. Public Health Service Clinical Guidelines on treating tobacco use and dependence recommends that tobacco dependence be looked at as a chronic disease, that clinicians consistently identify and document tobacco use, and that clinicians encourage every patient to make a quit attempt utilizing effective counseling interventions and medications (Fiore et al.,). Given the morbidity and mortality associated with smoking and tobacco use and the health benefits of cessation, it is essential that all health care providers incorporate smoking cessation counseling into their practice (D'Ambrosio, 2007) The Agency for Healthcare Research and Quality (2008) has published a guideline for clinicians on helping smokers quit. This brief intervention should be offered to every patient who uses tobacco:

- **Ask.** Systematically ask about tobacco use at every visit.
- **Advise.** In a clear, strong, and personalized manner, urge every tobacco user to quit. The benefits of tobacco cessation should be individualized for each user.
- **Assess.** Ask every smoker if he or she is willing to quit. If unwilling to quit at this time, help motivate the patient by employing a supportive manner and build confidence in the patient's ability to quit.
- **Assist.** Assist the patient in developing a quit plan by setting a date, anticipating challenges, and giving advice on successful quitting; consider use of medications; and provide resources. Patients can call toll-free the national access number to state-based quitline services at 1-800-QUIT-NOW (800-784-8669).
- **Arrange.** Schedule follow-up visits to assess the patient's progress and provide motivational support.

Posttraumatic Stress Disorder

Posttraumatic stress disorder (PTSD) results from exposure to an overwhelmingly stressful event (American Psychiatric Association, 2000). An affected person may have intrusive memories of the traumatic event (such as flashbacks or nightmares), avoidant or numbing behaviors (which may include substance abuse), and hyperarousal (which may lead to episodes of rage). These symptoms may develop immediately after the traumatic event, or they may not appear until years later.

Anyone of any age can get PTSD, including war veterans and survivors of physical and sexual assault, accident, and natural or human-made disasters (Box 22-8). Individuals may experience this disorder soon after the event or after a delay of many years, with repeated trauma, or when other vulnerabilities of aging lower emotional defenses and resiliencies. It is not uncommon that many older people make it through adult life with minimal difficulties despite earlier trauma in life until years later when facing another major stressor. Most of the research on PTSD in older adults has focused on reactions to combat, natural and human-made disasters, and the Holocaust (Falk, Hersen, & Van Hasselt, 1994; Joffe, Brodaty, Luscombe, & Erlich, 2003). There is some research linking the experience of trauma to the development of cognitive disorders in late life (Cook, Cassidey, & Ruzek, 2001; Golier et al., 2002; Mittal, Torres, Abashidze, & Jimerson, 2001). However, not everyone with PTSD has been through a dangerous event. Some people get PTSD after a friend or family member experiences danger or is harmed. The sudden, unexpected death of a loved one can also cause PTSD.

There has been increasing interest in the study of PTSD in aging veterans who functioned well during their adult life and in later life with retirement

BOX 22-8 Mental Health in Aging Veterans

There are currently 23.4 million veterans in the United States, including more than 1.6 million women (U.S. Census Bureau, 2010). A substantial percentage of people age 65 and older are veterans (see Fig. 3-8 in Chapter 3). A veteran is defined as someone who has served in the U.S. Armed Forces but is not currently serving. In general, veterans have better health, less dependence, and a lower death rate than the general population, possibly in part because the military only accepts people who are relatively fit and healthy (Xian, 2006).

Similar to the general population, however, older veterans may have mental health disorders. Indeed, military service—especially combat service—may raise the risk of certain mental health disorders, particularly posttraumatic stress disorder (PTSD), depression, anxiety, substance abuse, and traumatic brain injury. If a judge and panel decide that a veteran's mental health disorder is a service-related disability, the veteran may receive monthly financial aid.

Posttraumatic Stress Disorder

PTSD was originally known as combat fatigue, shell shock, or war neurosis. The lifetime prevalence of PTSD among the general population is about 3.6% for men and 9.7% for women (Gradus, 2007). In contrast, the U.S. government estimates the rate of PTSD among veterans at:

- More than 30% for Vietnam veterans
- About 10% for Gulf War and Afghanistan veterans
- About 20% for Iraq war veterans (National Institutes of Health, 2009)

Veterans of World War II developed PTSD as well, sometimes years after returning home. Delayed-onset PTSD may develop when a veteran receives initial support and appreciation, followed later in life by difficult losses, physical challenges, traumatic situations, or the reemergence of unresolved conflicts about wartime service.

Depression

The National Alliance on Mental Illness estimates that about 14% of veterans are diagnosed with depression, a condition known to be more prevalent than established diagnoses would indicate (National Alliance on Mental Illness, 2009). Diagnosis is significantly less likely if an older veteran also has dementia (U.S. Department of Veterans Affairs, 2008). Among head-injured veterans, the lifetime prevalence of major depression is considerably higher—more like 18.5% (Holsinger et al., 2002). As in the general population, depressed veterans have an increased risk of suicide. The risk appears to be higher among younger and older veterans than among middle-aged veterans (Zivin et al., 2007).

Successful treatment for depression requires more than a prescription or psychotherapy. Indeed, one in three older veterans may not fill an antidepressant prescription, and many older adults stop antidepressant therapy prematurely (U.S. Department of Veterans Affairs, 2008). Veterans commonly respond best to a clinician who is also a veteran and who has been exposed to the trauma of combat. Collaboration among health care providers is critical. The TIDES model (**T**ranslating **I**nitiatives for **D**epression into **E**ffective **S**olutions) provides an example of how collaborations can be implemented (U.S. Department of Veterans Affairs, 2010). A key feature of TIDES is use of a depression care manager to coordinate care between mental health specialists and primary care providers.

Anxiety

Everyone has a certain amount of anxiety from time to time. However, veterans have an increased risk for *acute anxiety,* especially if they experienced combat. The state of acute anxiety is commonly triggered by an event that challenges a person's sense of security. Seeing a fellow soldier severely wounded or killed naturally creates anxiety about one's own mortality, a condition that may resurface as an older veteran develops serious or chronic physical or mental conditions.

Substance Abuse

Younger veterans are more likely than older veterans to have serious psychological distress or issues with substance abuse. However, as a group, veterans of all ages have slightly higher usage of alcohol (including heavy use and driving under the influence), tobacco, marijuana, and other illicit drugs, although they may have lower rates of serious dependence (U.S. Department of Health and Human Services, 2008b).

Issues for Women Veterans

Mental health issues for women veterans include PTSD, depression, and military sexual trauma. These conditions are often hidden or ignored and possibly worsened by the general assumption by civilians that women are not placed directly in harm's way.

Because women soldiers often serve alone in mainly male units, they may feel isolated and unsafe, feelings that may continue when they return home. Rarely do these women reach out to veterans services because many do not believe that the Veterans Administration and other veterans organizations recognize women's unique needs (Cave, 2009). In recent years, services specific to women have become more readily available.

Mental Health Resources for Veterans

- Center for Women Veterans (http://www1.va.gov/womenvet/) is a program of Veterans Affairs specific to the needs of women.
- My HealtheVet (http://www.myhealth.va.gov/) allows the veteran to create a personal health record and provides links to screening tools for depression, PTSD, substance abuse, and suicide; wellness reminders, VA benefits, and prescription refills.
- Substance Abuse and Mental Services Administration (http://www.samhsa.gov/) is part of a collaborative effort to address the epidemic of suicide among veterans. Veterans who are having thoughts of self-harm can call 1-800-273-TALK.

Continued

BOX 22-8 Mental Health in Aging Veterans—cont'd

- The Veterans Affairs mental health website (http://www.mentalhealth.va.gov) helps veterans and their families better understand mental health issues among veterans and provides information about prevention and treatment strategies.
- Telehealth (http://www.carecoordination.va.gov/telehealth/) is a service through which veterans can receive care for medical and/or mental conditions over the phone. It is particularly useful for aging veterans who may not be easily able to receive care outside their homes. Unlike traditional telemedicine, which focuses on curative services, Telehealth addresses preventive, promotive, and curative services in a coordinated manner.
- The Vet to Vet Program (http://www.vettovetusa.com/) is a national veteran support program established in 2002 by Moe Armstrong, a Vietnam veteran with mental health illness (Armstrong, 2010). Vet to Vet is a group of veterans who help other veterans overcome mental illness and substance abuse in a format similar to that of Alcoholics Anonymous.
- The National Alliance on Mental Illness (http://www.nami.org/) is a grassroots mental health advocacy organization helping to educate Americans about mental illness. The organization has a Veterans Resource Center specific to the needs of veterans, active-duty troops, and their families.
- The National Center for Health Promotion and Disease Prevention (http://www.prevention.va.gov/) is a program of the Veterans Health Administration whose goals include providing, evaluating, and improving preventive health care services for veterans.

Doris Troth Lippman, APRN, EdD, FAAN

may reflect back on their wartime experience and experience stress-related symptoms. The take-home message for nurses is get to know something about the personal history of your patients even before a crisis hits.

Summary and Conclusions

I believe that the stories of living a long life are inherently interesting and that we can learn so much from our patients. Health care professions need insight into the complex nature of aging. We all have heard the expression, "Don't judge a person until you have walked a mile in their shoes." As health care professionals working with the elderly, we can't possibly have experienced what they have, but we can develop understanding of their challenges and empathy for their experiences and struggles. We do this by developing good communication skills and good listening skills and incorporating psychosocial context in our assessment and treatment. An easy-to-use algorithm for providing a therapeutic interventions in the context of an office visit is the BATHE technique. It uses the acronym BATHE, which is a five-step process to enhance communication about psychosocial issues. It consists of four questions followed by an empathic response (Lieberman & Stuart, 1999):

- **Background.** What is going on in your life? How is everything else going?
- **Affect.** How do you feel about this? What are you feeling right now?
- **Troubling.** What about this issue troubles you most?
- **Handling.** How are you handling this? What are your options? How do you think I can help you?
- **Empathy.** This must be very difficult for you. I can understand how that would make you feel.

It is important to remember that any algorithm is a simplification and that the BATHE tool is not diagnostic of mental illness, but it can start a conversation to address personal and emotional issues. Health care for older adults requires a broad perspective with equal weight given to the psychosocial aspects as to the medical issues that may present. Nurses and other health care professionals must be aware of the risks and challenges that compromise not only physical health but mental health as well. Social and psychological aspects of aging impact physical well-being and physical problems and disabilities can impair psychological functioning.

KEY POINTS

- Mental wellness and psychological resilience in aging is as important to successful aging as the prevention of physical disease.
- Older adults are among the most stable and mentally healthy of all age groups and typically report a high level of well-being.
- Erikson defined life in terms of developmental tasks to be mastered: generativity versus stagnation

in middle adulthood and integrity versus despair in later years.

- The Selective Optimization with Compensation theory focuses on optimizing one's strengths.
- Helping adults focus on healthy behaviors in earlier years increases the likelihood of good physical and mental health in later years.
- Impairment in cognitive function, although statistically more common in late life, should not be considered a natural or inevitable consequence of aging.
- Regular exercise, a healthy diet, managing stress, adequate sleep, not smoking, a strong support system, and emotional resilience promote cognitive functioning.
- Psychological well-being in late life is a function of multiple factors: resourcefulness, strong social supports, meaningful engagement in social activities, psychological hardiness and resilience, and relative physical health.
- Older adults face challenges such as retirement, declining health and independence, and loss of pets friends, siblings, and spouses. It is important for health care professionals to understand the experience of loss and grief and its impact on the emotional health of older adults.
- Normal grieving may be experienced and expressed through many different emotions, physical ailments, and disrupted routines.
- Prolonged grief, withdrawal, feelings of helplessness, exaggerated anger or guilt, low self-esteem, or suicidal ideation require psychological referral.
- Depression and anxiety, although not a normal part of aging, are underrecognized and treated among older adults, especially those in residential care settings.
- Depression doubles the risk of significant cognitive impairment and places older adults at higher risk of suicide: Elderly white men have the highest suicide rate.
- Health care providers need to be aware of symptoms of depression and use screening tools to identify and refer those at risk.
- Clinical depression requires treatment with medication and/or therapy by a trained mental health professional.
- Dementia, caused by diseases of the brain, is characterized by a chronic and progressive loss of intellectual function severe enough to interfere with everyday life.
- Alzheimer's disease is the most common cause of dementia, and Americans fear its diagnosis more than heart disease, stroke, or diabetes.
- Alzheimer's disease is a progressive, chronic, irreversible, organic brain disorder affecting memory, judgment, verbal and organizational skills, problem-solving ability, behavior, and emotions.
- Medication and care management strategies are often effective in treating the behavioral problems associated with Alzheimer's disease.
- Drug interactions, mental health issues, metabolic problems, sensory losses, poor nutrition, brain tumors, infections, substance abuse, or vascular issues may produce similar symptoms.
- The Alzheimer's Association defines disease progression in stages that can be helpful when speaking with patients, family members, and other caregivers.
- Because behavioral disturbances and total dependency are typical in the later stages, caregivers of these patients require education, support group referrals, and respite care to prevent distress and burnout. Support groups or psychotherapy may also be helpful for patients in the early stage of Alzheimer's disease.
- Delirium is common in hospitalized older patients and is characterized by an abrupt change in mental status.
- Risk factors for delirium include age, dementia, impaired functional status, sensory impairment, pain, poor nutritional status, and coexisting medical conditions.
- Delirium superimposed on dementia may be overlooked when behavioral problems are attributed to dementia.
- The Confusion Assessment Method is a standardized method for quick and accurate identification of delirium for nonpsychiatrically trained clinicians.
- Management of patients with delirium includes assessment and treatment of the underlying cause and ensuring the patient's safety from behavioral symptoms.
- Generalized anxiety disorder is the most common type of anxiety among older adults, characterized by persistent, excessive, unrealistic worry about ordinary things.
- Symptoms of anxiety may differ in older adults than in younger adults and be difficult to diagnose in patients with dementia and because symptoms may mimic other health problems.

- Substance abuse among older adults is often overlooked. Although alcohol is the most prevalent substance abused by older adults, misuse of psychoactive or over-the-counter medications or illicit drugs may also be a concern.
- Alcohol abuse increases the risk for injury, sleep problems, stroke, poor nutrition, memory disturbance, dementia, and depression.
- The National Institute on Alcohol Abuse and Alcoholism's recommended daily limit is more conservative for older adults because alcohol sensitivity increases with age and medications may further enhance the effects of alcohol.
- Depression, loneliness, and lack of social support are the greatest risk factors for both early-onset and late-onset alcohol abuse.
- Illicit use of such substances as marijuana, heroin, or cocaine, although rare in the elderly, is expected to rise as the Baby Boomers age. Abuse of prescribed drugs, particularly tranquilizers and sleeping pills, is more common.
- Clinicians should be aware of the signs and symptoms of abuse and the screening tools that are available.
- Older adults are more likely to have a long history of tobacco use that reduces their quality of life and places them at risk for chronic diseases.
- Counseling patients about health risks, cessation programs, and medications should be incorporated into the practice of all health care professionals.
- Depression, anxiety disorders, and PTSD are more prevalent among veterans than among the general populations and increase the risk factor of substance abuse.
- PTSD may occur soon after a stressful event or years later when facing another major stressor.
- BATHE is an acronym for a five-step process to enhance communication about psychosocial issues.

CRITICAL THINKING ACTIVITIES

1. As a beginning professional, it is difficult to accumulate experience with older adults in a short period of time. One suggestion is to enhance clinical experience with older adults with personal experience. You can start by interviewing a relative or neighbor, friend, teacher, or mentor older than 65. Ask them questions about their lives. Find out what has given them the most satisfaction in life, how they coped with difficult times and loss, and what their fears and their strengths are. You can also ask about high points and low points, challenges, loss, and turning points in their lives. The Foley Center for the Study of Lives has guidelines and structured questions to ask (http://www.sesp.northwestern.edu/foley/).
2. Another exercise to enhance learning and understanding of late life is to watch full-length motion pictures that portray a relevant theme of aging. The American Psychological Association provides a list of selected motion pictures that would be interesting to watch for clinicians (http://apadiv20.phhp.ufl.edu/cinema.doc). Another list of films on aging can be found on the *New York Times* blog *The New Old Age* in an article entitled "Silver Hair on The Silver Screen" http://newoldage.blogs.nytimes.com/2008/07/31/silver-hair-on-the-silver-screen/. As you are watching these movies, think about whether the portrayal of the older adults is realistic and what the film maker is conveying about aging (negative or positive).
3. Lastly, I suggest you imagine yourself growing older. What will you be like at age 70, 80, or 90? How would you describe your aging self? Think about what your older self might say about what has given you the most satisfaction in life. Describe your personal strengths. Describe how you believe you coped with difficult times and challenges, and what you hope for at this time in your life. Think about your older self and how the health care professionals you encountered have treated you. Are you content with your interactions with them? Do you have a health care professional you would feel comfortable talking to about personal concerns? What do you want from your health care providers?
4. Attend an outpatient PTSD group to hear veterans share their experiences.
5. Watch *Saving Private Ryan, WWII Battaan March,* or *The Hurt Locker* and discuss the potential mental health implications for these veterans.
6. Screen a classmate using the Primary Care PTSD instrument available at http://ptsd.va.gov/professional/pages/assessments/pc-ptsd.asp. This four-question tool is used in primary care settings to screen veterans for possible PTSD.

CASE STUDY | *MR. RODRIQUEZ*

Mr. Rodriquez was a 68-year-old unmarried Hispanic man diagnosed with PTSD, as well as lung cancer that had metastasized to his bones. A former medic during the Vietnam war, Mr. Rodriquez, while "in country," was exposed to *Agent Orange,* which many believed was directly related to the development of cancer and birth defects in returning soldiers' children. The patient was referred to the VA hospice unit by his primary care provider. On admission, he denied any psychiatric history or problems but did admit having difficulty with alcohol abuse. Shortly after his admission, Mr. Rodriquez began having trouble sleeping and admitted that he was experiencing nightmares and flashbacks, which he connected to his time in Vietnam. He also stated that he was having feelings of being stalked by the North Vietnamese enemy. On the basis of these symptoms, his nurse decided to refer Mr. Rodriquez for a psychiatric consultation. When a mental health exam was performed by the psychiatric nurse practitioner at the hospice unit, Mr. Rodriquez was diagnosed with depression and PTSD.

A male nursing student assigned to care for Mr. Rodriquez thought that it might help create rapport with this patient if the student revealed that his father had also served in Vietnam. The patient, who had previously refused to talk about his service in Vietnam, was able to open up a bit and share some of his experiences with the student. "When I came home people threw things at me and often called me a baby killer. My wife divorced me and I lost my job. I was homeless for many years until I was able to connect with a Vet Center and meet other Vietnam vets." Over the last few weeks of his life, Mr. Rodriquez continued to share his experiences with the nursing students and staff who cared for him. The patient died several weeks after admission to the hospice unit.

1. How might Mr. Rodriquez's experiences be linked to his mental health diagnoses?
2. How did the male nursing student help Mr. Rodriquez?
3. What impact might the opportunity to reveal war experiences have had on Mr. Rodriquez's dying experience?
4. What other interventions might have been helpful in this situation?

Doris Troth Lippman APRN, EdD, FAAN

REFERENCES

Abeles, N., Cooley, S, Deitch, I., et al. (1998). *What practitioners should know about working with older adults.* Washington, DC: American Psychological Association. Retrieved December 17, 2010, from http://www.apa.org/pi/aging/resources/guides/practitioners.pdf

Adams WL (1993) Alcohol-related hospitalizations of elderly people: Prevalence and geographic variation in the United States. *JAMA, 270,* 1222–1225.

Adams, W. L., Barry, K. L., & Fleming, M. F. (1996). Screening for problem drinking in older primary care patients. *Journal of the American Medical Association, 276*(24), 1964–1967.

Administration on Aging. (2001). *Older adults and mental health: Issues and opportunities.* Rockville, MD: Department of Health and Human Resources. Retrieved December 17, 2010, from http://www.globalaging.org/health/us/mental.pdf

Agency for Healthcare Research and Quality. (2008). *Helping smokers quit: A guide for clinicians.* Washington, DC: U.S. Department of Health and Human Services. Retrieved December 17, 2010, from http://www.ahrq.gov/clinic/tobacco/clinhlpsmksqt.htm

Alexopoulos, G. S., Raue, P., & Areán, P. A. (2003). Problem-solving therapy versus supportive therapy in geriatric major depression with executive dysfunction. *American Journal of Geriatric Psychiatry, 11*(1), 46–52.

Alzheimer's Association. (2007). *Stages of Alzheimer's disease.* Chicago, IL: Author. Retrieved December 17, 2010, from http://www.alz.org/national/documents/topicsheet_stages.pdf

Alzheimer's Association. (2010a). Alzheimer's disease facts and figures. *Alzheimer's & Dementia* (Vol. 6). Chicago, IL: Alzheimer's Association. Retrieved December 17, 2010, from http://www.alz.org/documents_custom/report_alzfactsfigures2010.pdf

Alzheimer's Association. (2010b). *Know the 10 signs.* Chicago, IL: Author. Retrieved December 17, 2010, from http://www.alz.org/alzheimers_disease_know_the_10_signs.asp

American Psychiatric Association. (2000). *Diagnostic and statistical manual of mental disorders* (4th ed., text rev.). Washington, DC: Author.

American Psychological Association. (2004). Guidelines for psychological practice with older adults. *American Psychologist, 59*(4), 236–260. Retrieved December 17, 2010, from http://www.apa.org/practice/guidelines/older-adults.pdf

Anxiety Disorders Association of America. (2010). *Older adults.* Retrieved December 17, 2010, from http://www.adaa.org/living-with-anxiety/older-adults

Areán, P., Hegel, M. A., Vannoy, S., Fan, M. Y., & Unuzter, J. (2008). Effectiveness of problem-solving therapy for older, primary care patients with depression: Results from the IMPACT project. *Gerontologist, 48*(3), 311–323.

Armstrong, M. (2010). *The vet to vet program.* Retrieved December 17, 2010, from http://www.nami.org/Template.cfm?Section=Issue_Spotlights&template=/ContentManagement/ContentDisplay.cfm&ContentID=26957

Arnold, E. (2004). Sorting out the 3 D's: Delirium, dementia, depression. *Nursing 34*(6), 36–42.

Baltes, P. B., & Baltes, M. M. (1993). Psychological perspectives on successful aging: The model of selective optimization with compensation. (pp 1-33). In P. B. Baltes & M. M. Baltes (Eds.), *Successful aging.* Cambridge, UK: University of Cambridge Press.

Bartels, S. J., & Smyer, M. A. (2002). Mental disorders of aging: An emerging public health crisis? *Generations, XXVI*(1), 14–20.

Belleville, S., Gilbert, B., Fontaine, F., et al. (2006) Improvement of episodic memory in persons with mild cognitive impairment and healthy older adults: Evidence from a cognitive intervention program. *Dementia and Geriatric Cognitive Disorders, 22*(5–6), 486–499.

Benson, H. (2007). *'Brain gym' may exorcise Boomers' fears about aging.* San Francisco, CA: San Francisco Chronicle. Retrieved December 17, 2010, from http://www.feldenkraisinstitute.org/articles/1213_BrainGym.pdf

Billig, N. (1993). *Growing older and wiser: Coping with expectations, challenges and change in the later years.* New York, NY: Lexington Books.

Birrer, R. B., & Venuri, S. P. (2004). Depression in later life: A diagnostic and therapeutic challenge. *American Family Physician, 69*(10), 2375–2382.

Blazer, D. G. (2003). Depression in late life: Review and commentary. *Journal of Gerontology, 58A*(3), 249–265.

Blazer, D. G. (2006). Successful aging. *American Journal of Geriatric Psychiatry, 14*(1), 2–5.

Blow, F. (1998). *Substance abuse among older adults.* Rockville, MD: U.S. Department of Health and Human Services.

Blow, F. C., Oslin, D. W., & Barry, K. L. (2002). Misuse and abuse of alcohol, illicit drugs, and psychoactive medication among older people. *Generations, XXVI*(1), 50-54. Retrieved December 17, 2010, from http://www.asaging.org/publications/dbase/GEN/GEN.26_1.Blow.pdf

Blow, F.C., Barry, K.L., Fuller, B.E., & Booth, B.M. (2008). Analysis of the National Health and Nutrition Examination Survey (NHANES): Longitudinal analysis of drinking over the life span. *In Substance Abuse by Older Adults: Estimates of Future Impact on the Treatment System.* Rockville, MD: Office of Applied Studies, SAMHSA.

Bonifas, R. (2008). *Grief, loss and bereavement in older adults: Reactions to death, chronic illness, and disability.* Alexandria, VA: CSWE Gero-Ed Center. Retrieved December 17, 2010, from http://www.cswe.org/CentersInitiatives/GeroEdCenter/Programs/MAC/GIG/Arizona/37528.aspx

Boss, P. (1999). Ambiguous loss: Learning to live with unresolved grief. Cambridge, MA: Harvard University Press.

Boss, P. (n.d.). *About ambiguous loss.* Retrieved December 17, 2010, from http://www.ambiguousloss.com/about_ambiguous_loss.php

Brody, J. (2010, April 6). The pain of losing a spouse is singular. *New York Times.* Retrieved December 17, 2010, from http://www.nytimes.com/2010/04/06/health/06cases.html

Bromley, D. B. (1966). *The psychology of human aging.* Baltimore, MD: Penguin.

Bruce, M. (2010). Subdromal depression and service delivery. *American Journal of Geriatric Psychiatry, 18*(3), 189–192.

Butler, R. N. (1975). *Why survive? Being old in America.* New York, NY: Harper Row.

Carpenter, B. D., Xiong, C., Porensky, E., et al. (2008). Reaction to a dementia diagnosis in individuals with Alzheimer's disease and mild cognitive impairment. *Journal of the American Geriatrics Society, 56*(3), 405–412.

Carstensen, L. (2009). *Myths and challenges.* Stanford Center on Longevity. Retrieved December 17, 2010, from http://longevity.stanford.edu/mymind/mythsandchallenges

Cavanaugh, J., & Blanchard-Fields, F. (2006). *Adult development and aging* (5th ed.). Belmont, CA: Wadsworth.

Cave, D. (2009). A combat role, and anguish, too. *New York Times,* October 31, 2009. Available at: http://www.nytimes.com/2009/11/01/us/01trauma.html.

Centers for Disease Control and Prevention. (2009). *Improving health literacy for older adults.* Atlanta, GA: U.S. Department of Health and Human Services. Retrieved December 17, 2010, from http://www.cdc.gov/healthmarketing/healthliteracy/reports/olderadults.pdf

Centers for Disease Control and Prevention. (2010). *Smoking & tobacco use.* Atlanta, GA: Author. Retrieved December 17, 2010, from http://www.cdc.gov/tobacco/data_statistics/fact_sheets/adult_data/cig_smoking/index.htm#overview

Cole, M. G., & Dendukuri, N. (2003). Risk factors for depression among elderly community subjects: A systematic review and meta-analysis. *American Journal of Psychiatry, 10*(6), 1147–1156.

Colliver JD, Compton WM, Gfroerer JC, Condon T. (2006). Projecting drug use among aging baby boomers in 2020. *Annals of Epidemiology 16(4)*,257-65

Cook, J. M., Cassidey, E. L., & Ruzek, J. I. (2001).Aging combat veterans in long term care. *National Center for PTSD Clinical Quarterly, 10,* 25–29.

D'Ambrosio, J. A. (2007). Tobacco use in older adults: Oral health consequences and cessation guidelines. *Health care and Aging,* 14 (1).

Didion, J. (2005) *The year of magical thinking.* New York, NY: Knopf.

Dorsey, E. R., Rabbini, A., Gallagher, S., Conti, R. M., & Alexander, G. A. (2010). Impact of FDA black box advisory on antipsychotic medication use. *Archives of Internal Medicine, 170*(1), 96–103.

Downs, M. G. (1999). How to tell? Disclosing a diagnosis of dementia. American Society on Aging, *Generations, XXIII*(2), 30-34. Retrieved December 17, 2010, from http://www.asaging.org/publications/dbase/GEN/Gen.23_3.Downs.pdf

Downs, M., Clibbens, R., Rae, C., Cook, A., & Woods, R. (2002). What do general practitioners tell people with dementia and their families about the condition? *Dementia, 1*(1), 47–58.

Dyehouse, J., Howe, S., & Ball, S. (1996). Silence Hurts: *Alcohol Abuse and Violence Against Women*, Module 6, Brief Interventions. Rockville, MD: Substance Abuse & Mental Health Services Administration http://pathwayscourses.samhsa.gov/vawp/vawp_supps_pg17.htm

Erikson, E. H. (1963). *Childhood and society* (2nd ed., p. 267). New York, NY: Norton.

Erikson, E. H. (1982). *The life cycle completed.* New York, NY: Norton.

Falk, B., Hersen, M., & Van Hasselt, V. B. (1994). Assessment of post-traumatic stress disorder in older adults: A critical review. *Clinical Psychology Review, 14*(5), 133–415.

Fernandez, A. (2008, June 3). *Brain training: Fact or fiction?* Huffington Post. Retrieved December 17, 2010, from http://www.huffingtonpost.com/alvaro-fernandez/brain-training-fact-or-fi_b_104986.html

Fiore, M. C., Jaén, C. R., Baker, T. B., et al. (2008). *Treating tobacco use and dependence: 2008 update.* Washington, DC: U.S. Department of Health and Human Services. Retrieved December 17, 2010, from http://www.surgeongeneral.gov/tobacco/treating_tobacco_use08.pdf

Freud, S. (1976). On psychotherapy. In J. B. Strachey (Ed.), *The complete psychological works of Sigmund Freud* (standard ed.). New York, NY: Norton. (Original work published 1905)

Geerlings, S. W., Beekman, A. T., Deeg, D. J., Twisk, J. W., & Van Tilburg, W. (2002). Duration and severity of depression predict mortality in older adults in the community. *Psychological Medicine, 32*(4), 609–618.

Gellis, Z. D., McClive-Reed, K., & McCracken, S. G. (2008). Depression in older adults with dementia. In *Mental health and older adults.* CSWE Gero-Ed Center, Master's Advanced Curriculum Project. Retrieved December 17, 2010, from http://www.cswe.org/File.aspx?id=23560

Gfroerer, J.C., Penne, M.A, Pemberton, M.R., & Folsom, R.E. (2008). The aging baby boom cohort and future prevalence of substance abuse. In *Substance Abuse by Older Adults: Estimates of Future Impact on the Treatment System*. Rockville, MD: Office of Applied Studies, SAMHSA.

Gleason, O. (2003). Delirium. *American Family Physician, 67*(5), 1027–1034.

Golier, J. A., Yehuda, R., Lupien, S. J., et al. (2002) Memory performance in Holocaust survivors with posttraumatic stress disorder. *American Journal of Psychiatry, 159,* 1682–1688.

Gradus, J. L. (2007). *Epidemiology of PTSD.* Washington, DC: U.S. Department of Veterans Affairs, National Center for PTSD. Retrieved December 17, 2010, from http://www.ptsd.va.gov/professional/pages/epidemiological-facts-ptsd.asp

Greene, K. (2009). The latest in mental health: Working out at the 'brain gym.' *Wall Street Journal,* March 28, 2009. Retrieved December 17, 2010, from http://online.wsj.com/article/SB123819562420161343.html

Gwyther, L. (2001). *Caring for people with Alzheimer's disease: A manual for facility staff.* Washington, DC: American Health Care Association. To order please call the Western Carolina Chapter of Alzheimer's Association (800-888-6671).

Hafner, K. (2008). Exercise your brain, or else you'll ... uh .... *New York Times,* May 3, 2008. Retrieved December 17, 2010, from http://www.nytimes.com/2008/05/03/technology/03brain.html

Herschbach, P. (2002). The "well-being paradox" in quality-of-life research. *Psychotherapie Psychosomatik Medizinische Psychologie, 52*(3–4), 141–150.

Hill, R. D. (2006). *Positive aging: A guide for mental health professionals and consumers.* New York, NY: Norton.

Hill, R. D. (2008). *Seven strategies for positive age.* New York, NY: Norton.

Holsinger, T., Steffens, D. C., Phillips, C., et al. (2002). Head injury in early adulthood and the lifetime risk of depression. *Archives of General Psychiatry, 59*(1), 17–22.

Hospice Education Institute. (n.d.). *Grief.* Retrieved December 17, 2010, from http://www.hospiceworld.org/book/grief.htm

Hoyl, M. T., Alessi, C. A., Harker, J. O., et al. (1999). Development and testing of a five-item version of the Geriatric Depression Scale. *Journal of the American Geriatrics Society, 47*(7), 873–878.

Inouye, S. K. (2000). Prevention of delirium in hospitalized older patients: Risk factors and targeted intervention strategies. *Annals of Medicine, 32,* 257–263.

Inouye, S. K. (2003). *The confusion assessment method (CAM) training manual and coding guide.* New Haven, CN: Yale University of Medicine.

Inouye, S. K. (2006). Delirium in older persons. *New England Journal of Medicine, 354,* 1157–1165.

Inouye, S. K., Bogardus, S. T., Charpentier, P. A., et al. (1999) A multicomponent intervention to prevent delirium on hospitalized older patients. *Journal of the American Medical Association, 340*(9), 669–676.

Inouye, S. K., & Charpentier, P. A. (1996). Precipitating factors for delirium in hospitalized elderly persons. *Journal of the American Medical Association, 275*(11), 852–857.

Inouye, S. K., Van Dyck, C., Alessi, C., et al. (1990). Clarifying confusion: The confusion assessment method. *Annals of Internal Medicine, 113*(12), 941–948.

Institute of Medicine. (2008). *Retooling for an aging America: Building the health care workforce.* Washington, DC: The National Academies Press. Retrieved December 17, 2010, from http://www.fhca.org/news/retooling.pdf

Jeste, D. V., Alexopoulos, G. S., Bartels, S. J., et al. (1999). Consensus statement on the upcoming crisis in geriatric mental health. *Archives of General Psychiatry, 56*(9), 848–853.

Joffe, C., Brodaty, H., Luscombe, G., & Ehrlich, F. (2003). The Sydney Holocaust study: Posttraumatic stress disorder and other psychosocial morbidity in an aged community sample. *Journal of Traumatic Stress, 16*(1), 39–47.

John A. Hartford Institute for Geriatric Nursing. (2001). *Best nursing practices in care for older adults: Curriculum guide incorporating essential gerontological content into baccalaureate nursing education and staff development.* New York: Author.

Kaplan, M. S., Adamek, M. E., & Calderon, A. (1999). Managing depressed and suicidal geriatric patients: Differences among primary care physicians. *Gerontologist, 39*(4), 417–425.

Kisley, M. A., Wood, S., & Burrows, C. L. (2007). Looking at the sunny side of life: Age-related change in an event-related potential measure of the negativity bias. *Psychological Science, 18*(9), 838–843.

Klap, R., Unroe, K. T., & Unutzer, J. (2003). Caring for mental illness in the United States: A focus on older adults. *American Journal of Geriatric Psychiatry, 11*(5), 517–524.

Kleinfield, N. R. (2002). More than death, fearing a muddled mind. *New York Times,* November 11, 2002. Available at: http://www.nytimes.com/2002/11/11/nyregion/more-than-death-fearing-a-muddled-mind.html

Lang, R. (1999). *The impact of Alzheimer's disease on the family caregiver: Course workbook.* Rocky Hill, CT: Alzheimer's Association, Connecticut Chapter.

Lang, R. (2003). *Dementia handout for family caregivers.* Center for Healthy Aging, Greenwich, CT: Greenwich Hospital.

Lavretsky, H., Zheng, L., Weiner, M. W., et al. (2010). Association of depressed mood and mortality in older adults with and without cognitive impairment in a prospective naturalistic study. *American Journal of Psychiatry, 167,* 589–597.

Lebowitz, B. D. (1997). Diagnosis and treatment of depression in late life: Consensus statement update. *Journal of the American Medical Assoociation, 278*(14), 1186–1190.

Liberto, J.G., & Oslin, (1995). D.W. Early versus late onset of alcoholism in the elderly. *International Journal of the Addictions* 30:1799-1818.

Lieberman, J. A., & Stuart, M. R. (1999). The BATHE method: Incorporating counseling and psychotherapy into the everyday management of patients. *Primary Care Companion to the Journal of Clinical Psychiatry, 1,* 35–38.

Lewis, C. S. (1961). *A grief observed.* New York, NY: Harper Collins.

Lichtenberg, P. A., Murman, D. L., & Mellow, A. M. (Eds.). (2003). *Handbook of dementia.* Hoboken, NJ: Wiley.

Lyness, J. M., Bruce, M. L., Koenig, H. G., et al.(1996). Depression and medical illness in late life: Report of a symposium. *Journal of the American Geriatric Society, 44*(2), 198–203.

Lyness, J. M., Yu, Q., Tang, W, Tu, X., & Conwell, Y. (2009). Risks for depression onset in primary care elderly patients: Potential targets for preventive interventions. *Am J Psychiatry, 166*(12), 1375–1383.

Mace, N., & Rabins, P. (2006). *The 36 hour day: A family guide to caring for people with Alzheimer disease, other dementias, and memory loss in later life* (4th ed.). Baltimore, MD: The John's Hopkins University Press.

Menninger, J.A. (2002). Assessment and treatment of alcoholism and substance-related disorders in the elderly. *Bulletin of the Menninger Clinic, 66,* 166-184.

Met Life Foundation. (2006). *MetLife Foundation Alzheimer's survey: What America thinks.* Retrieved December 17, 2010, from http://muskrat.middlebury.edu/lt/cr/faculty/shalpern-lt/Memory/20538296421147208330V1FAlzheimersSurvey.pdf

Mittal, D., Torres, R., Abashidze, A., & Jimerson, N. (2001). Worsening of post-traumatic stress disorder symptoms with cognitive decline: Case series. *Journal of Geriatric Psychiatry and Neurology, 14*(1), 17–20.

Naegle, M. A. (2007). Alcohol use screening and assessment for older adults. *Hartford Institute for Geriatric Nursing: Try This,* Issue 17. Retrieved December 17, 2010, from http://consultgerirn.org/uploads/File/trythis/try_this_17.pdf

Naegle, M. A. (2008). Screening for alcohol use and misuse in older adults: Using the short Michigan alcoholism screening test - geriatric version. *American Journal of Nursing, 108*(11), 50–58.

National Alliance on Mental Illness. (2009). *Depression and veterans. Fact sheet.* Arlington, VA: Author. Retrieved December 17, 2010, from http://www.nami.org/Template.cfm?Section=Depression&Template=/ContentManagement/ContentDisplay.cfm&ContentID=88939

National Institute on Aging. (2008). *Older adults and alcohol: you can get help.* Bethesda, MD: Department of Health and Human Resources. Publication Number 08-7350. Available at: http://www.nia.nih.gov/NR/rdonlyres/28DDEE88-38FB-4ED7-BD6C-4738381E1659/0/NIAAlcoholBooklet218final.pdf

National Institute of Mental Health. (2003). *Older adults: Depression and suicide facts.* Washington, DC: Author. Pub. No. 03-4593. Retrieved December 17, 2010, from http://www.nimh.nih.gov/health/publications/older-adults-depression-and-suicide-facts-fact-sheet/index.shtml

National Institute of Mental Health. (2010). *Anxiety disorders.* Washington, DC: Author. Retrieved December 17, 2010, from http://www.nimh.nih.gov/health/topics/anxiety-disorders/index.shtml

National Institutes of Health. (n.d.). *Cognitive and emotional health: The healthy brain workshop.* Washington, DC: National Institutes of Neurological Disorders and Stroke, Mental Health, and Aging. Retrieved December 17, 2010, from http://trans.nih.gov/cehp/NINDSSummary.pdf

National Institutes of Health. (2009). PTSD: A growing epidemic. *Medline Plus,* Winter 2009. Retrieved December 17, 2010, from http://www.nlm.nih.gov/medlineplus/magazine/issues/winter09/articles/winter09pg10-14.html

NIH Senior Health. (2010). *Anxiety disorders.* Washington, DC: National Institute on Aging. Retrieved December 17, 2010, from http://nihseniorhealth.gov/anxietydisorders/aboutanxietydisorders/01.html

O'Conner, K., Koeske, G., & Brown, C. (2009). Racial differences in attitudes toward professional mental health treatment: The mediating effect of stigma. *Journal of Gerontological Social Work, 52*(7), 695–712.

Patterson, T. L., & Jeste, D. V. (1999). The potential impact of the baby-boom generation on substance abuse among elderly persons. *Psychiatric Services, 50,* 1184–1188.

Pfizer, Inc. (2009). *Patient health questionnaire.* Retrieved December 17, 2010, from http://www.depression-primarycare.org/clinicians/toolkits/materials/forms/phq9/

Plassman, B. L. (2007). Prevalence of dementia in the United States. *Neuroepidemiology, 29*(1–2), 125–132. Published online: October 29, 2007. DOI: 10.1159/000109998

Post, S. G. (1995). *The moral challenge of Alzheimer's disease.* Baltimore, MD: John Hopkins University Press.

Qato DM, Alexander GC, Conti RM, Johnson M, Schumm P, Lindau ST. (2008). Use of prescription and over-the-counter medications and dietary supplements among older adults in the United States. *Journal of the American Medical Association, 300,* 2867-2878.

Qualls, S. H. (2002). Defining mental health in later life. *Generations, XXVI*(1), 9–13.

Quinn, R. (2009). 'Brain gyms' offer grey matter workouts. *Newser,* March 28, 2009. Retrieved December 17, 2010, from http://www.newser.com/story/54621/brain-gyms-offer-grey-matter-workouts.html

Rando, T. A. (1984). *Grief, dying, and death: Clinical interventions for caregivers.* Champaign, IL: Research Press.

Rando, T. A. (1986). Comprehensive analysis of anticipatory grief: Perspectives, processes, promises, and problems. In T. A. Rando (Ed.), *Loss and anticipatory grief* (pp. 3–37). Lexington, MA: Lexington Books.

Rathier, M. O., & McElhaney, J. (2005). Delirium in elderly patients: How you can help. *Psychiatric Times.* Retrieved December 17, 2010, from http://www.psychiatrictimes.com/geriatric-psychiatry/content/article/10168/56711.

Reagan, R. (1994). *Letter to the American people.* Retrieved December 17, 2010, from http://www.americanpresidents.org/letters/39.asp

Rosenberg, P., Mielke, M. M., Xue, Q., & Carlson, M. C. (2010). Depressive symptoms predict incident cognitive impairment in cognitively healthy older women. *American Journal of Geriatric Psychiatry, 18*(3), 204–211.

Ross, S. (n.d.) Alcohol use disorders in the elderly. *Psychiatry Weekly,* New York, NY. From: http://www.psychweekly.com/aspx/article/ArticleDetail.aspx?articleid=19

Rowe, J. W., & Kahn, R. L. (1998). *Successful aging.* New York, NY: Pantheon.

Rowe, S. K., & Rapaport, M. H. (2006). Classification and treatment of sub-threshold depression. *Current Opinion in Psychiatry, 19,* 9–13.

Salthouse, T. A. (1996). The processing speed theory of adult age differences in cognition. *Psychological Review, 103,* 403–428.

Salthouse, T. A. (2010). *Major issues in cognitive aging.* New York, NY: Oxford University Press.

Schaie, K. W., & Willis, S. L. (2005). *Intellectual functioning in adulthood: Growth, maintenance, decline and modifiability.* Washington, DC: American Society on Aging and Metlife Foundation.

Schofield, W. (1964). *Psychotherapy: The purchase of friendship.* New York, NY: Prentice-Hall.

Schonfeld, L., & Dupree, L. (1991). Antecedents of drinking for early-and late-onset elderly alcohol abusers. *Journal of Studies on Alcohol,* 52(6), 587-593.

Schuckit, M. A., & Pastor, P. A. (1979). Alcohol-related psychopathology in the aged. In O. J. Kaplan (Ed.), Psychopathology of Aging (pp.211-227). New York: Academic Press.

Schultz, R., Beach, S. R., Ives, D. G., et al. (2000). Association between depression and mortality in older adults: The cardiovascular health study. *Archives of Internal Medicine, 160*(12), 1761–1768.

Scogin, F., & Shah, A. (2006). Screening older adults for depression in primary care settings. *Health Psychology, 25*(6), 675–677.

Seligman, M., & Csikszentmihalyi, M. (2000). Positive psychology: An introduction. *American Psychologist,* 55, 5–14.

Sherman, F. T. (2001). Functional assessment: Easy-to-use screening tools speed initial office work-up. *Geriatrics, 56,* 36–40.

Singh, A., & Misra, N. (2009). Loneliness depression and sociability in old age. *Industrial Psychiatry Journal, 18*(1), 51–55.

Solomon, A. (2001). *The noonday demon: An atlas of depression* (p. 16) New York, NY: Scribner.

Snowden, M., Steinman L., & Frederick J. (2008). Treating depression in older adults: Challenges to implementing the recommendations of an expert. panel. *Preventing Chronic Disease, 5*(1), A26.

Sullivan, K. A., & O'Conor, F. M. (2001). Should a diagnosis of Alzheimer's disease be disclosed? *Aging and Mental Health, 5*(4), 340–348.

Styron, W. (1990). *Darkness visible: A memoir of madness.* New York, NY: Random House.

Tai-Seale, M., McGuire, T., Colenda, C., Rosen, D., & Cook, M. A. (2007). Two-minute mental health care for elderly patients: Inside primary care visits. *Journal of the American Geriatrics Society, 55*(12), 1903–1911.

Tampi, R. J. (2010, March 23). *Treating behavioral disturbances in dementia in the era of black box warnings.* Presented at the Alzheimer's Educational Conference, Cromwell, CT.

Teresi, J., Abrams, R., Holmes, D., Ramirez, M. C., & Eimicke, J. (2001). Prevalence of depression and depression recognition in the nursing home. *Social Psychiatry and Psychiatric Epidemiology, 36*(12), 613–620.

Thibault, J., & Steiner, R. (2004). Efficient identification of adults with depression and dementia. *American Family Physician, 70*(6), 1101–1110.

Tullman, D. F., Mion, L. C., Fletcher, K., & Foreman, M. D. (2008). *Nursing standard of practice protocol: Delirium: Prevention, early recognition, and treatment.* Hartford Institute for Geriatric Nursing. Retrieved December 17, 2010, from http://consultgerirn.org/topics/delirium/want_to_know_more

Unitzer, J., Katon, W,. Callahan, C., et al. (2002). Collaborative care management of late-life depression in the primary care setting. *Journal of the American Medical Association, 288,* 2836–2845.

Unitzer, J., Patrick, D. L., Marmon, T., Simon, G. E., & Katon, W. J. (2002). Depressive symptoms and mortality in a prospective study of 2,558 older adults. *American Journal of Geriatric Psychiatry, 10*(5), 521–530.

U.S. Census Bureau. (2010). *Facts for features: Veterans Day 2010.* Retrieved December 17, 2010, from http://www.census.gov/newsroom/releases/archives/facts_for_features_special_editions/cb10-ff21.html

U.S. Department of Health and Human Services. (2008). *Veterans.* Washington, DC: Substance Abuse and Mental Health Services Administration. Retrieved December 17, 2010, from http://www.oas.samhsa.gov/veterans.htm#Use

U.S. Department of Health and Human Services. (2009). *Illicit drug use among older adults. The NSDUH Report, December 29, 2009.* Washington, DC: Author. Retrieved

December 17, 2010, from http://oas.samhsa.gov/2k9/168/168OlderAdults.htm

U.S. Department of Veterans Affairs. (2008). *Depression and suicide in aging veterans: SMITREC initiatives.* HSR&D Forum, April 2008. Retrieved December 17, 2010, from http://www.hsrd.research.va.gov/publications/forum/Apr08/Apr08-5.cfm

U.S. Department of Veterans Affairs. (2010). *Collaborative care improves treatment for depression.* Washington, DC: Quality Enhancement Research Initiative. Retrieved December 17 2010, from http://www.queri.research.va.gov/about/impact_updates/MH.pdf

Vahia, I. V., Meeks, T. W., Thompson, W. K., et al. (2010). Subthreshold depression and successful aging in older women. *American Journal of Geriatric Psychiatry, 18*(3), 212–220.

Vaillant, G. S. (2002). *Aging well: Surprising guideposts to a happier life from the landmark Harvard study of adult development.* Boston: Little, Brown.

Wagenaar, D., Colenda, C. C., Kreft, M., et al. (2003). Treating depression in nursing homes: Practice guidelines in the real world. *Journal of the American Osteopathic Association, 103*(10), 465–469.

Wallace, M. (2006). *Healthy minds.* Interview on WLIW with Borenstein, J. MD, episode 103 accessed online November 10, 2009, from http://wliw.org

Waszynski, C. M. (2007). How to try this: Detecting delirium. *American Journal of Nursing, 107*(12), 50–60.

Weil, A. (2005). *Healthy aging.* New York, NY: Knopf.

Whitbourne, S. K. (2008). *Adult development and aging: A biopsychosocial approach* (3rd ed.). Hoboken, NJ: Wiley.

Whooley, M. A., Avins, A., Miranda, J., & Browner, W. (1997). Case-finding instruments for depression: Two questions are as good as many. *Journal of General Internal Medicine, 12*(7), 439–445.

Wolin, S.J.Bennett, L.A. & Jacobs, A.S. (2003). Assessing family rituals in alcoholic families. In E. Imber-Black, J. Roberts, & R.A. Whiting, *Rituals in Family and Family Therapy*, pp. 253-279.

Worden, J. W. (2001). *Grief counseling and grief therapy: A handbook for the mental health practitioner* (3rd ed.). New York, NY: Springer.

Xian, L., Engel Jr., C., Han, K., & Armstrong, D.W. (2006). Veterans and functional status transitions in older Americans. *Military Medicine, 171 (10),* 943-949.

Yesavage JA, Brink TL, Rose TL, Lum O, Huang V, Adey M, Leirer VO. (1983). Development and validation of a geriatric depression screening scale: A preliminary report. *Journal of Psychiatric Research, 17*(1), 37–49. Retrieved December 17, 2010, from http://www.stanford.edu/~yesavage/GDS.html.

Zivin, K., Kim, H. M., McCarthy, J. F., et al. (2007). Suicide mortality among individuals receiving treatment for depression in the Veterans Affairs health system: Associations with patient and treatment setting characteristics. *American Journal of Public Health, 97*(12), 2193–2198.

Chapter 23

Spirituality in Aging

Martha Meraviglia, PhD, RN, CNS, Carol D. Gaskamp, PhD, RN, and Rebecca Sutter, RN, CNS

LEARNING OBJECTIVES

- Identify theories that include spirituality used in the disciples of medicine, psychology, social work, and nursing.
- Explain the role of spirituality in coping with aging and chronic illness.
- Discuss strategies for assessing spirituality in the older adult.
- Describe effective interventions for enhancing spirituality in older adults.

Unlike the physical and mental dimensions of life, the spiritual dimension continues to grow and develop in later years. Even older adults who have Alzheimer's disease keep early memories of the rituals and activities of their faith community. A recent poll indicates that religion and spirituality were deemed very important to 77% of adults age 75 and older and 72% of those ages 65 to 74 (Gallup Poll, 2009).

Unlike the physical and mental dimensions of life, the spiritual dimension continues to grow and develop in later years.

Understanding spirituality and the importance of the human spirit on one's health, illness, and aging will enhance nursing and health care. This chapter explores some important aspects of spirituality, including definitions and theories of spirituality, assessment tools, spiritual coping strategies, and effective nursing interventions.

Defining Spirituality

Spirituality has been described in numerous ways that reflect a holistic understanding of the term. Most writings conceptualize spirituality as an ongoing, dynamic process that reflects and expresses the human spirit. Personal spirituality is derived from individual experiences that are unique to each person. Faith is seen as an attribute of spirituality representing a belief in God or a Supreme Being that provides a basis for positive meaning and hope in life. The spiritual dimension is thought to integrate all human dimensions—mind, body, and spirit—for a sense of wholeness and well-being (Meraviglia, 2004).

Spirituality is defined broadly as all the experiences and expressions of one's spirit reflecting faith in God or a Supreme Being; connectedness with oneself, others, nature, or God; and integration of the human dimensions. One aspect of spirituality is religion, which is described as an organized system of beliefs, practices, and symbols that facilitates closeness to God or a Supreme Being (Koenig, 2002).

A whole-person perspective views a human being as being integrated in the physical, emotional, social, and spiritual dimensions. An alteration of well-being in one dimension affects the other dimensions. As depicted in Figure 23-1, the spiritual dimension is the core of the person, and interventions directed at the spiritual dimension will affect the physical, emotional, and social dimensions. The ultimate goal for promoting spirituality is to support and enhance one's well-being and overall quality of life (Gaskamp, Sutter, & Meraviglia, 2004).

Theories That Include Spirituality

Numerous theories that include spirituality are used in the health care disciplines of medicine, psychology, social work, and nursing. Selected theories and their descriptions of spirituality are listed in Table 23-1.

Spirituality in medicine focuses mainly on the impact of spirituality and religion on physical and mental health. Larson, Swyers, and McCullough (1997) examined research concluding that spirituality

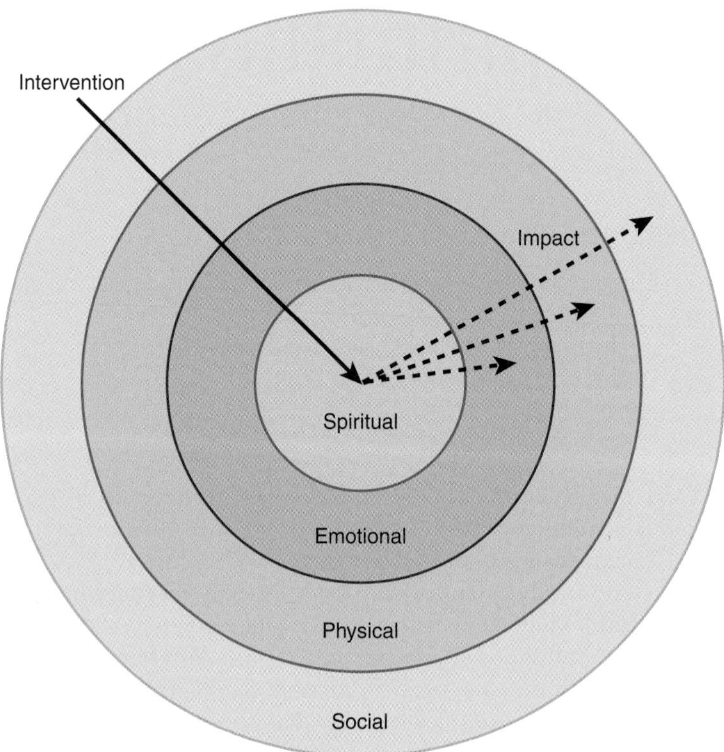

Figure 23-1 The holistic health model, in which an intervention directed at the spiritual dimension of life also affects the emotional, physical, and social aspects of life. *(From Gaskamp, C., Sutter, R., & Meraviglia, M. (2006). Evidence-based guideline: Promoting spirituality in the older adult. Journal of Gerontological Nursing, 32(11), 8–13.)*

TABLE 23-1 Theories with Spirituality Components

AUTHOR	THEORY	SPIRITUALITY DESCIPTION
Medicine		
Thomas		There is interaction between the dimensions of mind, body, and spirit.
Larson et al.	Spirituality/religion	Individual quest for understanding life's ultimate questions and meaning and purpose of life.
Psychology		
Frankl	Human motivation	The ultimate meaning in life is God. People are primarily motivated to find their meaning and purpose in life.
Farran		The mental processes for discovering what gives people meaning and where they look for guidance and authority.
Pargament	Religious coping	An expression of one's internal motives and desires concentrating on the self instead of God.
Sociology		
Russell		Internalized spirituality is described as the spiritual practices and rituals of groups of people as well as the social morality within personal relationships.

TABLE 23-1 Theories with Spirituality Components—cont'd

AUTHOR	THEORY	SPIRITUALITY DESCIPTION
Giddens	Reflexivity	Autonomous individual search for meaning and purpose is their responsibility; responsible for self, fate, and life choices, devoid of religious beliefs.
Nursing		
Reed	Spiritual perspective	Personal spiritual perspective, either horizontal toward others and/or vertical toward God or a Supreme Being.
Stoll	Spiritual interrelatedness	Interrelatedness via forgiveness, love, and trust resulting in meaning and purpose in life and hope.
Neuman	Systems model	Spirit can sustain body and promote wellness. Spiritual integrity is the primary need of the self-concept mode.
Watson	Human caring	Caring is a spiritual act that assists others to achieve greater sense of self and harmony with their mind, body, and spirit.

Adapted from McSherry, W. (2007). *Meaning of spirituality & spiritual care within nursing & health care practice.* London, England: Quay Books; and Taylor, E. J. (2002). *Spiritual care: nursing theory, research, and practice.* Upper Saddle River, NJ: Prentice Hall Pearson.

and religion are beneficial sources of coping strength and recovery from physical or emotional illness.

Spirituality in psychology includes one's ability to attain inward harmony and self-actualization. It has been broadly described as the way people choose to lead their lives. Frankl (1962) described spirituality more extensively than just psychologically when he incorporated theological thinking in his theory of human motivation. He emphasized that the ultimate meaning in life is God and that people are motivated mainly to find their meaning and purpose in life.

The sociology literature on spirituality examines the concept by studying groups of people. Within social sciences, people are viewed as being strongly influenced by other people and by the groups in which they live. Russell (1986) stated that in the past, religious groups have predominately influenced personal spirituality, but now an internalized spirituality is more prevalent.

McSherry (2007) identifies several nursing theorists (Neuman, Reed, Roy, and Watson), whose work explicitly includes spirituality. Most are grand theories with spirituality as one component. Reed (1987) analyzed spirituality in terms of one's spiritual perspective, either horizontal toward others, vertical toward God or a Supreme Being, or both. Stoll (1989) expanded on the holistic understanding of the spiritual dimension by incorporating concepts of forgiveness, love, and trust.

Role of Spirituality in Aging

Spirituality can help older adults cope with the challenges of aging and chronic disease. About 80% of older adults have at least one chronic condition, and 50% have two or more such conditions. This burden of chronic disease can negatively impact the aging process by increasing disability, emotional health, financial health, and quality of life (Centers for Disease Control and Prevention, 2010).

Older adults can maintain their health and quality of life, despite having chronic diseases, by maintaining or discovering their life meaning, sense of fulfillment, spiritual well-being, and closure at the end of life. Their spirituality is anchored in their community and reflects the importance of interpersonal relationships, thus providing a sense of belonging. Interconnection with others serves to counteract the effects of loneliness and despair older adults may experience.

Recent research demonstrates that spirituality increases in importance with aging and becomes extremely important for many as they cope with the multifaceted problems of chronic disease. For instance, people report using such spiritual forms of coping as prayer, faith, hope, and spiritual support. Religious coping strategies including reading religious materials and watching religious programs on television (Pargament, Koenig, & Perez, 2000).

PERSONAL PERSPECTIVE
Spirituality and Aging

Dominick, age 70 and disabled, still has the muscular build of the younger man who drove an 18-wheeler up and down the East Coast for 35 years. He shoots straight from the hip, his manner unpolished, his heart tender. Asked if his relationship with God has changed as he has aged, he responds with sincerity, purpose, and a great deal of animation. "I think my perception of God has gotten better than when I was younger," he says. "I always believed in the Lord. I'm a Christian. I believe in God immensely. There's no two ways about it. I'll get in arguments with people about it. They say, 'oh you're too overworked,' and I'll say, 'no I'm not too overworked.' I think as the years go on I'm getting more involved with the Lord. I go to Sabbath on Friday nights, and I'll go to the Catholic Mass. Not that I'm a Catholic, but even if it was a Protestant mass I would go, due to the fact that it's the Lord."

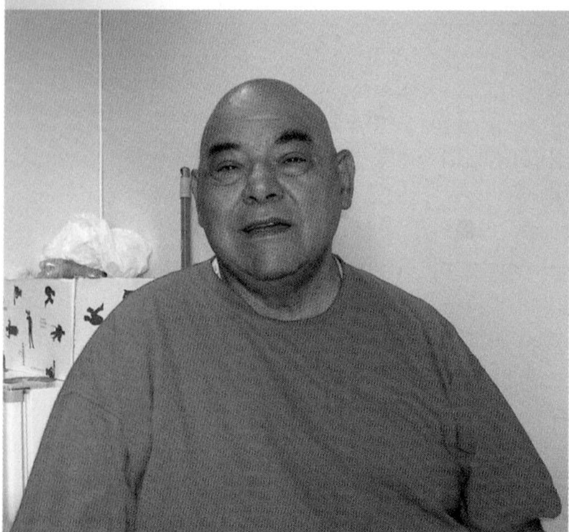

Asked why he goes to the Friday night Jewish Sabbath service, Dominick replies, "to have something to do, to be with other people, to pray to God. They've got the book, and I read the English part of it. I don't understand the Jewish part of it, but I'm praying to the Lord at the same time. It makes no difference if I'm in a Jewish church, a Catholic church, a Protestant church. There's only one God. You could be in a Muslim church. There's still only one God. He's the creator of heaven and earth. That's all there is to it. That's the way I believe."

"Sometimes I stop and think, 'What was my purpose in life? What did I accomplish?' I don't know what my purpose is. But I'm still living and who knows, somewhere down the future I may—BOOM—do just what the Lord intended me to do. I had to live all these years to do it. Looking forward I still don't see what I'm going to do, but the Lord has taken me and put me in different positions. He took me out of that house where I was, the condo, and put me here. Maybe it's something I'm going to do here. Maybe it's something I'm going to do after here. I don't know. Who are we to say?"

About Dominick Dominick Ferrara is the widowed father of three children, two of whom have passed away. He is very close with his surviving daughter. "I still look after her," he says, "and she looks after me." After the death of his other daughter, he took in his 5-year-old grandson and raised him until, as a teenager, the child returned to his father's home. During all those years of raising a family, Dominick drove an 18-wheeler from Canada to Richmond, Virginia. Asked about what he did in his free time during those years, Dominick responds, "I had no free time, and I regret it. I would have liked to spend more time with my kids." Today, Dominick has time and spends it visiting with his daughter and attending philosophy class, playing Wii golf, attending a *Let It Shine Journeys* Sage-ing program, and taking in a wide variety of other offerings at the assisted-living facility he calls home.

Lorri B. Danzig, MS, CSL

Older adults have the capacity to reorder their lives and make meaning of their experiences. This dynamic process enables them to translate an experience, even an experience of loss, crisis, or illness, and assign meaning to it on the basis of their personality traits, capacities, level of expectations, and spiritual perspective (Lawler-Row & Elliot, 2009).

Older adults have the capacity to reorder their lives and make meaning of their experiences.

Older adults can use spirituality to maintain their sense of fulfillment and quality of life. Spiritual well-being has been positively linked with physical and emotional well-being in many studies of older adults. In addition, having a strong sense of spiritual well-being is related to positive adjustment to illness and reduced feelings of uncertainty, anxiety, pain, depression, and loneliness among the chronically ill (Phillips, Paukert, Stanley, & Kunik, 2009).

Finally, spirituality is extremely important for closure at the end of life. There is an increasing awareness from recent research that sense of spiritual well-being positively impacts emotional health and adjustment to illness. Having a strong sense of spiritual well-being reduces feelings of hopelessness, despair, loneliness, depression, and desire to hasten death (McClain, Rosenfeld, & Breitbart, 2003).

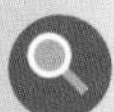

EVIDENCE FOR PRACTICE
Religion and Spirituality

Purpose: To examine the relationships between aspects of religiosity and spirituality with health and well-being in older adults, without consideration of religious affiliation.

Sample: The participants consisted of 425 adults (169 men and 243 women), ranging in age from 50 to 95, with a mean age of 63.4 years. Most participants (63%) were age 64 or younger, with 37% over age 65. In terms of religious affiliation, participants indicated their denomination as Protestant (36%), Baptist (30%), None (14%), Catholic (10%), or Other (10%).

Methods: The older adults completed questionnaires that addressed religiosity, spirituality, and health, plus healthy behaviors and social support. Relationships between the study variables were analyzed with multiple correlation and regression statistical analysis.

Results: Considering all participants, church members reported higher levels of healthy behaviors and social support. One's spirituality (existential well-being) was strongly related to all health measures (psychological well-being, subjective well-being, healthy behaviors, depression, and physical symptoms). Spiritual well-being (religious and existential well-being) and prayer significantly predicted psychological well-being and subjective well-being, as well as physical symptoms and depression. Healthy behaviors and social support were partial mediators of the influence of existential well-being and health measures. Interestingly, religious activities were not as important as spirituality for the older adults in the study and did not influence the health outcome measures as significantly.

Implications: Enhancing spirituality in older adults by promoting a sense of purpose and meaning in life and use of prayer can contribute to overall health and well-being.

Reference: Lawler-Row, K. A., & Elliott, J. (2009). The role of religious activity and spirituality in the health and well-being of older adults. *Journal of Health Psychology 14,* 43–53.

Assessing Spirituality

Assessment of spirituality beyond knowing a patient's denominational affiliation is now an expected aspect of care in health care facilities accredited by the Joint Commission (Staten, 2003). Various tools are available to assist nurses in assessing spirituality and identifying those at risk for spiritual distress.

Gaskamp, Sutter, and Meraviglia (2004) adapted several assessment guidelines into an assessment tool specific to older adults or to the caregiver if the older adult is unable to communicate. The assessment tool has six questions asking about their past and current spiritual resources and concerns (Box 23-1). In addition, Stranahan (2008) developed a screening tool to identify older adults experiencing spiritual distress. The tool is based on theories of behavioral development of older adults and assesses meaning and purpose, hope and coping, transcendence in relationships with God and others, and religious practices.

Several additional tools are available for assessing spirituality but are not designed specifically for older adults. These include the FACT spiritual history tool (Larocca-Pitts, 2008), Brief RCOPE (Pargament, Koenig, & Perez, 2000), and FICA (faith/beliefs, importance, community, and address) (Puchalski, 2002).

Interventions for Enhancing Spirituality

Spirituality may be supported and enhanced in older adults in a number of ways, some of which are outlined here. Paramount in all spiritually focused interactions with older adults is an acceptance of the other person's thoughts and feelings about his or her spiritual or religious beliefs and practice. Never is it acceptable to seek to influence or dissuade older adults away from their own traditions because you follow the tenets of a different spiritual or religious tradition.

BOX 23-1 Brief Assessment of Spiritual Resources and Concerns

Use the following questions as an interview guide with the older adult (or caregiver if the older adult is unable to communicate).

- Does your religion/spirituality provide comfort or serve as a cause of stress? (Ask to explain in what ways spirituality is a comfort or stressor.)
- Do you have any religious or spiritual beliefs that might conflict with health care or affect health care decisions? (Ask to identify any conflicts.)
- Do you belong to a supportive church, congregation, or faith community? (Ask how the faith community is supportive.)
- Do you have any practices or rituals that help you express your spiritual or religious beliefs? (Ask to identify or describe practices.)
- Do you have any spiritual needs you would like someone to address? (Ask what those needs are and if referral to spiritual professional is desired.)
- How can we (health care providers) help you with your spiritual needs or concerns?

Gaskamp, C., Sutter, R., & Meraviglia, M. (2004). Promoting spirituality in the older adult. Evidence-Based Protocol, Gerontological Nursing Interventions Research Center, University of Iowa College of Nursing: Iowa City, IA.

BOX 23-2 Nursing Diagnoses for Spirituality

The North American Nursing Diagnosis Association Definitions and Classification includes five diagnoses related to spirituality:

- *Spiritual distress* was introduced in 1978
- *Readiness for enhanced spiritual well-being* was accepted in 1994
- *Risk for spiritual distress* was added in 1998
- *Impaired religiosity,* both *risk for* and *actual,* were accepted in 2004

From NANDA International. (2009). Nursing diagnoses: Definitions & classification 2009-2011. Indianapolis, IN: Wiley-Blackwell.

Spiritual interventions must also be implemented with an awareness of the risk for feelings of loneliness and social isolation (McSherry, 2007). More than 40% of older adults experience occasional feelings of loneliness and over half of those age 80 and older report feeling lonely (Pinquart & Sorensen, 2001). Because of the high incidence of loneliness in older adults, it is especially important to assess older adults for feelings of loneliness and isolation in those who have been diagnosed with a chronic disease (Box 23-2).

Interventions proven to be effective in the aging population are presented here, as well as actions intuitively known to improve spirituality, starting with active listening. Actively listening to another person is very effective for meeting psychological and social needs. Moreover, active listening can enhance a person's spirituality when interventions are directed toward the spiritual dimension. For instance, by actively listening to the patient, the nurse is able to hear, understand, interpret, and synthesize what the person is saying about his or her spiritual beliefs and resources.

In addition, the nurse establishes a trusting relationship and provides sufficient time for patients to interpret their own spiritual feelings and experiences (Ackley & Ladwig, 2007). Spiritual care actions include being present for the patient, assisting the patient in finding the meaning of life events and purpose in life, encouraging reminiscence and life review, encouraging prayer, using caring touch, and encouraging the use of comforting religious practices. The use of expressive arts, such as art, music, and dramatics, may also enhance spirituality for older adults.

Presence

Presence is described as *being there* and *being with* a patient in meaningful ways. *Being there* encompasses much more than physical presence; it includes a relationship with sincere communication. In *being with* the patient, the nurse is fully available to hear and understand the patient's difficulty and suffering (Hessel, 2009).

As a nursing action for older adults, being present requires knowing and being comfortable with oneself. The nurse also connects with the person through affirmation, valuing, vulnerability, empathy, serenity, and silence.

Searching for Meaning

For the older adult, making meaning from critical life events or life itself can be a challenging process, one in which the nurse can have significant influence. The nurse can facilitate an older adult's search for meaning by asking probing questions, offering additional explanations, and reframing maladaptive interpretations of life events. In addition, the nurse can facilitate the older adult's search for purpose in life and a sense of personal worthiness at this point in life (Low & Molzahn, 2007).

Through the process of finding meaning in an illness, the death of a loved one, or the loss of independence, the older adult grows spiritually.

Through the process of finding meaning in an illness, the death of a loved one, or the loss of independence, the older adult grows spiritually. Research has shown that older adults who experience difficulty finding meaning have a higher incidence of depression.

Reminiscence and Life Review

Reminiscence and life review are the recalling and sharing with another person one's past life events. The process of reminiscence can facilitate successful aging and improve meaning and purpose by giving the person opportunities to rethink, reframe, clarify, and make meaning of previous experiences. Reminiscence through storytelling encourages the person to discover spiritual links between inner resources and how he or she lived through difficult life events. Reminiscence has positive benefits, such as successful adaptation to growing old and decreasing depression (Stinson, 2009). Nurses are in a unique position to facilitate reminiscence by developing long-term relationships with their older patients (Bephage, 2009).

To assist with the process of reminiscence, the nurse can encourage older adults to develop their genogram, which is a family tree for identifying and understanding patterns in one's family history. Additionally, the nurse can encourage patients to write or journal about their lives to discover spiritual experiences and concerns that support and reflect their spirituality. The nurse can validate spiritual concerns, providing support as the older adult processes these concerns to grow spiritually. Also, nurses can help older adults create and review scrapbooks as another method for sharing one's history to integrate one's life (Taylor, 2002).

Prayer

Prayer is a devout petition to, or any form of spiritual communion with, God or an object of worship. Prayers may include adoration and expressions of love, confession, thanksgiving, or supplication and asking for help. Specific nursing actions of prayer include offering to pray, meditate, or read a spiritual text with the older adult; arranging for another member of the health care team to do so; and respecting a person's time for quietness and prayer.

For an older adult who finds prayer meaningful, there are numerous benefits when prayer is included in nursing care. For instance, older adults are vulnerable to feelings of social isolation and loneliness, which can be relieved through supporting their prayer beliefs and practices. Nurses can participate in prayer with older adults to enhance their trust, self-worth, and hope. Additionally, research has shown a positive relationship between the practice of prayer and feelings of general well-being, psychological well-being, and quality of life (Meraviglia, 2004).

Caring Touch

Caring touch is an important nursing action for promoting spirituality in older adults. As a foundational aspect of nursing practice, touch, such as hand holding or touching an arm or shoulder, facilitates communication between nurse and patient. As a nursing action for older adults, personal touch conveys acceptance, concern, comfort, and reassurance, especially during stressful periods (Gaskamp, Sutter, & Meraviglia, 2006). Research has shown that personal touch relieves feelings of loneliness, provides comfort, and shows caring concern.

The effects of music, massage, and aromatherapy may be similar to those of touch and can be used therapeutically to provide relaxation and reduce feelings of stress (Hemming & Maher, 2005). Music has long been associated with calming effects not only for individuals but also for family dynamics. A key to using music to enhance relaxation is to have the individual select music that is personally meaningful or important. Massage with or without aromatherapy can be used to ease anxiety in older adults, especially residents of long-term care facilities and those with dementia. Massage can be provided by massage therapists, physical therapists, or nurses.

Religious Practices

Encouraging involvement in religious communities and practicing religious activities are appropriate nursing interventions for enhancing the spirituality of older adults. Involvement in religious communities provides social support and connection with family and friends. Religious practices and activities may include attending worship services, respecting dietary guidelines, using religious objects (e.g., prayer beads, undergarments, lockets, pendants, icons, mandalas), acknowledging holy days, and following healing or dying rituals (Taylor, 2002). Nurses need to be aware of the similarities and differences between major religions to provide appropriate spiritual care for older adults.

Practicing religious traditions influences all human dimensions: spiritual, emotional, social, and physical. Older adults who engage in religious practices may experience such benefits as improved mental health and social connection. Many older adults report that their religious beliefs and practices are very important to them and help them cope with the physical changes of aging or chronic disease (Phillips, Paukert, Stanley, & Kunik, 2009).

Expressive Arts

Nurses can use expressive arts to enhance the spirituality of older adults. Expressive arts include any creative or artistic endeavor, such as painting, knitting, dancing, crafts, poetry, music, dramatics, literature, and sewing. The spiritual benefits of artistic expressions are healing, self-awareness, resolution, connection, and tranquility (Taylor, 2002).

KEY POINTS

- Unlike the physical and mental dimensions, the spiritual dimension of life continues to grow and develop in later years.
- Assessment of spirituality is an expected aspect of health care.
- Spirituality is defined as all the experiences and expressions of one's spirit reflecting faith in God or a Supreme Being; connectedness with oneself, others, nature or God; and integration of the human dimensions.
- The spiritual dimension is the core of each human being and interventions directed at the spiritual dimension will affect one's physical, emotional, and social dimensions.
- Numerous theories including spirituality are used in the health care disciplines of medicine, psychology, social work, and nursing.
- Spirituality can assist older adults to cope with the challenges of aging and chronic disease by maintaining their health and quality of life.
- Older adults have the capacity to reorder their life and make meaning of their experiences of loss and crisis through spiritual coping.
- Assessment tools assist nurses in identifying those at risk for experiencing spiritual distress.
- Actively listening to another person can facilitate meeting their spiritual, psychological, and social needs.
- Interventions proven to be effective for older adults include being present, assisting their search for meaning and purpose in life, encouraging reminiscence, facilitating prayer, providing caring touch, encouraging religious activities, and promoting use of expressive arts.

CRITICAL THINKING ACTIVITIES

1. Explore your thoughts and feelings about spirituality and how it differs from religiousness.
2. Use one of the spiritual assessment tools to interview an older adult about his or her spirituality. How does the person use spirituality to cope with the aging process?
3. Examine regional and local spiritual resources to which you can refer patients for their spiritual needs.
4. Select a spiritual intervention you are interested in learning more about, and explore two related websites on the Internet. What did you discover about the intervention? How will you use this information with an older adult?

CASE STUDY | *BRENDA HENSON*

Brenda Henson is a 65-year-old retired school teacher from Montana who has recently relocated to her son's city to be closer to family members. She has a long history of type 2 diabetes and osteoarthritis that are well controlled with medications. Mrs. Henson is being seen at the health clinic today with complaints of difficulty walking upstairs because of the pain in her knees.

While you are conducting your assessment you ask Mrs. Henson about her medical conditions, feelings about relocating, and making new friends. She begins to cry as she expresses her sadness and loneliness from having no friends or church family in this city.

1. What other assessment questions would you want to ask at this time?
2. On the basis of what you have learned about spirituality, how do you think this patient is coping with her relocation?
3. What implications does this have for your nursing care?
4. Identify two interventions you could implement to address Mrs. Henson's spiritual needs.

REFERENCES

Ackley, B. J., & Ladwig, G. B. (2007). *Nursing diagnosis handbook.* (8th ed.) St. Louis, MO: Elsevier Health Sciences.

Bephage, G. (2009). Care approaches to spirituality and dementia. *British Journal of Healthcare Assistants, 3*(1), 43–46.

Centers for Disease Control and Prevention (2010). *Improving and extending quality of life among older Americans: At a glance 2010.* Retrieved on November 22, 2010, from http://www.cdc.gov/chronicdisease/resources/publications/aag/aging.htm

Frankl, V. E. (1962). *Man's search for meaning.* New York, NY: Pocket Books.

Gallup Poll. (2009). *Religion in America 2009.* Retrieved on December 3, 2010, from http://www.gallup.com/poll/1690/religion.aspx

Gaskamp, C., Sutter, R., & Meraviglia, M. (2004). *Promoting spirituality in the older adult lowa City, IA:* Evidence-Based Protocol, Gerontological Nursing Interventions Research Center, University of Iowa College of Nursing.

Gaskamp, C., Sutter, R., & Meraviglia, M. (2006). Evidence-based guideline: Promoting spirituality in the older adult. *Journal of Gerontological Nursing, 32*(11), 8–13.

Hemming, L., & Maher, D. (2005). Complementary therapies in palliative care: A summary of current evidence. *British Journal of Community Nursing, 10*(10), 414–418.

Hessel, J. A. (2009). Presence in nursing practice: A concept analysis. *Holistic Nursing Practice, 23*(5), 276–281.

Koenig, H. G. (2002). *Spirituality in patient care: Why, how, when, what?* Philadelphia, PA: Templeton Foundation Press.

Larocca-Pitts, M. A. (2008). FACT: Taking a spiritual history in a clinical setting. *Journal of Health Care Chaplaincy, 15,* 1–12.

Larson, D. B., Swyers, J. P., & McCullough, M. E. (Eds.). (1997). *Scientific research on spirituality and health: A consensus report.* Rockville, MD: National Institute for Healthcare Research.

Lawler-Row, K. A., & Elliott, J. (2009). The role of religious activity and spirituality in the health and well-being of older adults. *Journal of Health Psychology, 14,* 43–53.

Low, G., & Molzahn, A. E. (2007). Predictors of quality of life in old age: A cross-validation study. *Research in Nursing & Health, 30*(2), 141–150.

McClain, C. S., Rosenfeld, B., & Breitbart, W. (2003). Effect of spiritual well-being on end-of-life despair in terminally-ill cancer patients. *Lancet, 361,* 1603-1607.

McSherry, W. (2007). *The meaning of spirituality and spiritual care within nursing and health care practice.* London, England: Quay Books.

Meraviglia, M. G. (2004). The effects of spirituality on well-being of people with lung cancer. *Oncology Nursing Forum, 31*(1), 89–94.

NANDA International. (2009). *Nursing diagnoses: Definitions & classification 2009-2011.* Indianapolis, IN: Wiley-Blackwell.

Pargament, K. I., Koenig, H. G., & Perez, L. M. (2000). The many methods of religious coping: Development and initial validation of the RCOPE. *Journal of Clinical Psychology 56,* 519–543.

Phillips, L., Paukert, A., Stanley, M., & Kunik, M. (2009). Incorporating religion and spirituality to improve care for anxiety and depression in older adults. *Geriatrics, 64*(8), 15–18.

Pinquart, M., & Sorensen, S. (2001). Influences on loneliness in older adults: A meta-analysis. *Basic and Applied Social Psychology, 23,* 245–266.

Puchalski, C. M. (2002). Spirituality and end-of-life care: A time for listening and caring. *Journal of Palliative Medicine, 5,* 289–294.

Reed, P. (1987). Spirituality & well-being in terminally ill hospitalized adults. *Research in Nursing & Health, 10,* 335–344.

Russell, A. (1986). Sociology and the study of spirituality. In C. Jones, G. Wainwright, & E. Yarnold (Eds.), *The study of spirituality* (pp. 33–38). New York, NY: Oxford University Press.

Staten, P. (2003). Spiritual assessment required in all settings. *Hospital Peer Review, 28*(4), 55–57.

Stinson, C. K. (2009). Structured group reminiscence: An intervention for older adults. *Journal of Continuing Education in Nursing, 40*(11), 521–528.

Stoll, R. (1989). The essence of spirituality. In V. B. Carson (Ed.), *Spiritual dimensions of nursing practice* (pp. 4–23). Philadelphia, PA: Saunders.

Stranahan, S. (2008). A spiritual screening tool for older adults. *Journal of Religion and Health, 47,* 491–503.

Taylor, E. J. (2002). *Spiritual care: Nursing theory, research, and practice.* Upper Saddle River, NJ: Prentice Hall Pearson.

Chapter 24

Planning for the End of Life

Jean W. Lange, RN, PhD, FAAN

LEARNING OBJECTIVES

- Distinguish end-of-life care from palliative care.
- Describe barriers to quality care at the end of life.
- Discuss the biological, psychosocial, cultural, and spiritual dimensions of end-of-life care.
- Identify resources to assist families and patients in the terminal stages of illness.
- Explain team members' roles on a palliative care team.
- Discuss guidelines and expected nurse competencies regarding end-of-life care.
- List common symptoms present in the final months, days, and hours of life.
- Discuss nursing interventions to support dying patients and their families.
- Consider the ethical and legal dilemmas surrounding death and dying.

Life ends for everyone, suddenly and without warning for some, or at the end of a protracted illness for others. Most people begin to contemplate what the end of their lives might be like at some point. Ideally, as people approach their later years or are nearing the end of an incurable illness, they have thought about what they would prefer if they should need treatments such as dialysis, mechanical ventilation, medically provided hydration and nutrition, or resuscitation in order to survive. Considering questions about who should make decisions on one's behalf if one is no longer able to do so, planning for future care needs, and making financial arrangements for surviving dependents are important matters when preparing for the end of life. Discussing preferences with significant others and health care providers and putting these advance directives in writing will help to ensure that one's wishes are known.

Since 1991, the Patient Self-Determination Act has required health care agencies to inform patients of their right to make treatment choices through advance directives such as living wills, medical or durable power of attorney, or do-not-resuscitate (DNR) orders (Robert Wood Johnson Foundation, 2002). Out-of-hospital DNR orders are valid in most states and can be given to emergency medical personnel to prevent an undesirable resuscitation. Advance directives are designed to communicate the type of care patients want when they cannot speak for themselves and to appoint someone to make treatment decisions on their behalf. (See Chapter 18 for more information.)

Quality Care at the End of Life

Quality care at the end of life involves freedom from uncomfortable physical symptoms, adjusting to functional limitations, feeling supported through personal relationships, and being at ease with one's self and place within the larger world or universe (Sulmasy, 2002). Although not everyone lives to old age, most deaths do occur among older adults. Erikson, Erikson, and Kivnick (1986) describe the central tasks in late adulthood as threefold:

- Evaluating life's accomplishments
- Coping with physical, functional, and social losses
- Preparing for death

They theorized that people who master these challenges emerge with integrity, while those who somehow fall short feel a sense of despair. Terminal illness presents a final opportunity to complete these life tasks.

PERSONAL PERSPECTIVE

Doing the Heart Work of Life Completion

The work of life completion encompasses both the practical tasks of end-of-life planning and the acts from the heart that serve to complete us spiritually. Ellsworth, age 74 (and pictured in Chapter 10), has taken important steps toward completing the tasks of the heart. For many people, these are the hardest steps of all. Ellsworth talks about his relationship to death and the tasks of life completion: "I know," he says, "death is not something we want to talk about, but I know I'm not going to live forever. Death doesn't bother me because I live today. I'm not concerned about when I leave here. There's nothing I can do about it. When I go, I go. I just don't want to suffer. I don't want my family to suffer, watching me suffer. I feel good about life. I'm not going to say I've accomplished everything I wanted to, or even if I live to be one hundred that I will. But I feel good about what I've done, and if I went today, I would have no regrets."

"Ten years ago," he continues, "when my mom passed at the age of eighty-six, I started taking an inventory of myself and one of the things I came up with was the fact that there were things I wanted to say to her and never did say, or [I didn't] show my love for her as much as I should have, and I knew that I would never be able to do it. Then, two years ago, when my brother passed, the same frightening thought came to me. When he was first diagnosed with cancer, I didn't communicate with him as much as I should have, and I thought 'oh my God this is ridiculous'. I realized I didn't tell my children I love them as much as I should have. But in the last two years particularly, every time I see or talk to one of my children or someone in my family, I tell them I love them. And I give them a hug when I see them. And I feel better, and I know they feel better. So, I think by the time I leave this earth I will have fulfilled that promise I made to myself when my mom passed away."

About Ellsworth Ellsworth Lindsey is the divorced father of five children, and he now has seven grandchildren. Before retiring he had a varied career that included work as a head waiter at the Woodbridge Country Club, furniture salesperson, manager of a senior center lunch program, and line dancing teacher. After retirement, Ellsworth actively gave back to his community taking on the role of manager of the soup kitchen at his church. At the assisted-living complex where he now resides, Ellsworth leads an exercise class and is affectionately referred to as "The Mayor" because of his readiness to help, be involved, and get things done.

Lorri B. Danzig, MS, CSL

A team of health care professionals is often required to enable patients and their families achieve an optimal end-of-life care experience. Commonly, the nurse is the provider closest to the dying patient and his or her family and is in the best position to identify when the services of other disciplines are necessary. Patients experiencing uncomfortable physical symptoms may require the coordinated approach of a pain management team. A trained counselor or chaplain may assist the patient and family in dealing with the reality of impending death. Physical and occupational therapists can help patients accommodate to functional losses. Trained volunteers can offer social support to patients with insufficient interpersonal resources. Community resources to support physical care needs and provide financial assistance can often be negotiated by social workers. The capacity to manage common problems at the end of life, such as mental or cognitive changes, immobility, or social isolation, is greatly enhanced through a patient- and family-centered team approach.

Commonly, the nurse is the provider closest to the dying patient and his or her family and is in the best position to identify when the services of other disciplines are necessary.

End-of-Life and Palliative Care

End-of-life care is often confused with the broader term, *palliative care.* Similar to end-of-life care, palliative care incorporates interdisciplinary strategies designed to relieve physical and mental suffering and to enhance the quality of remaining life for persons of all ages. Likewise, palliative care considers spiritual needs and supports families during bereavement. Unlike end-of-life care, however, palliative care may begin in the *early* phases of a life-limiting or debilitating illness and *coexist* with life-prolonging treatment. Thus, in patients with chronic illness, palliative care may continue for many years. Guidelines for palliative care encompass end-of-life care, are patient centered, and involve multiple health care disciplines working together as a team (End-of-Life Nursing Education Consortium, 2006; National Consensus Project for Quality Palliative Care, 2009; World Health Organization, 2009).

End-of-life care takes place in the hours, days, weeks, or months leading up to and including death itself. End-of-life care is often considered to begin when the patient, family, and provider agree that medical treatment is no longer desired or beneficial. At this point, the goal is to optimize the patient's comfort and to facilitate a dignified and peaceful death that respects patient and family preferences (National Institutes of Health, 2004).

The Role of Hospice Care

The hospice movement began in Europe and was introduced in the United States in the 1970s. The goal of this movement was to enable more patients to die at home by providing the care, support, and comfort services that were otherwise unavailable (Kovacs, Bellin, & Fauri, 2006). Hospice services are designed to optimize the end-of-life care experience. The hospice philosophy empowers patients and families to be active participants and decision makers in the dying process. From a hospice perspective, family includes "all those in loving relationships with the person who is dying, the people who can be counted on for caring and support, regardless of blood or legal ties" (Lattanzi-Licht, Mahoney, & Miller, 1998, p. 29). This definition includes birth families, as well as adoptive or chosen families, and is consistent with the diversity of family structures seen in our society today (Kovacs, Bellin, & Fauri, 2006).

Hospice services encompass physical, psychosocial, emotional, and spiritual needs at the end of life. Family bereavement services are also included and may continue for up to 1 year after the patient's death if needed. An interprofessional team typically includes social workers, bereavement counselors, spiritual leaders, nurses, physicians, nursing assistants, trained volunteers, and pharmacists who collaborate to deliver services that are consistent with patient and family preferences. Hospice services can be provided in any setting of care, including private residence, nursing home, assisted-living facility, or hospice facility.

In the United States, Medicare pays for hospice care of all residents over the age of 65 with a life expectancy of 6 months or less if the focus of treatment is comfort rather than cure (End-of-Life Nursing Education Consortium, 2002). In addition, the Older Americans Act, amended in 2006, provides family members caring for older relatives at home with respite services, training, counseling, and education. These services are coordinated by a national network of state and area Agencies on Aging (Administration on Aging, 2009).

Dying in America

Most of the dying patients you will care for as a nurse will be older adults. With an average life expectancy in the United States of nearly 78 years, most deaths occur among adults over age 65 (Heron et al., 2009). In addition, the number of older adults in their 80s, 90s, and beyond who are living with chronic disease and in need of palliative care is on the rise. The end-of-life experience of many older adults, however, is often inconsistent with their wishes. The data show that although most people prefer to die comfortably at home after a brief illness and surrounded by loved ones, more than three quarters actually die in hospitals or nursing homes after a prolonged illness (Robert Wood Johnson Foundation, 2002). Most patients who die in hospitals and nursing homes would not require this institutional care if adequate resources were arranged in their homes (Emanuel, von Gunten, & Ferris, 2000).

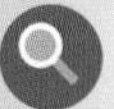

EVIDENCE FOR PRACTICE
Advance Directives

Purpose: To examine the role of advance directives 10 years after passage of the Patient Self-Determination Act.

Sample: A nationwide sample of 1,587 bereaved family members or knowledgeable informants about the advance directives of a patient who had recently died in a nursing home, hospital, or at home was recruited.

Methods: A descriptive design was used to conduct telephone interviews with survivors regarding the existence of written advance directives, use of life-sustaining treatment, and quality of care (whether symptom relief was sufficient, the patient's wishes were respected, and care was coordinated and included adequate family information and support).

Results: Nearly 71% of patients had some form of advance directive. Persons who died at home with hospice or in a nursing home were more likely to have an advance directive. Patients with advance directives were less likely to use life-sustaining treatment, such as mechanical ventilation (11.8% versus 22.0%) or an artificial feeding via a tube (17% versus 27%). Patients with advance directives were also less likely to die in a hospital and more likely to seek hospice care. Family members of decedents with written advance directives felt better informed about what to expect as part of the dying process, whereas those without advance directives were less satisfied with physician communications. Regardless of whether or not a patient had written advance directives, 25% of family members reported undertreated pain, 50% reported inadequate emotional support of the patient, and 33% stated that emotional support of the family was inadequate.

Implications: These results suggest that patient and family care needs at the end of life are often unmet. Preparation of advance directives may increase the likelihood that patient wishes about life-sustaining treatments are respected, that patient-family-physician communication is improved, and that a hospice-supported death occurs outside of a hospital setting.

Reference: Teno, J. M., Gruneir, A., Schwartz, Z., Nanda, A., & Wetle, T. (2007). Association between advance directives and quality of end-of-life care: A national study. *Journal of the American Geriatric Society, 55*(2), 189–194.

In addition to in-home resources, geography and social factors play a role in how one dies. Dying at home is more likely among Caucasians, those dying of cancer, and those who have strong social support systems. By contrast, lower education and minority status are associated with a greater likelihood of dying in a hospital. Older adults who have long-term care insurance are more likely to die in nursing homes (Grunier et al., 2007). Patients living in less populated areas such as Alaska, Oregon, or Utah are more likely to die at home (30+%) than patients living urban in areas such as Washington, DC, where than less than 12% die at home (Center for Gerontology and Health Care Research at the Brown Medical School, 2004).

Given the discrepancy between patient wishes and the actual circumstances surrounding most deaths, it is not surprising that patients and families report dissatisfaction with end-of-life care. Central concerns include inadequate management of symptoms, poor care coordination, inconsistent communication with health care providers, lack of respect, and insufficient support (Teno, Gruneir, Schwartz, Nanda, & Wetle, 2004). In a nationwide sample, Teno and colleagues reported that across all care settings, nearly one fourth of 1,578 survivors believed that their deceased relative received insufficient relief from pain (24.2%) or dyspnea (22.4%), half reported inadequate emotional support, and one fourth had concerns about physician communication regarding decision making. Family members of patients who received hospice services, however, reported greater satisfaction with all aspects of their end-of-life care experience.

Given the discrepancy between patient wishes and the actual circumstances surrounding most deaths, it is not surprising that patients and families report dissatisfaction with end-of-life care.

Barriers to Quality End-of-Life Care

One barrier to optimal end-of-life care is the inadequate education of health care providers regarding the management of dying patients. Two studies reveal that hospital nurses often feel unprepared to discuss death concerns with their patients (Thacker, 2008; White, Coyne, & Patel, 2001). The End-of-Life Nursing Education Consortium (2002) and the Toolkit for Nursing Excellence at End of Life Transitions (Wilkie et al., 2001) were designed to address this need by providing detailed curricula, case studies, and resources for faculty and students. Information about how to access these programs is included in the CD-ROM accompanying this text. The Hospice and Palliative Nurses Association (HPNA) also offers educational programs on palliative care and certification as a Hospice and Palliative Nurse by examination. A similar certification is available to physicians. Unfortunately, numbers of certified nurses and physicians continue to be well below numbers of these providers who practice in hospice and palliative care settings (Metzger & Kaplan, 2001).

Lack of access to palliative care services also contributes to suboptimal end-of-life care. In a survey of American hospitals in 2000, only 42% reported having a formalized pain management program (American Hospital Association, 2002). Pain management teams can help providers make better decisions about appropriate selection and dosing of pain medication and reduce the incidence of over- and under-medication (Ferrell, McCaffery, & Grant, 1991). Inadequate treatment of pain occurs at an alarming rate among nursing home residents. More than 40% of residents in one study failed to receive relief of documented pain within a 6-month period (Miller, Mor, Wu, Gozalo, & Lapone, 2002; Teno et al., 2004). Similarly, studies of cancer patients in intensive care units reveal that half to three quarters of participants experienced untreated moderate to severe pain, discomfort, anxiety, sleep disturbance, or unsatisfied hunger or thirst. Many patients also receive life-supporting treatments that are inconsistent with their advance directives (Fagerlin & Schneider, 2004; Kish, Martin, Shaw, & Price, 2001; Nelson et al., 2001; Schwartz et al., 2002). In a study of more than 1,100 patients across 12 nursing homes, advance care planning among residents, families, and health care providers was rarely discussed (Reynolds, Hanson, Henderson, & Steinhauser, 2008). From these studies, it appears that patient preferences are not routinely known or considered by health care providers in making end-of-life care decisions.

Guidelines and Competencies in End-of-Life Care

Clearly, there is a large gap between optimal end-of-life care and the current reality. Standards designed to guide practitioners in providing optimal end-of life care have been published by specialty groups as well as national and international organizations (Truog et al., 2008; U.S. National Consensus Project for Quality Palliative Care, 2009; World Health Organization, 2004). These documents state that patients and families should be central to end-of-life care. Other key recommendations include

- Respecting patient and family preferences
- Ensuring equal access to quality end-of-life care
- Providing care that is continuous across settings
- Using an interprofessional team approach
- Providing comfort measures
- Planning care consistent with the patient and family's cultural beliefs
- Supporting patients' and families' spiritual needs
- Addressing patients' and families' financial and bereavement concerns (Truog et al., 2008; U.S. National Consensus Project for Quality Palliative Care, 2009; Table 24-1).

TABLE 24-1 Clinical Practice Guidelines for Quality Palliative Care

DOMAIN	GUIDELINE
DOMAIN 1 Structure and processes of care	1.1 The timely plan of care is based on a comprehensive interdisciplinary assessment of the patient and family. 1.2 The care plan is based on the identified and expressed preferences, values, goals, and needs of the patient and family and is developed with professional guidance and support for decision making. 1.3 An interdisciplinary team provides services to the patient and family consistent with the care plan. In addition to nursing, medicine, and social work, other therapeutic disciplines with important assessment of patients and families include physical therapists, occupational therapists, speech and language pathologists, nutritionists, psychologists, chaplains, and nursing assistants. For pediatrics, this should include child-life specialists. Complementary and alternative therapies may be included. 1.4 The use of appropriately trained and supervised volunteers within the interdisciplinary team is strongly encouraged. 1.5 Support for education and training is available to the interdisciplinary team. 1.6 In its commitment to quality assessment and performance improvement, the palliative care program develops, implements, and maintains an ongoing data driven process that reflects the complexity of the organization and focuses on palliative care outcomes. 1.7 The palliative care program recognizes the emotional impact on the palliative care team of providing care to patients with life-threatening illnesses and their families.

TABLE 24-1 Clinical Practice Guidelines for Quality Palliative Care—cont'd

DOMAIN	GUIDELINE
	1.8 Palliative care programs should have a relationship with one or more hospices and other community resources to ensure continuity of the highest-quality palliative care across the illness trajectory. 1.9 The physical environment in which care is provided should meet the preferences, needs, and circumstances of the patient and family to the extent possible.
DOMAIN 2 Physical aspects of care	2.1 Pain, other symptoms, and side effects are managed based on the basis of the best available evidence, with attention to disease-specific pain and symptoms, which is skillfully and systematically applied.
DOMAIN 3 Psychological and psychiatric aspects of care	3.1 Psychological status is assessed and managed based on the basis of the best available evidence, which is skillfully and systematically applied. When necessary, psychiatric issues are addressed and treated. 3.2 A grief and bereavement program is available to patients and families on the basis of the assessed need for services.
DOMAIN 4 Social aspects of care	4.1 Comprehensive interdisciplinary assessment identifies the social needs of patients and their families, and a care plan is developed to respond to these needs as effectively as possible.
DOMAIN 5 Spiritual, religious, and existential aspects of care	5.1 Spiritual and existential dimensions are assessed and responded to on the basis of the best available evidence, which is skillfully and systematically applied.
DOMAIN 6 Cultural aspects of care	6.1 The palliative care program assesses and attempts to meet the needs of the patient, family, and community in a culturally sensitive manner.
DOMAIN 7 Care of the imminently dying patient	7.1 Signs and symptoms of impending death are recognized and communicated in developmentally appropriate language for children and patients with cognitive disabilities with respect to family preferences. Care appropriate for this phase of illness is provided to patient and family. 7.2 Post-death care is delivered in a respectful manner. Cultural and religious practices particular to the post-death period are assessed and documented. Care of the body post-death is delivered with respect to these practices, as well as in accordance to both organizational practice and local law. 7.3 A post-death bereavement plan is activated. An interdisciplinary team member is assigned to the family in the post-death period to help with religious practices, funeral arrangements, and burial planning.
DOMAIN 8 Ethical and legal aspects of care	8.1 The patient's goals, preferences and choices are respected within the limits of applicable state and federal law, within current accepted standards of medical care, and form the basis for the plan of care. 8.2 The palliative care program is aware of and addresses the complex ethical issues arising in the care of people with life-threatening debilitating illness. 8.3 The palliative care program is knowledgeable about legal and regulatory aspects of palliative care.

Reprinted with permission from U.S. National Consensus Project for Quality Palliative Care. (2009). *Clinical practice guidelines for quality palliative care* (2nd ed.). Retrieved December 10, 2010, from http://www.nationalconsensusproject.org/guideline.pdf

Nurses are often called upon to help patients and families prepare for a patient's final hours. The American Association of Colleges of Nursing (AACN) published 15 competencies (Box 24-1) asserting that "nurses have a unique and primary responsibility for ensuring that individuals at the end of life experience a peaceful death" (American Association of Colleges of Nursing, 2004). The primary goal of nurses caring for terminally ill patients involves helping families and patients realize the best possible quality of life in the time remaining. Accomplishing this requires addressing the physical, spiritual, psychological, and emotional needs of patients and their families. This includes providing comfort measures, ensuring that patients and families have the necessary medical information to make informed decisions about their care, facilitating meaningful conversations between family members to achieve closure, dispelling misconceptions, accessing resources to enable completion of end-of-life tasks, addressing spiritual needs, and supporting patients and families as they say their goodbyes and begin to grieve their loss. Facilitating active communication among the interprofessional team, families, and patients throughout the dying period is a critical role of the nurse.

Dimensions of End-of-Life Care

Identifying end-of-life care needs can be complex because it encompasses multiple dimensions (psychosocial, biological, cultural, and spiritual). A first step is to ascertain the patient's and family's understanding of and expectations about the patient's illness. Are they realistic and consistent with the prognosis? Do the patient and family share similar or diverse perspectives? When discrepancies are present, a conversation about differing perspectives can be helpful in revealing the values and wishes of the patient and family. Involving the physician in this discussion can aid in clarifying the prognosis and helping the physician gain a clearer understanding of advance directives.

Psychosocial Dimension

Sometimes it is difficult to decide when to approach patients or families about end-of-life concerns. Questions such as asking for more information about a terminal prognosis, how to manage the care needs of a dying relative at home, or how to safeguard a surviving loved one after a patient's death provide clues that the patient or family are ready to begin a discussion about end-of-life care planning. In the absence of overt cues, you may sense that the patient and family

BOX 24-1 Competencies Needed for Nurses to Provide Quality Care to Patients and Families at the End of Life

- Recognize dynamic changes in population demographics, health care economics, and service delivery that necessitate improved professional preparation for end-of-life care.
- Promote provision of comfort care to the dying as an active, desirable, and important skill and an integral component of nursing care.
- Communicate effectively and compassionately with the patient, family, and health care team about end-of-life issues.
- Recognize one's own attitudes, feelings, values, and expectations about death and the individual, cultural, and spiritual diversity existing in these beliefs and customs.
- Demonstrate respect for the patient's views and wishes during end-of-life care.
- Collaborate with interdisciplinary team members while implementing the nursing role in end-of-life care.
- Use scientifically based standardized tools to assess symptoms (e.g., pain, dyspnea, constipation, anxiety, fatigue, nausea/vomiting, and altered cognition) experienced by patients at the end of life.
- Use data from symptom assessment to plan and intervene in symptom management using state-of-the-art traditional and complementary approaches.
- Evaluate the impact of traditional, complementary, and technological therapies on patient-centered outcomes.
- Assess and treat multiple dimensions, including physical, psychological, social, and spiritual needs, to improve quality at the end of life.
- Assist patient, family, colleagues, and self to cope with suffering, grief, loss, and bereavement in end-of-life care.
- Apply legal and ethical principles in the analysis of complex issues in end-of-life care, recognizing the influence of personal values, professional codes, and patient preferences.
- Identify barriers and facilitators to patients' and caregivers' effective use of resources.
- Demonstrate skill at implementing a plan for improved end-of-life care within a dynamic and complex health-care delivery system.
- Apply knowledge gained from palliative care research to end-of-life education and care.

Reprinted with permission from American Association of Colleges of Nursing. (1998). Competencies necessary for nurses to provide high-quality care to patients and families during the transition at the end of life. Retrieved July 15, 2009, from http://www.aacn.nche.edu/Publications/deathfin.htm

are having difficulty starting a conversation about the recent news of a poor prognosis. If so, you may decide to facilitate that discussion by asking the patient or family about their reactions to the news.

Knowing that one's life will soon end is daunting for most patients and their families, so it is not surprising that many will need help in dealing with this reality. Psychosocial considerations include:

- Evaluating how the patient and family are coping
- Determining whether the patient is experiencing mental status changes, anxiety, or depression that may warrant intervention
- Evaluating family dynamics, support systems, and resources
- Appraising the adequacy of communications with the medical provider
- Discussing whether advance directives exist

Many patients do not complete living wills or converse with their provider and family about their wishes. In cases where the patient can no longer communicate his or her wishes, decisions are often based on the medical provider's views regarding the treatment benefit versus the potential cost and burden to the patient and family. Nurses are in a unique position to explore patient preferences and to facilitate discussions with the family and medical provider so that patient and family preferences are part of the decision-making process. Determining the availability of financial and social supports can also help the nurse decide what additional resources may be necessary. Access to resources such as caregiver or bereavement support groups, hospice services, or respite programs can greatly enhance patient and family experiences.

Biological Dimension

Many patients have unpleasant symptoms near the end of life that are undertreated and prevent a peaceful death (Box 24-2). Adverse symptoms commonly experienced near the end-of-life include breathlessness, anorexia, nausea or vomiting, coughing, constipation, dry mouth, thirst, skin breakdown, urticaria, pain, insomnia, fatigue, confusion, anxiety, and depression (Field & Cassel, 1997). Older adults are more likely to be undertreated than younger adults (Reynolds, Hanson, Henderson, & Steinhauser, 2008). Cognitive impairment, the inability to speak English, or a history of substance abuse also increases the risk of inadequate treatment (End-of-Life Nursing Education Consortium, 2002). Unrelieved symptoms may lead to other serious problems, such as depression, social isolation, disturbed sleep, decreased mobility, falls, difficulty in thinking clearly, and loss of appetite (Robert Wood Johnson Foundation, 2002). It is important therefore to note the occurrence and severity of adverse symptoms and the context in which they occur. Assess what treatments have already been prescribed, if they are effective, or whether the patient is experiencing any side effects. Inquire if the patient has found anything else that helps to alleviate the symptoms and the patient and family's preferences regarding symptom management. The point at which symptom relief occurs is often subjective; therefore, the goal of symptom management in dying patients should be to achieve "adequate" relief as determined by the patient rather than the provider.

BOX 24-2 Common Symptoms at the End of Life

Anorexia/cachexia is commonly found in patients with advanced disease. *Anorexia* is a lack of appetite, and *cachexia* is a disease-related loss of weight and muscle.

Constipation occurs in up to 50% to 78% of terminally ill adults.

Coughing and cough-related problems (pain, fatigue, vomiting, insomnia) are experienced by 39% to 80% of patients in palliative care.

Diarrhea is less common in the palliative-care setting than constipation but is especially problematic in patients with HIV/AIDS.

Dyspnea (breathlessness) is most common in patients with lung or heart disease, stroke, dementia, end-stage renal disease, or metastatic cancer. Fifty percent of the general outpatient cancer population and 70% of advanced cancer patients report dyspnea.

Fatigue is common in end-stage coronary artery disease, cancer, HIV/AIDS, rheumatoid arthritis, and renal disease.

Nausea is present in up to 70% of terminally ill patients. Vomiting occurs in about 30% of patients.

Psychological symptoms include fear, loss of independence or control, changes in body image, and depression. *Depression* is estimated to affect 25% to 77% of terminally ill patients.

Sources of some of the symptoms common at the end of life may include:

- Adverse drug effects from such medications as amphetamines, analgesics, antidiabetics, antihypertensives, antimicrobials, antiparkinsonian drugs, benzodiazepines, chemotherapy drugs, cimetidine, ethanol, hormones, levodopa, phenothiazines, and steroids
- Radiation
- Metabolic and endocrine abnormalities

Adapted with permission from End-of-Life Nursing Education Consortium. (2002). Training program. Duarte, CA: City of Hope and the American Association of Colleges of Nursing.

The point at which symptom relief occurs is often subjective; therefore, the goal of symptom management in dying patients should be to achieve "adequate" relief as determined by the patient rather than the provider.

Most physical symptoms that cause discomfort at the end of life can be managed effectively; however, many symptoms are overlooked or discounted among older adults. Pain is one of the most frequent yet undertreated symptoms experienced at the end of life. The World Health Organization (2008) suggests a three-step approach to pain management called the pain ladder (World Health Organization, 2010). In this approach, management begins with milder nonopioid medications such as aspirin, nonsteroidal anti-inflammatory drugs, or acetaminophen. Adjuvant drugs and increasingly potent opioids are added as needed to control the patient's pain. Adjuvant drugs that are useful in pain management include some steroids, antihistamines, antidepressants, and anticonvulsants. Complementary therapies such as relaxation techniques, massage, heat or cold, or exercise can generally be used at any stage and may be useful in controlling other symptoms as well as pain (Box 24-3). The analgesic ladder is considered to be the model for effective pharmacological management of pain. Intractable pain may be treated with sedation and is best managed by an interprofessional team.

Cultural Dimension

Studies have shown that cultural beliefs, values, and traditions can influence patient preferences about how symptoms are managed. Culture can also affect a person's openness to discussions about death, how decisions are made about treatment, filial expectations about the care and support of a dying family member, and the preferred circumstances surrounding death (Allen, Allen, Hilgeman, & DeCoster, 2008; Kagawa-Singer & Blackhall, 2001; Valente &

BOX 24-3 Physical and Psychological Modalities for Symptom Management

Active listening may reduce the stress of hospitalization or illness.

Cold causes vasoconstriction that reduces muscle spasm, bleeding, inflammation, and edema and increases peristalsis of the stomach, small bowel, and colon. Beneficial effects last longer than those from heat.

Controlled breathing increases oxygenation and improves elimination of carbon dioxide. This is a useful technique when transferring patients in or out of a bed or chair.

Distraction reduces pain intensity but does not eliminate symptoms. The mode of distraction needs to be interesting to the patient and consistent with the patient's energy level and ability to concentrate and may include television, games, music, imagery, visiting with friends and family, and so on.

Exercise activities that are of interest to patients can help to reduce their fatigue. Exercise programs need to be carefully planned with medical oversight to ensure compatibility with the patient's capabilities.

Heat helps to reduce striated muscle spasm, relax smooth muscles, reduce peristalsis, and reduce gastric acidity. Warm blankets, electric heating pads, moist hot packs, or shower or bath may be used, but care must be taken to protect the skin from being injured by prolonged heat exposure or intensity.

Massage can decrease muscle tension and pain for a short period after treatment, and it facilitates mental and physical relaxation.

Patient education may be beneficial in reducing the patient's anxiety level. Patient questions should guide the extent of information given.

Positioning can increase patient comfort and decrease anxiety. Examples include ensuring appropriate body alignment, supporting extremities, changing positions periodically, and placing items within reach.

Reinforcing or modifying symptom-control behaviors used by the patient (e.g., rubbing, positioning, splinting).

Relaxation strategies reduce muscle tension and may include progressive muscle relaxation, visualization, and biofeedback.

Specialty beds are often overlooked as a pain control strategy. Mattress options include fluidized, air, and foam overlays. Wrinkled bedding can be irritating. Pillows can be used to stabilize a joint, prevent deformity, or splint an incision. A pillow from home may provide psychological comfort.

Support services may be helpful from such consultants as social workers, psychologists, psychiatrists, massage therapists, biofeedback therapists, therapeutic touch practitioners, music therapists, and physical therapists

Adapted with permission from End-of-Life Nursing Education Consortium. (2002). Training program. Duarte, CA: City of Hope and the American Association of Colleges of Nursing.

Haley, n.d.; Werth, Blevins, Toussaint, & Durham, 2002). Blackhall and colleagues (1999) surveyed 800 Americans from European, African, Mexican, and Korean descent about their end-of-life beliefs and preferences. Korean and Mexican Americans were less likely to believe that a patient should be told of a terminal diagnosis and prognosis than African and European Americans and more likely to believe that families rather than patients should make decisions about life-sustaining treatment. Ethnicity was more important than religion, gender, or age in shaping these participants' attitudes. Other studies have found a relationship between ethnicity and the likelihood of having advance directives or wanting life-sustaining treatment during the terminal phase of an illness (Degenholtz, Arnold, Meisel, & Lave, 2002).

These studies help us to understand that culture can affect end-of-life preferences; however, it is important to recognize that individual differences exist within cultural groups. Seeking answers to the following questions can help you to understand your patient's preferences for end-of-life care:

- How open are the patient and family to discussions about end-of-life concerns?
- How much do they want to know about the patient's illness?
- To whom is full disclosure about the diagnosis and prognosis acceptable?
- Who do the patient and family feel should be included in end-of-life discussions?
- Who makes end-of-life care decisions?
- What role does the family wish to play in end-of-life care?
- Do community healers or spiritual leaders have a role in decision making?
- How are death and dying perceived in the culture?
- What are the beliefs and values regarding continuation or withdrawal of curative treatment?
- What rituals regarding dying, death, and grieving are followed?

Assessing the role of culture in end-of-life care helps to provide insight about patient and family preferences and patterns of bereavement, promote trust, improve communication, and prevent misunderstandings.

Spiritual Dimension

Approaching the end of life often leads people to review their accomplishments and consider what they will leave behind as a legacy. It also may raise larger questions about the meaning of life; purpose of human existence; possibility of afterlife; and connectedness to a higher being, power, or consciousness. Such questions are central to a person's spirituality.

Spirituality is an expression of how people relate to a larger whole or something greater than themselves, and how they find meaning in the midst of their suffering (End-of-Life Nursing Education Consortium, 2002).

Spirituality encompasses one's religious beliefs but is a broader concept that also involves the way people understand their lives to have meaning and value (McClain, Rosenfeld, & Breitbart, 2003). Purpose and meaning in life can be expressed through religious commitment, family bonds, nature, art, music, or in other ways that are uniquely personal (Puchalski, 2002).

Scholars suggest that spiritual expression contributes to emotional well-being among older adults and those with terminal illness (Morales, Lara, Kington, Valdez, & Escarce, 2002). Recent studies report that spiritual well-being strengthens psychological functioning and one's ability to cope with illness (Dingley & Roux, 2003; Hampton & Weinert, 2006; McClain et al., 2003). Patients dealing with terminal illness credit spirituality with being a source of comfort, solace, understanding, and support that strengthens their ability to transcend their illness (Hampton & Weinert, 2006). Feeling connected to a greater whole and believing in a higher purpose in life have also contributed to positive feelings of well-being and hopefulness among some patients (McClain et al., 2003).

It is clear that spiritual expression can be beneficial in dealing with illness and that providing opportunities for that expression is an important role of the nurse in caring for a dying patient and his or her family. Achieving a peaceful death may mean grappling with spiritual questions about life, such as

- What does life mean? Is it more than biological functioning?
- Can one cease being a person while still in some sense being alive?
- What meaning do we give to dependency on others? To decline and aging, to pain and suffering, to illness and death? (End-of-Life Nursing Education Consortium, 2002).

Offering patients the opportunity to discuss their thoughts and concerns about these issues can help patients and their families become more accepting of imminent death. Puchalski and Romer (2000) have developed some useful questions to help open this dialogue. Spiritual and religious leaders such as clergy, chaplains, parish nurses, and spiritual advisors are important resources for patients who are exploring these central questions. Parish nurses are trained registered nurses that support members of a congregation undergoing stressful situations, such as a dying family member. Their services include health education, counseling, support groups, and linkages to needed community resources. Spiritual and religious leaders can help patients plan their preferred death and support family members throughout the grieving process.

The Final Hours

Dying is unique for each of us. The role of the nurse during this time is to comfort and support the patient and family in a manner consistent with their personal, cultural, and spiritual beliefs. Most patients know where, with whom, and how they want to die (End-of-Life Nursing Education Consortium, 2006).

When patients cannot die at home, bringing meaningful belongings to a patient's room, such as favorite photographs, a pillow or blanket, or arranging visits from grandchildren or pets can make an institutional setting feel more familiar. Providing a single room where family members may remain as long as needed offers the space and privacy for closure and last goodbyes.

The nurse balances a watchful, caring presence with sensitivity to the patient and family's need to be alone. Questions about what to anticipate should be answered honestly and with compassion rather than with false hope. Focusing the patient and family's thoughts on a shared hope, such as to see one more sunrise together, to greet a distant son en route to the patient's bedside, or to spend the final hours of life pain-free, may help to ease the dying process.

Although no one can predict the exact time of death, there are typical signs and symptoms. Anxiety and fear about the unknown or in anticipation of life's end is not uncommon (Deeken, 2009; Valente, n.d.). Studies show that patients may sense when death is near and begin to withdraw from their surroundings (Lowey, 2008; Sand, Olsson, & Strang, 2009). Physical symptoms may include cognitive changes such as confusion, disorientation, delirium, restlessness, or agitation. Patients may tire more easily, sleep for longer periods, lose the desire for food or drink, and experience changes in bowel patterns, including incontinence. Periods of somnolence may alternate with times of alertness (Field & Cassel, 1997). Families may misinterpret these latter periods as a sign that the patient is recovering. These signs and symptoms of approaching death can appear hours to months before death occurs.

When death is within hours or days, symptoms include decreased urine output, cold and mottled extremities, decreasing heart rate and blood pressure, changes in breathing patterns, respiratory congestion, and sometimes hallucinations (Lichter & Hunt, 1990). Families and caregivers of dying patients may find it helpful to learn about these signs and symptoms so that they know what to expect and can anticipate imminent death.

Families may fear not knowing what to do when the end is near, being alone with the patient at the moment of death, causing discomfort by touching the patient, or hastening the death of a homebound patient by giving medication (End-of-Life Nursing Education Consortium, 2002). It is important to discuss these fears with families and dispel misconceptions ahead of time. Explain that physical touch, such as hand holding, stroking, light massage, or lying with the patient, is likely to console both the patient and family member, and that giving medication as prescribed promotes the patient's comfort (Bush, 2001). Playing favorite music, reading or praying, performing customary rituals, giving mouth care, or repositioning can also be sources of comfort (Henricson, 2008). Hospice services can be a significant support to families during these final stages.

Families may also fear that they will not recognize when their loved one has died. In addition to the absence of a heartbeat or respirations, the release of urine and stool, fixed pupils, unresponsiveness, pallor, and cool extremities can be expected. Eyes may remain open and the jaw may also relax and open. A sighing sound may be heard from air escaping the lungs when the body is turned. This can be alarming if unexpected. Rigor or stiffness typically occurs 2 to 4 hours after death (Field & Cassel, 1997; Lichter & Hunt, 1990).

Although a patient may be clinically dead, the finality of death for families is difficult to grasp. Spending time with the deceased member can help them to accept their loss and begin the grieving process; therefore, families should be afforded whatever time they desire to say goodbye to their loved one. When death occurs in the home, the family should notify the nurse or physician so that death can be confirmed. Once death is pronounced, the caretaker chosen by the family can be contacted for removal of the body. In cases where the cause of death is questionable, a coroner may need to be notified.

The nurse can help the family notify appropriate people, destroy unused medication in the home, remove medical equipment, and support the family in their grief. Grieving happens in many ways and can vary from a vast number of family members attending a death to patients who die alone. A death ritual is often the first step in a grieving process that may last months to years. Many cultures and religious groups have special rites surrounding the death of a group member that may range from solemnly mourning the loss to a festive celebration of the loved one's life. Mourning may be a very public or private event that occurs in the presence or absence of the deceased person's body. Personal expressions of grief vary from stoic containment of feelings to wailing, hugging, and sobbing. Special rules regarding attendance at or participation in death rituals may apply to small children and pregnant women. Rituals such as bathing, praying, singing, or anointing may be part of cultural or religious practices. When cremation is planned, bathing and dressing the deceased may be a last opportunity to be with a loved one and is an act that for some families expresses their respect (Ferrell & Coyle, 2006). Respecting family rituals and traditions is an important part of the nurse's role in facilitating bereavement.

Ethical and Legal Considerations

Advances in medical science and technology have made it possible to sustain life beyond what many consider to be quality living. The issue of whether or not patients have the right to end their lives when faced with a terminal illness has received significant attention in the media and in the legal system. Currently, only the Netherlands has legalized assisted suicide and euthanasia. Decisions about when to forgo further treatment, however, are challenging for patients and their families and providers. Providers who fear that family members will litigate may choose to continue futile treatments. In contrast, patients and families often find it difficult to abandon the hope that ongoing treatment may prolong life.

The current era of spiraling health care costs raises other concerns about who should receive limited health-care resources. For example, should terminally ill patients continue to receive expensive treatments that are unlikely to significantly delay their death? Should patients with a potential for living longer have priority over patients who have a limited life expectancy? Opponents argue that this latter view constitutes ageism. The financial impact of choosing palliative care over treatment that prolongs life is also a consideration because life-prolonging treatment, although often more expensive, may be reimbursed at a higher rate than palliative and hospice care services. This poses a dilemma for families for whom discrepancies in coverage will cause a significant financial burden. There are no easy answers to these debates. Nurses must advocate to ensure that patients and families clearly understand their options and that their preferences are respected by the health care team.

As the proportion of older adults has grown, issues about death have transitioned from a taboo topic to one that is increasingly open to discussion. As a result, society is experiencing a heightened awareness of death and dying concerns. Key issues affecting nursing practice include the insufficient support for and numbers of family and community caregivers to enable more patients to die in their homes, the ethics of medical futility (interventions that are unlikely to achieve a significant benefit), and a lack of provider knowledge that prevents adequate end-of-life care. Nurses with a better understanding about appropriate treatment at the end of life, the value of interprofessional collaboration, management of adverse symptoms, and ways to access needed resources will be better able to meet their dying patients needs and to help them achieve a more peaceful and dignified death.

KEY POINTS

- The Patient Self-Determination Act requires health care agencies to inform patients of their right to make treatment choices through advance directives such as living wills, power of attorney for finances or health care, and do-not-resuscitate (DNR) orders.
- Quality care at the end of life involves being free from uncomfortable physical symptoms, adjusting to functional limitations, feeling supported through personal relationships, and being at ease with one's self and place within the larger world or universe.
- Central tasks in late adulthood include evaluating life's accomplishments; coping with physical, functional, and social losses; and preparing for death.

- A team of health care professionals is often required to enable patients and their families to achieve an optimal end-of-life care experience.
- Palliative care may begin in the early phases of life-limiting or debilitating illness, can coexist with life-prolonging treatments, and can also encompass care at the end of life.
- The end-of-life period includes the hours to months before death and begins when medical treatment is no longer desired or beneficial. The goal of end-of-life care is a comfortable, dignified, and peaceful death consistent with patient and family preferences.
- Hospice teams address the physical, psychosocial, and spiritual needs of dying patients and their families in any setting of care.
- Medicare and the Older Americans Act include supportive services for dying patients, caregivers, and families.
- Most deaths occur in institutional settings and among adults over age 65.
- Central concerns regarding end-of-life care include inadequate management of adverse symptoms, uncoordinated care that may be inconsistent with patient and family wishes, and insufficient support resources.
- Barriers to quality in end-of-life care include inadequate education of health care providers regarding the management of dying patients and insufficient availability of palliative care services.
- The National Consensus Project and the American Association of Colleges of Nursing have published guidelines and nursing competencies for quality palliative care.
- Comprehensive end-of-life care involves psychosocial, biological, cultural, and spiritual dimensions.
- The World Health Organization's analgesic ladder is the preferred model for pain management.
- Cultural beliefs, values, and traditions can influence patients' willingness to discuss death, treatment decisions, family expectations, and grieving behavior.
- Spiritual expression can contribute to emotional well-being among those with terminal illness.
- During the final hours of a patient's life, the nurse strives to balance a watchful, caring presence with sensitivity to the patient and family's need for privacy.
- Typical signs and symptoms weeks to months before death include anxiety and fear of the unknown, introspection, cognitive changes, fatigue, anorexia, changes in bowel patterns, and alternating periods of somnolence and alertness.
- Imminent signs of death include decreased urine output, cold and mottled extremities, decreasing heart rate and blood pressure, changes in breathing patterns, respiratory congestion, and hallucinations.
- The nurse should discuss common fears about death with families and dispel any misconceptions ahead of time.
- Respecting family rituals and traditions is an important part of the nurse's role in facilitating bereavement.
- Ethical and legal issues surrounding the end of life include deciding what constitutes quality living, whether assisted suicide and euthanasia should be legalized, when treatment becomes futile, and how limited health care resources should be allocated to terminally ill patients.

CRITICAL THINKING ACTIVITIES

1. Visit the Center for Gerontology and Health Care Research at the Brown Medical School (http://www.chcr.brown.edu/dying/2001DATA.HTM) to research the statistics about the location of death in your home state. Review state policies regarding end-of-life care available in the Robert Wood Johnson Foundation (2002) report, "Means to a Better End: A Report on Dying in America Today," available at http://www.rwjf.org/files/publications/other/meansbetterend.pdf. How might these policies affect the death statistics in your state? What solutions might you propose?
2. Discuss your thoughts about your preferred death with a partner. What advance planning might you need to do in order to make your preferences a reality? What resources might be necessary for yourself and your family?
3. What experiences have you had with death? How did you feel about those experiences?
4. View the movie *Terms of Endearment* (Brooks, 1983). Why do you believe the mother lashes out at the nurses about getting her daughter pain medication? What resources are necessary to support the family in this situation? How might the nurse have helped the patient and family?
5. Choose a cultural group that interests you and explore its beliefs about death and dying and grieving rituals.

CASE STUDY | *MR. DIAZ*

Mr. Diaz had always been an active and independent person who handled the family finances, volunteered in his community, and could handle any home repair need that came along. Following his 80th birthday, Mr. Diaz began to contemplate the reality of his eventual death. He had quit smoking at age 55, but his emphysema continued to worsen and Mr. Diaz had already been hospitalized twice with pneumonia. He knew that he would never wish to be kept alive on a mechanical respirator and feared that he might die in pain and be unable to communicate his wishes. Mr. Diaz decided that it was important to express his wishes in writing and to share them with his two daughters, his wife, and physician. Included in his living will were directives to his family about his preference for cremation and a simple funeral at a location owned by a man he trusted. Next, he sought the counsel of an attorney to safeguard the financial security of his surviving spouse and arranged for long-term care insurance should the need arise in her old age.

Mr. Diaz continued to live an active life for the next 10 years until he was once again hospitalized for influenza complicated by pneumonia. After several weeks in intensive care and rehabilitation, Mr. Diaz was able to return home. Mrs. Diaz kept her promise to care for her husband and keep him from going into a nursing home. For the next 3 years, she provided companionship and care while Mr. Diaz became increasingly more dependent. On several occasions, he told his wife that he wanted to "go home." Mr. Diaz refused to have outside caregivers come into his home, and so Mrs. Diaz soon was unable to leave the house for more than a brief period of time. Mrs. Diaz became isolated and depressed and began to reach out to her friends by learning to use e-mail. Eventually, Mr. Diaz became very weak and fell when trying to go outside. He broke several ribs and was in severe pain. After several days, he agreed to go to the hospital, where he could receive adequate treatment to control his pain. His physician ordered morphine to manage Mr. Diaz's pain and conferred with the family about their wishes for recovery. Mr. Diaz's daughters and spouse agreed that the time had come to let Mr. Diaz die in peace, and he passed away several hours later.

1. What do you think Mr. Diaz meant when he told his wife that he wanted to "go home"?
2. Why do you think Mr. Diaz refused to have outside caregivers in the home?
3. What resources might have been helpful to Mrs. Diaz?
4. What role did Mr. Diaz's advance directives play in the decisions made about his care during his final hours?
5. How might hospice services have benefitted this family?

REFERENCES

Administration on Aging. (2009). *Older Americans Act.* Retrieved December 16, 2010, from http://www.aoa.gov/AOARoot/AoA_Programs/OAA/index.aspx

Allen, R. S., Allen, J. Y., Hilgeman, M. M., & DeCoster, J. (2008). End-of-life decision-making, decisional conflict and enhanced information: Race effects. *Journal of the American Geriatrics Society, 56,* 1904–1909.

American Association of Colleges of Nursing. (2004). *Peaceful death: Competencies and curricular guidelines for end-of-life nursing care.* Retrieved December 1, 2010, from http://www.aacn.nche.edu/Publications/deathfin.htm

American Hospital Association. (2002). *Hospital statistics.* Chicago, IL: Health Forum.

Blackhall, L. J., Frank, G., Murphy, S. T., Michel, V., Palmer, J. M., & Azen, S. P. (1999). Ethnicity and attitudes towards life sustaining technology. *Social Science & Medicine, 48,* 1779–1789.

Brooks, J. L. (Producer/Director). (1983). *Terms of endearment* [Motion picture]. Hollywood, CA: Paramount Pictures.

Bush, E. (2001). The use of human touch to improve the well-being of older adults. *Journal of Holistic Nursing, 19,* 256–270.

Center for Gerontology and Health Care Research at the Brown Medical School. (2004). *Facts on dying: Policy relevant data on care at the end of life.* Retrieved December 1, 2010, from http://www.chcr.brown.edu/dying/2001DATA.HTM

Deeken, A. (2009). An inquiry about clinical death—Considering spiritual pain. *Keio Journal of Medicine, 2,* 110–119.

Degenholtz, H. B., Arnold, R. A., Meisel, A., & Lave, J.R. (2002). Persistence of racial disparities in advance care plan documents among nursing home residents. *Journal of the American Geriatrics Society, 50,* 378–381.

Dingley, C., & Roux, G. (2003). Inner strength in older Hispanic women with chronic illness. *Journal of Cultural Diversity, 10,* 11–22.

Emanuel, L. L., von Gunten, C. F., & Ferris, F. D. (2000). Gaps in end-of-life care. *Archives of Family Medicine, 9,* 1176–1180.

End-of-Life Nursing Education Consortium. (2002). *Training program.* Duarte, CA: City of Hope and the American Association of Colleges of Nursing.

End-of-Life Nursing Education Consortium. (2006). *Promoting palliative care in advanced practice nursing.* Duarte, CA: City of Hope and the American Association of Colleges of Nursing.

Erikson, E., Erikson, J., & Kivnick, H. (1986). *Vital involvement in old age: The experience of old age in our time.* New York, NY: Norton.

Fagerlin, A., & Schneider, C. E. (2004). Enough: The failure of the living will. *Hastings Center Report, 34*(2), 30–42.

Ferrell, B. R., McCaffery, M., & Grant, M. (1991). Clinical decision making and pain. *Cancer Nursing, 14*(6), 289–297.

Ferrell, B. R., & Coyle, N. (Eds.). (2006). *Textbook of palliative nursing* (2nd ed.). New York, NY: Oxford University Press.

Field, M. J., & Cassel, C. K. (1997). *Approaching death: Improving care at the end of life.* Washington, DC: National Academies Press.

Gruneir, A., Mor, V., Weitzen, S., Truchil, R., Teno, J., & Roy, J. (2007). Where people die: A multilevel approach to understanding influences on site of death in America. *Medical Care Research and Review, 64,* 351–378.

Hampton, J. S., & Weinert, C. (2006). An exploration of spirituality in rural women with chronic illness. *Holistic Nursing Practice, 20,* 27–33.

Henricson, M. (2008). *Tactile touch in intensive care.* Unpublished doctoral dissertation. Karlstads University, Borås. Retrieved December 10, 2010, from http://bada.hb.se/bitstream/2320/1814/1/Maria%20Henricson_avh.pdf

Heron, M. P., Hoyert, D. L., Murphy, S. L., Xu, J., Kochanek, K. D., & Tejada-Vera, B. (2009). Deaths: Final data for 2006. *National Vital Statistics Report, 57*(14). National Center for Health Statistics. DHHS Publication No. (PHS) 2009-1120. 1-80.

Kagawa-Singer, M., & Blackhall, L. J. (2001). Negotiating cross-cultural issues at the end of life: "You got to go where he lives." *Journal of the American Medical Association, 286,* 2993–3001.

Kish, W. S., Martin, C. G., Shaw, A. D., & Price, K. J. (2001). Influence of an advance directive on the initiation of life support technology in critically ill cancer patients. *Critical Care Medicine, 29,* 2294–2298.

Kovacs, P. J., Bellin, M. H., & Fauri, D. P. (2006). Family-centered care: A resource for social work in end-of-life and palliative care. *Journal of Social Work in End-of-Life & Palliative Care, 2,* 13–27.

Lattanzi-Licht, M., Mahoney, J. J., & Miller, G. W. (1998). *The hospice choice: In pursuit of a peaceful death.* New York, NY: Fireside.

Lichter, I., & Hunt, E. (1990). The last 48 hours of life. *Journal of Palliative Care, 6*(4), 7–15.

Lowey, S. E. (2008). Letting go before a death: A concept analysis. *Journal of Advanced Nursing, 63,* 208–215.

McClain, C., Rosenfeld, B., & Breitbart, W. (2003). Effect of spiritual well-being on end-of-life despair in terminally-ill cancer patients. *Lancet, 361,* 1603–1607.

Metzger, M. & Kaplan, K. O. (2001). *Transforming death in America: A state of the nation report.* Washington, DC: Last Acts.

Miller, S. C., Mor, V., Wu, N., Gozalo, P., & Lapone, K. (2002). Does receipt of hospice care in nursing homes improve the management of pain at the end-of-life? *Journal of the American Geriatrics Society, 50,* 507–515.

Morales, L. S., Lara, M., Kington, R. S., Valdez, R. O., & Escarce, J. J. (2002). Socioeconomic, cultural, and behavioral factors affecting Hispanic health outcomes. *Journal of Health Care for the Poor and Underserved, 13,* 477–503.

National Consensus Project for Quality Palliative Care. (2009). *Clinical practice guidelines for quality palliative care* (2nd ed.). Retrieved December 12, 2010, from http://www.nationalconsensusproject.org/AboutGuidelines.asp

National Institutes of Health. (2004). *State-of-the-science conference statement on improving end-of-life care.* Retrieved December 12, 2010, from http://consensus.nih.gov/2004/2004EndOfLifeCareSOS024html.htm

Nelson, J. E., Meier, D. E., Oei, E. J., Nierman, D. M., Senzel, R. S., Manifredi, P. L., . . . Morrison, R. S. (2001). Self-reported symptom experience of critically ill cancer patients receiving intensive care. *Critical Care Medicine, 29,* 277–282.

Puchalski, C. M. (2002). Spirituality and end of life care. In A. M. Berger, R. K. Portenoy, & D. E. Weissman (Eds.), *Principles and practice of palliative care and supportive oncology* (2nd ed., pp. 799–812). Philadelphia, PA: Lippincott Williams & Wilkins.

Puchalski, C. M., & Romer, A. L. (2000). Taking a spiritual history allows clinicians to understand patients more fully. *Journal of Palliative Medicine, 3,* 129–137.

Reynolds, K. S., Hanson, L. C., Henderson, M., & Steinhauser, K. E. (2008). End-of-life care in nursing home settings: Do race or age matter? *Palliative & Supportive Care, 6,* 21–27.

Robert Wood Johnson Foundation. (2002). *Means to a better end: A report on dying in America today.* Washington DC: Author. Retrieved December 12, 2010, from http://www.rwjf.org/files/publications/other/meansbetterend.pdf

Sand, L., Olsson, M., & Strang, P. (2009). Coping strategies in the presence of one's own impending death from cancer. *Journal of Pain and Symptom Management, 37,* 13–22.

Schwartz, C. E., Wheeler, H. B., Hammes, B., Basque, N., Edmunds. J., Reed, G., . . . Yanko, J. (2002). Early intervention in planning end-of-life care with ambulatory geriatric patients. *Archives of Internal Medicine, 162,* 1611–1618.

Sulmasy, D. P. (2002). A biopsychosocial-spiritual model for the care of patients at the end of life. *Gerontologist, 42,* 24–33.

Teno, J. M., Clarridge, B. R., Casey, V., Welch, L.C., Wetle, T., Shield, R., . . . (2004). Family perspectives on end-of-life care at the last place of care. *Journal of the American Medical Association, 291,* 88–93.

Teno, J. M., Gruneir, A., Schwartz, Z., Nanda, A., & Wetle, T. (2007). Association between advance directives and quality of end-of-life care: A national study. *Journal of the American Geriatrics Society, 55,* 189–194.

Thacker, K. S. (2008). Nurses' advocacy behaviors in end-of-life nursing care. *Nursing Ethics, 15,* 174–185.

Truog, R. D., Campbell, M. L., Curtis, J. R., Haas, C.E., Luce, J.M., Rubenfeld, G.D., . . . Kaufman, D. C. (2008). Recommendations for end-of-life care in the intensive care unit: A consensus statement by the American College of Critical Care Medicine. *Critical Care Medicine, 36,* 953–963.

U.S. National Consensus Project for Quality Palliative Care. (2009). *Clinical practice guidelines for quality palliative care* (2nd ed.). Retrieved November 29, 2010, from http://www.nationalconsensusproject.org/guideline.pdf

Valente, S. (n.d.). *Fact sheet on end-of-life care.* Washington, DC: American Psychological Association. Retrieved December 1, 2010, from http://www.apa.org/pi/aids/programs/eol/end-of-life-factsheet.pdf

Valente, S., & Haley, B. (n.d.). *Culturally diverse communities and end-of life care.* Washington, DC: American Psychological Association. Retrieved December 5, 2010, from http://www.apa.org/pi/aids/programs/eol/end-of-life-diversity.pdf

Werth, J. L., Blevins, D., Toussaint, K. L., & Durham, M. R. (2002). The influence of cultural diversity on end-of-life care and decisions. *American Behavioral Scientist, 46,* 204–219.

White, K. R., Coyne, P. J., & Patel, U. B. (2001). Are nurses adequately prepared for end-of-life care? *Journal of Nursing Scholarship, 33,* 147–151.

Wilkie, D. J., Brown, M. A., Corless, I., Farber, S., Judge, K., & Shannon, S. (2001). *Toolkit for nursing excellence at end of life transition, nurse educators' (TNEEL-NE) CD ROM* (Version 1). Seattle, WA: University of Washington.

World Health Organization. (2004). *Palliative care: Symptom management and end-of-life care. Integrated management of adolescent and adult illness: Interim guidelines for first level facility health workers.* Geneva, Switzerland: Author. Retrieved December 10, 2010, from http://www.who.int/3by5/publications/documents/en/genericpalliativecare082004.pdf

World Health Organization. (2008). *Scoping document for WHO treatment guidelines on pain related to cancer, HIV and other progressive life-threatening illnesses in adults.* Geneva, Switzerland: Author. Retrieved December 1, 2010, from http://www.who.int/medicines/areas/quality_safety/Scoping_WHOGuide_malignant_pain_adults.pdf

World Health Organization. (2009). *WHO definition of palliative care.* Geneva, Switzerland: Author. Retrieved December 9, 2009, http://www.who.int/cancer/palliative/definition/en/

World Health Organization. (2010). *WHO's pain ladder.* Geneva, Switzerland: Author. Retrieved December 12, 2010, from http://who.int/cancer/palliative/painladder/en/

Chapter 25

International Perspectives on Aging

Jean W. Lange, RN, PhD, FAAN
AFRICA: Leana R Uys, D Soc Sc, ASSAf
NIGERIA: Timothy C. Okeke, PhD, PLCSW
CANADA: Joan Lindsay, PhD
GUATEMALA: Margaret A. Perkinson, PhD; Ellen Z. Navarro, *MA*
IRELAND: Kathy Murphy, PhD, RGN; Dympna Casey, PhD, RGN; Adeline Cooney, PhD, RGN, RNT Eamon O'Shea, PhD; Philip Larkin, PhD; Mary Keys, PhD
JAPAN: Christina E. Miyawaki, MA, MSW, Doctoral Candidate
NORWAY: Dagfinn Nåden, RN, HVD (Doctor in Health Care); Åshild Slettebø, RN, PhD

LEARNING OBJECTIVES

- Describe global demographic and health care trends influencing the care of older adults.
- Compare aging population trends among European, African, Asian, and North and South American nations.
- Describe national priorities with respect to older adults in selected countries.
- Identify global trends regarding end-of-life concerns.
- Discuss key issues surrounding aging and health care from a global perspective.
- Discuss future implications of aging populations from an international perspective.

Health has become an international concern. Members of the World Health Organization and the United Nations represent the wealthiest to poorest countries and work collectively to address global health problems, such as infectious diseases, that affect every nation. The Madrid International Plan of Action on Ageing is a collaborative effort to promote national policies that preserve the rights, dignity, and security of older adults worldwide and ensure that older adults are included in international agendas (Sodorenko & Walker, 2004; United Nations, 2002). The impact of global policy and trade affects the fiscal health of nations and resources available to promote health. The health of aging citizens is thus inextricably linked to national economy.

Demographic trends impact national priorities with respect to health and the allocation of resources. The demographics of aging vary greatly among developed and developing countries (Table 25-1). A country's developmental status is defined by the United Nations (UN) classification system on the basis of socioeconomic indicators. Developed countries include most of Europe, North America, Australia, Japan, and New Zealand. Least or less developed countries (LDC) have higher child mortality rates; lower incomes, educational attainment, and literacy rates; higher levels of malnutrition; and greater economic vulnerability (UN Office of the High Representative for the Least Developed Countries, Landlocked Developing Countries and Small Island Developing States, 2010).

Forty-nine countries are currently classified as *least developed countries,* including one in Latin America, 33 in Africa, and 13 in Asia or the Pacific. Poverty, malnutrition, lack of adequate sanitation infrastructures, and lack of education for citizens are common struggles. The populations in developing countries tend to be younger, poorer, and less educated. Only half can typically read and write. Most people in least developed countries live in rural areas on less than $1.25 (U.S. dollars) per day. Communication infrastructure is also limited so that, on

TABLE 25-1 Comparison of Health Indicators among Developed and Developing Nations

	DEATHS PER 1,000 POPULATION	NET MIGRATION RATE PER 1,000 POPULATION	INFANT MORTALITY RATE PER 1,000 LIVE BIRTHS	TOTAL FERTILITY RATE[a]	PERCENT OF POPULATION AGED 65+
More developed	10	2	6	1.7	16
Less developed	8	-1	50	2.7	6
Least developed	12	0	81	4.5	3

[a]Average number of children born to a woman during her lifetime.

From Population Reference Bureau. (2010). *World population data sheet.* Washington, DC. Retrieved December 15, 2010, from http://www.prb.org/pdf10/10wpds_eng.pdf

average, only 1 in 5 persons has telephone access and only 1 in 50 has Internet connectivity (Population Reference Bureau, 2010).

Birth rates in less developed and least developed countries are two to three times higher than in developed countries, respectively; however, 8% of newborns die in LDC on average compared with less than 1 percent of infants in developed countries (Box 25-1). As of 2008, the average life expectancy in LDC countries was 57 years of age, more than two decades below that of developed countries (Population Reference Bureau, 2010). Inadequate sanitation and the spread of infectious diseases are also major health concerns in LDC. Nearly 60% of the citizens in these countries lack adequate sanitation. Malaria, tuberculosis, and HIV infection account for a significant proportion of deaths versus the much more prevalent chronic diseases experienced by older adults in developed countries.

Urban migration for economic reasons has contributed to the spread of disease and also limited the availability of family caregivers for the rural-dwelling older adults who are left behind. Resources to address the needs of aging citizens are of lower priority in most LDC nations that have a proportionately younger population. Infant mortality and controlling the spread of infectious disease tend to take precedence.

In contrast, citizens in developed countries tend to be older and have lower birth rates. This means

BOX 25-1 Health Trends in 34 Developed Nations

- Life expectancy has increased for all ages and is, on average, 85 years for women and 82 years for men.
- Significant progress has been made in cancer survival rates and in decreasing mortality from cardiovascular diseases.
- Obesity and the prevalence of chronic diseases such as diabetes are on the rise.
- Use of medication is increasing in developed nations, particularly for treating diabetes and depression.
- Although the average hospital length of stay has shortened, readmissions for complications of many chronic diseases suggest the need for better control and prevention.
- Access to care and the quality of care varies with the availability and training of providers.
- The number of nurses and physicians has increased in most developed countries, but geographic distribution is uneven.
- Low-income and rural populations have less access to care.
- Public funds support most health care costs in most nations.
- The percentage of money allocated to health is increasing because of technological innovation and graying populations.
- Most developed countries have nationalized health care plans.
- Health care expenditure in the United States is mostly privatized and nearly 2.5 times that of other developed nations.

From Organization for Economic Co-operation and Development. (xxxx). OECD health data 2010. Retrieved December 15, 2010, from http://www.ecosante.fr/index2.php?base=OCDE&langh=ENG&langs=ENG&sessionid=

that the proportion of older adults is growing while the economic contributions to their care by working-aged citizens are declining. For example in Europe, Japan, and Canada there are fewer than 5 working-aged people for every elderly person as compared with 25:1 in many African and Middle Eastern nations (Population Reference Bureau, 2010). In more highly developed nations facing a graying population trend, funding the social, economic, and health care needs of an aging population have become a much higher priority.

Despite more favorable economic conditions in developed countries, dollars spent do not necessarily translate to better outcomes (Figs. 25-1, 25-2, and 25-3). As an example, the United States spends nearly twice as much money on health care as other developed nations (16% of its gross domestic product versus 8.9% among other nations), yet it ranks 24th in average life expectancy among 30 developed countries (Organization for Economic Co-operation and Development, 2009a). As individuals in developed nations live longer, the incidence of comorbidities from chronic disease is spiraling upward. Efforts to control health care costs in most developed countries are therefore focused on improving lifestyle habits to reduce the risk of developing chronic diseases such as diabetes, vascular diseases, and cancer. Optimizing quality of life for those suffering from chronic disease and providing for a peaceful, dignified death have also received a great deal of attention. This chapter gives an inside view of the aging demographics, health priorities, and issues in diverse regions around the world. The impact of population trends, economics, public infrastructure, cultural traditions, and national policy on the health of older adults is vividly contrasted in the following synopses and case studies written by natives of Canada, South Africa, Nigeria, Norway, Ireland, Guatemala, and Japan.

	AUS	CAN	GER	NETH	NZ	UK	US
Overall Ranking (2010)	3	6	4	1	5	2	7
Quality care	4	7	5	2	1	3	6
Effective care	2	7	6	3	5	1	4
Safe care	6	5	3	1	4	2	7
Coordinated care	4	5	7	2	1	3	6
Patient-centered care	2	5	3	6	1	7	4
Access	6.5	5	3	1	4	2	6.5
Cost-related problem	6	3.5	3.5	2	5	1	7
Timeliness of care	6	7	2	1	3	4	5
Efficiency	2	6	5	3	4	1	7
Equity	4	5	3	1	6	2	7
Long, healthy, productive lives	1	2	3	4	5	6	7
Health expenditures/capita, 2007	$3,357	$3,895	$3,588	$3,837*	$2,454	$2,992	$7,290

Country Rankings
- 1.00–2.33
- 2.34–4.66
- 4.67–7.00

Note: *Estimate. Expenditures shown in SUS PPP (purchasing power parity).
Source: Calculated by The Commonwealth Fund based on 2007 International Health Policy Survey; 2008 International Health Policy Survey of Sicker Adults; 2009 International Health Policy Survey of Primary Care Physicians; Commonwealth Fund Commission on a High Performance Health System National Scorecard; and Organization for Economic Cooperation and Development, *OECD Health Data, 2009* (Paris: OECD, Nov. 2009).

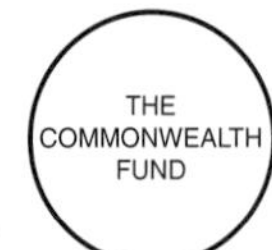

Figure 25-1 Expenditures versus outcomes of care across selected developed countries. *(Reprinted with permission from The Commonwealth Fund. (2010). Mirror mirror on the wall: How the performance of the U.S. health care system compares internationally, 2010 update charts. Retrieved December 15, 2010, from http://www.commonwealthfund.org/Content/Charts/Report/Mirror-Mirror-on-the-Wall-2010-Update/Overall-Ranking.aspx)*

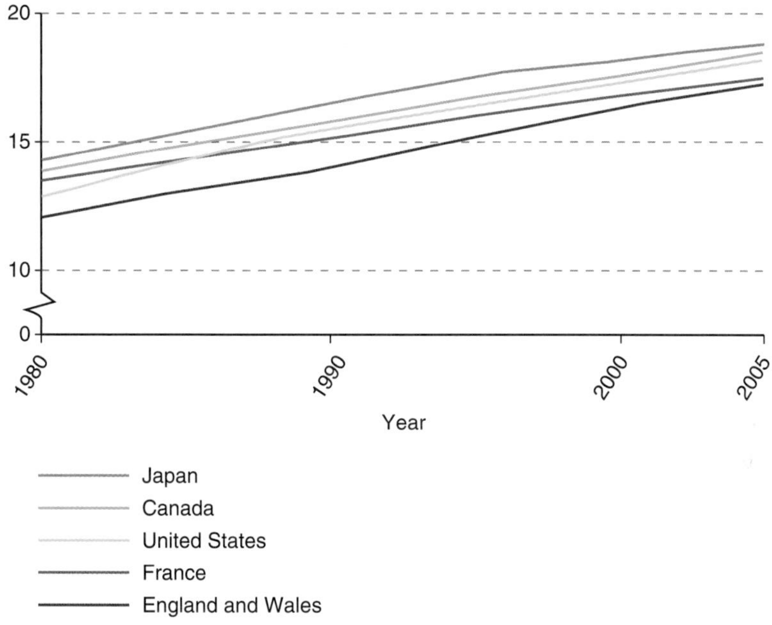

Figure 25-2 *(From Centers for Disease Control and Prevention, National Center for Health Statistics, United States. [2009].)*

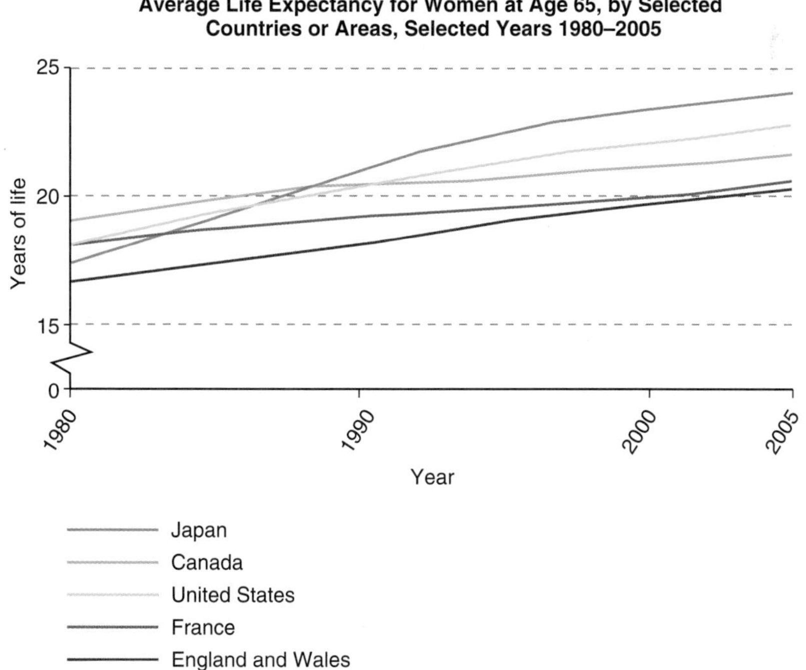

Figure 25-3 *(From Centers for Disease Control and Prevention, National Center for Health Statistics, United States. [2009].)*

Africa

The countries in Africa are roughly divided into sub-Saharan Africa (SSA), which falls into the World Health Organization's African region (AFRO), and Africa North of the Sahara, which falls into the Eastern Mediterranean Region (EMRO). Another division is the language divide, which is in many ways stronger than the geographical divide: The majority of the countries speak French, while a smaller group speaks English, and the smallest groups speak Portuguese or Arabic. Even within countries, people speak many different languages, leading to marginalization of small language groups.

In most African countries the primary health care (PHC) approach where patients are first seen is a primary health care clinic for diagnosis and treatment. These services are mostly provided by registered nurses, midwives, or physician assistants. Africa is experiencing a severe shortage of nurses and midwives because too few are trained and many who are trained then migrate to other countries. There is also a maldistribution of nurses and many die as a result of the HIV/AIDS pandemic.

Demographic Trends

Africa has the lowest proportion of older persons (5.3%) among the UN countries, namely (United Nations Department of Economic and Social Affairs, 2007). Because the African population is very large, however, this percentage translates to as many older adults as in the United States (50.1 million as compared to 52 million). Southern Africa has the highest proportion of older people at 6.2%.

There are racial disparities with respect to life expectancy in South Africa. Whites live about 5 years longer than Asians and between 8 and 10 years more than Colored and African groups (Mostert, Hofmeyer, & Oosthuizen, 1997, cited in Charlton, 2000). Apartheid limits access to education, work opportunities and health care to all but the white population. Gender differences in South Africa's life expectancy are also evident: 52.7 years for men compared with 56.3 years for women (Fathers for Life, 2010).

Aging Issues

In Africa, few countries have policies on aging. Of 25 countries surveyed in 2003, only 7 had national aging policies and 9 had pending policies (Kowal, Chapati Rao, & Mathers, 2003).

Most older adults living in Africa reach age 60 without health insurance and are dependent on the National Health Services. In South Africa, only 17% over age 60 have health insurance (Statistics South Africa, 2008, p. 77). Older adults often live in rural areas where access to health care is limited. In addition, younger family members often migrate to cities where work is more readily available. This leaves rural-dwelling older adults with fewer family members who can care for them. In South Africa, 42.5% live in rural areas (Statistics South Africa, 2001, p.7).

Unlike other African nations, South Africa provides a pension for about 60% of adults over age 60 (Kinsella & Ferreira, 1997). This is a significant safety net for the elderly, and these pensions are usually shared with family members living in the same household. Often, they are the sole source of income. This practice often leads to elder neglect as needs of the rest of the family take precedence (Charlton, 2000; Moller & Sotshongaya, 1996).

National Priorities

Transition from Infectious to Chronic Disease

Four of the top five leading causes of death in the African Region are infectious diseases:

- HIV/AIDS
- Lower respiratory infections
- Malaria
- Diarrheal disease
- Perinatal conditions (WHO, 2010)

Among older adults, however, chronic diseases are the principle causes of death:

- Ischemic heart disease
- Cerebrovascular disease
- Lower respiratory disease
- Chronic obstructive pulmonary disease
- Diarrhea-related diseases (Kowal et al., 2003)

Although ischemic heart disease and stroke accounts for almost 33% of deaths in older African adults, cancer is also a significant problem (Joubert & Brandshaw, 2008). Lung cancer is the primary cause of death among men, followed by prostate and esophageal cancer. In women, breast cancer is the most prevalent, followed by lung and cervical cancer. Africa is in transition from a disease pattern dominated by infectious diseases to one of chronic diseases that require lifestyle changes. Prevention programs to address chronic diseases must be increased drastically, especially because resources for treatment are so limited (Arogundade & Barsoun, 2008; Smith & Mensah, 2003).

Africa is in transition from a disease pattern dominated by infectious diseases to one of chronic diseases that require lifestyle changes.

HIV/AIDS Pandemic

HIV/AIDS has reduced life expectancy in sub-Saharan Africans by an estimated 6 years (Kowal et al., 2003). Infection rates range from 9% to 28% (Nicolay, 2008). HIV-infected older adults are more prone than younger adults to hospitalization because of interactions between antiretrovirals and other drugs (Mehta et al., 2008). Uninfected older adults are often caregivers for their infected adult children, as well as for their grandchildren (Zimmer & Dayton, 2003). Twenty-three percent of grandparents live with grandchildren whose parents are not living in the household (Zimmer & Dayton, 2003). Lack of parental income to support these grandchildren can lead to poverty and a poor quality of life for the elderly (Table 25-2).

Urbanization and Changes in Family Structure

In Africa, many younger adults have moved from rural agrarian areas to cities, where job opportunities are more favorable. Older family members are often left behind (Zimmer & Dayton, 2003). Balancing the separation of younger and older generations is a tradition that if an elderly parent needs assistance, a grandchild is sent to live with his or her as a helper. One respondent to a study in rural South Africa describes this tradition as follows: "They said that my grandson must stay with me and help me with some difficult jobs, for example going to fetch water, because we walk for kilometers to fetch water. He also protects me and

TABLE 25-2 Selected Characteristics of Older Adults in Africa Surveys

COUNTRY	PERCENT FEMALE	PERCENT MEN LIVING WITH SPOUSE	PERCENT WOMEN LIVING WITH SPOUSE	PERCENT MEN WITH SOME SCHOOLING	PERCENT WOMEN WITH SOME SCHOOLING
Total[a]	49.8	84.8	44.1	37.9	16.1
East Africa					
Ethiopia	48.1	90.3	39.3	9.8	1.2
Kenya	53.9	80.1	43.3	63.6	29.8
Madagascar	52.2	82.2	45.6	64.3	44.8
Mozambique	51.2	82.3	43.8	49.3	14.4
Tanzania	50.5	80.9	38.5	52.2	18.2
Uganda	52.8	74.3	38.2	59.5	21.9
Zambia	51.1	85.9	46.0	71.9	35.4
Zimbabwe	53.4	73.1	40.6	75.4	56.6
West Africa					
Benin	52.7	78.9	43.1	21.9	8.3
Burkina Faso	50.8	91.5	63.7	4.2	1.2
Ghana	55.5	67.5	27.9	52.7	21.9
Guinea	49.1	88.8	55.0	11.4	4.8
Mali	46.3	93.1	60.9	9.2	3.6
Niger	48.7	93.5	53.5	4.6	2.6
Nigeria	46.9	86.9	47.6	46.6	27.0
Togo	58.9	76.1	40.4	33.4	8.3

[a] Weighted average across counties.

From Zimmer, Z., & Dayton, J. (2003). *The living arrangements of older adults in sub-Saharan Africa in a time of HIV/AIDS.* No 169. New York, NY: Population Council, Policy Research Division.

the house" (Schatz, 2007, p. 151). Coresidence of older adults with children is less common in Africa than in Latin America and Asia, despite the fact that Africa is the poorest region in the world (Bongaarts & Zimmer, 2002).

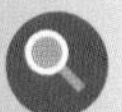

EVIDENCE FOR PRACTICE
Diet in Urban South Africa

Purpose: To describe quality and adequacy of diet in older adults living in an urban area in Sharpeville, South Africa.

Sample: 170 elderly respondents randomly selected.

Method: A 24-hour recall questionnaire and anthropometric and biochemical measurements were used. A dietary diversity score and a food variety score were calculated. To estimate nutrient adequacy at a 70% cut-off, a food variety score had to be at least 8 and the dietary variety score had to be at least 6.

Results: 58.6% had three meals a day, 28.9% had two meals a day, and the rest had one meal or less. The dietary diversity score was 3.41 (±1.34) and food variety score was 4.77 (±2.2) for this group.

Implications: Food variety and dietary diversity scores give a fairly good assessment of the adequacy of the diet, which in this case indicates a general problem of dietary inadequacy.

Reference: Oldewage-Theron, W. H., & Kruger, R. (2008) Food variety and dietary diversity as indicator of the dietary adequacy and health status of an elderly population in Sharpeville, South Africa. *Journal of Nutrition for the Elderly, 27*(1–2), 101–133.

A study of households in 16 African countries revealed that nearly half are composed of nuclear families (Zimmer & Dayton, 2003). There was a significant difference between men and women, however. Although almost 70% of women lived in extended families, only about 43% of men did. Further, men were more likely to live with adult children, while women were more likely to live with grandchildren, perhaps because women tend to live longer and are more likely to be caretakers than men.

Nurses in the Care of the Aged

Because of a shortage and uneven distribution of physicians, nurses in Africa have taken over many responsibilities that are traditionally the physician's domain. Gerontological nursing, however, has not emerged as a specialization, and there is little interest in nursing care for older adults. With the rapid growth in Africa's aging population, this hopefully will change in the near future.

Nurses in Africa need to educate older and younger adults about chronic illnesses. Currently there is little information available about prevention, treatment, and symptom management of chronic conditions. In addition, many people cannot read and, even for the literate, material is often unavailable in one's home language. Nurses must also be aware of what community support services are available in order to link patients to needed resources. In many communities and especially rural environments, community resources are nonexistent. Nurses working in settings where patients lack money or family support must be creative in addressing their needs.

Conclusion

Caring for older adults in Africa is in some ways the same as caring for older adults in other parts of the world. Yet crucial differences also exist. Because geriatrics has yet to be identified as a specialty, and national policies prioritize controlling infectious diseases, little attention is paid to research about the elderly population. Evidence for practice therefore is limited and is rarely focused on older adults. Another major difference is the number of older adults in Africa who provide the sole source of income for grandchildren and their ailing parents. The limited infrastructure in rural areas leaves many older adults without access to health care and the social supports they need. The Nigerian experience in caring for its older adults illustrates some of these issues.

Nigeria

Demographic Trends

Nigeria's population of 151 million is exploding and is projected to reach 264 million by 2050 (United Nations Statistics Division, 2009). Nigeria is the eighth most populated country in the world and, with 3% or 4.7 million residents over age 65, has the largest number of older adults in Africa (Central Intelligence Agency, 2010). Although the average life expectancy is currently 51 years, increasing numbers of adults are surviving to old age.

CASE STUDY | *MRS. LINDIWE NGCOBO*

Mrs. Lindiwe Ngcobo is 69 years old and a widow. She and her husband raised four children in Greytown, a small rural village in the Province of KwaZulu-Natal, South Africa. She was a primary school teacher and retired on pension when she was 63 years old. She has two surviving adult sons and moved to Durban when her youngest son started his university studies so that he could study from home. He has now graduated and is working in another city, where his brother lives.

Lindiwe is a small, rotund woman who lives alone in her own small house. She has a domestic worker who comes in every day to do the cleaning and cooking. Lindiwe says she can now do very little because shortness of breath makes it difficult for her to walk. She has no family nearby and, because she moved to the area after retiring, when her mobility was already reduced, she has no friends in the area. She says she reads a lot and watches television.

She is attending a specialist geriatric clinic at a tertiary hospital in Durban, where she is seen mainly by a specialist physician. Care and medication are free because she is a state pensioner. She is being treated for mitral valve disease, atrial fibrillation, and hypertension.

1. If you were Lindiwe's primary care nurse, which issues would you explore further?
2. How will you address the issue of exercise for this patient?

Leana Uys, D Soc Sc, ASSAF

Aging Issues

In Nigeria, there is a tangible shift away from the traditional extended family to a more nuclear one. Economic conditions have caused many rural youth to relocate into the cities. This urban migration has reshaped the population distribution and led to decreased familial care and support of aging elders. Rather than being revered and encouraged to live with their children until they die, older Nigerians are often seen as a burden. Being referred to as old, retired, or a pensioner is considered undesirable. Because of society's negative view of aging, getting old is feared among Nigerian youth today (Williams, 2009). Aging adults often try to postpone the stigma of being seen as old by staying active. For example, one can see older adults walking long distances, bicycling heavy loads to market, or doing heavy farm labor to stay healthy and strong (Hartford Institute Geriatric Nursing Forum, 2009).

In addition to ageism, gender bias is pronounced in Nigeria, particularly with respect to gay, lesbian, and transgender groups. According to a 2007 estimate, 2.6 million adults were living with HIV/AIDS, of which 170,000 died (Central Intelligence Agency, 2010). Those with HIV/AIDS typically are regarded as outcasts and a disappointment to their families. These stereotypical attitudes toward those diagnosed with HIV/AIDS stem from society's negative attitude toward homosexuality. In a culture where heterosexist and ageist values are dominant, the stigma of HIV/AIDS becomes a burden not only for those infected but also their families (Adisa, Agunbiade, & Akanmu, 2008).

Abuse and neglect are a daily occurrence in Nigerian society, especially among older adult women, because such abuse is taboo and seldom reported to law enforcement agencies. In addition, there is no legislation prohibiting elder abuse. However, public awareness of abuse as a health and societal concern has intensified since the first Nigerian World Elder Abuse Awareness Day in 2006 (Ajomale, 2009). Awareness is the first step toward change. Future policies must reflect current demographic changes in a society where every third person will soon be over age 60 and entering the retirement pool.

National Priorities

Nigeria is experiencing a significant increase in the number of people living and dying from chronic illness and communicable diseases (Aboderin, 2009; World Health Organization, 2006). There is no national payment or insurance system to support retiree living or to pay for health care; thus, those who cannot afford to pay must do without. Older adults living in urban areas are often homeless or live in the poorest neighborhoods. Rescue homes provide relief for some, but the need far surpasses availability. Less than 1% of adults over age 60 receive any government subsidy or pension. In addition to poor living conditions, many older adults also lack access to adequate health services (Adisa et al., 2008).

Policies to support the care of older adults in Nigeria are lacking in part because of a cultural tradition that caring for older adults is an individual or family responsibility (Iroegbu, 2007; Otuyelu, 2002). With Nigeria's high birth rate and proportionately younger population, issues such as reducing the high infant mortality rate and controlling the spread of such infectious diseases as HIV/AIDS, tuberculosis, cholera, polio, meningitis, and avian influenza take precedence over the housing and health care needs of older adults (World Health Organization, 2006).

Lack of a national agenda to improve the healthcare delivery system in Nigeria has caused the World Bank to advocate for privatization of public health services in developing countries such as Nigeria (Bretton Woods Project, 2009; Shittu, 2008). This movement has negatively impacted the public health system's responsiveness to infectious disease and promoted the spread of disease. Privatization of health care delivery has left more older adults without care when they cannot afford to pay for services.

Another barrier to adequate health care for older adults in Nigeria relates to the inadequate preparation and number of providers qualified to care for their needs. The top five causes of mortality in Nigeria are infectious diseases: HIV/AIDS, lower respiratory infections, malaria, diarrheal diseases, and measles. These five diseases account for half of all deaths, making death from infectious disease far more common than from chronic disease (World Health Organization, 2006). Training of Nigeria's health care practitioners therefore emphasizes acute communicable diseases. There is little emphasis on chronic disease; thus, many providers lack expertise in the treatment and prevention of chronic disease.

Low literacy rates among Nigeria's population compound its inadequate health care services by impeding access to health information. Only about half of adults can read and write; and only 13% of those over age 80 can do so. To improve the health of its citizens preventing chronic and infectious diseases, the ability to use written education materials is essential in a country with too few providers (Aboderin & Gachuhi, 2006; Omotola, Adesola, & Adenike, 2006).

End-of-Life Care

Culturally, death is not a taboo topic. Nigerians believe in an immortal soul and an afterlife. As a part of everyday life, death is sometimes the subject of jokes, anecdotes, and teasing because people accept its inevitability. Although death is considered to be a normal aspect of life, however, the manner of death can affect the quality of care and support received. When a person is dying of an illness that carries a social stigma, such as HIV/AIDS, he or she may fear that revealing the diagnosis may lead to rejection, abandonment, or embarrassment to his or her family (Alexander, Bank, & Perron, 2006). Because of societal stigma, families are seldom willing to care for relatives dying of AIDS in their home. It is not uncommon, therefore, for patients to withhold such diagnoses from their friends and family. This secrecy can preclude realization of patient and family wishes that are critical to experiencing a peaceful and dignified death. Better training of palliative care providers and traditional healers to address the multiple aspects of end-of-life care beyond merely pain control is necessary.

The pathway to better health in Nigeria is complex. Cultural traditions and biases embedded within society are deeply rooted. Reshaping national health care policies will require addressing socioeconomic and political challenges to improve provider training, literacy rates, housing, and access to care for its aging citizens.

Canada

Canada has 10 provinces and 3 territories. Although each has unique characteristics, we discuss Canada here from primarily a national perspective. Canada is officially English-speaking with the exceptions of New Brunswick, where French is an official language, and Quebec, where French is *the* official language. Twenty percent of Canada's total population and 30% of those age 65 and older emigrated from other countries (Statistics Canada, 2009a). Canada's birth rate has been below replacement level for quite some time, but its population continues to grow through immigration (Statistics Canada 2005, 2008).

Demographic Trends

The proportion of Canadians age 65 and over has increased steadily since 1921 (Fig. 25-4). This trend is expected to escalate during the next three decades as Baby Boomers born between 1946 and 1965 begin to turn 65 in 2011 (Statistics Canada, 1973, 2008). In 2006, those age 65 and older represented 13.7% of the population. It is estimated that the proportion of residents over age 65 will increase to 18.7% by 2021 (Fig. 25-5). By 2031, nearly one in four residents will be over age 65 (Statistics Canada,

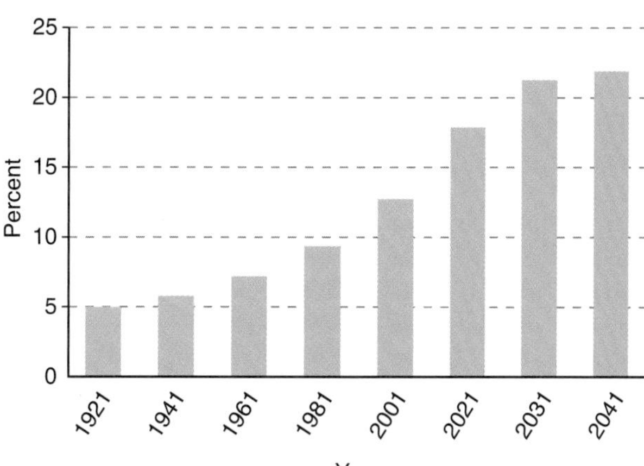

Figure 25-4 *(From Statistics Canada. [1973]. 1971 Census of Canada. Population. Catalogue no. 92-715 Vol: 1-Part: 2. Statistics Canada. Ottawa: Information Canada, Minister of Industry, Trade and Commerce; and Statistics Canada. [2008]. Projected population by age group and sex according to a medium growth scenario for 2006, 2011, 2016, 2021, 2026 and 2031 at July 1. CANSIM table 052-0004 and Population Projections for Canada, Provinces and Territories. Catalogue no. 91-520-X. Ottawa, Statistics Canada. Retrieved December 15, 2010, from http://www40.statcan.gc.ca/l01/cst01/demo23a-eng.htm)*

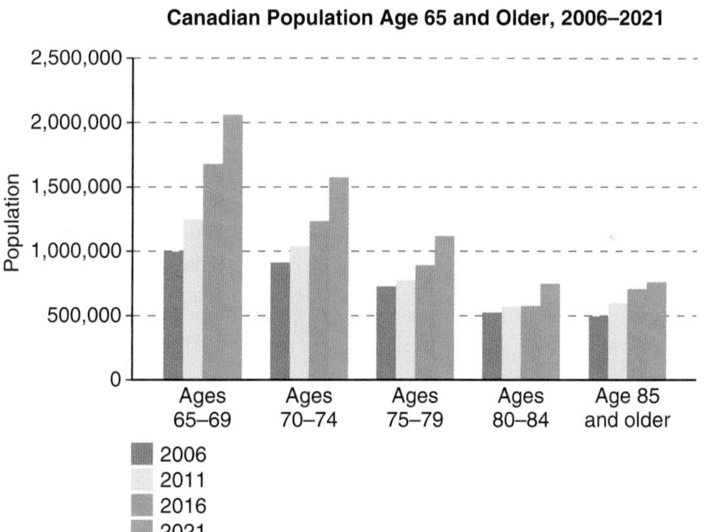

Figure 25-5 *(From Statistics Canada. [2007a]. Age and sex, 2006 counts for both sexes, for Canada, provinces and territories–100% data (table). Age and Sex Highlight Tables. 2006 Census. Statistics Canada Catalogue no. 97-551-XWE2006002. Ottawa, Statistics Canada. Retrieved December 15, 2010, from http://www12.statcan.ca/english/census06/data/highlights/agesex/index.cfm?Lang=E; Statistics Canada. [2007b]. Portrait of the Canadian population in 2006, by age and sex, 2006 Census. Ottawa: Minister of Industry. Retrieved December 15, 2010, from http://www.statcan.gc.ca/bsolc/olc-cel/olc-cel?lang=eng&catno=97-551-X2006001; and Statistics Canada. [2008]. Projected population by age group and sex according to a medium growth scenario for 2006, 2011, 2016, 2021, 2026 and 2031 at July 1. CANSIM table 052-0004 and Population Projections for Canada, Provinces and Territories. Catalogue no. 91-520-X. Ottawa, Statistics Canada. Retrieved December 15, 2010, from http://www40.statcan.gc.ca/l01/cst01/demo23a-eng.htm)*

2007a, 2007b, 2008). As in the United States, women tend to live longer than men. Current life expectancy is 78.4 years for men and 83.0 years for women. This represents an increase in longevity and a narrowing gap between men and women since the early 1980s (when life expectancy was 72 and 79 years, respectively).

Older residents tend to cluster in certain regions within Canada. In the provinces, Alberta has the youngest population, while Saskatchewan has the oldest. The Yukon, Northwest, and Nunavut territories have fewer elderly residents than the provinces. In part, this is because a fairly high percentage of the territories' population is Aboriginal. These individuals have a substantially shorter life expectancy and much higher birth rate. Canada's Aboriginal population is about 1 million, of which only 4.8% are age 65 or over (Statistics Canada, 2009a).

National Priorities

Policy

In the late 1980s and 1990s, with the impending increase in the population of those age 65 and over, the health of older Canadians became a matter of concern to the federal and provincial/territorial governments. This led to a nationwide series of consultations with seniors, senior organizations, and government officials that informed the publication, *Principles of the National Framework on Aging: A Policy Guide* (Health Canada, 1998). The report highlights five basic principles that should be considered when designing programs or polices for senior citizens: dignity, independence, participation, fairness, and security. A more recent publication, *Portrait of Seniors in Canada* (Turcotte & Schellenberg, 2007) is modeled after the principles enumerated in the *Policy Guide.*

Consistent with these guidelines, the initial priority focused on increasing the independence of older adults by reducing the proportion who live in long-term care facilities. In Canada, families tend to be nuclear rather than extended or multigenerational. Thus, many older adults live alone, particularly if they are widowed or, as is increasingly common, divorced. Until recently, community services to enable older people to remain in their homes were often poorly coordinated. Greater emphasis by legislators has improved service provision and coordination to allow more older adults to continue living at home.

Strategies to deal with various aspects of the aging population have been launched in several provinces. For example, Alberta has been a leader in developing residences that are particularly well suited to caring for people with dementia. Ontario has also devoted attention to dementia. In 2007, Ontario announced a new Aging at Home Strategy, which will expand community living options for older adults, with a wider range of home care and community support services available (Ontario Ministry of Health and Long-Term Care, 2007).

Research and Data Sources

In 1988, federal funding was earmarked for research on older adult health issues. Known as the Seniors Independence Research Program, initial money was allocated to studying the epidemiology of dementia (Lindsay, Sykes, McDowell, Verreault, & Laurin, 2004). Osteoporosis was also a designated priority (Berger et al., 2008). These funds led to two large multisite studies, one of which was the Canadian Multicentre Osteoporosis Study (CMOS). CMOS was a longitudinal study of more than 9,000 participants age 25 and older (Berger et al., 2008).

A second study, the Canadian Study of Health and Aging (CSHA) included 10,263 participants age 65 and over from 18 sites covering all 10 provinces. Three rounds of data collection were completed between 1991 and 2002. Results estimated that 8% of older adults had dementia. Of these, 64% were of the Alzheimer's type and 19% were vascular dementia (Canadian Study of Health and Aging Working Group, 1994). CSHA examined risk factors for Alzheimer's disease and vascular dementia and looked at patterns of caring for people with dementia (Canadian Study of Health and Aging Working Group, 1994, 2002). The study also identified a category called *cognitive impairment, not dementia (CIND),* which has become of increasing interest as researchers try to identify cognitive problems earlier in order to slow the decline. As the CSHA progressed to the second and third waves of data collection, it became considerably broader in scope, including topics such as healthy aging, factors affecting the risk of institutionalization, frailty, medication use, urinary incontinence, and norms for several neuropsychological tests (Lindsay et al., 2004).

Since these early studies, Statistics Canada has conducted a number of large, national surveys over the past several years that permit analyses of many aspects of older adults' health. One example is the National Population Health Survey (NPHS), a longitudinal analysis of the health of 40-year-olds (Orpana et al., 2009). The Canadian Institute for Health Information (CIHI) provides relevant data on health services utilization and addresses issues such as wait time for surgery or placement in another center of care (e.g., hospital to long-term care facility), and adequacy of health care personnel (Canadian Institute for Health Information, 2009a, 2009b).

A major new multicenter study, the Canadian Longitudinal Study on Aging (CLSA), has recently been funded by the Canadian Institutes of Health Research. The CLSA will follow 50,000 people, ages 45 to 85, for 20 years (Martin-Matthews & Mealing, 2009). The CLSA will become a rich data source for the study of complex interrelationships among biological, physical, psychosocial, and societal factors that affect healthy aging (Raina et al., 2009). Researchers will be able to link the data to the health administrative data in each province.

Aging Issues

The increasing size of the population of older adults has led to debate about the sustainability of Canada's nationalized health care system in the coming years. Leaders recognize the need for planning and adaptation of the current health care system in the immediate future to deal with an increasingly older population. Resources are necessary to prolong independence and provide more options for levels of care. Issues such as inadequate caregiver support, polypharmacy, fragmented service provision, and lack of geriatric training among health care providers are priorities in addressing the needs of Canada's aging population.

Issues such as inadequate caregiver support, polypharmacy, fragmented service provision, and lack of geriatric training among health care providers are priorities in addressing the needs of Canada's aging population.

Increasing Independence, Healthy Aging

Awareness about the benefits of healthy lifestyle choices has increased across all age groups in Canada. The Public Health Agency of Canada promotes physical activity for older adults on its website and provides recommendations to overcome common barriers, such as tiredness, joint pain, fear of overexertion or falling, temperature extremes, and being short of time (Public Health Agency of Canada, 2003). Greater emphasis is necessary, however, to promote the benefits of physical and mental activity, healthy diet, and weight control among older adults.

Caregiving

As of 2007, 25% of those providing informal care to older adults were older adults themselves. About one third of all caregivers were friends (14%), extended family (11%), and neighbors (5%). Caregiving does not always end when an older adult moves to a care facility. In one study, more than 20% of caregivers continued providing care to older adults living in facilities that provide custodial care (Carstairs & Keon, 2009; Cranswick & Dosman, 2008).

Informal caregivers may experience high levels of stress and require opportunities for relief or help navigating the health care system on behalf of the person for whom they are caring. A great deal of attention has been focused on the plight of these informal, unpaid caregivers, particularly as awareness has developed about the mental and physical challenges associated with caring for people with dementia (Canadian Study of Health and Aging Working Group, 1994, 2002). Most people with declining health prefer to remain in their communities rather than relocate to an institution. However, burnout is a reality when services to support family caregivers are inadequate. Respite programs are one example of services that can support caregivers and delay the need to move an older relative to a long-term care facility (Frederick & Fast, 1999). The 2003 First Ministers' Accord on Health Care Renewal provides home care following a hospital stay for a limited time, and the Employment Insurance compassionate care benefits provide income support and job protection for workers caring for gravely ill family members in their final days. These programs provide limited, short-term support to caregivers; however, more resources are necessary to support caregivers on a long-term basis (Carstairs & Keon, 2009).

Community Health and Social Services

Recent increases in the number and type of services available vary by province/territory. Little has been done to address the lack of service coordination, gaps in service, or barriers in navigating the health care system (Carstairs & Keon, 2009). Although, as of 2003, 15% of older adults received home care, it is not known to what extent this level of service met the actual need (Rotermann, 2006).

Long-Term Care Facilities

The number of people age 65 and older living in health care institutions rose from about 173,000 in the early 1980s to more than 263,000 in 2001. Projections estimate that, in 20 years, more than twice as many people will require long-term care (Ramage-Morin, 2006). There is a distinction between long-term care facilities, where people have more extensive care requirements, and assisted-living facilities. Assisted-living facilities are less regulated than long-term care facilities, and the recent Senate Committee recommended that this situation needs to be monitored to ensure that assisted living facilities do not become unregulated long-term care facilities with extra charges for extra care (Carstairs & Keon, 2009). A second issue is that there is no standard terminology for long-term care facilities nationwide. They may be called special care homes, nursing homes, continuing care centers, personal care homes, government manor homes, private manor homes, homes for the aged, or residential continuing care facilities (Carstairs & Keon, 2009). These concerns need to be addressed to facilitate placement of an increasing number of older adults who will require residential care services.

Medication Use

Polypharmacy is defined as taking five or more different drugs within a 2-day period. This is common among older adults and is a health concern because of possible drug interactions, which increase exponentially the risk of an adverse reaction. In a national survey, multiple medication use was reported by 53% of older adults living in residential care facilities and 13% of community dwellers. Medication use was associated with a greater number of chronic conditions and the presence of chronic pain. One exception was among institutionalized older adults with dementia (Ramage-Morin, 2009). Better training is necessary among prescribers about the increased risk of adverse effects among older adults who take multiple medications.

Alternate Level of Care

A significant financial burden to the health care system in Canada is linked to the problem of placement. Acute-care hospital beds are frequently occupied by people who no longer need these limited and costly services but are awaiting placement in a more appropriate setting. *Alternate level of care* is the term used to describe these nonacute hospital days (Canadian Institute for Health Information, 2009b). In 2007–2008, alternate level of care patients accounted for 5% of hospitalizations and 14% of hospital days. The median age of patients with alternate level of care status was 80 years. These patients were also more likely to have a diagnosis of dementia or stroke or to have sustained trauma. Most alternate level of care patients were waiting for placement in long-term care or rehabilitation facilities. Alternate level of care patients are also more likely to be rehospitalized after discharge (Canadian Institute for Health Information, 2009b).

The capacity of each province and territory to provide care in the most appropriate setting is unknown. Another question is whether increasing community services and post-acute facilities will reduce health care costs (Canadian Institute for Health Information, 2009b). Given a lack of service coordination, there is no information about the effect of family or friend advocacy on the incidence of alternate level of care. Better tools for system navigation, as well as adequate numbers of assisted living, long-term care, and rehabilitative beds, are priorities in Canada's aging population.

Education and Training

The need for more providers educated to care for older adults is well documented. More geriatricians are necessary, as are nurses specializing in geriatric care. Gerontology is not well paid when compared with doctors and nurses working in other fields; this needs to be addressed to attract more qualified professionals. The contribution of home-care workers to helping older adults remain longer in their homes is also underrecognized. These individuals would benefit from specialized training about the care needs of older adults (Carstairs & Keon, 2009).

End-of-Life Care

More than 220,000 Canadians die each year (Statistics Canada, 2009d). Not surprisingly, 75% of all deaths occur in older adults. Most die in hospitals or long-term care facilities, despite the fact that most Canadians would prefer to die at home (Cartstairs & Keon, 2009). Only 25% of Canadians who require hospice care are able to access these services. There is evidence that many older people suffer unnecessarily due to inadequate assessment and treatment of their palliative care needs (Carstairs & Keon, 2008). Recommendations have been made at the federal level to improve this situation with the aim of providing integrated quality end-of-life care for all Canadians (Carstairs & Keon, 2009). The extent to which these recommendations become reality remains to be seen, but it is hoped that pressure can be applied by the Baby Boomer generation to further the development of integrated end-of-life health care services in time for the greater demands this cohort will place on the health care system.

Advance Directives

Advance directives are designed to facilitate communication between an individual and his or her providers and significant others. Ideally, directives provide guidance to those who must make difficult decisions regarding treatment at a time when patients cannot advocate for themselves (Carstairs &

Beaudoin, 2000). In Canada, there is no federal legislation on the use of advance directives; provincial legislation is not uniform and is absent altogether in the province of New Brunswick.

Research in End-of-life Care

Canada is fortunate to have rich sources of data that inform many aging issues. One area where there is limited research, however, is end-of-life care. Existing studies tend to be in a single region and do not therefore lend themselves to addressing end-of-life care needs across the nation (e.g., Burge, Lawson, & Johnston, 2005; Heyland et al., 2006). One national study analyzed factors associated with the likelihood of having completed an advance directive. Cognitively intact women and those with more education were more likely to have thought about or discussed their preferences. Those who had thought about or discussed their preferences were also more likely to have formalized them in a document (Garrett, Tuokko, Stajduhar, Lindsay, & Buehler, 2008). To gain better insight into end-of-life care needs, one proposal has been to integrate questions about end of life within Canada's ongoing Community Health Survey. Whether the public response to such questions would be favorable, however, is uncertain (Singer & Wolfson, 2003).

Guatemala

Guatemala is a Central American country bordered on the north and west by Mexico, on the east by Belize and the Caribbean Sea, on the southwest by Honduras and El Salvador, and on the southwest by the Pacific Ocean. A mountainous country with narrow coastal plains, it is approximately the size of Tennessee and is divided into 22 departments or provinces. It is now a democratic republic but endured a violent, 36-year civil war in its relatively recent past. A predominantly agrarian society, its major exports include coffee, sugar, bananas, and flowers. A majority of the population (about 60%) speaks Spanish; the rest speak one of its 23 Mayan languages.

In contrast to most of the countries discussed in this chapter, Guatemala's population is relatively young, poised at the very beginning of a demographic and epidemiological transition. As such, it has a window of opportunity to prepare for the social, health, and economic issues that tend to accompany aging populations. Whether it can take advantage of this opportunity is an open question, given its general level of poverty, extreme social stratification, and ethnic segregation. Concentrated in the rural, less fertile north and western highlands, impoverished indigenous Mayans represent about 41% of the total population. The nonpoor, urban *ladinos* or *mestizos* (persons of mixed Amerindian-Spanish descent) represent 59% of the population and cluster in metropolitan areas in the south and east (De Broie & Hinde, 2006). The social, economic, and health disparities experienced throughout their lives would seem to ensure dramatically different experiences of old age for members of the two groups.

Demographic Trends

With about 14 million inhabitants (U.S. Department of State, 2009), Guatemala has the largest population in Central America. Its age distribution is that of a young population: 39.4% are between birth and age 14, 56.8% are ages 15 to 64, and 3.8% are age 65 or older. The median age is 19.4 years (Central Intelligence Agency, 2010). Overall mortality rates are declining, however, and fertility rates continue to be among the highest in Latin America. The current aggregate total fertility rate, 3.47 births per woman (2009 estimate; Central Intelligence Agency, 2010), reflects a sharp recent drop in fertility among *ladinos* but masks exceptionally high rates among rural Mayans, exceeding an average of six births per woman in rural Guatemala and close to eight births per woman in the rural frontier region of the Petén (Grandia & Schwartz, 2001). Guatemala ranks the third lowest in the Americas in its use of contraception (World Health Organization, 2007), which is used by only 6% of rural Mayans (Bertrand, Seiber, & Escudero, 2001). With an annual growth rate of 2.066% (Central Intelligence Agency, 2010), Guatemala's population remains young and rapidly expanding. Its dependency ratio is 0.9, the highest in Latin America (U.S. Department of State, 2009).

Average life expectancy at birth has increased and now averages 70.29 years (68.49 years for men and 72.19 years for women) (Central Intelligence Agency, 2010). Infectious diseases remain the main causes of death; however, mortality due to noncommunicable diseases such as cardiovascular disease, chronic respiratory disease, cancer, and diabetes is on the rise (Pan American Health Organization, 2007b).

More than half of Guatemalan families (and 76% of indigenous families) live in poverty (Gragnolati & Marini, 2003; Pan American Health Organization,

2007a). Nevertheless, Guatemala is classified as a lower-middle income country (World Bank, 2009). Extreme disparities in its distribution of land, wealth, and health resources make it one of the most socially and economically stratified countries in the Western Hemisphere (Gragnolati & Marini, 2003). Two percent of the population owns between 65% and 70% of all arable land (Green, 1999). In 2009, the wealthiest 10% of households received almost 50% of the nation's income, while the poorest 40% of households received 8% (U.S. Department of State, 2009). Thirty-two percent of Guatemalan families live on less than $2 per day; 13.5% live on less than $1 per day (Gragnolati & Marini, 2003). Only 69% of households have potable running water. Forty-seven percent of the total population has access to adequate sewage disposal (77% of urban dwellers versus 17% of those in rural areas) (World Health Organization, 2007). About 49% of Guatemalan children under age 5 (68% of indigenous children) are chronically malnourished (World Health Organization, 2007).

Literacy rates (defined as percent of population age 15 and over who can read and write) differ significantly by sex and age. In 1981, 68.7% of men ages 25 to 54 could read and write compared with 21% of women in that age group. Only 16.8% of men and 2.8% of women aged 60 or older were literate (Gragnolati & Marini, 2003). Current literacy rates for the total population are 69% (Central Intelligence Agency, 2010). In 2003, approximately half of the indigenous population remained illiterate (Gragnolati & Marini, 2003), although recent studies indicate improved rates of education for select villages (Maluccio, Melgar, Mendez, Murphy, & Yount, 2005).

There is relatively little information about the marital status and living arrangements of Guatemalan elders. For persons aged 60 and over in 1986–1987, 50% of men and 28% of women were married; 15.6% of men and 49% of women were widowed. According to a 1981 survey, 18% of Guatemalan households were headed by an older adult. Of those elder-headed households, 37% were nuclear families, 49% were extended families, and 9.9% were single-person households (De Blois, 1991). More recent data indicate that 6% of persons aged 60 and over live alone with no support from family networks (Pan American Health Organization, 2002). Given the current lack of geriatric services and residential care options, this does not bode well for a substantial subset of older Guatemalans.

National Priorities

Guatemala's spending on public health is among the lowest in the Americas. Government per capita health expenditure is $93 (Pan American Health Organization, 2007a). Health service provision is fragmented and segregated. Less than 60% of the population has access to health care (defined as residing within 1 hour's transportation to health services) (Pan American Health Organization, 2001). Health services sponsored by the government are covered by the Ministry of Public Health and Social Assistance (MPSAS), which provides services for all at little or no charge in its 1,304 health facilities (Pan American Health Organization, 2007a), and the Guatemalan Social Security Institute (IGSS), which runs its own 139 facilities and provides retirement benefits and health services for the 17% of the population that this program covers (U.S. Department of State, 2009). The Medical Care Center for Retired State Employees (CAMIP) provides health care and social services for former government workers who are retired, widowed, or disabled and their dependent children and orphans. Approximately 30,000 retirees are eligible for these services. Private voluntary groups run by religious associations, international NGOs (Non-governmental organizations associated with the United Nations) with local affiliates, or national NGOs are additional sources for health care and social services. Public-sponsored care is regarded as generally inferior (Berry, 2008). Given a choice, most would opt for care from private for-profit or nonprofit groups.

Guatemala suffers a severe shortage of trained health care providers. For every 10,000 Guatemalans, there are 9 physicians, 3 nurses, 11 nurses' aides, and 1.3 dentists. Health professionals cluster in a few major cities: 80% of physicians, 56% of nurses, and 50% of nurses' aides work in metropolitan areas (Pan American Health Organization, 2007a). The high-risk rural populations rely on nurses' aides, rural health technicians, midwives, community health promotion volunteers, and traditional healers for their health care. A relatively recent program, the Comprehensive Health Care System (*Sistema Integral de Attencion de Salud,* SIAS), was initiated in 1997 to extend basic health care to Mayan populations in remote rural areas. It relies on local volunteers, trained and supported by a medical team that works closely with the community to provide specific, ongoing health services. The current focus of SIAS is on prenatal care; services to infants, children, and women of reproductive age; family planning; sanitation; and emergency care. Nevertheless, the model would seem amenable to providing services to older care recipients as well.

The two most influential organizations for Guatemalan aging policy are the Gerontological Association of Guatemala, a private group of physicians and social workers started in 1980, that advocates for rights and services for older adults, and the National Committee for the Protection of the Elderly, which was formed in 1981 by representatives of various public institutions (e.g., the Ministry of Health) and some private groups (e.g., the Gerontological Association of Guatemala, the Medical Association, and the Association of Retired State Employees). The National Programme for Older Persons in Guatemala (Economic Commission for Latin America and the Caribbean [ECLAC], 2004), focuses on provision of food (with plans to open meal programs and provide food allowances), health (promoting eye and dental medical days), and culture and recreation (providing craft classes, fairs, and literacy training). The National Programme includes a plan to open a shelter and dining rooms for indigent elders in Guatemala City.

The State lacks resources and facilities to provide adequate geriatric care, even for current numbers of elderly Guatemalans. There is one 130-bed government-run long-term care facility that has a long waiting list. Most Guatemalan long-term care facilities are supported by religious groups or are privately owned. Almost all are in urban centers. Since 2005, there has been a strong push to develop such facilities in the capital, Guatemala City, to accommodate growing numbers of abandoned elders who have nowhere else to go.

The Plan for Education Aging in Guatemala, which is part of the National Plan, calls for gerontological training for university undergraduate and graduate students, students in nursing, and nursing assistants. Although implementation has been slow, departments of physical and occupational therapy in some of the major universities, such as San Carlos University and University Mariano Galvez de Guatemala, have included gerontological classes in their curriculum.

Guatemala's Alzheimer's Association, the *Asociación Grupo ERMITA,* initiated and currently run by a local geriatrician and his wife, is a member of Alzheimer's Disease International. It provides family support groups, monthly activities for people with dementia, training for care providers who work in residential care homes for older adults, medical evaluations, courses in nutrition, occupational therapy, and access to a library of resources on dementia (Garcia, 2009).

Aging Issues

Health disparities for older adults loom large, especially for the elder indigenous poor in remote rural areas. Guatemala's underdeveloped and fragmented system of health and social services provides an unreliable safety net at best, and families, for the most part, play a major role in elder care. However, the impact of recent historic events and current social conditions has proven especially harsh for the current cohort of middle-aged, those expected to provide care for the current cohort of older adults. Displacement as an after-effect of the civil war or result of internal migration patterns and large-scale emigration to the United States has undermined the strength of traditional family support systems.

Lasting from 1960 to 1996, the violent clash between Guatemalan army and guerilla fighters was the longest civil war in Latin American history. It officially ended with the signing of the 1996 Peace Accords. During that war, some 200,000 Guatemalans were killed or disappeared, and an estimated 1.5 million (about 20% of the population) became displaced refugees (Worby, 1999). About 200,000 fled the country, most to Mexico. After the 1996 Peace Accords, many returned and resettled in remote jungle areas. In 1988, a group of indigenous women whose husbands, sons, and daughters were either killed or disappeared during the war formed The National Coordination of Widows of Guatemala (*Coordinadora Nacional de Viudes de Guatemala,* CONAVIGUA) to help each other meet basic needs. They continue work to promote human rights, especially the rights of women, children, and the indigenous, to honor those killed in the war, and to provide psychological and social support to survivors. Posttraumatic stress from war experiences is still keenly felt and represents a major mental health issue for survivors, many of whom are in old age.

Internal seasonal migration, in which indigenous workers migrate from the western highlands to work in the plantations (*fincas*) of the south, represents another blow to traditional family support networks. In 2004, about 881,300 temporary workers migrated south. A 1996 survey of migrant workers revealed that 98% were male and 80% were under age 40. Migrant workers encounter numerous threats to health, including inadequate housing, lack of health services, exposure to pesticides, alcoholism, malnutrition, exposure to AIDS, and high incidences of respiratory and gastrointestinal infections (Gragnolati & Marini, 2003). Adverse health effects, coupled with disruption of education and attenuation of family ties from long periods of absence, diminish the ability of a significant number of indigenous men to contribute to the care of their older relatives. The negative impact on family structure eventually places these men at a similar risk for an old age bereft of family support.

Persons who travel to the United States for work opportunities to support families left behind represent another large group of displaced Guatemalans. Nearly 15% of the Guatemalan population migrates to the United States (Moran-Taylor, 2008) with the hope of sending money back to their relatives. In 2007, Guatemalans in the United States sent home more than $4 billion. In spite of the financial benefits, transnational families who attempt transnational caregiving run the risk of conflict, especially when acculturation alters family caregiving expectations and norms (Zechner, 2007). Mayan traditions of family caregiving fall heavily on adult children, especially sons and their spouses, who are expected to provide support, in both financial and personal care (Harman, 2001). As more adult sons and daughters leave home to work, they leave elderly parents home to fend for themselves. A growing number of older adults who are no longer able to live alone have joined the ranks of abandoned elders and moved to local *hogars* or old age homes, when that option is available.

End-of-Life Care

In general, Guatemalans attach strong significance to ceremonies that commemorate and mourn their dead. The proper execution of such rituals is critically important in helping survivors come to terms with the death (Gonzalez & Hereira, 2008). A proper burial entails the involvement of both family members and members of the larger community. Neighbors assist with the preparation of the body, which is displayed for public viewing in the family home. Relatives and friends assemble to mourn, view the body, show their respect to the deceased, and celebrate his or her life.

Strong ties to the land are reflected in the desire to be buried in the homeland, regardless of current place of residence. Even if most family members emigrated to the United States, families will go to great expense to send a body back to Guatemala for a proper funeral and burial (Moran-Taylor, 2008). Although the costs are significant (involving the procurement of notarized documentation, consulate fees, a hermetically sealed casket shipped in a special container, and the fees to transport the body), American Airlines estimated that it ships approximately 3,000 bodies per year from the United States to Latin America (Farrar, 2007). Brandes (2001) describes the anguish of a Guatemalan family whose son, after immigrating to the United States, was denied proper burial. The son was killed in a car accident in San Francisco and was accidentally cremated by the county morgue when workers confused him with another *ladino* man. In his family's view, the absence of the intact corpse made it impossible to carry out traditional funeral customs in an appropriate manner. It was believed that the failure to properly fulfill end-of-life traditions had implications for the man's destiny in the afterlife and for the family's status in their community.

The significance of traditional burial ceremonies also is reflected in recent widespread movements to exhume the bodies of persons who had been executed during the civil war from their mass graves. Each body is identified, if possible, and receives a proper reburial accompanied by traditional funeral rites, "so they could rest in peace" (Lykes, Blanke, & Hamber, 2003, p. 82). Various communities have erected monuments to honor those killed in the civil war, fulfilling spiritual practices and at the same time challenging the Guatemalan army's official version of history (Gidley & Roberts, 2003).

Future Trends

Despite fledgling attempts to address the needs of older adults, Guatemala's limited health resources continue to target the young rather than the old. National short-term health priorities focus on prenatal care, reproductive health, infants and children, and the treatment and prevention of infectious and parasitic diseases. Recent experiments in health reform, specifically attempts at decentralization through community-based health care under the SIAS program, would seem to mesh with indigenous traditions that address problems through local group involvement. This model, adapted to address the needs of older adults, could provide effective solutions to the challenges of a future changing demographic. An emergent movement of ethnic pride in Mayan identity (Hale, 2006) also may contribute to enhanced status for elders knowledgeable about cultural traditions and reinforce their traditional roles (Harman, 2001) as respected guardians of Mayan values and life ways.

CASE STUDY | *DON PEDRO*

Don Pedro is a 68-year-old indigenous Mayan farmer who lives in the department of El Peten, Guatemala, with his 61-year-old wife and 3-year-old grandson. Don Pedro had 2 years of school and, although he can speak Spanish, his primary language is K'iche. He was originally from the western highland town of Santa Cruz del Quiche, but he fled to Southern Mexico with his family in the early 1980s when Guatemala was gripped by violent civil war. After the Peace Accords were signed in 1996, Don Pedro returned to Guatemala with his family and was offered a small plot of land in El Peten, the largest department in the country, as part of a government resettlement program. He supports himself and his family by raising corn, beans, and chickens and tending a small vegetable garden. Two of his children stayed in Mexico, but his older daughter made the journey back with her parents. However, last year she crossed the border into the United States to join her husband and left her son to live with Don Pedro and his wife.

Don Pedro has various health problems related to his career in agriculture. As a young man, he traveled to the coastal plantations of Guatemala at harvest time to work as a hired hand. One season, he was bitten by a *Barba Amarilla* (fer-de-lance) snake while cutting bananas and part of his hand was amputated as a result. In later years, he developed asthma and a chronic cough from years of slash and burn agricultural practices and direct application of pesticides on his own plot of land in the highlands.

Lately, Don Pedro's wife has noticed that her husband is forgetting simple things on a daily basis. Currently, there are no services for people with memory problems in El Peten, although access to health care has improved over the past 15 years.

1. How are the family dynamics of transnational families likely to differ from those of more traditional families? What are the implications of these differences for the experience of old age within transnational families? What types of assistance or support might be necessary?
2. How might encounters with extreme violence in youth or middle-age manifest as symptoms of posttraumatic stress in later life? What are some culturally appropriate ways for dealing with posttraumatic stress in older indigenous Guatemalans?
3. What advice would you give to Don Pedro's wife to help her deal with his memory problems?
4. How might one efficiently distribute health information to populations with high rates of illiteracy?

Ellen Z. Navarro, MA, and Margaret A. Perkinson, PhD

Ireland

Demographic Trends

Ireland has seen a significant demographic shift over the past 20 years. There has been an increase in the overall population, particularly among those over age 65, and a decline in young adults between ages 20 and 25 (Central Statistics Office, 2006). Those age 65 and over make up 11% of the population, a percentage that is steadily increasing. In 2006, there were 54,000 more people over age 65 than there were in 1996. Fahey (1995) estimated that there would be a 26% increase in those over 65 from 1995 to 2011.

Increasing longevity is one reason for the growing number of older adults in Ireland. The percentage of those living to age 75 has increased by 8.2% for men and 10.4% for women (Department of Health and Children, 2001). The average life expectancy in 2005 was 77.3 for men and 83.7 for women (Central Statistics Office, 2006). Because women tend to live longer, they constitute an increasing percentage of the older population. Of the 25 countries in the European Union, the longevity of the men in Ireland was ranked 12th and women 16th (Centre for Aging Research and Development in Ireland, 2009) .

The distribution of older adults in Ireland is uneven, with most living in western and lower eastern regions. Western Ireland is relatively rural, with many people living 3 to 4 hours from the nearest city. The mid-east and midland areas have the highest life expectancy for men (77.2 years), and the west has the highest life expectancy for women (82.7 years) (Centre for Aging Research and Development in Ireland, 2009).

Aging Issues

Most older people in Ireland are active, fit, and healthy and live independently in their own homes. About 5% of older adults live in long-stay residential care while another 15% to 20% receive varying levels of care in the community (Mercer Limited, 2002). Because of an increasing number of people over age 65, it is expected that more will become dependent on others for their care in the future (Central Statistics Office, 2006). Almost 394,000 people (9.3% of the total population) report having a long-lasting health problem or disability (Census of Population, 2006). Nearly one in three adults age 65 and over have a reported disability. This percentage rises with age, reaching 59% of those 85 and over.

In Ireland, as with many countries in Europe, families traditionally have provided care for relatives who become dependent (Timonen & Doyle, 2008). In the future, however, the health care system will bear greater responsibility for meeting the care needs of most older adults because many elderly will not have family or friends to care for them. Three factors contributing to this change include a significant numbers of today's aging adults who chose to remain single, relocation of youth to find jobs, and women entering the workforce. Ireland in the early years of the 20th century had an exceptionally high rate of nonmarriage. Twenty percent of women and 24% of men in now ages 75 to 79 never married (Layte, Fahey, & Whelan, 1999). Because families are often the main carers of their relatives or spouses, this high level of nonmarriage has resulted in many older people being unable to find care support at home when their health fails (Layte et al., 1999). Emigration has also had a dramatic effect on families in rural areas of Ireland. During the 1960s and 1970s many young people left rural areas to find work elsewhere in Ireland or abroad. In addition, it became more common during the 20th century for women to work. Reduced marriages, economic-induced migration, and more women working outside the home has greatly reduced familial caregiving resources for the elderly. As people age without a strong support system, many become isolated and vulnerable (Western Health Board, 2000).

Today's health care system is not well prepared to care for its increasingly older population. Community care services include home care and nursing services; however, the demand far exceeds current resources (National Economic and Social Forum, 2005). These services are critical in allowing older people to remain in their own homes and in providing needed support to informal caregivers. Unfortunately, however, home help services are often a substitute for rather than a complement to family caregiving, so familial caregivers do not always get the support they need (Bolin, Lindgren, & Lundborg, 2008). In addition, services are fragmented and uneven, thereby placing a greater burden on families.

Recently, "home-care packages" have been designed for older people living at home. These packages provide services such as rehabilitation that are in addition to the typical community-based services. Home-care packages target people on the brink of needing long-stay care and are designed to keep them at home for as long as possible. Data suggest that about 8,000 people benefited from a home-care package at any one time in 2007, at a cost of €110 million (about $147 million) per annum (Parliamentary Question 15143-08). Unfortunately no clear guidelines exist about who is eligible for what services. Thus, service provision is determined more by the needs of the providers than the actual needs of the older person.

For highly dependent older people who cannot continue living at home, residential care in Ireland is currently provided through a combination of private and public facilities. There are a total of 24,253 nonacute beds in long-stay facilities, or 52 beds per 1,000 older people. Current bed availability is unlikely to meet the needs of 394,000 people with long-lasting health problems or disabilities who may require long-term care in the future . Most residents in long-stay care (39.6%) are categorized as maximally dependent. However, 9% of long-stay care residents are in the low-dependency category because community-based resources are inadequate to meet their social needs, such that these residents cannot remain at home.

National Priorities

Health and social policy for older people in Ireland has evolved over the past 40 years. A 1988 report, *The Years Ahead: A Policy for the Elderly,* highlighted the need for more home-based care services and coordination between the public, private, and voluntary or informal care providers (Report of the Working Party on Services for the Elderly, 1988). The report called for the development of a model to keep older people in their homes when possible, or to provide high-quality long-stay care and rehabilitation when required. The importance of the *Years Ahead* report was recognized in 1993, when it was adopted as official government policy.

In 1997, the National Council on Ageing and Older People (NCAOP) evaluated the *Years Ahead* achievements against stated objectives and found a number of shortcomings. In particular, community services were deemed to be fragmented, with little coordination among services or between health boards and local authorities, public and private sectors, and community and residential care. Fragmented care continues to be a significant problem today (National Economic and Social Forum, 2005). In their report, *Care for Older People,* the National Economic and Social Forum suggested that much more needs to be done to make community care provision a reality in Ireland. The problem is partly underfunding for community care and partly failure to make the best use of existing resources to support people living in their own homes.

Ireland spent approximately 0.62% of its gross domestic product on long-term care for older people in 2005. It is estimated that Ireland will need to spend an additional €500 million (about $668 million) (National Economic and Social Forum, 2005). The government is about to introduce *Fair Deal,* a controversial new funding model for long-stay care (Department of Health and Children, 2008). The aim of Fair Deal is to streamline long-stay care financing so that it is equitable, transparent, and biased toward care in the community. The goal is to institute a more formalized and comprehensive assessment of care needs so that only maximally dependent older people receive financial support for residential care. A cost-sharing model would require the older person to contribute a portion of their pension and 5% of housing assets per each year of care. The latter payment is deferred until after one's death and is capped at 3 years of care or 15% of housing assets (Department of Health and Children, 2008). Fair Deal is highly contested because of its cost-sharing from housing assets. However, this new model has the potential to bring greater efficiency and equity into residential care services. A key question is whether Fair Deal will also provide more resources for community care. Some argue that a social insurance system would be more likely to generate the reforms needed for improved community-based care (O'Shea, 2007b).

The Irish Office for Older People is currently developing a National Positive Ageing Strategy on the basis of the United Nation's Principles for Older Persons: independence, dignity, self-fulfillment, participation, and care (United Nations, 1991). Inclusion of key stakeholders was sought in order to design a comprehensive strategy that addresses aging issues such as "participation in society, the ways in which programs and services for older people are organized and utilized; and the determinants of quality of life for older people such as income, health and social care, housing, transport, education and employment, or any other issue of relevance to older people" (Department of Health and Children, 2009). A strategic investment in the aging population, particularly with regard to community-based care, will yield rich dividends for Irish society in the coming decades.

End-of-Life Care

Recent research suggests that almost two thirds of Irish elderly would prefer to be cared for at home if they were dying (Weafer, 2004). However, only 20% of older people actually die at home (Central Statistics Office, 2006). In reality, people are more likely to die in acute hospital settings, private or public nursing homes, or other public long-stay care facilities. Apart from the work by O'Shea et al. (2008), there is very little evidence regarding end-of-life care across these different settings.

A nationwide study funded by the National Council on Ageing and Older People and the Irish Hospice Foundation examined service provision and care for older people dying in acute hospitals and long-stay settings (O' Shea et al., 2008). A total of 592 acute and long-term care facilities were surveyed. Qualitative interviews were then carried out in six randomly selected sites, chosen to reflect the range of care facilities where older people die. Interviews with staff and dying patients revealed a number of concerns. Concerns included lack of advanced health care directives, staff unprepared to provide good end-of-life care, limitations to providing optimal care because of the physical environment, and a lack of resources.

Advance Health Care Directives

An advanced health care directive is an oral or written statement that is intended to go into effect under stated conditions anticipated in the future. Although advance directives are not confined to end-of-life issues, they are discussed in that context in this chapter. At present there is no legislation in Ireland regarding advance health care directives. The English common law decisions on advance directives are useful and are relevant to the Irish context, where it is anticipated that the introduction of a statutory basis for such decision making will take time. In the interim, it seems, based on the right to consent recognized in Irish medical ethics and law, that (a) where the evidence is unequivocal that capacity was present at the time the decision was made, (b) it was voluntary, and (c) it was made in anticipation of the circumstances in question, then the Irish legal system would be supportive of such action. However, there is as yet no clear legal decision on the matter and no statutory basis for advance directives.

Education and Training: Palliative Care and Cultural Diversity

To provide optimal care for the dying, nurses must be educated and skilled in palliative and end-of-life care. O' Shea and colleagues (2008) reported, however, that most nurses have not received any formal education in palliative care, and less than one third of all facilities report nurse employees with post-registration certification or training in palliative care. Staff reported reluctance to openly discuss death and dying with dying patients because of their lack of knowledge. Instead, a system of closed awareness exists around death, where everyone knows a patient is dying, but it is not openly discussed. Strategies such as keeping cheerful, reassuring a patient that he or she will be fine, or using distraction techniques are often used to avoid discussions about death.

> *Culturally inappropriate care or a lack of awareness of people's cultural beliefs and traditions surrounding death and dying may profoundly affect the experience of patients and their families.*

Nursing staff must also be educated to deliver culturally appropriate end-of-life care. Indeed, culturally inappropriate care or a lack of awareness of people's cultural beliefs and traditions surrounding death and dying may profoundly affect the experience of patients and their families (Lothian & Philp, 2001). Traditionally, Ireland was predominantly Roman Catholic; however, given the recent influx of migrant workers, Ireland is rapidly becoming a multicultural society. The last census (Central Statistics Office, 2006) reveals that the number of non-Irish people living in Ireland almost doubled to 420,000 since 2002. The largest group is British nationals, followed by Poles, Lithuanians, Nigerians, and Latvians. In the future therefore, Ireland's elderly will include people from diverse backgrounds that have cultural and spiritual beliefs different from those of native Irish. Few guidelines exist to illuminate the needs of people from ethnic minority groups (O' Shea et al., 2008). Health care providers therefore require education and training in cultural awareness and an understanding of the diverse traditions and beliefs around death and dying, including an awareness of religious practices other than the Catholic tradition (Tracey & Ling, 2005). One trend that is helping to address the lack of understanding about various cultures is the increasing number of health care workers from diverse backgrounds (Irish Nursing Home Organisation, 2006). Better training about end-of-life care will promote better understanding about the needs of dying patients and their families and a respect for cultural traditions that are critical to a dignified death.

Physical Environment and Resources

Despite the fact that most people in Ireland die in acute or long-stay settings, availability of designated palliative care beds is extremely low (O'Shea et al., 2008). Lack of privacy by having a single room is particularly a concern in private nursing homes. Access to consultant-led palliative care teams is also limited, especially in long-stay facilities. Such low levels of provision reflect existing resource constraints but may also reflect the sequestration of dying people from living people by health care professionals. Older dependent people receiving end-of-life care may not only be physically separated from the rest of society through admission to long-stay care facilities but may be further isolated through the work practices and work patterns of health care providers. The needs of patients nearing the end of life are often unmet. Resources to address health care profession training, policies, and the physical environment are crucial to ensuring that older people at the end of life in Ireland receive the highest standard of care that nurses can provide.

CASE STUDY | *MRS. MARY DALY*

Mrs. Mary Daly, age 84, moved into a public nursing home 6 months ago. She is grateful to be here because it was getting to be too much of a struggle at home. However, it is very different than what she was used to. Here, she shares a room with five other women. It is good to have company, and certainly there were times when she was lonely at home, but it can be overwhelming. The noise is sometimes overpowering, televisions blaring and people shouting. There does not seem to be anywhere to go for some peace and quiet. Sometimes Mary misses her own little room and her own things around her. She feels lucky, though; she can walk with the help of a walking aid and can get to the toilet or go for a stroll on the corridor. She is much more independent than the others, but she does need help with washing and dressing. It is important to her to remain as independent as possible.

Mary lived at home until she moved here. She cared for her husband until he died 10 years ago. They bought their home 30 years ago and raised their three children there. There were a lot of memories bound up in that house. She managed well, the house was always shining, and people admired her garden. She met her friends once or twice a week and joined a local horticultural group. It was nice meeting people with a shared interest, and they swapped tips and plants. She was grateful that she learned to drive. Living in the country was lovely but had its challenges. She lived 10 miles from the nearest town and had to drive everywhere. That all changed when she had a stroke. It left her with a weakness in her arm and leg, and it stopped her driving. She depended on the kindness of friends and neighbors to do her shopping and take her to Mass at the Catholic church. Keeping the house and garden the way she liked was impossible. It upset her greatly seeing her garden turn into a wilderness. The Public Health Nurse (a community-based nurse) came to visit and suggested that Mary consider having home help. It was a hard decision because it meant accepting she needed help, but in the end she decided it was the only option. The alternative was a nursing home and she did not want that. Her children tried to help, but they lived too far away. The home help came twice a week for an hour. She was good, but it was not enough, and Mary struggled to manage. She was going to the bathroom one night when she tripped and fell. She could not get up and lay on the floor for hours. Luckily a friend called in, and she was rushed to hospital. She was diagnosed with a fractured hip and had a hip replacement. She did well after the operation but everybody said she could not go home again. She reluctantly agreed to move into long-stay care.

Mary thinks it is good here, the nurses are very kind, the food is good, and she has made friends with two of the women in her ward. However, she really misses her home and garden. She would love if she could still do a little gardening; a few pots would do, but that does not seem possible. The nurses are so busy she would not like to ask. They have to make sure that everybody is up and washed and dressed. There is a huge rush to get everybody up in the morning and then a lull and another rush at lunch time and then a lull and a rush in the evening to get everybody into bed. Mary goes to bed earlier than she used to. Everybody seems to because there are so few staff on at night time. Every day seems the same, and sometimes it is hard to tell one day from another. Someone did ask her if she would like to go to the main hall to play bingo, but she never played bingo and doesn't feel she could start now. There is a trip out next week, and she is really looking forward to a break in the routine.

1. Consult the literature on transition; focus on transition from home to long-stay care. Drawing on what you have learned, what are the priorities for Mary's care?
2. How can you (and the wider team) generate a sense of home for Mary in the long-stay care setting?
3. Consider the impact of the routine of this care home on Mary. What changes would you make to how care is delivered? When answering this question consider the impact of the organization and philosophy or approach to care on the person's experience.
4. How would you support Mary to meet her goal of staying as independent as possible? Use the literature to support your answers.

Japan

Demographic Trends

According to the White Paper published by the Cabinet Office in May 2009, Japan has more than 127 million people, of which almost 29 million are over age 65 (Naikakufu, 2009). Those age 65 and older represent 22.7% of the total population, an increase of 0.6% from October 2008. Of these, 13.22 million (10.4% of the total population) are over age 75 and considered old-olds. In 2009, the proportion of old-olds reached 10% for the first time in history. This upward trend is expected to increase to 25.2% (1 in 4) in 2013, to 33.7% (1 in 3) in 2035, and to 40.5% (1 in 2.5) in 2055. If realized, Japan will have the greatest percentage of citizens over age 75 in the world (Kōseirōdōshō, 2009c).

Part of the reason for the increasing proportion of older adults in Japan is its low fertility rate (Fukawa, 2007). There were 17.18 million children younger than age 14 as of October 2008. At the current fertility rate (1.32 in 2006), the child population will be less than 10 million in 2039 and 7.52 million (less than half the 2008 figure) in 2055. With a declining birth rate, the working-age population (ages 15 to 64) will also decline, leaving fewer young adults to care for their aging elders (Kōseirōdōshō, 2009c).

A second reason for the increasing proportion of older adults in Japan is an increasing life expectancy. In 2007, the male and female life expectancies were 79.2 years and 86 years, respectively. In 2055, men are anticipated to live 83.67 years, on average, and women more than 90 years (Kōseirōdōshō, 2009c). On the basis of these figures, Japan is indeed an aging country.

Along with an aging trend, the structure of families and households in Japan has also changed. As of 2007, 40% of Japanese households included one or more residents over age 65. Of these, 4.33 million (22.5%) were one-person households, 5.73 million (29.8%) were households with couple only, and 3.53 million (18.3%) were three-generation households. The proportions of one-person households and households with couples have only increased seven-fold in the past 30 years, while the number of three-generation families (elderly living with their children and grandchildren) has not grown (Kōseirōdōshō, 2009c). Increasing numbers of older persons are living alone or separated from their younger family members. The responsibility of caring for aging citizens is therefore shifting from the family to society.

Most older adults report that they do not have adequate finances (Kōseirōdōshō, 2009c). It is not surprising, therefore, that labor participation rates among older people are quite high. Half of men and more than 28% of women ages 65 to 69 work. In recent years, there has been a drastic growth in labor participation among persons in their early 60s who postpone their retirement or are rehired after reaching their retirement (Kōseirōdōshō, 2009c).

National Priorities

New Long-Term Care Insurance and Its Expenditures

Japan's social security system consists of pensions, health insurance, and long-term care. This system universally covers the whole population in Japan (Morioka, 2007). Japan's universal health insurance system was established in 1961 and operates through a combination of tax and insurance systems, ensuring free access to medical institutions. The Organization for Economic Co-operation and Development (OECD) provides comparable health statistics across 30 developed countries worldwide. OECD's Health Data 2009 shows that Japan's health expenditure as a percentage of its gross domestic production (8.%) is less than average (8.9%; Organization for Economic Co-operation and Development, 2009). This percentage has increased since 2005 and is expected to continue to grow in keeping with Japan's aging population.

As a consequence of Japan's rapidly aging population and the growing number of families living separately from their elder parents, the number of physically and cognitively impaired elderly and the percentage of the elderly who live alone or only with an aging spouse has increased. The availability of younger family caregivers is declining as more women work outside the home, thus leaving elder care to an elderly spouse. In addition to these demographic changes in recent years, medical expenses for the elderly have increased. These conditions have threatened sustainability of social security systems; hence, how to finance health expenditures of the elderly has become one of Japan's major concerns (Fukawa, 2007). In response, the Japanese government implemented the Long-Term Care Insurance (LTCI) program for the elderly in April 2000 (Asahara, Momose, & Murashima, 2003; Fukawa, 2007).

LTCI is part of the social security system, offering universal coverage. It is run by local municipalities. Those age 40 and over, as well as service providers, pay premiums that are set by each municipality. Eligibility is determined by age (65 and over) and an assessment by care managers of the degree of physical or mental disability. Those who qualify to use the LTCI services pay 10% of the cost of home services or institutional care. Cost is based on the level of care and the kind of institution within each region (Asahara et al., 2003). Demand for institutional care has been high and waiting lists are common among these facilities. The idea of the LTCI was to share the burden of elderly care among all members of society to lessen the burden on individual family caregivers (Fukawa, 2007). The increasing expense of this program, however, led to a 2006 amendment that increased the elder's copayment, promoted lifestyle change to prevent disease, created a new medical system with insurance premiums for the old-olds, adopted a facility fee for room and board, and created small-scale home and institutional care options within communities (Morioka, 2007).

Healthy Japan 21

Older people in Japan are generally healthy, employed, and engaged in activities, although they have become less connected and involved with other generations of family members and neighbors. Japan also faces some challenges because of its aging population, the poor financial status of many older citizens, and the isolation of older adults from potential family caregivers. Japan has taken measures to overcome these challenges with some success.

As health care costs have spiraled upward, Japan is experimenting with various approaches to health reform. How to control and finance health and long-term care expenditures of the elderly has become a more serious issue in recent years due to Japan's aging population (Fukawa, 2007). One way to reduce the financial burden is to reduce the number of service users and to deliver services more efficiently and effectively. In response to this national concern, the Cabinet Office started a national movement called, "National Health Promotion Movement in the 21st Century (Healthy Japan 21)" in 2000 (Box 25-2). Evaluating what impact this movement and its recommended changes will make on the lives of older persons in an aging society is critical to the future health of Japanese citizens.

BOX 25-2 Healthy Japan 21

The central motto of the Healthy Japan 21 movement is "to promote citizens' health throughout life with goals to improve lifestyles, eliminate risk factors, enhance health check-ups and decrease diseases." Initiatives under this movement include:

- Promotion of health and welfare
- Employment and management of long-term care service providers
- Securing direct care workers
- More education among health care providers about dementia and long-term care
- Social engagement among older adults
- The establishment of regional comprehensive support centers for older persons in their communities (Kōseirōdōshō, 2009a)

Aging Issues

Japan has the world's longest average life expectancy. A survey in 2006 revealed that 64 percent of Japanese elderly reported feeling healthy despite a high frequency of medical service use (56.8%) as compared with other developed countries (e.g., 26.7% in the United States, Kōseirōdōshō, 2009c). Japan's high use may be due in part to its universal coverage that makes medical care easily accessible to all residents regardless of income level.

The large numbers of aging adults means that more people are needing support to remain in their communities. As of 2009, nearly 4.8 million people over age 65 required care support, more than twice the number requiring support in 2000 (Inoue, 2009; Kōseirōdōshō, 2009c). Most caregivers are women who live in the same household and are a spouse, child, or in-law (Kōseirōdōshō, 2007a, 2007c). More than half of today's caregivers are themselves over age 60. This is a consequence of Japan's overall aging population, low birth rate, increased number of younger women in the work force, and a trend toward nuclear versus extended family households.

The increasing need for care among older adults prompted the Japanese government to create a new long-term care plan for the elderly in 2000. There are currently several levels of care service: long-term "preventive" care (visiting nurse or outpatient day care for individuals certified as requiring assistance), long-term nursing care that provides a higher level of care (in-home or outpatient day care), and residential nursing homes

(Kōseirōdōshō, 2007a, 2007b, 2007c, 2009b, 2009d). Use of these services is rapidly expanding. Another level of care, community-based services, is designed to help older adults remain in their homes. Community-based services include overnight care and care for patients with dementia. The use of these services showed a significant increase from 2007 to 2009 (186,600 people in 2007 to 240,000 in 2009). The need for dementia care service also increased from 128,100 to 141,600 (Kōseirōdōshō, 2007a, 2007b, 2007c, 2009b, 2009c). The projected number of elderly with dementia is estimated to double by 2025 (Yoshida, Ogawa, & Kai, 2009).

Continuing to meet the expanding health-care needs of an aging Japanese population will be a significant challenge in the future. Like other developed countries, Japan is now focusing more of its efforts on prevention and health promotion. Healthy Japan 21 addresses the issue of lifestyle-related diseases and their possible causes. Lifestyle changes that promote better nutrition, physical activity, mental health, smoking and alcohol cessation or moderation, and dental care will help decrease the incidence of preventable or chronic illnesses (Morioka, 2007). The educational initiatives of Healthy Japan 21 are designed to maximize and prolong independence to reduce health care service use and long-term care expenditures (Fukawa, 2007; Morioka, 2007).

End-of-Life Care

In Japanese culture, death is considered a natural event that should be a positive ending to someone's life (Masuda et al., 2003). Discussing death, however, is considered to be a taboo subject (Kimura, 1998). Japanese tradition also views the individual as part of a social group in which the group makes decisions on behalf of individuals (Davis & Konishi, 2000). Therefore, the death of an individual is considered not only a personal concern but also a familial, communal, and societal matter (Kimura, 1998).

Japanese tradition is also influenced by Confucianism, which emphasizes a hierarchical model for social and political order, where the concept of filial piety is embedded into the social framework. Hence, a hierarchical order of responsi bility, duty, and personal interaction has been established. This hierarchy also prescribes autho rity for decision making. However, this authority is highly ambiguous with respect to decisions about end-of-life preferences (Matsui, Braun, & Karel, 2008). According to the Confucianism model, a person in a superior position is responsible for the care of persons in a lower position. Those in a lower position are to be loyal and obey their superiors. In the case of a physician-patient relationship, Japanese people typically place complete and unquestioning trust in their physicians. Japanese believe that neither the patient nor family members, rather only the physician, should make decisions on behalf of the patient (Kimura, 1998). Matsui et al. (2008) reported that more than half the Japanese participants in their study believed that someone else should decide on end-of-life preferences. In regard to life-sustaining treatment, between 38% and 47% of Japanese thought that it was up to the physicians and between 13% and 17% thought it was up to the family to decide.

Loss of face (how others view the family and its actions) is another cultural influence that seriously influences decision making. Potentially negative reactions from outsiders when a family's decision is not in line with traditional Japanese values may have a significant impact on a family's choices. Loss of face sometimes results in decisions that are not in the best interests of patients or their family members (Davis & Konishi, 2000). These cultural traditions often affect whether a terminal diagnosis is disclosed to patients (Davis & Konishi, 2000). In Japan, traditionally, the true diagnosis is not explained to terminally ill patients because this is considered the best and most compassionate way to proceed (Kimura, 1998; Davis & Konishi, 2000). Because decisions are made by the family unit, a terminal diagnosis is usually disclosed to the family first, and it is up to the family to decide whether or not to tell the patient.

Living Will and Advance Directives

Japanese traditions do not, however, appear to be entirely consistent with Japanese preferences or current medical practice. A recent study concerning Japanese views about disclosing a terminal diagnosis, end-of-life preferences, or living will revealed that the vast majority (73%) were in favor of disclosing a fatal illness, and 81% expressed a desire to learn about their end-of-life care options. Eighty-two percent indicated a positive attitude toward preparing a living will; however, more than half did not believe that these wills should be legally binding. About one third did not consider a written end-of-life documentation necessary at all. When living wills are presented to physicians, it appears that patient and family wishes expressed in these documents are usually respected. Since 1976, *Nihon Songenshi Kyokai* (the Japan Society for Dying with Dignity) has campaigned to promote public and health officials' awareness about living wills. According to a 2002 survey of *Nihon Songenshi* members experiencing the death of a relative, 70% reported having presented a living will to the physician when end-of-life decisions had to be made. Nearly all (96%) responded that the living will was respected by physicians and considered when making decisions about end-of-life care (Onda, 2005).

Despite this evidence in support of advanced directives, they are not widely used in Japanese society (Masuda et al., 2003). *Nihon Songenshi Kyokai*'s work is beginning to raise awareness, but living wills are not legally recognized and the concept of advance directives is not widely endorsed by Japanese society (Kimura, 1998; Matsui, 2007). Long-standing cultural traditions about decision making, social influences, and the dying process are slow to change (Long & Chihara, 2000).

Contrary to a reluctance to embrace advance directives, hospice and palliative care is more widely integrated in Japan for selected diagnoses. By the early 1970s, the possibility of starting hospice practice and home hospice had been explored by a number of medical professionals. By the late 1980s, the Ministry of Health, Labor, and Welfare decided to develop hospice programs and, in 1990, the Ministry established standards and issued regulations governing reimbursement of hospice and palliative care units connected with hospitals or licensed medical facilities (Long & Chihara, 2000).

National health insurance covers the cost of hospice care at licensed palliative care hospitals. Patients younger than age 70 pay a 10% copayment, and patients age 70 and above pay a 30% copayment of ¥11,340 (about $126) per day. When available, a private room surcharge must be paid in addition to the regular copayment (Long & Chihara, 2000). A lack of private rooms and insufficient numbers of hospice beds are barriers to optimal end-of-life care. Home hospice care is not covered by insurance (Imamura, 2007). Because Japanese universal health insurance, in general, provides generous hospital coverage for treatable illness, including the best available technology and medical staff, some patients believe that it is less costly to stay in the hospital than to stay at home and pay for hospice care (Long & Chihara, 2000).

Additional barriers to receiving optimal palliative care services are imposed by the Ministry's criteria for admission and staffing and space regulations. Unfortunately, these criteria limit payment for hospice and palliative care to terminally ill patients with cancer or AIDS. Facilities offering palliative care services must meet the high standards of staffing and space requirements required of acute care hospitals and employ at least one full-time physician trained in palliative care (Long & Chihara, 2000). The number of licensed and unlicensed palliative care hospitals in Japan has increased in recent years but is still far below current needs. Due to a lack of palliative care hospital beds, most terminally ill AIDS or cancer patients die in regular hospital wards (Hayashi, 2008). There are no reimbursable palliative care beds available for Japanese dying from other illnesses. This means that families and patients who desire such care must pay privately.

Japan's traditions and government policies surrounding palliative care and reimbursable healthcare services have complicated end-of-life care. Concepts such as advance directives, hospice, and palliative care are still new to many in Japanese society. Given limited fiscal resources, resolving individual, government, health professional, and societal perspectives regarding end-of-life care is a formidable challenge. From a family perspective, it is difficult to decide when to stop treatment in favor of respecting a loved one's personal wishes and dignity. Given the long embedded traditions of Japanese culture, changes affecting end-of-life care are likely to come very slowly.

Norway

Demographic Trends

The Norwegian population is expected to increase from 4.8 million in 2009 to 6.9 million in 2060. This represents a 44% increase in the general population; however, the percentage of those over age 67 is estimated to increase by 140% during the same period. Growth in Norway's senior population is a consequence of high birth rates during the 1930s and 1940s, an increasing life span, and high

CASE STUDY | *DR. YAMADA*

Dr. Yamada is a 78-year-old retired professor who lives at home with his son in Tokyo. Dr. Yamada and his wife own the house, have lived there for more than 40 years, and raised their only son, who is a 40-year-old unmarried man who works for a computer company. Retired for several years, Dr. Yamada has physical disabilities. He can walk continuously for only about 30 minutes because of an injured leg.

Dr. Yamada and his 75-year-old wife of 50 years traveled quite a bit within Japan after his retirement and enjoyed personal time together. Two years ago, Mrs. Yamada fell while riding a bicycle to go shopping. She hit her head so badly that her cognition was severely affected. She was hospitalized, recovered from a month-long coma and was eventually institutionalized in a nursing home on the outskirts of Tokyo. Mrs. Yamada is able to recognize her family members, but she cannot sustain conversations because she no longer can follow a train of thought. This unexpected misfortune devastated both Dr. Yamada and the couple's son and changed their lifestyle, because Mrs. Yamada had played a major role in their everyday life.

Typical of Dr. Yamada's generation in Japan, Japanese men were discouraged from doing household or kitchen work and were held in esteem as the breadwinner of the household. Until her accident, Mrs. Yamada took care of all household chores, including cooking, shopping, cleaning, and raising a child while her husband worked. Therefore, when she was hospitalized, Dr. Yamada and his son had no idea how to take over her duties.

It took more than a year for both Dr. Yamada and his son to accept the fact that Mrs. Yamada would no longer return to perform these duties, and they had no one to provide the joy of physical and psychological help normally provided by Mrs. Yamada. In the 2 years that have passed, they have just started to adjust to their new lifestyle. The son prepares breakfast and Dr. Yamada's lunch before going to work, and then he cooks dinner after work, which is around 10 o'clock in the evening. Dr. Yamada washes dishes, cleans the house, and does the laundry.

Six months ago, Dr. Yamada decided to join a ceramics class at a local senior center while waiting for his son to come home rather just watching television. He enjoyed the class at the beginning, but once class members found out that Dr. Yamada had been a professor at a prestigious university, their attitude changed because professors are highly esteemed in Japan's tradition of a hierarchical society. Dr. Yamada felt uncomfortable and decided not to continue with the class. Now he spends most of his time reading books, watching television, and not socializing outside of the home because Mrs. Yamada had been his main connection to the outside world.

It has been almost 2 years since the son began preparing their daily meals and doing the shopping. In Japan, it is customary to do the grocery shopping every day because living space is very limited, especially in Tokyo. Therefore, in addition to his work, the son has to buy food every evening after work and then cook and share an evening meal with Dr. Yamada, which puts a lot of pressure on both the son and Dr. Yamada. The son feels pressure not to have Dr. Yamada wait for a long time for his dinner, and Dr. Yamada feels uneasy that he cannot help his son with the cooking.

One year ago, as Dr. Yamada qualified to receive house chore help under the national health insurance plan, he suggested that he would have a home helper once a week for basic housework and have meals delivered every day so that these services would ease the son's daily burden. However, the son was not agreeable to the idea. Receiving outside help and "welfare" assistance while the family is still resourceful does not appear good and would cause the family to lose face *(Sekentei)*. Dr. Yamada is very much concerned about the possibility of his son's burnout, but Dr. Yamada understands his son and accepts his proposal

CASE STUDY | *DR. YAMADA*—cont'd

that he will continue his role as a son, fulfilling his filial obligation in Japanese tradition for as long as possible despite Dr. Yamada's wishes to ease the living condition of the son, as well as his own.

1. Considering the Japanese traditions and customs, are there any other ways to take care of Dr. Yamada and his son's living situation?
2. When, if ever, is it time to accept outside help, such as a home helper or meal delivery service?
3. As Dr. Yamada gets older and more frail, he will most likely need more assistance in his activities of daily living. What are the signs to take different approaches for their living conditions, if there are any?
4. How can the son accept the concept that receiving outside help is not a sign of abandoning his filial obligation?
5. How can Dr. Yamada be encouraged to connect with outside society such as attending classes?
6. What other outside sources can he approach and how?

Christina E. Miyawaki, MA, MSW, Doctoral Candidate

immigration rates. Life expectancy is projected to significantly increase from 78.3 to 87.1 years for men and from 83 to 93.4 years for women by 2060 (Statistics Norway, 2009).

With an increasing life expectancy, it is not surprising that the number of adults over age 80 will nearly double in the next 35 years (Norwegian Ministry of Health and Care Services, 2006). The greatest growth in this age group will take place around 2020 (Norwegian Directory of Health and Social Affairs, 2007a). At the same time, there will be fewer working adults and fewer middle-aged adults to care for these elderly. Women have traditionally cared for aging relatives, but men have been more participatory in recent years. The greatest potential resource for future family care is through an increased participation by men (Norwegian Ministry of Health and Care Services, 2006).

The financial burden to provide health care for an increasingly older population is significant. Cost projections for nursing and health care estimate a 6.1% increase over the next 40 years. Adding to the fiscal burden is the fact that more older adults will receive pensions that are supported by a smaller workforce. As life expectancy increases, so does the time during which pensions must be paid. Estimates from the Pension Commission (NOU 2009:13) show that expenditures for retirement pensions are expected to nearly triple by 2050. The financial impact will be felt sooner in the pension sector than in the long-term care sector. Addressing these financial burdens is one of Norway's greatest challenges.

National Priorities

In Norway, the Patients' Rights Act guarantees health care services regardless of age or location (Norwegian Ministry of Health and Care Services, 2009). Some of the rights conferred by this Act are the right to needed health care, to choose which hospital to be treated at, and to have an individualized plan of care for complex needs (such as services from several health care professionals or from different levels in the health care system). One professional is responsible for coordinating services and implementing the individualized plan.

Nordic health care, or its welfare model, is characterized by well-developed health and social services that include long-term care (LTC). LTC services support family caregivers who also need to continue working. Services are determined on the basis of the individual's wishes and needs regardless of social status, personal finances, place of residence, or way of living. Long-term care includes in-home care, as well as municipal or community-based care housing services. Nearly 80% of services are provided in the home, and there has been a twofold increase in the number of users under age 67 since 1996.

With the increased number and proportion of older adults in Norway over the past several years, there has been a corresponding growth in demand for health care services. This has placed an economic burden on the nation such that Norway is currently reevaluating the capacity and adequacy of its community and hospital services with regard to future LTC service needs (Norwegian Ministry of Health and Care Services, 2006). Care Plan 2015, proposed in 2006, charges communities, the government, and citizens to engage in long-term planning for the nation's health-care needs. The plan includes investment in buildings, personnel, training, and adaptation of the physical and social environment. This planning work must be carried out at both municipal and national levels and requires a close interaction between national authorities and the municipal sector. It is envisioned that the future welfare state will require everyone to contribute toward health care costs. The Norwegian government has challenged its citizens to become involved in planning and designing new community structures and services for the future (Norwegian Ministry of Health and Care Services, 2006).

Aging Issues

Care of the aged in Norway is facing increasing demand, as well as the need for reform of its service delivery. Nursing homes constitute more than 60% of all registered institutions in Norway (Vigran, 2000). The average age of Norwegian residents in nursing homes is 84 years. Each resident averages four to five medical diagnoses, and 80% have cognitive decline or dementia (Engedal, Kirkevold, Eek, & Nygård, 2002; Lafortune & Balestat, 2007). One goal is that all people in elderly care have single rooms and, in 2008, more than 96% of all rooms in institutions for persons with a disability were private rooms. In the past two decades, there has been greater emphasis on adapted housing for those who have disability but are still fairly independent. These houses or apartments are often built near nursing homes where residents can access more assistance if necessary.

Despite these efforts, there remains a shortage of nursing home beds and adapted housing. The Norwegian Directory of Health and Social Affairs has estimated the need for rebuilding nursing homes and new construction of adapted housing at 37,000 dwelling units from 2006 until 2030 (Norwegian Ministry of Health and Care Services, 2007). Surveys also indicate that current LTC services do not meet the social and cultural needs of residents (Werntoft, Hallberg, & Edberg, 2007b). It is important for LTC services to include more than just physical care of the elderly. Small-scale communal living arrangements and wards with programmed activities and direct access to adapted outdoor areas provide opportunities for engagement not possible in multistory structures with large units and long corridors. More emphasis on the patient's perspective as a central focus and better integration of multidisciplinary services are necessary to provide optimal care.

An increasing number of patients with dementia places additional demands on personnel and services and underscores the need to customize care to meet individual needs (Norwegian Ministry of Health and Care Services, 2006). The occurrence of dementia increases with age:

- 0.9% among those ages 65 to 69
- 17.6% among those ages 80 to 84
- 40.7% for those age 90 and above

With life expectancy in Norway approaching the eighth and ninth decades, it is estimated that numbers of persons suffering from dementia could double by the year 2040. More than 80% of nursing home residents have a dementia illness, but only about half of patients diagnosed with dementia live in a nursing home. The remainder live in their own homes. Public policy firmly supports the right to receive services that will allow patients to live at home for as long as possible. Adjusted housing is another option for patients who can live independently with modifications to their physical environment. Unfortunately, as stated previously, housing availability is far below demand.

Dementia illnesses already represent the largest group of illnesses in the care services. By 2020, the estimated annual cost for dementia illnesses is expected to be 18 billion crowns ($2.9 billion), a 50% increase since 1995 (Norwegian Directory of Health and Social Affairs, 2007a). To address the increasing incidence of dementia illness and associated care needs, Dementia Plan 2015 was published in 2007. The Dementia Plan recognized that current care services are inadequately developed and adapted to persons with dementia. The primary goal of this plan is that persons with dementia and their families receive accurate information and individually adjusted services without regard to their address of residence (Norwegian Directory of Health, 2010). The plan also recognized the need for better provider training, organizational care models that promote patient-centered care, and structural designs that optimize quality living in a safe environment.

For patients who stay at home, day programs are necessary to support family caregivers. Day programs are a missing link in the current levels of service. These programs are meant to occupy and stimulate patients, be enjoyable, and provide a meaningful daily existence. At the same time, they can provide some relief for immediate family from care tasks during the day, helping to enable spouses and other family members to cope with the demands of caring for a loved one with dementia. Only 4% of those who live at home with a dementia disorder in 2006 had a program to attend during the day (Norwegian Ministry of Health and Care Services, 2007).

Several reports have shown that a person's age may affect treatment (Larsson, Schlundt, Patel, McClellan, & Hargreaves, 2007; McCabe, Hertzog, Grasser, & Walker, 2005; Werntoft, Hallberg, & Edberg, 2007a, 2007b). In 2001, a Norwegian study reported that persons age 70 and over had to wait longer for medical treatment or surgery (Arnesen, Erikssen, & Stavem, 2001). In 2005, investigators reported that older adults with myocardial infarction had been excluded from some clinical studies and received less than optimal treatment. For example, Eritsland, Kløw, Westheim, Bendz, and Mangschau (2005) reported that older people were less likely to receive antithrombolytic treatment or angiography than younger people despite the fact that the success rate of revascularization is shown to be similar between older (mean age 80) and younger patients. Melberg, Thoresen, Hansen, and Westheim (2005) similarly reported that older adults suffering from a stroke did not receive the same quality of treatment and care as younger patients (Center for Medical Method Assessment, 2002). Age, comorbidities, and cognitive decline have been cited as reasons why older adults sometimes do not receive health-care services (Førde, Pedersen, Nortvedt, & Aasland, 2006). Despite federal documents stating that entitlement to health care services should not be based on age but rather on severity of disease, treatment efficacy, and cost versus benefit, it appears that older age may negatively impact the treatment and care of older adults (Norges Offentlige Utredninger, 1987, 1997).

Better education of patients with dementia and their families about municipal and social services is a key focus of Norway's Dementia Plan (Norwegian Ministry of Health and Care Services, 2007). "School for family caregivers" is designed to teach family members caring for a relative with a dementia disease increased knowledge about the disease, as well as coping skills in dealing with friends, other family members, and staff in LTC settings (http://www.nasjonalforeningen.no/no/Demens/Parorende/Parorendeskole/).

End-of-Life Care

About 80% of Norwegians today die in hospitals or nursing homes, compared with 100 years ago when 90% of deaths occurred at home. Death has moved from the place of the family and home to an institutional environment where the values and views of elderly people, their family members, health care staff, the organization, and society intersect (Schaffer 2007, p. 242). Although 40% of Norwegians die in nursing homes, Husebø and Husebø (2005) state that nursing homes may be suitable places for good end-of-life care if the dying patient is met with the necessary competence and recourse for alleviating adverse symptoms. Unfortunately, this is often not the case. They propose that alleviating unnecessary treatment and hospitalizations at the end of life ought to be a declared goal in Norwegian nursing homes (Husebø & Husebø, 2005).

The development of palliative care in Norway started in the early 1970s but did not become an official part of the national health care system until the early 1990s. A report on symptom control and overall care of the seriously ill and dying patient identified a number of neglected problem areas and proposed a package of measures to improve palliative care in Norway. Free-standing hospice units were deemed unrealistic in the Norwegian health care system. Dedicated units within the existing nursing care and hospital departments were recommended as an alternative. To facilitate provider education, training, and clinical research, hospice units were recommended in all university hospitals. The first university-based palliative unit was established in Trondheim in 1992. Since then, palliative medical units with designated beds and expert teams have been established at several local hospitals and nursing homes (Kaasa, Breivik, & Jordhøy, 2002). Because the size of Norwegian municipalities varies considerably, in small municipalities one alternative to a palliative care unit is to designate one or two beds for palliative treatment and make use of these as required (Norwegian Directory of Health and Social Affairs, 2007b).

The increasing number of elderly in Norway creates challenges in recruiting sufficient numbers of health care professionals trained in palliative care and in providing enough beds to meet the demand for institutional end-of-life care (Kaasa, Breivik, & Jordhøy, 2002). Increasing resources have been allocated to palliative care over the past few years, including the establishment of an academic chair in palliative medicine. In 2001, the Norwegian Society of Palliative Medicine was recognized as a specialist society within the Norwegian Medical Association (Kaasa et al., 2002).

In 2003, Norway had the least number of palliative care units in northern Europe relative to its population, while today there are five competence centers for alleviating treatment in Norway (Husebø & Husebø, 2003). There is also more focused interest and awareness of the need for palliative care in society at large so that, despite this progress, health professionals, older adults, and family members have criticized the government for not allocating more resources to improve the quality of health care for its aging citizens (Kaasa, et al., 2002; Schaffer, 2007).

The issue of medical futility at the end of life is complex. The Norwegian Directory of Health and Social Affairs (2009) recently published a guide for making decisions about when to restrict life-prolonging treatment in seriously ill and dying patients. The purpose of this guide is to ensure the quality of the decision-making process. Most patients, however, do not prepare advance directives such as health care proxies or living wills (Life Testament) to express their wishes about treatment when they become terminally ill (Box 25-3).

BOX 25-3 Norway's Life Testament

Norway's living will, called a Life Testament, is legally recognized but not legally binding. Requirements for the Life Testament in Norway include the following:

- Physicians must have a reasonable time in which to consider the injury and prognosis before deciding whether to start or continue active treatment.
- Patients with a Life Testament must annually sign and carry a card in their wallet affirming that the Life Testament is still valid (Slettebø, 2009).

Research shows that the intention of not wanting active treatment often changes in relation to changes in condition (Ruyter, Nortvedt, & Førde, 1993), and this makes it difficult for providers to decide whether to follow the intention in the Life Testament or not. Despite greater public awareness about palliative care, the Life Testament is not commonly used by Norwegians.

Although quality of life in Norway is high, conditions may still be humiliating for people living in nursing homes, in their own homes, and in hospitals (Lillestø, 1998; Nåden & Sæteren, 2006; Slettebø, 2002). To address the issue, the Norwegian Ministry of Health and Care Services (2009) released a discussion document proposing regulations about dignified care of the elderly. It asserts the right of all citizens to receive care within a system of integrity and that respect for an individual's dignity is a fundamental element in reasonable health care services. The document also raises questions concerning what constitutes justifiable and secure living arrangements and existential topics such as the value and meaning of life. Hopefully this discussion document will generate new regulations that support its assertions. Attending to a patient's need for dignity is regarded as one of the primary objectives of the health professions (Edlund, 2002; Eriksson, 1996; Gonzales, 2000).

Conclusion

Challenges in meeting the needs of older adults are faced by all nations, whether developing or developed. Policies and structures that provide care to those who are poor, living in rural areas, or living without family support are struggles many nations have yet to resolve. Adequate community resources and housing for aging citizens who can no longer care for themselves or live safely alone is also lacking in many countries around the globe. Helping older adults achieve health habits that prevent disease empowers them to achieve a better quality of life, yet resources and infrastructures to support healthy living and prevent disease have yet to be optimized.

Attitudes and misperceptions held by providers, policymakers, and leaders affect how national priorities are determined and the allocation of resources. Understanding that successful aging is multifaceted, with physical, psychological, spiritual, and social dimensions, requires a holistic perspective. Globally, insufficient numbers of providers specialize in gerontology and articulate what change is necessary to those in leadership. Better education about the needs of older adults in health care curricula is an essential first step toward greater understanding. Optimization of health among older citizens is a global challenge. Through international collaboration, better solutions and the sharing of proven, cost-effective models of care are possible.

CASE STUDY | *MRS. ANNA ANDERSEN*

Mrs. Anna Andersen, age 70, is hospitalized in a local hospital because of a stroke. She has arm and foot paralysis and difficulties talking. She improves after some weeks and is able to walk with a walker. Her language has improved as well but still causes her some difficulty. Her friend and next of kin, Mrs. Jensen, also 70 and an educated nurse, accompanied her to the hospital and has visited Mrs. Andersen in the hospital several times a week.

During her hospital stay, Mrs. Andersen has benefited from physiotherapy and speech therapy.

The staff discuss what to do with Mrs. Andersen. Her continual improvement is due to her hospital stay, yet other patients have more acute needs for hospital care. They tell Mrs. Jensen that they don't know what to do with Mrs. Andersen. Mrs. Jensen argues that Mrs. Andersen's wish is to either stay in the hospital until she has gained more mobility and improved her speech or move to a specialist rehabilitation clinic. She also informs the staff that both she and Mrs. Andersen wish to attend the meeting when the patient's future is to be discussed.

One day when Anna Andersen's friend sits together with her in her room, the physician and head nurse enter the room. They remain standing when they inform Mrs. Andersen that they have decided to move her to a nursing home. The head nurse emphasizes that this will be a better situation for Mrs. Andersen because it will be quieter and calmer than the hospital. The two women are shocked. They had hoped that the staff would listen to the patient's wish.

Mrs. Andersen's friend asks whether a nursing home is the right place for rehabilitation and would like to know whether there is physiotherapy and speech therapy. The physician says that there may be physiotherapy, but he doubts that there is speech therapy.

You are a nurse on this ward, and you have taken part in the staff's discussions. You also observe the situation in Mrs. Andersen's room.

1. What are your reactions to the situation? What do you do?
2. How would you describe the communication among the patient, the next of kin, and the health care personnel?
3. How is human life valued in this situation?
4. How can the patient's dignity and autonomy be restored after this episode?
5. What are the patient's civil rights in a situation like Mrs. Andersen's (from the perspective of the laws in the respective country)?

Dagfinn Nåden, RN, HVD (Doctor in Health Care) and Åshild SlettebØ, RN, PhD

KEY POINTS

Demographic Trends

- The average life expectancy has increased around the world but is greater among developed than developing nations.
- Among developed nations, the population is increasingly composed of older adults due to declining fertility or birth rates and a longer life expectancy.
- Classically, in developing countries the disease pattern is dominated by infectious diseases, while in developed countries the issues are chronic diseases of lifestyle.
- Factors such as the displacement effects of war, urbanization, seasonal migration in agrarian nations, and emigration of breadwinners have distanced family members from one another, leaving many older adults with limited familial support.
- Women are traditionally the primary familial caregivers in most nations.

Health Trends and Priorities

- Developed nations are ramping up health promotion programs to limit disease and disability in an attempt to control upwardly spiraling health care costs.
- Health priorities in developing countries are more focused on controlling infectious diseases, reducing infant and maternal mortality, improving sanitation, and reducing malnutrition.

- Nearly all developed countries have nationalized health care insurance programs.
- With limited resources, developing countries with predominantly younger populations tend to target the young rather than the old.
- Movement from extended to nuclear families undermines traditional family support systems and increases social responsibility for the care of older adults.

Aging Issues

- Health expenditures do not necessarily translate to better health and greater longevity.
- The United States spends more than any other developed nation on health care and also has the highest percentage of privatized health care insurance.
- Many developing countries lack nationalized health care policies or coverage.
- The underserved poor and uninsured remain concerns in developed and developing nations.
- In developed nations, trends such as adults remaining single, economic migration, and more women in the workforce have resulted in fewer family caregivers for an increasingly older population.
- Developed nations struggle with inadequate social support services and insufficient rehabilitation services or residential beds to meet the needs of their aging populations.
- Declining birth rates in many developed countries mean that there are fewer working aged adults to support retirement, health, and custodial care costs of increasingly older populations.
- Worldwide, there are insufficient numbers of health care providers who are trained in geriatrics.
- All nations struggle with inadequate prevention programs and inadequate and poorly coordinated community support services for older adults.
- Ageism continues to be a factor in allocating health care resources.

End-of-Life Care

- Most countries, whether developed or developing, lack adequate end-of-life care resources.
- Culture and tradition play a large role in end-of-life preferences and decision making.
- Most people would prefer to be cared for at home if they were dying; however, many people in developed countries die in hospitals or nursing homes.
- End-of-life concerns include the frequent lack of advance directives, staff who are uneducated in providing good end-of-life care, and limitations in providing optimal care because of unsuitable physical environments and lack of resources.

CRITICAL THINKING ACTIVITIES

1. What influence might nurses have over national policies on aging?
2. How might you motivate specialist training for nurses in gerontology?
3. What role can community and faith-based organizations have in meeting the care and support needs of older persons in the community?
4. How can the dominant myths about growing older in Africa among policymakers and politicians be addressed?
   a. "No specific care is necessary, since African families look after their own older people."
   b. "We do not have a problem in terms of older people because we have a young population."
5. Explore the traditions of death and dying in a culture that is different from your own.

REFERENCES

Africa

Arogundade, F. A., & Barsoum, R. S. (2008). CKD prevention in sub-Saharan Africa: A call for governmental, nongovernmental, and community support. *American Journal of Kidney Diseases, 51*(3), 515–523.

Bongaarts, J., & Zimmer, Z (2002). Living arrangements of the elderly in the developing world: An analysis of DHS household surveys. *Journal of Gerontology: Social Sciences, 57*(1), S145–S157.

Charlton, K. E. (2000). Nutrition, health and old age: The case of South African urban elderly. *SA Journal of Clinical Nutrition, 13*(1), 1–8.

Fathers for Life. (2010). *Differences in the life expectancies of the sexes in various countries in the world.* Retrieved December 15, 2010, from http://www.fathersforlife.org/health/lifeexpw.htm

Joubert, J. D., & Bradshaw, D. (2008). Population ageing and health challenges in South Africa. In K. Steyn, J. Fourie, & N. Temple (Eds.), *Chronic diseases of lifestyle in South Africa: 1995-2005. Technical Report.* Cape Town: South African Medical Research Council.

Kinsella, K., & Ferreira, M. (1997). *International brief. Aging trends: South Africa.* Washington, DC: U.S. Department of Commerce Economics and Statistics, Bureau of Census.

Kowal, P. R., Chalapati Rao, P. V., & Mathers, C. (2003). *Minimum data set on ageing in sub-Saharan Africa: Report on a WHO Workshop.* Pretoria, South Africa, February, 12–14, 2003.

Mehta, U., Durrheim, D. N., Blockman, M., Kredo, T., Gounden, R., & Barnes, K. I. (2008). Adverse drug reactions in adult medical inpatients in a South African hospital serving a community with a high HIV/AIDS prevalence: Prospective observational study. *British Journal of Clinical Pharmacology, 65*(3), 396–406.

Moller, V., & Sotshongaye, A. (1996). My family eats this money too: Pension sharing and self-respect among Zulu grandmothers. *South African Journal of Gerontology, 5*(2), 9–19.

Nicolay, N. (2008). *Summary of: provincial HIV and AIDS statistics for South Africa.* Retrieved December 15, 2010, from http://www.metam.co.za/documents_v2/File/RedRibbon_2009/Provincial%20HIV%20and%20AIDS%20statistics%20for%202008.pdf

Oldewage-Theron,W. H., & Kruger, R. (2008). Food variety and dietary diversity as indicators of the dietary adequacy and health status of an elderly population in Sharpeville, South Africa. *Journal of Nutrition for the Eldery, 27*(1–2), 101–133.

Schatz, E. J. (2007). Taking care of my own blood: Older women's relationships to their households in rural South Africa. *Scandinavian Journal of Public Health, 35*(69), 147–154.

Smith, S. M., & Mensah, G. A. (2003). Population aging and implications for epidemic cardiovascular disease in sub-Saharan Africa. *Ethnicity and Disease, 13*(2), S77–S80.

Sodorenko, A., & Walker, A. (2004). The Madrid international plan of action on ageing: From conception to implementation. *Ageing & Society, 24,* 147–165.

Statistics South Africa. (2001). *Census 2001. Investigation into appropriate definitions of urban and rural areas for South Africa.* Report no. 03-02-20. Pretoria: Author.

Statistics South Africa. (2008). *General household survey 2007.* Statistical release P0318. Pretoria: Author. Retrieved December 15, 2010, from http://www.statssa.gov.za/publications/P0318/P0318July2007.pdf

United Nations. (2002). *Madrid international plan of action on ageing, 2002.* Retrieved December 12, 2010, from http://www.un.org/ageing/madrid_intlplanaction.html

United Nations: Department of Economic and Social Affairs. (2008). *World population aging: 2007.* New York: Author.

Zimmer, Z., & Dayton, J. (2003). *The living arrangements of older adults in sub-Saharan Africa in a time of HIV/AIDS.* No 169. New York, NY: Population Council, Policy Research Division. Retrieved December 15, 2010, from http://www.popcouncil.org/pdfs/wp/169.pdf

Nigeria

Aboderin, I. (2009). *Advancing health services provision for older persons and age-related non-communicable diseases in sub-Saharan Africa.* Oxford Institute of Aging, Oxford University.

Aboderin, I., & Gachuhi, M. (2006). *First East African policy-research dialogue on aging. AFRAN Policy Research Series no. 1. African research on aging.* Oxford Institute of Aging, University of Oxford.

Adisa, A. I., Agunbiade, M., & Akanmu, O.E. (2008). House ownership as a well-being index among retirees in Ogun state, Nigeria. *Journal of International Social Research, 1*(5), 1–46.

Alexander, S. C., Bank, A., & Perron, M. (2006). Medical care at the end of life. In J. F. O'Neill, P. A. Selwyn, & H. Schietinger (Eds.), *A clinical guide to supportive and palliative care for HIV/AIDS, 2003.* Merrifield, VA: Health Resources and Services Administration, U.S. Department of Health and Human Services.

Ajomale, O. (2009). *Country report: ageing in Nigeria—current state, social and economic implications.* Madrid, Spain: International Sociological Association, Research Committee II, Sociology of Aging of the International Sociological Association. Retrieved December 12, 2010, from http://www.eldis.org/go/country-profiles&id=42024&type=Document

Bretton Woods Project. (2009). *World Bank health work flawed: Still pushing for privatisation of services.* Retrieved December 5, 2010, from http://www.brettonwoodsproject.org/art-564820

Central Intelligence Agency. (2010). *The world factbook: Nigeria.* Washington, DC: Author. Retrieved December 15, 2010, from https://www.cia.gov/library/publications/the-world-factbook/geos/ni.html

Hartford Institute Geriatric Nursing Forum. (2009). The epidemiology of independence in older people in Nigeria: Prevalence, determinants. *Journal of the American Geriatrics Society, 3*(8), 2.

Iroegbu, S. (2007). *Nigeria: Caring for the aged . . . Task before Nigeria.* New York, NY: Global Action on Aging. Retrieved December 15, 2010, from http://www.globalaging.org/elderrights/world/2007/nigeria.aged.htm

Omotola, I., Adesola, O., & Adenike, O. (2006). Family nursing education and family nursing practice in Nigeria. *Journal of Family Nursing, 12*(4), 442–447.

Otuyelu, S. A. (2002, April 10). *Nigeria statement.* Madrid, Spain: Second World Assembly on Ageing. Retrieved December 15, 2010, from http://www.un.org/swaa2002/coverage/nigeriaE.htm

Shittu, H. (2008, March 10). *Nigeria: World bank, government partner on health-care delivery.* Retrieved December 15, 2010, from http://allafrica.com/stories/200803101260.html

United Nations Statistics Division. (2009). *World statistics pocketbook 2009.* New York, NY: Author.

Williams, R. (2009). *The hardships of being an elder in Nigeria.* Retrieved December 15, 2010, from http://www.associatedcontent.com/article/1332504/the_hardships_of_being_an_elder_in.html

World Health Organization. (2006). *Mortality country fact sheet 2006: Nigeria.* Geneva, Switzerland: Author. Retrieved December 15, 2010, from http://www.who.int/whosis/mort/profiles/mort_afro_nga_nigeria.pdf

Canada

Berger, C., Langsetmo, L., Joseph, L., Hanley, D. A., Davidson, K. S., Josse, R., . . . Goltzman, D. (2008). Change in bone mineral density as a function of age in women and men and association with the use of antiresorptive agents. *CMAJ, 178*(13), 1660–1668.

Burge, F. I., Lawson, B., & Johnston, G. (2005, January 27). Home visits by family physicians during the end-of-life: Does patient income or residence play a role? *BMC Palliative Care, 4.* 1. Retrieved December 15, 2010, from http://www.biomedcentral.com/1472-684X/4/1

Canadian Institute for Health Information. (2009a). *Health care in Canada 2009: A decade in review.* Ottawa: Author.

Retrieved December 15, 2010, from http://secure.cihi.ca/cihiweb/products/HCIC_2009_Web_e.pdf

Canadian Institute for Health Information. (2009b). *Analysis in brief. Alternate level of care in Canada.* Ottawa: Author. Retrieved December 15, 2010, from http://secure.cihi.ca/cihiweb/products/ALC_AIB_FINAL.pdf

Canadian Study of Health and Aging. (1994). Patterns of caring for people with dementia in Canada. *Canadian Journal on Aging, 13*(4), 470–487.

Canadian Study of Health and Aging Working Group. (1994). Canadian Study of Health and Aging: Study methods and prevalence of dementia. *CMAJ, 150*(6), 899–913.

Canadian Study of Health and Aging Working Group. (2002). Patterns and health effects of caring for people with dementia: The impact of changing cognitive and residential status. *Gerontologist, 42*(5), 643–652.

Carstairs, S., & Beaudoin, G. A. (2000). *Quality end-of-life care: The right of every Canadian. Subcommittee to update "Of Life and Death" of the standing senate committee on social affairs, science and technology. Final Report.* Ottawa: Senate of Canada. Retrieved December 15, 2010, from http://www.parl.gc.ca/36/2/parlbus/commbus/ senate/com-e/upda-e/rep-e/repfinjun00-e.htm

Carstairs, S., & Keon, W. J. (2008). *Issues and options for an aging population. Special senate committee on aging second interim report.* Ottawa: Senate of Canada. Retrieved December 15, 2010, from http://www.parl.gc.ca/39/2/parlbus/commbus/senate/com-e/agei-e/rep-e/repfinmar08-e.pdf

Carstairs, S., & Keon, W. J. (2009). *Canada's aging population: Seizing the opportunity. Special Senate committee on aging final report.* Ottawa: Senate of Canada. Retrieved December 15, 2010, from http://www.parl.gc.ca/40/2/parlbus/commbus/senate/com-e/agei-e/rep-e/AgingFinalReport-e.pdf

Cranswick, K., & Dosman, D. (2008). Eldercare: What we know today. *Canadian Social Trends, 86,* 48–56. Retrieved December 15, 2010, from http://www.statcan.gc.ca/pub/11-008-x/2008002/article/10689-eng.pdf

Frederick, J. A., & Fast, J. E. (1999). Eldercare in Canada: Who does how much? *Canadian Social Trends, 54,* 26–32. Retrieved December 15, 2010, from http://www.statcan.gc.ca/pub/11-008-x/1999002/article/4661-eng.pdf

Garrett, D. D., Tuokko, H., Stajduhar, K. I., Lindsay, J., & Buehler, S. (2008). Planning for end-of-life care: Findings from the Canadian Study of Health and Aging. *Canadian Journal on Aging, 27*(1), 11–21.

Health Canada. (1998). *Principles of the national framework on aging: A policy guide.* Cat. no. H88-3/21-1998E. Ottawa: Minister of Public Works and Government Services Canada. Retrieved December 15, 2010, from http://www.phac-aspc.gc.ca/seniors-aines/publications/pro/healthy-sante/nfa-cnv/index-eng.php

Heyland, D. K., Dodek, P., Rocker, G., Groll, D., Gafni, A., Pichora, D., . . . Lam, M. (2006). What matters most in end-of-life care: Perceptions of seriously ill patients and their family members. *CMAJ, 174*(5). DOI:10.1503/cmaj.050626.

Lindsay, J., Sykes, E., McDowell, I., Verreault, R., & Laurin, D. (2004). More than the epidemiology of Alzheimer's disease: Contributions of the Canadian Study of Health and Aging. *Canadian Journal of Psychiatry, 49*(2), 83–91.

Martin-Matthews, A., & Mealing, L. (2009). Editorial: Realizing the vision. The Canadian Longitudinal Study on Aging as a strategic initiative of the Canadian Institutes of Health Research. *Canadian Journal on Aging, 28*(3), 209–214.

Ontario Ministry of Health and Long-Term Care. (2007, August 28). News Release: McGuinty government transforming community living to help seniors live independently at home. Retrieved December 15, 2010, from http://www.health.gov.on.ca/english/media/news_releases/archives/nr_07/aug/nr_20070828.html

Orpana, H. M., Ross, N., Feeny, D., McFarland, B., Bernier, J., & Kaplan, M. (2009). The natural history of health-related quality of life: A 10-year cohort study. *Health Reports, 20*(1), 1–7.

Public Health Agency of Canada. (2003). *Canada's physical activity guide to healthy active living for older adults.* Retrieved December 15, 2010, from http://www.phac-aspc.gc.ca/pau-uap/paguide/older/index.html

Raina, P., Wolfson, C., Kirkland, S. A., Griffith, L. E., Oremus, M., Patterson, C., . . . Brazil, K. (2009). The Canadian longitudinal study on aging (CLSA). *Canadian Journal on Aging, 28*(3), 221–229.

Ramage-Morin, P. L. (2006). Successful aging in health care institutions. *Health Reports, 16*(Suppl.), 47–56.

Ramage-Morin, P. L. (2009). Medication use among senior Canadians. *Health Reports, 20*(1), 1–8.

Rotermann M. (2006). Seniors' health care use. *Health Reports, 16*(Suppl.), 33–45.

Singer, P. A., & Wolfson, M. (2003). The best places to die. *British Medical Journal, 327,* 173–174.

Statistics Canada. (1973). *1971 Census of Canada.* Population. Catalogue no. 92-715 Vol: 1-Part: 2. Statistics Canada. Ottawa: Information Canada, Minister of Industry, Trade and Commerce.

Statistics Canada. (2005). *Population and growth components (1851–2001 Censuses). 2001 Census of Population.* Ottawa: Statistics Canada. Retrieved October 9, 2009 from http://www40.statcan.gc.ca/l01/cst01/demo03-eng.htm

Statistics Canada. (2007a). *Age and sex, 2006 counts for both sexes, for Canada, provinces and territories–100% data (table). Age and Sex Highlight Tables. 2006 Census.* Statistics Canada Catalogue no. 97-551-XWE2006002. Ottawa, Statistics Canada. Retrieved December 15, 2010, from http://www12.statcan.ca/english/census06/data/highlights/agesex/index.cfm?Lang=E

Statistics Canada. (2007b). *Portrait of the Canadian Population in 2006, by Age and Sex, 2006 Census.* Ottawa: Minister of Industry. Retrieved December 15, 2010, from http://www.statcan.gc.ca/bsolc/olc-cel/olc-cel?lang=eng&catno=97-551-X2006001

Statistics Canada. (2008), *Projected population by age group and sex according to a medium growth scenario for 2006, 2011, 2016, 2021, 2026 and 2031 at July 1.* CANSIM table 052-0004 and Population Projections for Canada, Provinces and Territories. Catalogue no. 91-520-X. Ottawa, Statistics Canada. Retrieved December 15, 2010, from http://www40.statcan.gc.ca/l01/cst01/demo23a-eng.htm

Statistics Canada. (2009a). *Selected demographic, cultural, educational labour force and income characteristics, mother tongue, age groups and sex for the population of Canada, provinces, territories, census divisions and census subdivisions, 2006 census – 20% sample data.* 2006 Census of Population. Catalogue no. 97-555-XCB2006057. Retrieved December 15, 2010, from http://www12.statcan.gc.ca/census-recensement/2006/dp-pd/tbt/Rp-eng.cfm?LANG=E&APATH=3&DETAIL=0&DIM=0&FL=A&FREE=0&GC=0&GID=837928&GK=0&GRP=1&PID=99016&PRID=0&PTYPE=88971,97154&S=0&SHOWALL=0&SUB=0&Temporal=2006&THEME=70&VID=0&VNAMEE=&VNAMEF=

Statistics Canada. (2009b). *Life expectancy at birth, by sex, by province.* Catalogue no 84-537-XIE. Ottawa, Statistics Canada. Retrieved December 15, 2010, from http://www40.statcan.gc.ca/l01/cst01/health26-eng.htm

Statistics Canada. (2009c). *Life expectancy at birth and at age 65 by sex and by geography.* CANSIM, table 102-0511 and Catalogue no. 84-537-XIE. Ottawa, Statistics Canada. Retrieved December 15, 2010, from http://www40.statcan.gc.ca/l01/cst01/health72a-eng.htm

Statistics Canada. (2009d). *Deaths, estimates, by province and territory. CANSIM* table 051-0004 and Catalogue no. 91-215-X. Ottawa: Statistics Canada. Retrieved December 15, 2010, from http://www40.statcan.gc.ca/l01/cst01/demo07a-eng.htm

Turcotte, M., & Schellenberg, G. (2007) *A portrait of seniors in Canada 2006.* Cat. no. 89-519-XPE. Ottawa: Minister of Industry. Retrieved December 15, 2010, from http://www.statcan.gc.ca/bsolc/olc-cel/olc-cel?lang=eng&catno=89-519-X

Guatemala

Berry, N. S. (2008). Who's judging the quality of care? Indigenous Maya and the problem of "not being attended". *Medical Anthropology, 27*(2), 164–189.

Bertrand, J., Seiber, E., & Escudero, G. (2001). Contraceptive dynamics in Guatemala: 1978-1998. *International Family Planning Perspectives, 27*(3), 112–118, 136.

Brandes, S. (2001). The cremated Catholic: The ends of a deceased Guatemalan. *Body & Society,* 7, 111–120.

Central Intelligence Agency. (2010). *The world factbook: Guatemala.* Washington, DC: Author.

De Blois, J. A. (1991). *Aging in Guatemala.* International Institute on Aging (United Nations - Malta), 1-63. Retrieved December 15, 2010, from http://www.cicred.org/Eng/Publications/pdf/c-d12.pdf

De Broie, S., & Hinde, A. (2006). Diversity in fertility patterns in Guatemala. *Population, Space and Place, 12,* 435–459.

Economic Commission for Latin America and the Caribbean. (2004). *Report of the meeting of experts on aging: Second Central American and Caribbean forum on policies for older persons.* Economic Commission for Latin America and the Caribbean, 1-28.

Farrar, L. (2007). It can take a village to send Hispanics to final home. *The Boston Globe,* August 19, 2007.

Garcia, S.C. (2009). *Enfemedad de Alzheimer en Guatemala.* Report from Universidad del Valle de Guatemala, Departamento de Ciencias Sociales.

Gidley, R., & Roberts, H. (2003). Setting the truth in stone: Guatemala's monuments to the dead. *Medicine, Conflict, and Survival, 19*(2), 148–157.

Gonzalez, F., & Hereira, M. (2008). Home-based viewing (*el velorio*) after death: A cost-effective alternative for some families. *American Journal of Hospice and Palliative Care, 25,* 419–420.

Gragnolati, M., & Marini, A. (2003). *Health and poverty in Guatemala.* The World Bank, 1-65.

Grandia, L., & Schwartz, N. (2001). *Peten: Salud, migracion, y recuros naturals, Technical report.* Guatemala, Instituto Nacional de Estadistica.

Green, L. (1999). *Fear as a way of life.* New York, NY: Columbia University Press.

Hale, C. (2006). *Mas que un indio.* Santa Fe, NM: School of American Research.

Harman, R. C. (2001). Activities of contemporary Mayan elders. *Journal of Cross-Cultural Gerontology, 16,* 57–77.

Lykes, M. B., Blanche, M. T., & Hamber, B. (2003). Narrating survival and change in Guatemala and South Africa: The politics of representation and a liberatory community psychology. *American Journal of Community Psychology, 31*(1), 79–90.

Maluccio, J. A., Melgar, P., Mendez, H., Murphy, A., & Yount, K. M. (2005). Social and economic development and change in four Guatemalan villages: Demographics, schooling, occupation, and assets. *Food and Nutrition Bulletin, 26*(2 Suppl. 1), S25–S45.

Moran-Taylor, M. J. (2008). Guatemala's ladino and maya migra landscapes: The tangible and intangible outcomes of migration. *Human Organization, 67*(2), 111–124.

Pan American Health Organization. (2001). *Guatemala. Promoting health in the Americas* (pp. 294–302). Geneva, Switzerland: World Health Organization.

Pan American Health Organization. (2002). *Carmen country profiles: Guatemala.* Pan American Health Organization, 1-3.

Pan American Health Organization. (2007a). *Health in the Americas.* Pan American Health Organization, 375-393.

Pan American Health Organization. (2007b). *Survey of diabetes, hypertension and chronic disease risk factors: Villa Nueva, Guatemala 2007.* Pan American Health Organization, 1-80.

U.S. Department of State. (2009). *Guatemala: Country specific information.* Retrieved December 15, 2010, from http://travel.state.gov/travel/cis_pa_tw/cis/cis_1129.html

Worby, P. (1999) *Lessons learned from UNHCR's involvement in the Guatemala refugee repatriation and reintegration programme (1987-1999).* Office of the United Nations High Commissioner for Refugees, 1-15.

World Bank. (2009). *Guatemala at a glance.* Retrieved December 15, 2010, from http://devdata.worldbank.org/AAG/gtm_aag.pdf

World Health Organization. (2007). *Country cooperation strategy at a glance.* World Health Organization, 1-2.

Zechner, M. (2008). Care of older persons in transnational settings. *Journal of Aging Studies, 1,* 32–44.

Ireland

Bolin, K., Lindgren, B., & Lundborg, P. (2008). Your next of kin or your own career? Caring and working among the 50+ of Europe. *Journal of Health Economics, 27*(3), 718–738.

Census of Population. (2006). Dublin, Ireland: Stationery Office.

Central Statistics Office. (2006). *Population and labour force projections.* Dublin, Ireland: Author.

Centre for Aging Research and Development in Ireland. (2009) *Latest CSO figures confirm the need for older carers' strategy.* Retrieved December 15, 2010, from http://www.cardi.ie/

Department of Health and Children. (2001). *Quality and fairness: A health system for you.* Dublin, Ireland: Stationery Office.

Department of Health and Children. (2008). *A fair deal: The nursing home care support scheme,* 2008. Government of Ireland.

Department of Health and Children. (2009). *National positive ageing strategy: Frequently asked questions.* Retrieved December 15, 2010, from http://www.dohc.ie/consultations/closed/positiveageing/faqs.html

Fahey, T. (1995). *Health service implication of population ageing in Ireland.* Dublin, Ireland: National Council for the Elderly.

Irish Nursing Home Organisation. (2006) *Annual private nursing home survey 2006.* Dublin, Ireland: Author.

Layte, R., Fahey, T., & Whelan, C. (1999) *Income, deprivation and well-being among older Irish people.* Report 55. Dublin, Ireland: National Council on Ageing and Older People.

Lothian, K., & Philp, I. (2001). Care of older people: Maintaining the dignity and autonomy of older people in the health care setting. *British Medical Journal, 322,* 668–670.

Mercer Limited. (2002). *Study to examine the future of long-term care in Ireland.* Dublin, Ireland: Stationary Office.

National Economic and Social Forum. (2005). *Care for older people. NSEF Report No. 32.* National Economic and Social Development Office. Retrieved December 3, 2010, from http://www.nesf.ie/dynamic/pdfs/No-32-Care-for-Older-People.pdf

O'Shea, E. (2007). Towards a strategy for older people in Ireland. *Irish Medical Journal, 100,* 8.

O'Shea, E., Murphy K., Larkin P., Payne, S., Froggatt, K., Casey D., . . . Keys, M. (2008), *End of life care for older people in acute and long-stay settings in Ireland.* Dublin, Ireland: Hospice Friendly Hospitals Programme, National Council on Ageing and Older People.

Report of the Working Party on Services for the Elderly. (1988). *The years ahead: A policy for the elderly.* Dublin, Ireland: Stationery Office.

Timonen, V., & Doyle, M. (2008). From the workhouse to the home; Evolution of domiciliary care policies in Ireland. *International Journal of Sociology and Social Policy, 28,* 3–4.

Tracey, G., & Ling, J., 2005, Multicultural Ireland: Weaving the fabric of diversity. In J. Ling & L. O'Siorain (Eds.), *Palliative care in Ireland.* Maidenhead, England: Open University Press.

United Nations. (1991). *United Nations principles for older persons.* Geneva, Switzerland: Author. Retrieved December 15, 2010, from http://www.un.org/ageing/un_principles.html

Weafer, J. A. (2004). *Nationwide study of public attitudes and experiences regarding death and dying.* Dublin, Ireland: The Irish Hospice Foundation.

Western Health Board. (2000). *Services for older people: A strategy for health and wellbeing 2001-2006.* Western health Board, Services for Older People.

Japan

Asahara, K., Momose, Y., & Murashima, S. (2003). Long-term care insurance in Japan. *Disease Management and Health Outcomes, 11*(12), 769–777.

Davis, A. J., & Konishi, E. (2000). End-of-life ethical issues in Japan. *Journal of Geriatric Nursing, 21*(2), 89–91.

Fukawa, T. (2007). Health and long-term care expenditures of the elderly in Japan using a micro-simulation model. *Japanese Journal of Social Security Policy, 6*(2), 199–206.

Hayashi, A. (2008). *Kanwakea no nihon no genjō ni tsuite* [The current state of palliative care in Japan]. Symposium on Gan shumakki no iryotaisei wo kangaeru [Medical care for the terminal cancer patients], Tokyo, Japan.

Imamura, M. (2007). *Kanwakea ni okeru nichibei hikaku* [Palliative care: A comparison between Japan and the U.S.]. *Hitotsubashi Hōgaku* [The Hitotsubashi Journal of Law and International Studies], *6*(1), (2), (3), 473–508, 919–963, 1393–1415.

Inoue, C. (Ed.). (2009). *Kaigo no kihon* [Caregiving basics]. Kyoto, Japan: Meibun Publisher.

Kimura, R. (1998). Death, dying, and advance directives in Japan: Socio-cultural and legal point of view. In H-M. Sass, R. M. Veatch, & R. Kimura (Eds.), *Advance directives and surrogate decision making in health care* (pp. 187–208). Baltimore, MD: Johns Hopkins University Press.

Kōseirōdōshō (Ministry of Health, Labor and Welfare). (2007a). *Heisei 19 nen kaigo sābisu shisetsu & Jigyosho chosakekka no gaikyo* [2007 Summary of long-term care facilities and services]. Tokyo: Tōkeijōhōbu (Statistics and Information Section), Daijin Kanbō (Minister's Secretariat), Kōseirōdōshō.

Kōseirōdōshō (Ministry of Health, Labor and Welfare). (2007b). *Kaigo hoken jigyojyokyo hōkoku no gaiyō heisei 19 nendoban* [2007 Report on the status of long-term care insurance]. Tokyo: Tōkeijōhōbu (Statistics and Information Section), Daijin Kanbō (Minister's Secretariat), Kōseirōdōshō.

Kōseirōdōshō (Ministry of Health, Labor and Welfare). (2007c). *Kaigo kyofuhi jittaichosa geppo Heisei 19 nen 8 gatsu shinsabun* [2009 Ministry of Health: Monthly survey of long-term care payment FY 2007 minute 8]. Tokyo: Tōkeijōhōbu (Statistics and Information Section), Daijin Kanbō (Minister's Secretariat), Kōseirōdōshō.

Kōseirōdōshō (Ministry of Health, Labor and Welfare). (2009a). *Heisei 20 nen kōreisha no kenkō ni kansuru ishiki chōsa kekka* [2008 Results of survey on the health of the elderly]. Tokyo: Tōkeijōhōbu (Statistics and Information Section), Daijin Kanbō (Minister's Secretariat), Kōseirōdōshō.

Kōseirōdōshō (Ministry of Health, Labor and Welfare). (2009b). *Kaigo kyofuhi jittaichosa geppo Heisei 21 nen 8 gatsu shinsabun* [2009 Ministry of Health: Monthly survey of long-term care payment FY 2009 minute 8]. Tokyo: Tōkeijōhōbu (Statistics and Information Section), Daijin Kanbō (Minister's Secretariat), Kōseirōdōshō.

Kōseirōdōshō (Ministry of Health, Labor and Welfare). (2009c). *Kōrei shakai hakusho, heisei 21 nenban* [2009 White paper on aging society]. Tokyo: Tōkeijōhōbu (Statistics and Information Section), Daijin Kanbō (Minister's Secretariat), Kōseirōdōshō.

Kōseirōdōshō (Ministry of Health, Labor and Welfare). (2009d). *Nenndobetsu rōjiniryo jukyotaishosū, Rōjiniryo jigyo hōkoku* [Chart of annual medical care elderly recipient 2009 in Report of medical care among the elderly]. Tokyo: Hokenkyoku (Health Service Bureau), Daijin Kanbō (Minister's Secretariat), Kōseirōdōshō.

Long, S. O., & Chihara, S. (2000). Difficult choices. In S. O. Long (Ed.), *Caring for the elderly in Japan and the U.S.* (pp. 146–171). New York, NY: Routledge.

Masuda, Y., Fetters, M. D., Hattori, A., Mogi, N., Naito, M., Iguchi, A., . . . (2003). Physicians' report on the impact of living wills at the end of life in Japan. *Journal of Medical Ethics, 29,* 248–252.

Matsui, M. (2007). Perspectives of elderly people in advance directives in Japan. *Journal of Nursing Scholarship, 39*(2), 172–176.

Matsui, M., Braun, K. L., & Karel, H. (2008). Comparison of end-of-life preferences between Japanese elders in the United States and Japan. *Journal of Transcultural Nursing, 19*(2), 167–174.

Morioka, S. (2007). Challenges of productive aging in Japan. In M. Robinson, W. Novelli, C. Pearson, & L. Norris (Eds.). *Global health & global aging.* (pp. 128–139). San Francisco, CA: Jossey-Bass.

Naikakufu (The Cabinet Office, Government of Japan). (2009). *Kourei Shakai Hakusho, Heisei 21 Nenban* [White paper on aging society 2009 edition]. Tokyo: Kyoseishakaiseisaku (Cabinet General for Policy Planning).

Onda, H. (2005). *Anrakushi to makkiiryo* [Euthanasia and end-of-life care]. Issue Brief No. 472. *National Diet Library.*

Organization for Economic Co-operation and Development. (2009). *Health at a glance 2009: OECD indicators* (5th ed.). Retrieved December 15, 2010, from http://www.oecd.org/document/14/0,3343,en_2649_34631_16502667_1_1_1_1,00.html

Yoshida, S., Ogawa, T., & Kai, I. (2009). *Projection of the elderly with dementia and those needing care.* Retrieved December 15, 2010, from http://www.jarc.net/int/?p=140

Norway

Arnesen, K. E., Erikssen, J., & Stavem, K. (2001). Factors influencing physicians' assessment of urgency for inpatient surgery. *Journal of Health Services Research, 6*(4), 214–219.

Center for Medical Method Assessment. (2002). *Helsetjenester og gamle – hva er kunnskapsgrunnlaget?* [Health care services and elderly persons—The knowledge basis]. Oslo, Norway: Report no. 11.

Edlund, M. (2002). *Människans värdighet – ett grundbegrepp inom* vårdvetenskapen [Human dignity—A fundamental concept in caring science]. Akademisk avhandling (Doctoral thesis). Åbo, Norway: Åbo Akademi University Press.

Engedal, K., Kirkevold, Ø., Eek, A., & Nygård, A. M. (2002). *Makt og avmakt: Rettighetsbegrensninger og bruk av tvangstiltak i institusjoner og boliger for eldre* [Power and powerlessness]. Sem, Norway: Nasjonalt kompetansesenter for aldersdemens.

Eriksson, K. (1996). Om människans värdighet [About human dignity]. In T. Bjerkreim, J. Mathisen, R. Nord (Eds.), *Visjon, viten og virke* [Vision, knowledge and work]. Oslo, Norway: Universitetsforlaget.

Eritsland, J., Kløw, N. E., Westheim, A., Bendz, B., & Mangschau, A. (2005). Primær angioplastikk ved akutt ST-hevningsinfarkt hos eldre. *Tidsskrift for den Norske Lægeforening, 125*(21), 2922–2924.

Førde, R., Pedersen, R., Nortvedt, P., & Aasland, OG. (2006). Får eldreomsorgen nok ressurser? [Does geriatric care receive enough resources?]. *Tidsskrift for den Norske Lægeforening, 126*(15), 1913–1916.

Gonzales, B. (2000). Palliative medicine in oncology. *Anales de la Real Academia de Medicina, 117*(2), 245–267.

Husebø, B. S., & Husebø, S. (2003). *The final days and hours: Treatment and care in the final days of life.* Bergen, Norway: Red Cross Nursing Home.

Husebø, B. S., & Husebø, S. (2005). Sykehjemmene som arena for terminal omsorg – hvordan gjør vi det i praksis? [Nursing homes as arena of terminal care—How do we do it in practice?]. *Tidsskrift for Den norske legeforening, 125*(10), 1352–1354.

Kaasa, S., Breivik, H., & Jordhøy, M. (2002). Norway: Development of palliative care. *Journal of Pain and Symptom Management, 24*(2), 211–214.

Lafortune, G., Balestat, G., & the Disability Study Expert Group Members. (2007). *Trends in severe disability among elderly people: Assessing the evidence in 12 OECD countries and the future implications.* OECD Health Working Papers No. 26 DELSA/HEA/WD/HWP 2007; 2. Retrieved December 15, 2010, from http://www.oecd.org/dataoecd/13/8/38343783.pdf

Larson, C. O., Schlundt, D., Patel, K., McClellan, L., & Hargreaves, M. (2007). Disparities in perceptions of health care access in a community sample. *Journal of Ambulatory Care Management, 30*(2), 142–149.

Lillestø, B. (1998). *Når omsorgen oppleves krenkende* [When care is experienced as humiliating]. NFrapport 22/98. Bodø, Norway: Nordlandsforskning.

McCabe, B. W., Hertzog, M., Grasser, C. M. & Walker, S. N. (2005). Practice of health-promoting behaviors by nursing home residents. *Western Journal of Nursing Research, 27*(8), 1000–1016.

Melberg, T., Thoresen, M., Hansen, J. B., & Westheim, A. (2005). Hvordan behandles pasienter med akutt koronarsykdom i norske sykehus? [How are patients with acute coronary illness treated in Norwegian hospitals]. *Tidsskrift for den Norske Lægeforening, 125*(21), 2925–2928.

Nåden, D., & Sæteren, B. (2006). Cancer patients' perceptions of being or not being confirmed. *Nursing Ethics, 13*(3), 222–235.

Norges Offentlige Utredninger (Government Document). (1987). *Retningslinjer for prioriteringer innen norsk helsetjeneste* [Guidelines for prioritization for Norwegian health care services]. NOU 1987: 23 (Norwegian).Oslo, Norway.

Norges Offentlige Utredninger (Government Document). (1997). *Prioritering på ny* [Prioritization again]. NOU 1997:18 (Norwegian). Retrieved July 6, 2009, from http://www.regjeringen.no/en/dep/hod/documents/nouer/1997/nou-1997-18.html?id=140956

Norges Offentlige Utredninger (Government Document). (2009). *Brede pensjonsordninger* [Broad pension agreements]: NOU 2009: 13 (Norwegian). Oslo, Norway

Norwegian Directory of Health. (2010). *Årsrapport, Omsorgsplan 2015* [Annual report 2008, care plan 2015]. Report 15-1775. Oslo, Norway.

Norwegian Directory of Health and Social Affairs. (2007a). *Glemsk, men ikke glemt! Om dagens situasjon og framtidas utfordringer for å styrke tjenestetilbudet til personer med demens* [Forgetful but not forgotten!]. Report 15-1486. Oslo, Norway.

Norwegian Directory of Health and Social Affairs. (2007b). *Nasjonalt handlingsprogram med retningslinjer for palliasjon i kreftomsorgen* [National action program and guidelines for palliation in cancer care]. Report 15-1529. Oslo, Norway.

Norwegian Ministry of Health and Care Services. (2006). *Report No. 25 (2005-2006) to the Storting. Long term care–Future challenges. Care Plan 2015.* Oslo, Norway.

Norwegian Ministry of Health and Care Services. (2007). *Dementia Plan 2015. Sub-plan of Care Plan 2015.* Oslo, Norway.

Norwegian Ministry of Health and Care Services. (2009*). Høringsnotat [Discussion Document]. Endringer i kommunehelsetjenesteloven – et verdig tjenestetilbud. Forslag til ny forskrift om en verdig eldreomsorg* [Changes in the law of municipality health care—Dignified health service]: *Verdighetsgarantien* [The dignity guarantee]. Oslo, Norway.

Ruyter, K., Nortvedt, P., & Førde, R. (1993). Aktiv dødshjelp – en medisinsk oppgave? [Active euthanasia—A medical task?]. *Nytt Norsk Tidsskrift, 2,* 129–143.

Schaffer, M. A. (2007). Ethical problems in end-of-life decisions for elderly Norwegians. *Nursing Ethics, 14*(2), 242–256.

Slettebø, Å. (2002). *Strebing mot pasientens beste* [Striving towards the best of the patient]. Doctoral thesis. Oslo, Norway: Universitetet i Oslo (Norwegian).

Slettebø, Å. (2009). *Sykepleie og etikk* [Nursing and ethics]. Oslo, Norway: Gyldendal Akademisk (Norwegian).

Statistics Norway. (2009). *High growth in population.* 12.06.2009. Oslo, Norway.

Vigran, Å. (2000). *Pleie og omsorgstjenestene.* Oslo, Norway: Statistics Norway.

Werntoft, E., Hallberg, I. R., & Edberg, A. K. (2007a). Older people]s reasoning about age-related prioritization in health care. *Nursing Ethics, 14*(3), 399–412.

Werntoft, E., Hallberg, I. R., & Edberg, A. K. (2007b). Prioritization and resource allocation in health care: The views of older people receiving continuous public care and service. *Health Expectations, 10*(2), 117–128.

Other References

Organization for Economic Co-operation and Development. (2009a). *OECD health data: Statistics and indicators.* Retrieved December 15, 2010, from http://www.oecd.org/health/healthdata

Organization for Economic Co-operation and Development. (2009b). *Health at a glance 2009: OECD indicators* (5th ed.). Retrieved December 15, 2010, from http://www.oecd.org/document/14/0,3343,en_2649_34631_16502667_1_1_1_1,00.html

Population Reference Bureau. (2010). *World population data sheet.* Washington, DC: Author.

Sodorenko, A., & Walker, A, (2004). The Madrid international plan of action on ageing: From conception to implementation. *Ageing & Society, 24,* 147–165.

United Nations Department of Economic and Social Affairs. (2007). *World economic and social survey 2007: Development in an ageing world.* New York, NY: United Nations. Retrieved December 15, 2010, from http://www.un.org/esa/policy/wess/wess2007files/wess2007.pdf

United Nations. (2002). *Madrid international plan of action on ageing.*. Retrieved December 15, 2010, from http://www.un.org/ageing/madrid_intlplanaction.html

United Nations Office of the High Representative for the Least Developed Countries, Landlocked Developing Countries and Small Island Developing States. (2010). *Criteria for identification of LDC.* Retrieved December 15, 2010, from http://www.unohrlls.org/en/ldc/related/59/

World Health Organization. (2010). *The African Regional Health Report.* Geneva, Switzerland. Author.

Index

Page numbers followed by f indicate figures; t, tables; b, boxes.